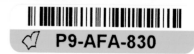

PRINCIPLES OF
MANUAL MEDICINE

Second Edition

PRINCIPLES OF MANUAL MEDICINE

Second Edition

Philip E. Greenman, D.O., F.A.A.O.
Professor of Biomechanics
College of Osteopathic Medicine
Michigan State University
East Lansing, Michigan

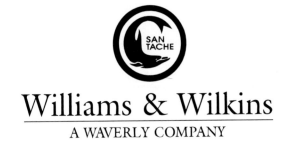

Williams & Wilkins

A WAVERLY COMPANY

BALTIMORE • PHILADELPHIA • LONDON • PARIS • BANGKOK
BUENOS AIRES • HONG KONG • MUNICH • SYDNEY • TOKYO • WROCLAW

Editor. John P. Butler
Managing Editor. Linda S. Napora
Production Coordinator. Peter J. Carley
Book Project Editor. Jennifer D. Weir
Copy Editor. Pam Goehrig
Designer. Maria Karkucinski
Typesetter. Maple-Vail
Printer. Maple-Vail
Binder. Maple-Vail

351 West Camden Street
Baltimore, Maryland 21201-2436   USA

Rose Tree Corporate Center
1400 North Providence Road
Building II, Suite 5025
Media, Pennsylvania 19063-2043   USA

Accurate indications, adverse reactions, and dosage schedules for drugs are provided iin this book, but it is possible that they may change. The reader is urged to review the package information data of the manufacturers of the medications mentioned.

Printed in the United States of America

Library of Congress Cataloging in Publication Data

Greenman, Ph. E., 1928–
   Principles of manual medicine / Philip E. Greenman. — 2nd ed.
      p.   cm.
   Includes index.
   ISBN 0-683-03558-4
   1. Manipulation (Therapeutics)   2. Medicine. Physical.   I. Title.
   [DNLM: 1. Physical Medicine.   2. Manipulation, Orthopedic.   WB
460 G814p   1996]
RM724.G74   1996
615.8′2—dc20
DNLM/DLC   95-9178
for Library of Congress   CIP

The Publishers have made every effort to trace the copyright holders for borrowed material. If they have inadvertently overlooked any, they will be pleased to make the necessary arrangements at the first opportunity.

96 97 98 99
2 3 4 5 6 7 8 9 10

Reprints of chapters may be purchased from Williams & Wilkins in quantities of 100 or more. Call Isabella Wise in the Special Sales Department, (800) 358-3583.

DEDICATION

This second edition is dedicated to the memory of John F. Bourdillon, a friend, colleague, and major contributor to the field of manual medicine in the medical profession worldwide. He was one of the original faculty members of the Continuing Medical Education Manual Medicine Courses at Michigan State University, and continued longer than any other, giving his time, energy, and talent so future generations of practitioners could provide enhanced care to their patients. His death in 1992 occurred as he was preparing to teach another class. He is missed by all who were privileged to know him.

Since the publication of the first edition of this text in 1989, a number of changes have occurred in the field of Manual Medicine. The North American Academy of Manipulative Medicine has merged with the American Association of Orthopaedic Medicine, becoming the representative for the United States and Canada to the International Federation of Manual Medicine. A Congress on the Role of the Sacroiliac Joint in Low Pain was held in 1992. This Congress documented the significant role of sacroiliac joint dysfunction in low back pain. The American Academy of Physical Medicine and Rehabilitation has annually cosponsored a course on the Principles of Manual Medicine at their annual meeting, and the American Academy of Neurology has, for the first time, included presentations on Manual Medicine at their annual meeting.

The number of colleges of osteopathic medicine has increased from 15 to 17, and three more schools are in stages of development. After an extensive study of the research literature, the federal government has acknowledged the efficacy of manipulation in treating acute back pain. There is an ever-increasing number of continuing education offerings for health professionals involved in manipulative medicine. Current Procedural Terminology (CPT) 1995 changed the coding for osteopathic manipulative procedures performed by a physician. Despite these advances, there continues to be a deficit in understanding manual medicine by the orthodox medical community. There is, however, an increasing desire by many to learn more about the field. This book is an attempt to elevate the knowledge base of the student and introduce the uninitiated to the basic concepts.

Goals of this new edition are to provide additional and enhanced visual demonstration of the art of manual medicine today, update material throughout, and expand by including new material in the form of clinical correlations and integration.

Principles of Manual Medicine, second edition, continues to support the continuing education series sponsored by the College of Osteopathic Medicine (D.O.) and supported by the College of Human Medicine (M.D.) at Michigan State University. It provides basic concepts, principles, and technique procedures of the current state of the art in the field. It is intended to be a student-friendly resource in the field of manual medicine. The book is organized in three sections: Section I deals with the principles in the field; Section II finds the specific techniques in the various systems; and Section III deals with adjunctive diagnostic and therapeutic topics and correlations.

With the current focus on cost containment in the health care system, and with back pain continuing to be a high-cost item in terms of lost time compensation and medical cost, manual medicine may well turn out to be an efficient and cost-effective way to deal with the problem. Knowledge about what manual medicine is and is not can be helpful in this dilemma. The reader is urged to keep an open mind when reading this and other texts in the field. Try it, you might like it.

Philip E. Greenman, D.O., F.A.A.O.

ACKNOWLEDGMENTS

Principles of Manual Medicine, second edition, continues to be the effort of a single author to convey his understanding of manual medicine after 43 years of study and experience. Many people have contributed to the accumulation of the information provided. I am extremely privileged to have had the opportunity to study with many mentors willing to share their extensive knowledge and experience. In the osteopathic profession, the list reads like a Who's Who. Included are C.G. Beckwith, A.G. Cathie, D. Heilig, P.E. Kimberly, P.T. Lloyd, F.L. Mitchell, Sr., R.M. Tilley, E.D. Tucker, and P.T. Wilson. In the medical profession, the list includes J. Bourdillon, J. Fossgreen, S. Haldeman, V. Janda, K. Lewit, J. Mennell, R. Maigne, and H.D. Neumann. Drs. Bourdillon and Mennell were instrumental in the development and implementation of the Manual Medicine Continuing Education Series at Michigan State University. They have passed on since the publication of the first edition and are sorely missed.

I am indebted to my colleagues in the osteopathic profession, particularly at Michigan State University: M.C. Beal, B. Briner, L. Brumm, J. Goodridge, R. Hruby, W. Johnston, F.L. Mitchell, Jr., S. Sutton, D.F. Stanton, E.G. Stiles, and R.C. Ward.

My thanks to John Williamson for photographic assistance and to Jacob Rowan for serving as the model. We spent many happy hours together.

Appreciation is expressed to Brenda Robinson for the many hours spent typing the manuscript and to Linda Napora for her advice, counsel, and encouragement in the project.

To my wife goes my everlasting love and thanks for her support and tolerance through the many months of the effort.

CONTENTS

SECTION III.   CLINICAL INTEGRATION AND CORRELATION

Section **1**

PRINCIPLES AND
CONCEPTS

1

MANIPULATIVE MEDICINE

HISTORY

Manual medicine is as old as the science and art of medicine itself. Strong evidence exists of the use of manual medicine procedures in ancient Thailand, as shown in statuary at least 4000 years old. The use of the hands in treatment of injury and disease was practiced by the ancient Egyptians. Even Hippocrates, the father of modern medicine, was known to use manual medicine procedures, particularly traction and leverage techniques, in the treatment of spinal deformity. The writings of such notable historical figures in medicine as Galen, Celisies, and Oribasius refer to the use of manipulative procedures. There is a void in the reported use of manual medicine procedures corresponding to the approximate time of the split of physicians and barber-surgeons. As physicians became less involved in patient contact and as direct hands-on patient care became the province of the barber-surgeons, the role of manual medicine in the healing art seems to have declined. This period also represents the time of the plagues, and perhaps physicians were reticent to come in close personal contact with their patients.

The 19th century found a renaissance of interest in this field. Early in the 19th century, Doctor Edward Harrison, a 1784 graduate of Edinburgh University, developed a sizable reputation in London by using manual medicine procedures. Like many other proponents of manual medicine in the 19th century, he became alienated from his colleagues by his continued use of these procedures.

Bonesetters

The 19th century was a popular period for "bonesetters" both in England and in the United States. The work of Hutton, a skilled and famous bonesetter, led such eminent physicians as James Paget and Wharton Hood to report in such prestigious medical journals as the *British Medical Journal* and *The Lancet* that the medical community should pay attention to the successes of the unorthodox practitioners of bonesetting. In the United States the Sweet family practiced skilled bonesetting in the New England region of Rhode Island and Connecticut. It has also been

reported that some of the descendants of the Sweet family emigrated west in the mid-19th century. Sir Herbert Barker was a well-known British bonesetter who practiced well into the first quarter of the 20th century and was of such eminence that he was knighted by the crown.

19th Century Controversy

The 19th century was a time of turmoil and controversy in medical practice. Medical history of the day is replete with many unorthodox systems of healing. Two individuals who would profoundly influence the field of manual medicine were products of this period of medical turmoil. Andrew Taylor Still, M.D., was a medical physician trained in the preceptor fashion of the day, and D.D. Palmer was a grocer turned self-educated manipulative practitioner.

Osteopathic Medicine

Andrew Taylor Still (1828–1917) first proposed his philosophy and practice of osteopathy in 1874. His disenchantment with the medical practice of the day led to his formulation of a new medical philosophy, which he termed osteopathic medicine. He appeared to have been a great synthesizer of medical thought and built his new philosophy on both ancient medical truths and current medical successes, while being most vocal in denouncing what he viewed as poor medical practice, primarily the inappropriate use of medications then in current use.

Still's strong position against the drug therapy of his day was not well received by his medical colleagues and is certainly not supported by contemporary osteopathic physicians. However, he was not alone in expressing concern about the abuse of drug therapy. In 1861 Oliver Wendell Holmes said, "If all of the MATERIA MEDICA were thrown into the oceans, it will be all the better for mankind, and worse for the fishes." Sir William Osler, one of Still's contemporaries, stated, "One of the first duties of the physician is to educate the masses not to take medicine. Man has an inborn craving for medicine. Heroic dosing for several generations has given his tissues a thirst for drugs. The desire to take medicine is one feature which distinguishes man, the animal, from his fellow creatures."

Still's new philosophy of medicine in essence consisted of the following:

1. The unity of the body.
2. The healing power of nature. He held that the body had within itself all those things necessary for the maintenance of health and recovery from disease. The role of the physician was to enhance this capacity.
3. The somatic component of disease. He believed that the musculoskeletal system was an integral part of the total body and alterations within the musculoskeletal system affected total body health and the ability of the body to recover from injury and disease.
4. Structure-function interrelationship. The interrelationship of structure-function had been espoused by Virchow early in the 19th century, and Still applied this principle within his concept of total body integration. He strongly believed that structure governed function and function influenced structure.
5. The use of manipulative therapy. This became an integral part of Still's philosophy because he believed that restoration of the body's maximal functional capacity would enhance the level of wellness and assist in recovery from injury and disease.

It is unclear when and how Dr. Still added manipulation to his philosophy of osteopathy. It wasn't until 1879, some 5 years after his announcement of the development of osteopathy, that he became known as the "lightning bonesetter." There is no recorded history that he met or knew any members of the Sweet family as they migrated west. Still never wrote a book on manipulative technique. His writings were extensive, but they focused on the philosophy, principles, and practice of osteopathy.

Still's attempt to interest his medical colleagues in these concepts was rebuffed, particularly when he took them to Baker University in Kansas.

As he became more clinically successful, and nationally and internationally well known, many individuals came to study with him and learn the new science of osteopathy. This led to the establishment in 1892 of the first college of osteopathic medicine at Kirksville, Missouri. In 1995 there were 17 colleges of osteopathic medicine in the United States, graduating over 2000 students per year. Osteopathy in other parts of the world, particularly in the United Kingdom and in the commonwealth countries of Australia and New Zealand, is a school of practice limited to

structural diagnosis and manipulative therapy, although strongly espousing some of the fundamental concepts and principles of Still. Osteopathic medicine in the United States has from its inception, and continues to be, a total school of medicine and surgery while retaining the basis of osteopathic principles and concepts and continuing the use of structural diagnosis and manipulative therapy in total patient care.

Chiropractic

Daniel David Palmer (1845–1913) was, like Still, a product of the midwestern portion of the United States in the mid-19th century. Although not schooled in medicine, he was known to practice as a magnetic healer and became a self-educated manipulative therapist. Controversy continues as to whether Palmer was ever a patient or student of Still's at Kirksville, Missouri, but it is known that Palmer and Still met in Clinton, Iowa early in the 20th century. D.D. Palmer moved about the country a great deal and founded his first college in 1896. The early colleges were at Davenport, Iowa and in Oklahoma City, Oklahoma.

Although D.D. Palmer is given credit for the origin of chiropractic, it was his son, Bartlett Joshua Palmer (1881–1961), who gave the chiropractic profession its momentum. Palmer's original concepts were that the cause of disease was a variation in the expression of normal neural function. He believed in the "innate intelligence" of the brain and central nervous system and believed that alterations in the spinal column (subluxations) altered neural function, causing disease. Removal of the subluxation by chiropractic adjustment was viewed to be the treatment. Chiropractic has never professed to be a total school of medicine and does not teach surgery or the use of medication beyond vitamins and simple analgesics. There remains a split within the chiropractic profession between the "straights," who continue to espouse and adhere to the original concepts of Palmer, and the "mixers," who believe in a broadened scope of chiropractic that includes other therapeutic interventions, such as physiotherapy, electrotherapy, diet, and vitamins.

In the mid-1970s the Council on Chiropractic Education (CCE) petitioned the U.S. Department of Education for recognition as the accrediting agency for chiropractic education. The CCE was strongly influenced by the colleges with a "mixer" orientation, which has led to increased educational requirements both before and during chiropractic education. Chiropractic is practiced throughout the world, but the vast majority of chiropractic education continues to be in the United States. The late 1970s found increased recognition of chiropractic in both Australia and New Zealand, and their registries are participants in the health programs in these countries.

MEDICAL MANIPULATORS

The 20th century has found renewed interest in manual medicine in the traditional medical profession. In the first part of the 20th century, James Mennell and Edgar Cyriax brought joint manipulation recognition within the London medical community. John Mennell continued his father's work and contributed extensively to the manual medicine literature and its teaching worldwide. As one of the founding members of the North American Academy of Manipulative Medicine (NAAMM), he was instrumental in opening the membership in NAAMM to osteopathic physicians in 1977. He strongly advocated an expanded role for appropriately trained physical therapists to work with the medical profession in providing joint manipulation in patient care.

James Cyriax is well known for his textbooks in the field and also fostered the expanded education and scope of physical therapists. He incorporated manual medicine procedures in the practice of "orthopedic medicine" and founded the Society for Orthopedic Medicine. In his later years James Cyriax came to believe that manipulation restored function to derangements of the intervertebral discs and spoke less and less about specific arthrodial joint effects. He had no use for "osteopaths" or other manipulating groups, and the influence of his dynamic personality will be felt long after his death in 1985. John Bourdillon, a British-trained orthopedic surgeon, first was attracted to manual medicine as a student at Oxford University. During his training, he learned to perform manipulation while the patient was under general anesthesia and subsequently used the same techniques without anesthesia. He observed the successful results of non-medically qualified manipulators and began a study of their techniques. A lifelong student and teacher in the field, the fifth edition of "Spinal Manipulation," with coauthors E.A. Day and M.A. Bookhout, was published in 1992 shortly before his death.

The NAAMM merged with The American Association of Orthopaedic Medicine in 1992 and continues to represent the United States and Canada in the International Federation of Manual Medicine.

PRACTICE OF MANUAL MEDICINE

Manual medicine should not be viewed in isolation or separate from "regular medicine," and clearly is not the panacea for all ills of humankind. Manual medicine considers the functional capacity of the human organism, and its practitioners are as interested in the dynamic processes of disease as those who look at the disease process from the static perspective of laboratory data, tissue pathology, and the results of autopsy. Manual medicine focuses on the musculoskeletal system, which comprises over 60% of the human organism and through which evaluation of the other organ systems must be made. Structural diagnosis not only evaluates the musculoskeletal system for its particular diseases and dysfunctions but also can be used to evaluate the somatic manifestations of disease and derangement of the internal viscera. Manipulative procedures are used primarily to increase mobility in restricted areas of musculoskeletal function and to reduce pain. Some practitioners focus on the concept of pain relief, whereas others are more interested in the influence of increased mobility in restricted areas of the musculoskeletal system. When appropriately used, manipulative procedures have been noted to be clinically effective in reducing pain within the musculoskeletal system, increasing the level of wellness of the patient, and in helping patients with a myriad of disease processes.

GOAL OF MANIPULATION

In 1983 a 6–day workshop was held in Fischingen, Switzerland, which included approximately 35 experts in manual medicine from throughout the world. They represented many different countries and schools of manual medicine with considerable diversity in clinical experience. The proceedings of this workshop (Dvorak J, Dvorak V, Schneider W (eds): Manual Medicine 1984. Heidelberg, 1985, Springer-Verlag) represent the state of the art in manual medicine of the day. That workshop reached a consensus on the goal of manipulation:

> The goal of manipulation is to restore maximal, pain-free movement of the musculoskeletal system in postural balance.

This definition is comprehensive but specific and is well worth consideration by all students in the field.

ROLE OF THE MUSCULOSKELETAL SYSTEM IN HEALTH AND DISEASE

It is indeed unfortunate that much of the medical thinking and teaching looks at the musculoskeletal system only as the coat rack on which the other organ systems are held and not as an organ system that is susceptible to its own unique injuries and disease processes. The field of manual medicine looks at the musculoskeletal system in a much broader context, particularly as an integral and interrelated part of the total human organism. Although most physicians would accept the concept of integration of the total body including the musculoskeletal system, specific and usable concepts of how that integration occurs and its relationship in structural diagnosis and manipulative therapy seem to be limited.

There are five basic concepts that this author has found useful. Because the hand is an integral part of the practice of manual medicine, and includes five digits, it is easy to recall one concept for each digit in the palpating hand. These concepts are as follows:

1. Holism;
2. Neurological control;
3. Circulatory function;
4. Energy expenditure; and
5. Self-regulation.

Concept of Holism

The concept of holism has different meanings and usage by different practitioners. In manual medicine the concept emphasizes that the musculoskeletal system deserves thoughtful and complete evaluation, wherever and whenever the patient is seen, irrespective of the nature of the presenting complaint. It is just as inappropriate to avoid evaluating the cardiovascular system in a patient presenting with a primary musculoskeletal complaint as it is to avoid evaluation of the musculoskeletal system in a patient presenting with acute chest pain thought to be cardiac in origin. The concept is one of a sick patient who needs to be evaluated. The musculoskeletal system comprises most of the human body, and alterations within it influence the rest of the human organism; diseases within the internal organs manifest themselves in alterations in the musculoskeletal system, frequently in the form of pain. It is indeed fortunate that holistic concepts have gained increasing popularity in the medical community recently, but the concept expressed here is one that speaks to the integration of the total human organism rather than a summation of parts. We must all remember that our role as health professionals is to treat patients and not to treat disease.

Concept of Neurological Control

The concept of neurological control is based on the fact that humans have the most highly developed and sophisticated nervous system in the animal kingdom. All functions of the body are under some form of control by the nervous system. A patient is constantly responding to stimuli from the internal and external body environment through complex mechanisms within the central and peripheral nervous systems. As freshmen in medical school, we all studied the anatomy and physiology of the nervous system. Let us briefly review a segment of the spinal cord (Fig. 1.1). On the left side of the figure are depicted the classic somaticosomatic reflex pathways with afferent impulses coming from skin, muscle, joint, and tendon. Afferent stimuli from the nociceptors, mechanoreceptors, and proprioceptors all feed in through the dorsal root and ultimately synapse, either directly or through a series of interneurons, with an anterior horn cell from which an efferent fiber extends to the skeletal muscle. It is through multiple permutations of the central reflex arc that we respond to external stimuli, including injury; orient our bodies in space; and accomplish many of the physical activities of daily living. The right side of the figure represents the classical viscero-visceral reflex arc wherein afferents from the visceral sensory system synapse in the intermediolateral cell column and then to the sympathetic lateral chain ganglion or collateral ganglia to

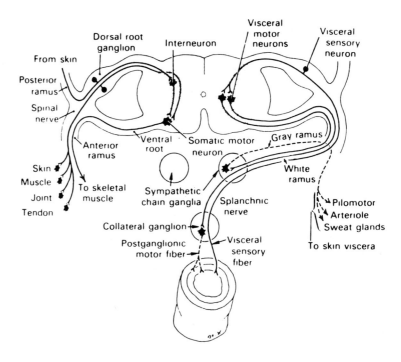

Figure 1.1.
Cross-section of spinal cord segment.

synapse with a postganglionic motor fiber to the target end organ viscera. Note that the skin viscera receive efferent stimulation from the lateral chain ganglion.

These sympathetic reflex pathways innervate the pilomotor activity of the skin, the vasomotor tone of the vascular tree, and the secretomotor activity of the sweat glands. Alteration in the sympathetic nervous system activity to the skin viscera results in palpatory changes that are identifiable by structural diagnostic means. Although this figure separates these two pathways, they are in fact interrelated so that somatic afferents influence visceral efferents and visceral afferents can manifest themselves in somatic efferents. This figure represents the spinal cord in horizontal section and it must be recalled that ascending and descending pathways from spinal cord segment to spinal cord segment, as well as from the higher centers of the brain, are occurring as well.

Another neurological concept worth recalling is that of the autonomic nervous system (ANS). The ANS is made up of two divisions, the parasympathetic and sympathetic. The parasympathetic division includes cranial nerves III, VII, VIII, IX, and X and the S2, S3, and S4 levels of the spinal cord. The largest and most extensive nerve of the parasympathetic division is the vagus. The vagus innervates all of the viscera from the root of the neck to the midportion of the descending colon and all glands and smooth muscle of these organs. The vagus nerve (Fig. 1.2) has an extensive distribution and is the primary driving force of the cardiovascular, pulmonary, and gastrointestinal systems. Many pharmaceutical agents alter parasympathetic nervous activity, particularly that of the vagus.

The sympathetic division of the ANS (Fig. 1.3) is represented by preganglionic neurons originating in the spinal cord from T1 to L3; the lateral chain ganglion, including the superior, middle, and inferior cervical ganglia; the thoracolumbar ganglia from T1 to L3; and the collateral ganglia. Sympathetic fibers innervate all of the internal viscera as do the parasympathetic division but are organized differently. The sympathetic division is organized segmentally. It is interesting to note that all of the viscera above the diaphragm receive their sympathetic innervation from preganglionic fibers above T4 and T5, and all of the viscera below the diaphragm receive their sympathetic innervation preganglionic fibers from below T5. It is through this segmental organization that the relationships of certain parts of the musculoskeletal system and certain internal viscera are correlated. Remember that the musculoskeletal system receives only sympathetic division innervation and receives no parasympathetic innervation. Control of all glandular and vascular activity in the musculoskeletal system is

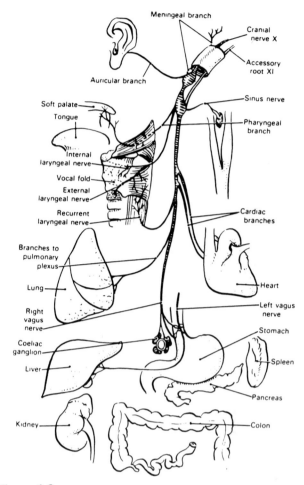

Figure 1.2.
Vagus nerve distribution.

mediated through the sympathetic division of the ANS.

Remember that all of these reflex mechanisms are constantly under the local and central modifying control of excitation and inhibition. Conscious and subconscious control mechanisms from the brain constantly modify activity throughout the nervous system, responding to stimuli. The nervous system is intimately related to another control system, the endocrine system, and it is useful to think in terms of neuroendocrine control. Recent advances in the knowledge of neurotransmitters, endorphins, enkephalins, and materials such as substance P have both enlightened us as to the detail of many of the mechanisms previously not understood and also begin to provide answers for some of the mechanisms through which biomechanical alteration of the musculoskeletal system can alter bodily function.

Emphasis has been placed on the reflex and neural transmission activities of the nervous system, but the nervous system has a powerful trophic function as well. Highly complex protein and lipid substances are transported antegrade and retrograde along neu-

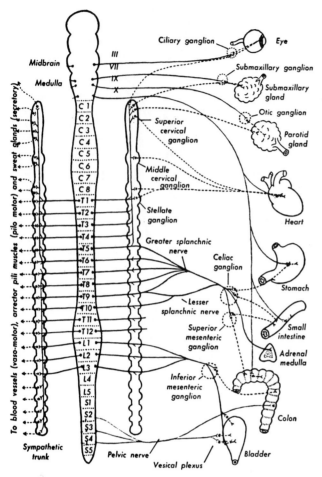

Figure 1.3.
Autonomic nervous system.

rons and cross over the synapse of the neuron to the target end organ. Alteration in neurotrophin transmission can be detrimental to the health of the target end organ.

Circulatory Function

The third concept is that of circulatory function. The concept can be simply described as the maintenance of an appropriate cellular milieu for each and every cell of the body (Fig. 1.4). Picture a cell, a group of cells making up a tissue, or a group of tissues making up an organ, resting in the middle of the "cellular milieu." That cell is dependent for its function, whatever its function is, on the delivery of oxygen, glucose, and all other substances necessary for its metabolism being supplied by the arterial side of the circulation. The arterial system has a powerful pump, the myocardium of the heart, to propel blood forward. Cardiac pumping function is intimately controlled by the central nervous system, particularly the ANS, through the cardiac plexus. The vascular tree receives its vasomotor tone control through the sympathetic division of the ANS. Anything that interferes with sympathetic ANS outflow, segmentally mediated, can influence vasomotor tone to a target end organ.

The arteries are also encased in the fascial compartments of the body and are subject to compressive and torsional stress that can interfere with the delivery of arterial blood flow to the target organ cell. Once the cell has received its nutrients and proceeded through its normal metabolism, the end products must be removed. The low pressure circulatory systems, the venous and the lymphatic systems, are responsible for the transport of metabolic waste products. Both the venous and lymphatic systems are much thinner walled than the arteries, and they lack the driving force of the pumping action of the heart,

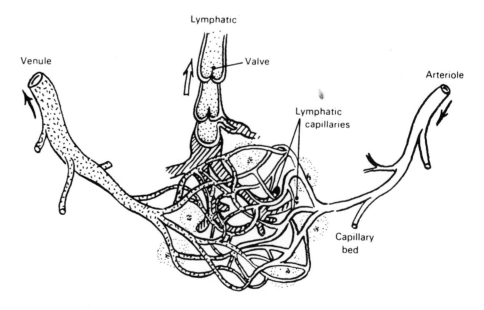

Figure 1.4.
Cellular milieu.

depending instead on the musculoskeletal system for their propelling action. The large muscles of the extremities contribute greatly to this activity, but the major pump of the low pressure systems is the diaphragm (Fig. 1.5).

The diaphragm has an extensive attachment to the musculoskeletal system, including the upper lumbar vertebra; the lower six ribs; the xiphoid process of the sternum; and through myofascial connections with the lower extremities, the psoas and quadratus lumborum muscles. The activity of the diaphragm modulates the negative intrathoracic pressure that provides a sucking action upon venous and lymphatic

return through the vena cava and the cisterna chyli. Because of the extensive attachment of the diaphragm with the musculoskeletal system and from its innervation via the phrenic nerve from the cervical spine, alterations in the musculoskeletal system at a number of levels can alter diaphragmatic function and, consequently, venous and lymphatic return. Accumulation of metabolic end products in the cellular milieu interferes with the health of the cell and its recovery from disease or injury. It should be pointed out that the foramen for the inferior vena cava is at the apex of the dome of the diaphragm. There is some evidence that diaphragmatic excursion has a di-

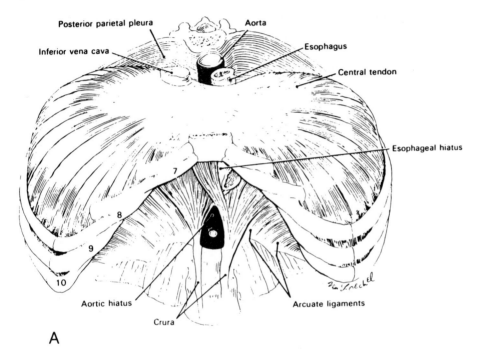

A

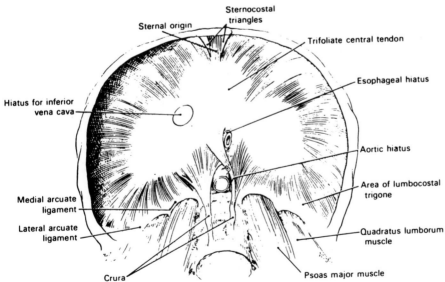

B

Figure 1.5.
A, B. Thoracoabdominal diaphragm.

rect squeezing and propelling activity on the inferior vena cava.

Another circulatory concept related to musculo-skeletal function concerns the lymphatic system (Fig. 1.6) and the location where it empties into the venous system. The lymph from the right side of the head, right side of the neck, and right upper extremity enters into the right subclavian vein at the thoracic inlet just behind the anterior end of the first rib and the medial end of the clavicle. The lymph from all of the rest of the body empties into the left subclavian vein at the thoracic inlet behind the anterior extremity of the left first rib and the medial end of the left clavicle. Alteration in the biomechanics of the thoracic inlet, particularly its fascial continuity, can affect the thin-walled lymph vessels as they empty into the venous system. Maximal function of the musculoskeletal system is an important factor in the efficiency of the circulatory system and the maintenance of a normal cellular milieu throughout the body.

Energy Expenditure

The fourth concept is that of energy expenditure primarily through the musculoskeletal system. The musculoskeletal system not only comprises over 60% of the human organism but is also the major expender of body energy. Any increase in activity of the musculoskeletal system calls upon the internal viscera to develop and deliver energy to sustain that physical activity. The greater the musculoskeletal activity, the greater the demand. If dysfunction alters the efficiency of the musculoskeletal system, there is an increase in demand for energy, not only for increased activity but for normal activity as well. If we have a patient with a compromised cardiovascular and pulmonary system who has chronic congestive heart failure, any increase in demand for energy delivery to the musculoskeletal system can be detrimental. For example, a well-compensated chronic congestive heart failure patient who happens to sprain an ankle and attempts to continue normal activity might well have a rapid deterioration of the compensation because of the increased energy demand by the altered gait of the sprained ankle. Obviously, it would make more sense to treat the altered musculoskeletal system by attending to the ankle sprain than to increase the dosage of medications controlling the congestive heart failure. Restriction of one major joint in a lower extremity can increase the energy expenditure of normal walking by as much as 40%, and, if two major joints are restricted in the same extremity, it can increase by as much as 300%. Multiple minor restrictions of movement of the musculoskeletal system, particularly in the maintenance of normal gait, can also have a detrimental effect upon total body function.

Self-Regulation

The fifth concept is that of self-regulation. There are literally thousands of self-regulating mechanisms op-

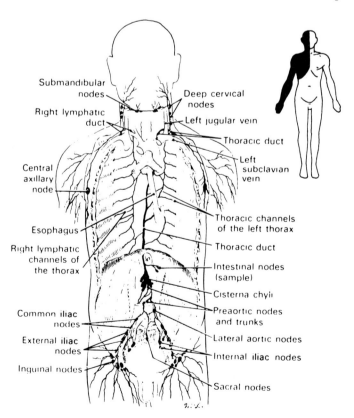

Figure 1.6.
Lymphatic system.

erative within the body at all times. These homeostatic mechanisms are essential for the maintenance of health, and if altered by disease or injury, they need to be restored. All physicians are dependent on these self-regulating mechanisms within the patient for successful treatment. The goal of the physician should be to enhance all of the body's self-regulating mechanisms to assist in the recovery from disease. Physicians should not interfere with self-regulating mechanisms more than absolutely necessary during the treatment process. All things that are done to, or placed within the human body, alter these mechanisms in some fashion. When any foreign substance is given to a patient, the beneficial and the detrimental potential of the substance must be considered. As modern pharmacology grows by leaps and bounds with evermore potent pharmacological effects, we must all recognize the potential for iatrogenic disease. Many patients are on multiple medications, particularly in the hospital environment, and the actions and interactions of each must be clearly understood to avoid iatrogenic problems. Only physicians cause iatrogenic disease. It has been reported that one in seven hospital days in the United States is due to adverse reaction to pharmacological intervention.

MANIPULABLE LESION

Manual medicine deals with the identification of the manipulable lesion and the appropriate use of a manual medicine procedure to resolve the condition. The field of manual medicine has suffered from multiple, divergent, and sometimes confusing definitions of the entity amenable to manipulative intervention. It has been called the "osteopathic lesion," "chiropractic subluxation," "joint blockage," "loss of joint play," "joint dysfunction," and other names. Currently the acceptable term for this entity is somatic dysfunction. It is defined as impaired or altered function of related components of the somatic (body framework) system; skeletal, arthrodial, and myofascial structures; and related vascular, lymphatic, and neural elements (Hospital Adaption of the International Classification of Disease, ed 2. 1973). Notice that the emphasis is on altered function of the musculoskeletal system and not on a disease state or pain

syndrome. Obviously, if a somatic dysfunction is present that alters vascular, lymphatic, and neural function, a myriad of symptoms might well be present, including painful conditions and disease entities. The diagnosis of somatic dysfunction can accompany many other diagnoses or can be present as an independent entity. The art of structural diagnosis is to define the presence of somatic dysfunction(s) and determine any significance to the patient's complaint or disease process presenting at the time. If significant, it should be treated by manual medicine intervention just as other diagnostic findings might also need appropriate treatment.

DIAGNOSTIC TRIAD FOR SOMATIC DYSFUNCTION

The diagnostic criteria for identification of a somatic dysfunction can be expressed by the mnemonic ART. "A" stands for asymmetry of related parts of the musculoskeletal system, either structural or functional. Examples are altered shoulder height, height of iliac crest, and contour and function of the thoracic cage, usually identified by palpation and observation. "R" stands for range of motion of a joint, several joints, or region of the musculoskeletal system. The range of motion could be abnormal either by being increased (hypermobility) or restricted (hypomobility). The usual finding in somatic dysfunction is restricted mobility, identified by observation and palpation using both active and passive patient cooperation. "T" stands for tissue texture abnormality of the soft tissues of the musculoskeletal system (skin, fascia, muscle, ligament, and so on). Tissue texture abnormalities are identified by observation and a number of different palpatory tests. By using these three criteria, one attempts to identify the presence of somatic dysfunctions, their location, whether they are acute or chronic, and particularly whether or not they are significant for the state of the patient's wellness or illness at that moment in time. In addition to the diagnostic value, changes in these criteria can be of prognostic value in monitoring the response of the patient, not only to manipulative treatment directed toward the somatic dysfunction but also to other therapeutic interventions.

2

Structural diagnosis in manual medicine is specifically directed toward evaluation of the musculoskeletal system with the goal of identification of the presence and significance of somatic dysfunction(s). It is a component part of the physical examination of the total patient. Most of the evaluation of the internal viscera takes place by evaluation of these structures through the musculoskeletal system. Therefore, it is easy to examine the musculoskeletal system while evaluating the internal viscera of the neck, chest, abdomen, and pelvic regions. Structural diagnosis uses the traditional physical diagnostic methods of observation, palpation, percussion, and auscultation. Of these, observation and palpation are the most useful. Structural diagnosis of the musculoskeletal system should never be done in isolation and should always be done within the context of a total history and physical evaluation of the patient.

The diagnostic entity sought by structural diagnosis is somatic dysfunction. It is defined as follows:

Somatic dysfunction: impaired or altered function of related components of the somatic (body framework) system; skeletal, arthrodial, and myofascial structures; and related vascular, lymphatic, and neural elements (Hospital Adaption of the International Classification of Disease, ed 2. 1973).

The three classical diagnostic criteria for somatic dysfunction can be identified with the mnemonic ART as follows:

"A" for asymmetry. Asymmetry of related parts of the musculoskeletal system either structural or functional. Examples might be the height of each shoulder by observation, height of iliac crest by palpation, and contour and function of the thoracic cage both by observation and palpation. Asymmetry is usually discerned by observation and palpation.

"R" for range-of-motion abnormality. Alteration in range of motion of a joint, several joints, or region of the musculoskeletal system is sought. The alteration may be either restricted or increased mobility. Restricted motion is the most common component of somatic dysfunction. Range-of-motion abnormality is determined by observation and palpation, using both active and passive patient cooperation.

"T" for tissue texture abnormality. Alteration in the characteristics of the soft tissues of the musculoskeletal system (skin, fascia, muscle, ligament) is ascertained by observation and palpation. Percussion is also used in identifying areas of altered tissue texture. A large number of descriptors are used in the literature to express the quality of the abnormal feel of the tissue.

HAND-EYE COORDINATION

In structural diagnosis it is important for the physician to maximize the coordinated use of the palpating hands and the observing eyes. When using vision for observation, it is important to know which eye is dominant so that it can be appropriately placed in relation to the patient for accuracy in visual discrimination. Because most structural diagnosis uses hand-eye coordination with the arms extended, it is best to test for the dominant eye at arm's length distance (Figure 2.1). The test is as follows:

1. Extend both arms and form a small circle with the thumb and index finger of each hand.
2. With both eyes open, sight through the circle formed by the thumbs and fingers at an object at the other end of the room. Make the circle as small as possible.
3. Close your left eye only. If the object is still seen through the circle, you are right-eye dominant. If the object is no longer seen through the circle, you are left-eye dominant.
4. Repeat the procedure closing the right eye and note the difference.

When looking for symmetry or asymmetry, it is important that the dominant eye be located midway between the two anatomical parts being observed and/or palpated. For example, when palpating each acromion process to identify the level of the shoul-

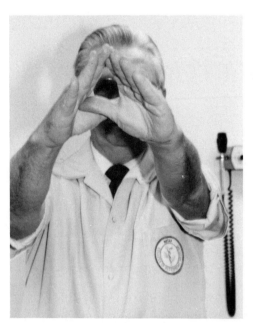

Figure 2.1.
Test for dominant eye.

1. The ability to detect tissue texture abnormality.
2. The ability to detect asymmetry of position, both visual and tactile.
3. The ability to detect differences of movement in total range, quality of movement during the range, and quality of sensation at the end of the range of movement.
4. The ability to sense position in space of both the patient and examiner.
5. The ability to detect change in palpatory findings, both improvement and worsening, over time.

It is important to develop coordinated and symmetrical use of the hands so that they may be linked with the visual sense. In developing palpatory skill, one must be aware that different parts of the hands are valuable for different tests. For example, the palm of the hands is best suited to sense contour through stereognosis; the dorsum of the hand is more sensitive to temperature variation; the fingerpad is best for fine discrimination of textural differences, finite skin contour, and so on; and the tip of the thumb is useful as a pressure probe for the assessment of difference in depth.

Three stages in the development and perception of palpatory sense have been described: reception, transmission, and interpretation. The proprioceptors and mechanoreceptors of the hand receive stimulation from the tissues being palpated. This is the reception phase. These impulses are then transmitted through the peripheral and central nervous system to the brain where they are analyzed and interpreted. During the palpation process, care must be exercised to assure efficiency of reception, transmission, and interpretation. Care must be taken of the examiner's hands to protect these sensitive diagnostic instruments. Avoidance of injury abuse is essential; hands should be clean and nails an appropriate length. During the palpation process, the operator should be relaxed and comfortable to avoid extraneous interference with the transmission of the palpatory impulse. To accurately assess and interpret palpatory findings, it is essential that the physician concentrate on the act of palpation, the tissue being palpated, and the response of the palpating fingers and hands. All extraneous sensory stimuli should be reduced as much as possible. Probably the most common mistake in palpation is the lack of concentration by the examiner.

Tissue palpation can be further divided into light touch and deep touch. In light touch the amount of pressure is very slight and the examiner attempts to assess tissue change both actively and passively. By simply laying hands on the tissue passively, the exam-

ders, the dominant eye should be in the midsagittal plane of the patient, equidistant from each palpating hand. In other words, the dominant eye should be on the midline of the two anatomical parts being compared. With a patient supine on the examining table, a right-eye-dominant examiner should stand on the right side of the patient and a left-eye-dominant examiner should stand on the left side of the patient. Remember that the hands and eyes should be on the same reference plane when one is attempting to determine whether paired anatomical parts are symmetrically placed. For example, when evaluating the height of the shoulders by palpating the two acromion processes and visualizing a level against the horizontal plane, the eyes should be on the same horizontal plane as the palpating hands. When palpating the two iliac crests to identify whether they are level against the horizontal plane, the eyes should be at the level of the iliacs crests in the same plane as the palpating hands. Whenever possible the eyes should be in the plane against which anatomical landmarks are being compared for symmetry or asymmetry.

All physicians use palpation in physical examination of the abdomen for masses, normal organs for size and position, point of maximum impulse of the heart, tactile fremitus of the lungs, and pulsations of the peripheral vessels. Palpation is also used to identify masses, normal and abnormal lymph nodes, and other changes of the tissues. In structural diagnosis palpation requires serious consideration and practice to develop high-level diagnostic skill. Palpatory skill affects:

iner is able to make tactile observation of the quality of the tissues under the palpating hand. By moving the lightly applied hand in an active fashion, scanning information of multiple areas of the body can be ascertained, both normal and apparently abnormal. Deep touch is the use of additional pressure to palpate deeper into the layers of the tissue of the musculoskeletal system. Compression is palpation through multiple layers of tissue and shear is a movement of tissue between layers. Combinations of active and passive palpation and light and deep touch are used throughout the palpatory diagnostic process.

It is useful to develop appropriate terms to describe the changes in the anatomy being palpated and evaluated. The use of paired descriptors such as superficial-deep, compressible-rigid, moist-dry, warm-cold, painful-nonpainful, circumscribed-diffuse, and rough-smooth, to name a few, are most useful. It is best to define in anatomical and physiological terms both normal and abnormal palpatory clues. Second, it is useful to define areas of altered palpatory sense by describing the state of the tissue change as either acute, subacute, or chronic in nature. Third, it is useful to develop a scale to measure the severity of the altered tissue textures being palpated. Are the tissues normal or are there changes that could be identified as mild, moderate, or severe? A 0, +1, +2, +3 scale is useful in diagnosing the severity of the problem and in monitoring response to therapeutic intervention over time. Try to use descriptive language that a colleague can comprehend.

LAYER PALPATION

The following describes a practice session that has been found helpful in learning skill in layer palpation of the tissues of the musculoskeletal system. Two individuals sit across from each other with their arms placed on a narrow table (Figure 2.2). Each individual's right hand is the examining instrument and the left forearm is the part for the partner to examine. Starting with the left palm on the table, each individual places the right hand (palms and fingers) over the forearm just distal to the elbow.

1. The right hand gently makes contact with the skin. No motion is introduced by the operator's right hand. The operator "thinks" skin. How thick is it? How warm or cold is it? How rough or smooth is it? The left forearm is now supinated and the examiner's right hand is placed on the volar surface of the forearm in the same fashion. Again, analysis of the skin is made and comparison made between the dorsal and volar aspects (Figure 2.3). Which is the thickest? Which is the smoothest? Which is the warmest? It is interesting to note the ability to identify significant difference between skin of one area and another by concentration on skin alone.

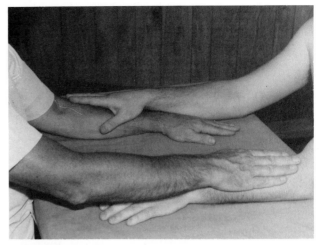

Figure 2.2.
Layer palpation dorsal forearm.

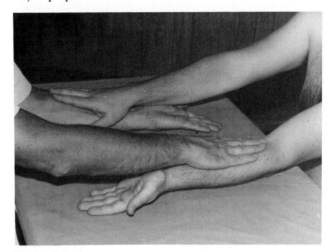

Figure 2.3.
Layer palpation volar forearm.

2. With the right hand firmly in contact with the skin, slight movement of the skin is made, both longitudinally and horizontally, to evaluate the subcutaneous fascia. You now concentrate on the second layer, the subcutaneous fascia. How thick is the layer? How loose is it? Note that movement in one direction that the tissues are more "loose" and in the other direction are more "tight." It is within this layer that many of the tissue texture abnormalities associated with somatic dysfunction are found.

3. Within the subcutaneous fascia layer are found the vessels, arteries, and veins. Palpate these structures for their identification and description.

4. Gently increase the pressure until you sense the deep fascia layer that envelops the underlying structures. Think deep fascia. It can be described as smooth, firm, and continuous. By palpating the deep fascia layer and moving the hand gently horizontally across the forearm, you can identify areas of thickening that form fascial compartments between

bundles of muscle. The ability to define these enveloping layers of deep fascia is helpful, not only in separating one muscle from another but as a means of getting deeper into underlying structures between muscle.

5. Palpating through the deep fascia, you now concentrate on the underlying muscle and, through concentration, identify individual fibers and the direction in which the fibers run. Move your hands both transversely and longitudinally, sensing for differences in smooth and rough. As you palpate across muscle fiber it feels rougher, but as you move in the direction of the muscle fiber it feels more smooth. While palpating muscle, both individuals slowly open and close their left hands, energizing the muscles of the forearm. Your right hand is now palpating contracting and relaxing muscle. Next, squeeze the left hand as hard as possible and palpate muscle during that activity. You are now palpating "hypertonic" muscle. This is the most common tissue texture abnormality feel at the muscle level in areas of somatic dysfunction.

6. While palpating at the muscle level, slowly course down the forearm until you first feel change in tissue and the loss of ability to discern muscle fiber. You have now contacted the musculotendinous junction, a point in muscle that is vulnerable to injury (Figure 2.4).

7. Continue to course down toward the wrist, beyond the musculotendinous junction, and palpate a smooth, round, firm structure called a tendon. Note the transition from muscle through musculotendinous junction to tendon.

8. Follow the tendon distally until you palpate a structure that binds the tendons at the wrist. Palpate that structure (Figure 2.5). It is the transverse carpal ligament. What are its characteristics? What direction

do its fibers traverse? How thick is it? How firm is it? Ligaments throughout the body feel quite similar.

9. Now return your palpating right hand to the elbow with your middle finger overlying the dimple of the elbow in the dorsal side and your thumb opposite it on the ventral side to palpate the radial head (Figure 2.6). Stay on bone and think bone. How hard it is? Is there any "life" in it?

10. Now move just proximal with your palpating thumb and index finger until you fall into the joint space. Underlying your palpating fingers is a structure that you should not be able to feel, namely, the joint capsule. Palpable joint capsules are present in pathological joints and are not usually found in somatic dysfunction. In fact, some individuals believe that a palpable joint capsule, with the limited exception of the knee joint, is a contraindication to direct-action manipulative treatment.

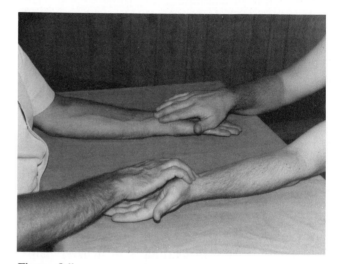

Figure 2.5.
Palpation of transcarpal ligament.

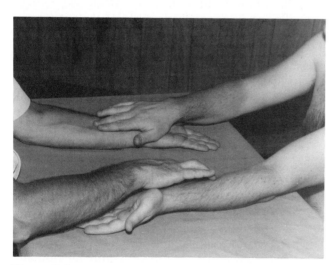

Figure 2.4.
Palpation of musculotendinous junction.

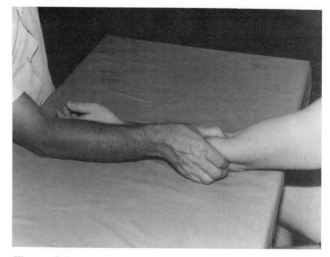

Figure 2.6.
Palpation of radial head.

You have now palpated skin, subcutaneous fascia, blood vessels, deep fascia, muscle, musculotendinous junction, tendon, ligament, bone, and joint space. After using the forearm as the model, these same structures are palpable throughout the body. Practice and experience can enhance your capability as a structural diagnostician.

Development of high level palpation skill requires considerable practice and is accumulated over time if a concentrated effort is made. It is also important to avoid the three most common errors in palpation, namely lack of concentration, too much pressure, and too much movement. As stated earlier, the most common error is the lack of concentration on the task at hand. The beginner frequently attempts to gain information rapidly and presses much too hard. Remember, the harder you press, the more stimulation you provide to your own mechanoreceptors, increasing the amount of sensory impulse being transmitted. The beginner is also prone to use too much movement in searching for anatomical landmarks and in identifying layers of tissue. This is called the "jiggling hands syndrome." One must remember that the more motion exerted by the hands, the more stimulation there is to the afferent system to be transmitted and interpreted by the nervous system. Therefore, concentrate, do not push too hard, and do not move too much.

MOTION SENSE

In identifying areas of somatic dysfunction by defining alterations in the diagnostic triad of asymmetry, altered range of motion, and tissue texture abnormality, a combination of observation and palpation is used. In palpation both static and dynamic dimensions are present. Statically, we look for levels of paired anatomical parts to identify asymmetry. Both by static and dynamic palpation, we look for alteration in tissue texture abnormality. In palpating tissues without movement, the examiner is interested in skin temperature, smoothness, thickness, and other qualifiers of the state of the tissue. In dynamic palpation, one evaluates, by compression and shear movement, the thickness of the tissue, the amount of normal tissue tone, and a sense of which tissues are abnormal. It is within the evaluation of the range of motion that the palpatory sense becomes highly refined. Because restoration of the maximal normal amount of motion possible in the tissue is the desired end point, it is essential that we be able to identify normal and abnormal ranges of motion within both soft tissue and arthrodial structures.

Motion sense is an essential component of the palpatory art in structural diagnosis. The examiner attempts to identify whether there is normal mobility, restricted movement (hypomobility), or too much movement (hypermobility). In motion testing, the examiner may put a region or part of the body through both active and passive movement to ascertain how that part complies with the motion demand placed on it. Information is sought as to whether the mobility is abnormal in a regional sense or confined to one segment. A wide variety of techniques can be used, both actively and passively, to test for motion.

The examiner must recognize that there is an inherent tissue motion that is continuous and palpable with practice. Return to the hand and forearms positions of Figure 2.2 with very light contact. Close your eyes and concentrate on the behavior of the tissues under your palpating hand. With practice you will note that the forearm is not static but is inherently, dynamically moving. This inherent motion is thought to be a compilation of motions from transmissions of the arterial pulse, effect of respiration, contraction and relaxation of muscle fibers during normal muscle tone, and the cranial rhythmic impulse.

It is essential that good contact be made with the examiner's hand(s) on the part(s) being palpated. As the part is taken through range of motion, either actively or passively, the examiner is interested in three elements, range of movement, quality of movement during the range, and "end feel." In determining range of movement, one is interested in the quantity of movement. Is it normal, restricted, or increased in range? Second, how does it feel during the movement throughout the range. Is it smooth? Is it "sticky" or "jerky" or "too loose?" There are a number of alterations in movement feel during the range that can be of assistance to the examiner in determining what factors might be altering the range of movement. Third, what is the feel at the end point of the range of movement? Is there symmetry to the range, and does each extreme of the range of movement feel the same? If there is alteration in the end feel, what are the qualities of the end point? Is it hard? Is it soft? Is it spongy? Is it jerky? There are a wide variety of characteristic end feels that experience will teach the examiner. The quality of the end feel is most helpful in determining what the cause of the restrictive movement might be and what type of manipulative therapy might be most effective.

Hypermobility

Manual medicine procedures are used to overcome restrictions of movement. Techniques that increase mobility should not be used in the presence of hypermobility. Hypermobility is present when there is an increase in the range of movement, a loose feeling throughout the range of movement, and loss of normal tissue resiliency at the end feel. Hypermobility might very well be normal in certain highly trained athletes, such as gymnasts and acrobats, but in most individuals it must be considered abnormal. In the vertebral complex it is not uncommon to find relative hypermobility of one vertebral motion segment adjacent to a vertebral motion segment that is restricted. This has been described as "compensatory hypermobility" and has been explained as the body's attempt to maintain mobility of the total mechanism in the presence of restricted mobility of a part of the vertebral axis. It is not infrequent to find that hypermobile segments are the areas of symptomotology. As such, they gain a great deal of attention from the examiner. Care must be exercised not to provide manual medicine procedures that increase the relative hypermobility of these segments rather than appropriately applying mobilizing techniques to the segment(s) with restricted mobility. Hypermobility can be taken to the stage that can best be described as instability. Instability occurs when the integrity of the tissues supporting the joint structure cannot maintain appropriate functional apposition of the moving parts so the relative stability of the motion unit is lost. The dividing line between hypermobility and instability is not always definite, and good objective measures to quantify instability are still not available. Nonetheless, the skilled clinician must develop some sense of normal motion, hypomobility, hypermobility, and instability of anatomical structures within the musculoskeletal system. It is for this reason that the development of a motion sense is worth the effort.

One must also develop the skill of motion sense to identify change in the range of motion, quality of movement during a range, and the end feel after a manual medicine intervention. It is useful in prognosis as well as diagnosis. It should be possible to identify change in range of motion, and its quality, if a manual medicine intervention has been successful. Retesting the range of motion available is always the last step in any manual medicine therapeutic intervention.

Motion sense is an essential component of the palpatory art in structural diagnosis. As in any art form, practice is the major requirement for mastery.

SCREENING EXAMINATION

The screening examination evaluates the total musculoskeletal system as part of patient examination. It answers the question, "is there a problem within the musculoskeletal system that deserves additional evaluation?" There are numerous formats for a screening examination. The following 12-step procedure is comprehensive in scope and can be accomplished rapidly.

Step 1. Gait analysis in multiple directions.
Step 2. Observation of static posture and palpable assessment of paired anatomical landmarks.
Step 3. Dynamic trunk sidebending.
Step 4. Standing flexion test.
Step 5. Stork test.
Step 6. Seated flexion test.
Step 7. Screening test of upper extremities.
Step 8. Trunk rotation.
Step 9. Trunk sidebending.
Step 10. Head and neck mobility.
Step 11. Respiration of thoracic cage.
Step 12. Lower extremity screening.

Step 1. Gait Analysis

1. Observe gait with patient walking toward you (Figure 2.7).

2. Observe patient walking away from you (Figure 2.8).

3. Observe patient walking from the side (Figures 2.9 and 2.10).

4. Observe length of stride, swing of arm, heel strike, toe off, tilting of the pelvis, and adaption of the shoulders.

5. One looks for the functional capacity of the gait, not the usual pathological conditions. Of particular importance is the cross-patterning of the gait and symmetry of stride.

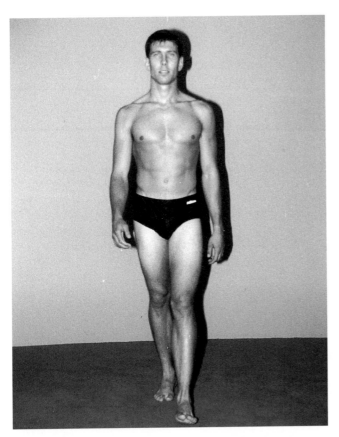

Figure 2.7.

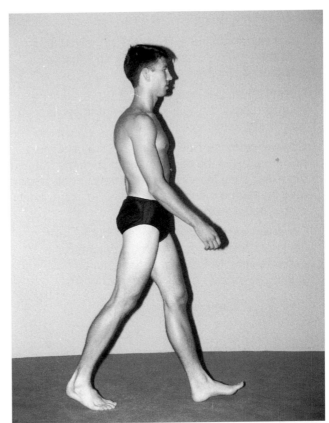

Figure 2.9.

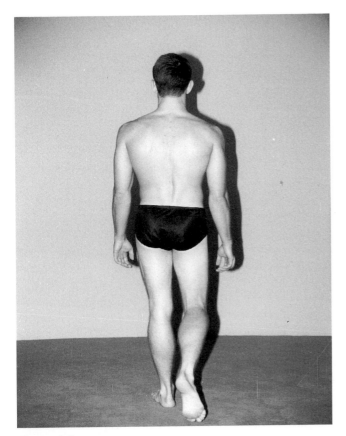

Figure 2.8.

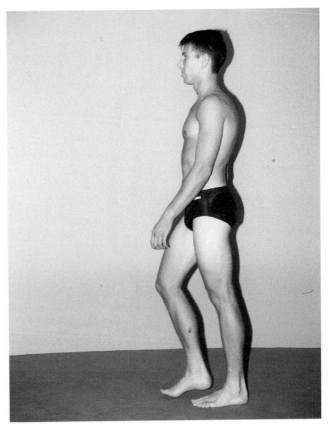

Figure 2.10.

Step 2A. Static Analysis Posture

1. Observe from the front (Figure 2.11), evaluating weight distribution, head carriage, shoulder level, and foot placement.

2. Observe from the back (Figure 2.12), evaluating head carriage, shoulder height, level of pelvis, and weight distribution on the feet.

3. Observe from the side (Figure 2.13), evaluating posture against the plumb line, which drops from the external auditory meatus to the tip of the acromion through the femoral trochanter to just in front of the medial malleolus.

4. Observe from the opposite side (Figure 2.14), again assesses plumb line and compares with opposite side. Note head carriage, anteroposterior spinal curves, and extent of knee extension.

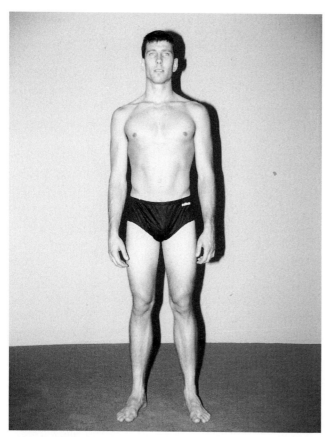

Figure 2.11.

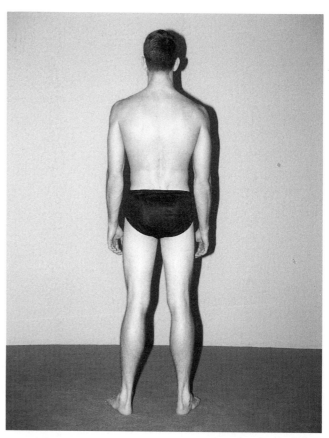

Figure 2.12.

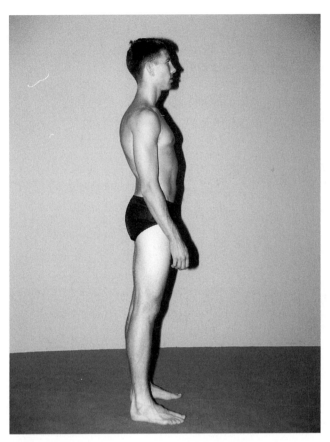

Figure 2.13.

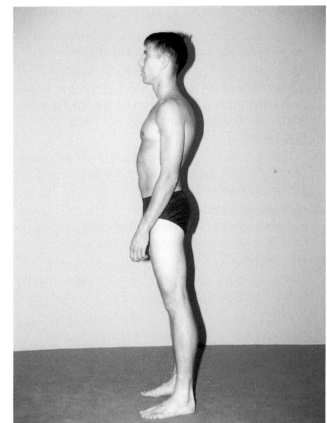

Figure 2.14.

Step 2B. Static Posture Anatomical Levels

1. Combined palpation and observation is made of the levels of the acromion process (Figure 2.15).

2. Palpation of the iliac crest (Figure 2.16) is performed by pushing soft tissue out of the way from below and placing proximal phalanges of the index fingers on similar portions of the right and left innominate.

3. Palpation and observation of the top of the greater trochanter requires lateral to medial compression of the soft tissues of the lateral hip (Figure 2.17).

4. Unleveling of the iliac crest and greater trochanter in the standing position is the first index of suspicion for a short leg, pelvic tilt syndrome.

5. Note that the eyes are on the same horizontal place as are the palpating fingers for better hand and eye coordination.

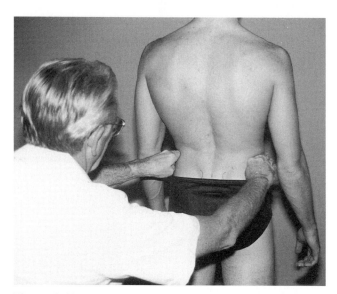

Figure 2.16.

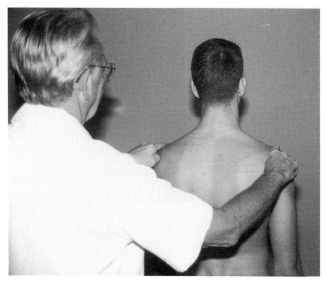

Figure 2.15.

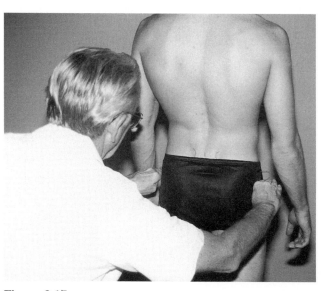

Figure 2.17.

STEP 3. Trunk Sidebending

1. Observation is made from the back.

2. Patient is asked to sidebend left (Figure 2.18) as far as possible without bending forward.

3. The patient repeats the sidebending to the right (Figure 2.19), again without bending forward.

4. Observation is made of the symmetry of range right to left as a reflection of fingertip distance on the lateral leg.

5. Observation is made of the induced spinal curve, which should be a smooth symmetrical C shape and with fullness on the side of the induced convexity. Straightening of segments of the induced curve and fullness on the side of the concavity are highly suggestive of significant vertebral motion segment dysfunction at that level.

6. Observation is made of the symmetry of the pelvic shift right to left during the sidebending effort and whether the loading of the lower extremities appear symmetric.

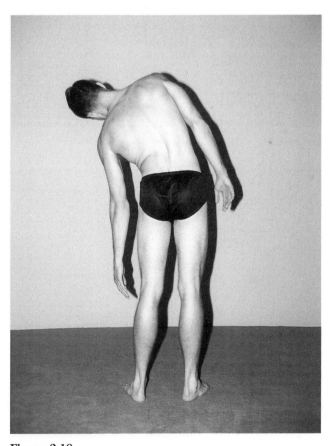

Figure 2.18.

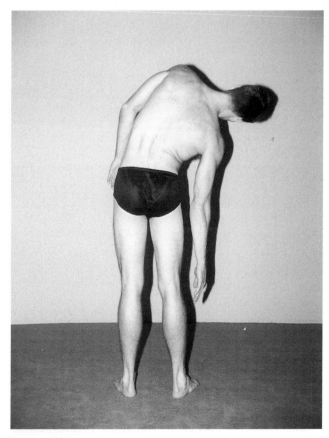

Figure 2.19.

Step 4. Standing Flexion Test

1. Patient stands with feet approximately 4 inches apart with weight under hip joints (Figure 2.20).

2. Operator palpates with pads of the thumbs the inferior slope of the posterior superior iliac spine.

3. Patient is instructed to bend forward as smoothly as possible attempting to touch the floor (Figure 2.21). Operator's thumbs follow the posterior superior iliac spines to see whether one appears to move more cephalward or ventral than the other.

4. The test is viewed as positive if one posterior superior iliac spine moves further than the other.

5. Observation is also made of the lower thoracic and lumbar spines for segmental rhythm and for the introduction of sidebending rotational curves.

6. This test is very sensitive to dysfunctions in the articulations of the bony pelvis and the fascias of the trunk and lower extremity. Its value is to lateralize dysfunction from one side to the other of the pelvis.

7. Repeating the standing flexion test beginning with the arms overhead (Figure 2.22) and forward bending with the arms in that position (Figure 2.23) alters the behavior of the pelvic girdle through loads through the fascias of the rib cage and upper extremity.

8. Different behavior of the posterior superior iliac spine in the two variations gives the examiner information as to whether major restrictors are above or below the pelvis.

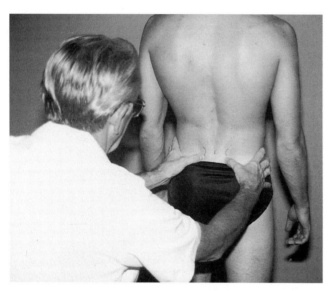

Figure 2.20.

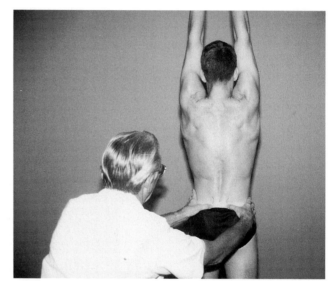

Figure 2.22.

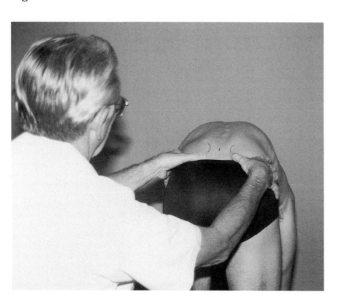

Figure 2.21.

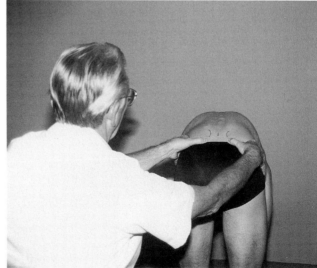

Figure 2.23.

Step 5. Stork Test

1. With the patient standing and the operator sitting behind, the operator's left thumb is placed over the most posterior portion of the left posterior superior iliac spine and the right thumb overlying the midline of the sacrum at the same level (Figure 2.24).

2. Operator asks the patient to flex the left hip and knee to a minimum of 90° hip flexion (Figure 2.25).

3. A negative test finds the left thumb on the posterior superior iliac spine moving caudad in relation to the right thumb on the sacrum.

4. The thumb placements are reversed, and the pa-

tient is asked to raise the right leg in similar fashion (Figure 2.26).

5. A positive finding occurs when the thumb on the posterior superior iliac spine moves cephalward in relation to the thumb on the sacrum.

6. This test is correlated with the standing flexion test. The stork test is more specific for sacroiliac joint restriction.

7. If the patient has difficulty in standing on one foot to perform the test, proprioceptive sensory motor balance deficit should be further evaluated.

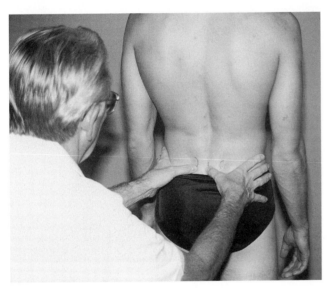

Figure 2.24.

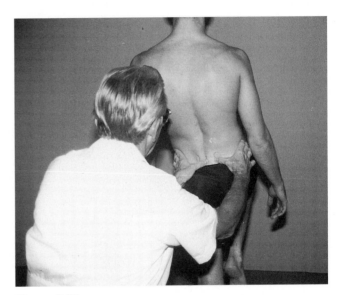

Figure 2.26.

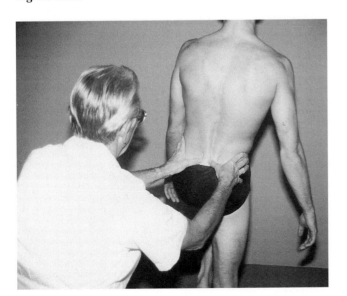

Figure 2.25.

Step 6. Seated Flexion Test

1. Patient sitting on examining stool with knees apart and feet flat on the floor.

2. Operator's two thumbs contact the inferior slope of each posterior superior iliac spine (Figure 2.27).

3. Patient is instructed to bend forward with the arms between the knees as far as possible (Figure 2.28).

4. Operator monitors the movement of the two posterior superior iliac spines (Figure 2.29). The one that moves the furthest in a cephalward or ventral direction is deemed positive, indicative of restricted mobility on that side of the pelvis.

5. Operator observes the behavior of the lower thoracic and lumbar spines for dysrhythmia and for the introduction of sidebending and rotational curves.

6. Comparison of findings with those of a standing flexion test evaluates the behavior of the pelvic girdle and vertebral complex without the influence of the lower extremities as the patient is sitting on the ischial tuberosities.

7. Unleveling of the iliac crest when seated to perform this test is presumptive evidence of inequality in size of the right and left innominates.

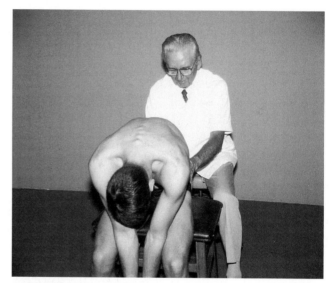

Figure 2.28.

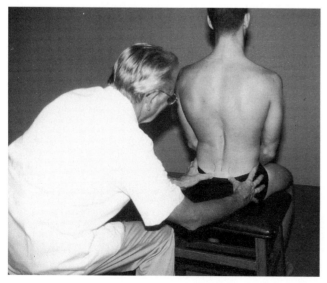

Figure 2.27.

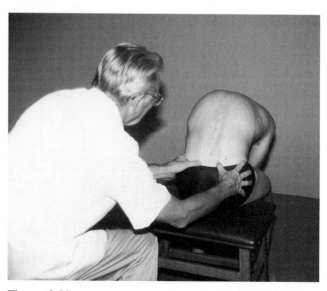

Figure 2.29.

Step 7. Upper Extremity Screen

1. Patient seated on examining stool or table.

2. Patient instructed to fully abduct both upper extremities in the coronal plane, reach to the ceiling, and turn the backs of the hands together (Figure 2.30).

3. Observation is made from the front.

4. Observation is also made from behind (Figure 2.31).

5. This maneuver requires mobility of the sternoclavicular, acromioclavicular, glenohumeral, elbow, and wrist joints.

6. Any asymmetry indicates additional evaluation necessary.

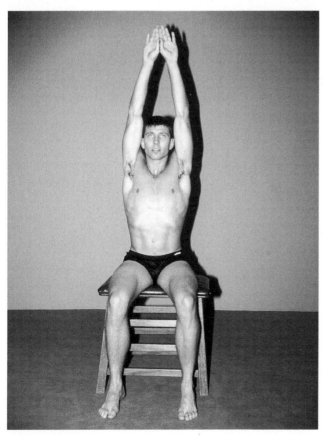

Figure 2.30.

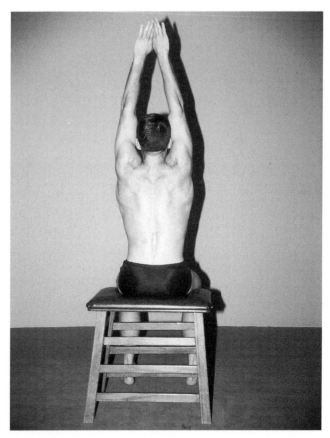

Figure 2.31.

Step 8. Trunk Rotation

1. Patient sitting on table with operator standing behind.

2. Operator grasps each shoulder (Figure 2.32).

3. Operator introduces trunk rotation through the shoulders (Figure 2.33) sensing for range, quality of movement, and end feel.

4. Operator rotates trunk to the left (Figure 2.34), comparing range, quality of movement, and end feel with right rotation.

5. Asymmetry of right to left rotation indicates additional diagnostic procedures for the vertebral column and thoracic cage.

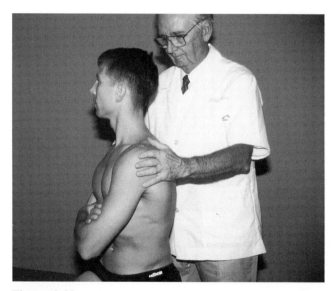

Figure 2.33.

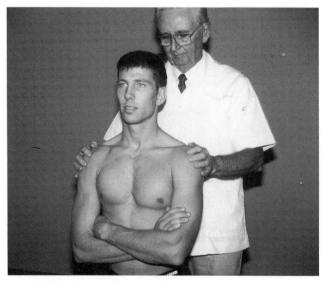

Figure 2.32.

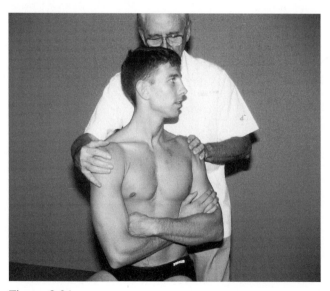

Figure 2.34.

Step 9. Trunk Sidebending

1. Patient sitting with operator standing behind.

2. Operator grasps each shoulder (Figure 2.35).

3. Operator presses downward on right shoulder by the right hand introducing right sidebending (Figure 2.36) sensing for range, quality of movement, and end feel.

4. Operator pushes left shoulder inferiorly to introduce left sidebending (Figure 2.37) sensing for range, quality of movement, and end feel.

5. Comparison is made of left and right sidebending for symmetry or asymmetry. Asymmetry demonstrates need for additional diagnostic evaluation of the vertebral column and the thoracic cage.

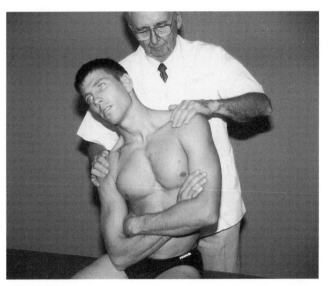

Figure 2.36.

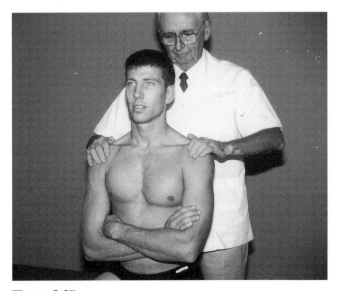

Figure 2.35.

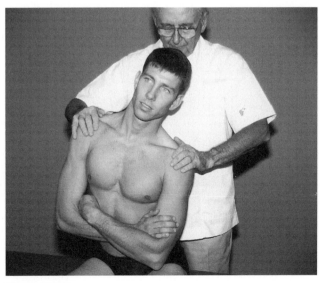

Figure 2.37.

Step 10. Mobility of The Head and Neck

1. Patient sitting on table with operator standing behind.

2. Operator grasps head between the two hands (Figure 2.38).

3. Operator introduces backward bending (Figure 2.39). Normal extension is 90°.

4. Operator introduces forward bending (Figure 2.40). Normal range is 45° of flexion.

5. Operator introduces right sidebending (Figure 2.41) and left sidebending (Figure 2.42). Normal range is 45° to each side.

6. Operator introduces rotation left (Figure 2.43) and to the right (Figure 2.44). Normal range is 80–90° each side.

7. Operator evaluates range, quality of movement during the range, and end feel looking for symmetry or asymmetry. If asymmetric, additional diagnostic evaluation of the cervical spine, upper thoracic spine, and rib cage is necessary.

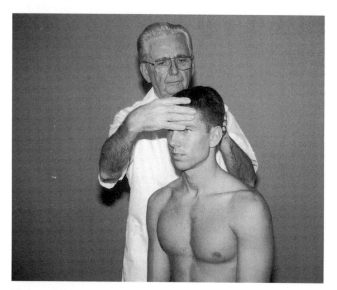

Figure 2.38.

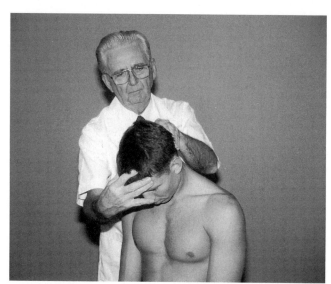

Figure 2.40.

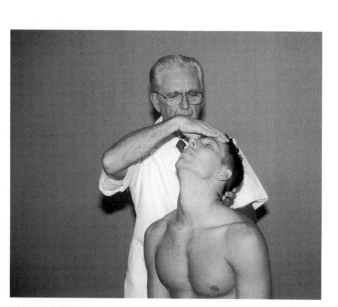

Figure 2.39.

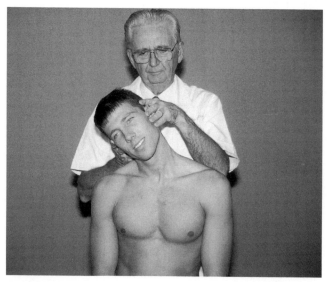

Figure 2.41.

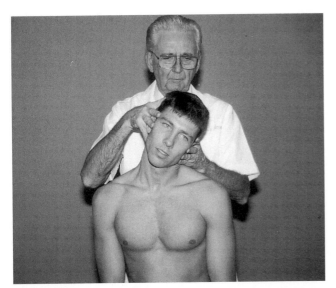

Figure 2.42.

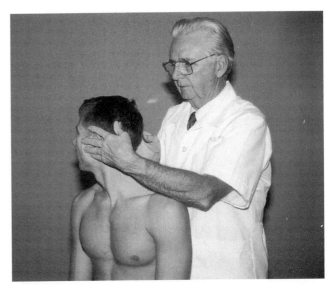

Figure 2.44.

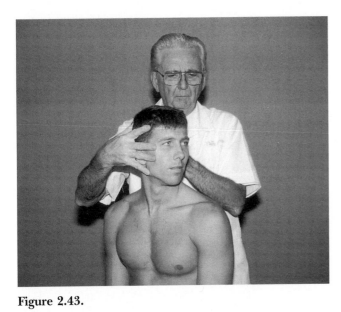

Figure 2.43.

Step 11. Respiratory Movement of Thoracic Cage

1. Patient supine on the table with operator standing at side with dominant eye over the midline of the patient.

2. Operator symmetrically places hands over the anterolateral aspect of the lower rib cage bilaterally (Figure 2.45).

3. Patient is instructed to deeply inhale and exhale while operator follows lower thoracic cage movement during respiration looking for symmetry or lack of same.

4. Operator places hands in intercostal spaces of the anterolateral aspect of the upper rib cage (Figure 2.46) to evaluate bucket handle movement of upper ribs during inhalation and exhalation by the patient.

5. Operator's hands are placed vertically over anterior aspect of the upper rib cage with the longest finger in contact with the cartilage of the first rib under the medial end of the clavicle (Figure 2.47) and assesses pump handle motion response of the upper rib cage to inhalation and exhalation.

6. Asymmetry of movement of inhalation and exhalation effort calls for more definitive diagnosis of the thoracic spine and rib cage.

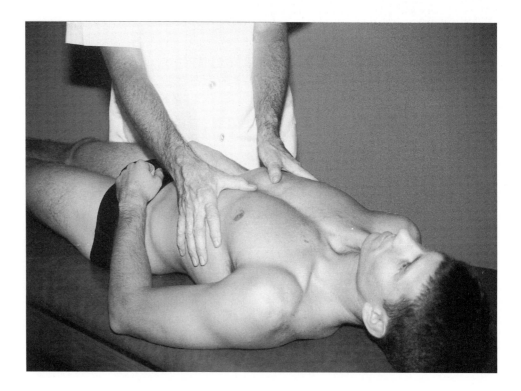

Figure 2.45.

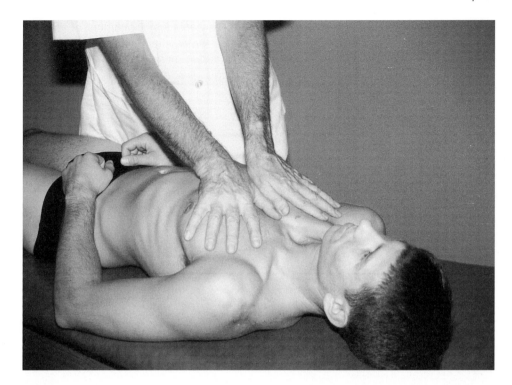

Figure 2.46.

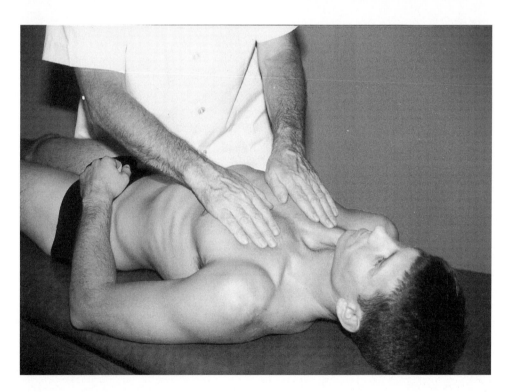

Figure 2.47.

Step 12. Lower Extremity Screen

1. Patient supine on table with operator standing at side.

2. Operator grasps left ankle while monitoring the right anterior superior iliac spine (Figure 2.48).

3. Operator lifts left leg until first movement of the right anterior superior iliac spine is felt, indicative of length of the hamstring muscle group (Figure 2.49).

4. Comparison is made with the opposite side for symmetry or asymmetry.

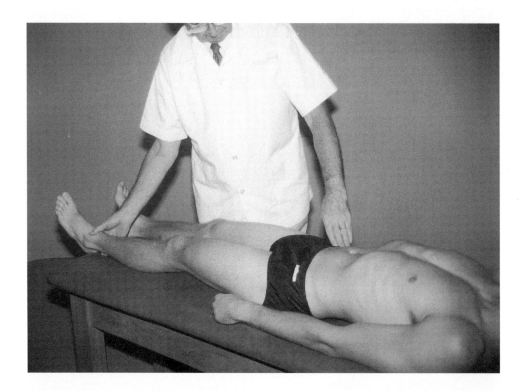

Figure 2.48.

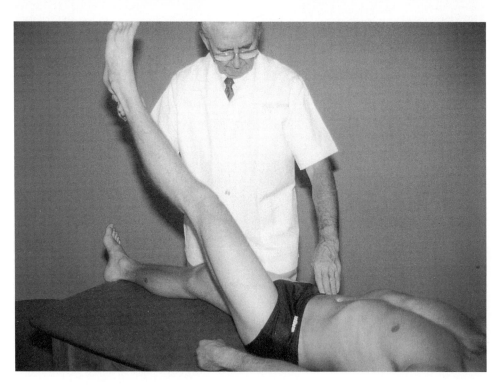

Figure 2.49.

5. Operator flexes, externally rotates, and abducts the patient's right hip (Figure 2.50). Comparison is made with the opposite side for symmetry or asymmetry. Restricted motion suggests dysfunction and pathology of the right hip joint.

6. Patient is instructed to do a deep knee bend maintaining the heels on the floor (Figure 2.51). This squat test requires mobility of the foot, ankle, knee, and hip joints bilaterally. Inability to perform the squat test indicates additional diagnostic evaluation of the lower extremities.

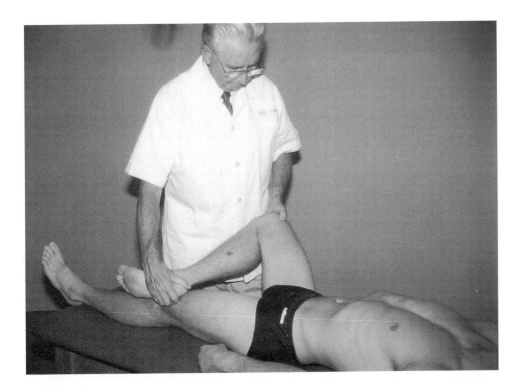

Figure 2.50.

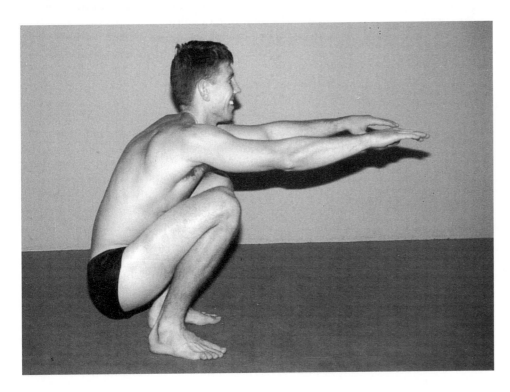

Figure 2.51.

SCANNING EXAMINATION

Once an area of the musculoskeletal system has been identified during the screening examination as being of sufficient abnormality for further investigation, a scanning procedure of that region is initiated. The scanning examination is designed to answer the question what part of the region and what tissues within the region are significantly dysfunctional? By using the analogy of a microscope, we have gone from low power (the screening examination) to high power (scanning examination). More definitive evaluation of soft tissue can be accomplished with active and passive light and deep touch. Thumbs or fingers can be used as a pressure probe searching for areas of tenderness or more specific signs of tissue texture change. Multiple variations of motion scanning can be introduced to look for alterations in symmetry of range, quality of movement, and sensations at end feel. Respiratory effort might be used to evaluate the response of the region to inhalation and exhalation efforts. Responses within the region to demands placed on it from more remote areas of the musculoskeletal system are frequently useful in better defining the area requiring specific attention.

SKIN ROLLING TEST

One valuable diagnostic test for scanning purposes is the skin rolling test. In this examination, a fold of skin is grasped between the thumb and index finger and rolled as if one were rolling a cigarette (Figure 2.52). Skin rolling can be accomplished symmetrically on each side of the body, testing for normal pain-free laxity of the skin and subcutaneous fascia. A positive finding is tenderness and pain provocation in certain dermatonal levels of skin with tightness

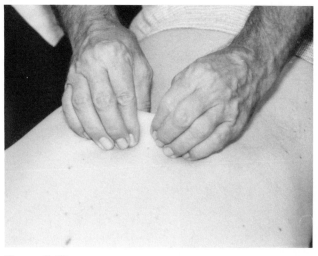

Figure 2.52.
Skin rolling.

and loss of resiliency within the skin and subcutaneous fascia. Frequently, tender nodules will be palpated while accomplishing this test. They are interpreted to represent alteration in dermatomal innervation from dysfunctions within the vertebral axis. In the examination of the thoracic and lumbar regions of the spine, it is recommended that the skin be rolled in the midline overlying the spinous processes and more laterally, coursing from below upward, comparing changes on one side to the other. Although defined as a scanning procedure, skin rolling can be quite specific in defining specific segmental dysfunction because of the clinically observable dermatomal relationship to altered vertebral motion segment function.

SEGMENTAL DEFINITION

The third element to the diagnostic process is segmental definition, used to identify the specific vertebral motion segment, or peripheral joint, that is dysfunctional. It is also used to determine the specific motion restriction that is involved. An attempt is made to identify the tissue(s) that are most involved in the dysfunctional segment.

One method of identifying the specific joint that is dysfunctional, and the motion that is lost, is to test for joint-play movements. This concept has been advocated for many years by Mennell. Joint-play movements are defined as being independent of the action of voluntary muscle and are found within synovial joints. The range of joint play is very small but very precise. Normal joint-play movement allows for easy, painless performance of voluntary movement. The amount of joint play is usually less than one-eighth of an inch in any one plane within a synovial joint. Mennell defines joint dysfunction as the loss of joint-play movement that cannot be recovered by the action of voluntary muscles. Once the precise system for identifying joint play is learned, very similar maneuvers can be used therapeutically in restoring anatomical and physiological function to the joint by restoring its normal joint play.

There are numerous diagnostic procedures that can specifically define within the vertebral motion segment, or within the synovial extremity joint, the specific dysfunction that is present. Subsequent chapters deal with the methods most commonly used by this author. The primary goal is to determine which specific vertebral motion segment is dysfunctional, which joint within that vertebral motion segment is dysfunctional, the direction of altered motion(s), and some estimate of the tissue involved in the restricted motion. Primary emphasis is placed on motion loss and its characteristics. Many diagnostic systems depend on localization of pain or provocation of pain by certain motion introductions. In the opinion of this author, motion loss and its characteristics are more valuable diagnostic criteria than the presence of pain and the provocation of pain by movement. Pain and its provocation can be of assistance in diagnosis, but they are not diagnostic in and of themselves.

These principles of structural diagnosis need to be studied extensively and mastered by the physician who wishes to be skilled in the field of manual medicine. An accurate and specific diagnosis is essential for successful results from manual medicine therapeutic interventions.

3

BARRIER CONCEPTS

Within the diagnostic triad of asymmetry, range of motion abnormality, and tissue texture abnormality, perhaps the most significant is alteration in the range of joint and tissue movement. Loss of normal motion within the tissues of the musculoskeletal system, or one of its component parts, responds most favorably to appropriate manual medicine therapeutic intervention. To achieve the goal of manual medicine intervention and restore maximal, pain-free movement to a musculoskeletal system in postural balance, we must be able to identify both normal and abnormal movement. In the presence of altered movement of the hypomobility type, an appropriate manual medicine intervention might be the treatment of choice. We must strive to improve mobility of all of the tissues of the musculoskeletal system, bone, joint, muscle, ligament, fascia, and fluid, with the anticipated outcome of restoring normal physiological movement and maximum functional physiology as well.

In the musculoskeletal system there are inherent movements, voluntary movements, and involuntary movements. The inherent movement has been described by some authors as relating to the recurrent coiling and uncoiling of the brain and longitudinal movement of the spinal cord, together with a fluctuation of the cerebral spinal fluid. Inherent motion is also the movement of the musculoskeletal system in relation to respiration. It has been observed that during inhalation the curves within the vertebral column straighten and with exhalation the curves are increased. With inhalation the extremities rotate externally, and with exhalation, internally. The voluntary movements of the musculoskeletal system are active movements resulting from contraction of muscle from voluntary conscious control. The involuntary movements of the musculoskeletal system are described as passive movements. Passive movement is induced by an external force moving a part of the musculoskeletal system through an arc of motion. The joint-play movements described by Mennell are also involuntary movements. They are not a component of the normal active or passive range of movement but are essential for the accomplishment of normal active and passive movement.

In structural diagnosis we speak of both normal and abnormal barriers to joint and tissue motion. The examiner must be able to identify and characterize normal and abnormal range of movement and normal and abnormal barrier to movement to make an accurate diagnosis. Most joints have motion in multiple planes, but for descriptive purposes we describe barriers to movement within one plane of motion for one joint. The total range of motion (Fig. 3.1) from one extreme to the other is limited by the anatomical integrity of the joint and its supporting ligaments, muscles, and fascia. Exceeding the anatomical barrier causes fracture, dislocation, or violation of tissue such as ligamentous tear. Somewhere within the total range of movement is found a midline neutral point.

Within the total range of motion there is a range of passive movement available that the examiner can extraneously introduce (Fig. 3.2). The limits to this passive range of movement have been described by some as the elastic barrier. At this point all tension has been taken within the joint and its surrounding tissues. There is a small amount of potential space between the elastic barrier and the anatomical barrier described by Sandoz as the paraphysiological space. It is within this area that the high-velocity low-amplitude thrust appears to generate the popping sound that results from the maneuver.

The range of active movement (Fig. 3.3) is somewhat less than that available with passive movement, and the end point of the range is called the physiological barrier. The normal end feel is due to resilience and tension within the muscle and fascial elements.

Frequently, there is reduction in available active motion due primarily to myofascial shortening (Fig. 3.4). This is often seen with aging, but it can occur at all ages. It is the stretching of this myofascial shortening that all individuals, particularly athletes, should do as part of physical exercise. Stretching exercise to

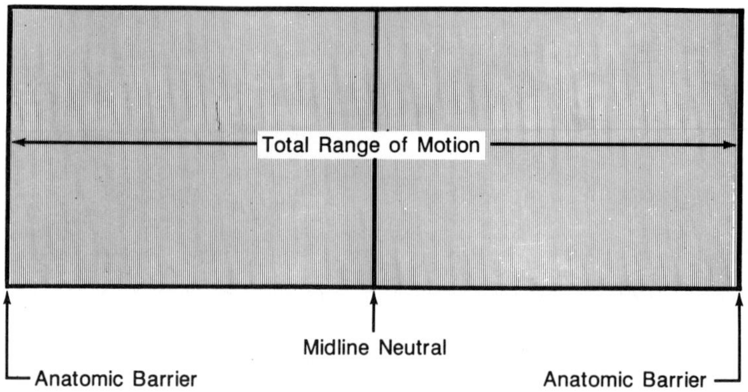

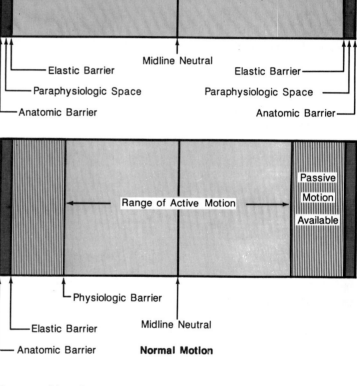

Figure 3.1.
Total range of motion.

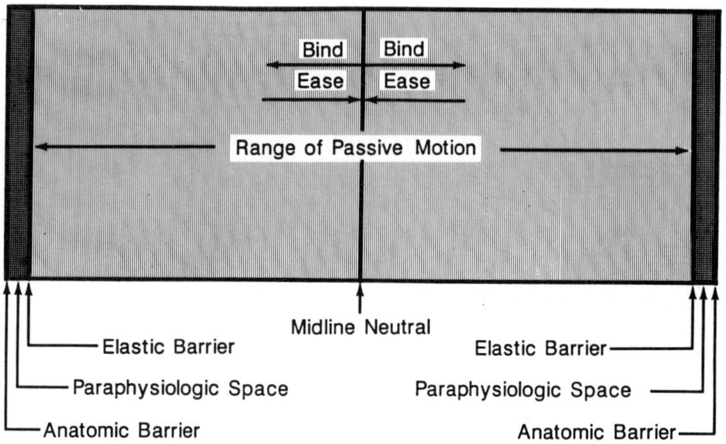

Figure 3.2.
Range of passive movement.

Figure 3.3.
Range of active movement.

the muscles and fascia enhances the active motion range available and the efficiency of myofascial function.

When motion is lost within the range, it can be described as major (Fig. 3.5) or minimal (Fig. 3.6). The barrier that prevents movement in the direction of motion loss is defined as the restrictive barrier. The amount of active motion available is limited on one side by the normal physiological barrier and on the opposite by the restrictive barrier. The goal of a manual medicine intervention would then be to move the restrictive barrier as far into the direction of motion loss as possible. Another clinically describ-

able phenomena associated with motion loss is the shifting of the neutral point from midline to the middle of the available active range. This is described as the "pathological" neutral and is usually, but not always, in the midrange of active motion available.

Each of the barriers described have palpable findings that can be described as either normal or abnormal end feel. Within a normal range of passive movement, the elastic barrier will have a normal sensation at the end point as a result of the passively induced tension within the joint and its surrounding structures. At the end of the range of active movement, the physiological barrier likewise has a charac-

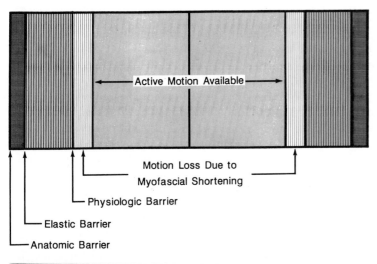

Figure 3.4.
Reduced range from myofascial shortening

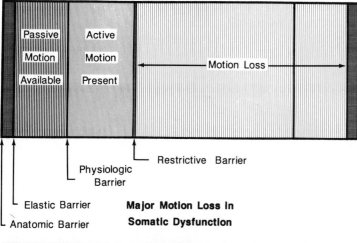

Figure 3.5.
Major motion loss.

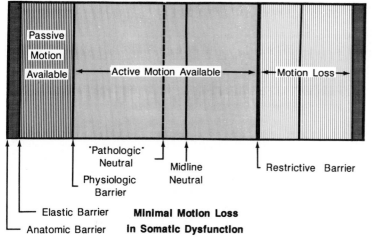

Figure 3.6.
Minimal motion loss.

teristic feel that results from the voluntary increase in resistance due to the apposition of the joints and the myofascial tension developed during voluntary muscular activity.

Let us return to the layer palpation exercise (see Chapter 2) and begin at the point where one examiner was evaluating the joint space at the proximal radiohumeral joint (Fig. 3.7). While palpating this joint with the thumb placed anteriorly and the index finger placed posteriorly, have the subject actively introduce pronation and supination (Fig. 3.8). You will note that the range is not symmetrical in pronation and supination and that the end feel is not the same at the terminal range of pronation and supination. Which range is greater? Which end feel seems tighter? Now grasp the subject's hand and wrist and passively introduce pronation and supination while monitoring at the proximal radiohumeral joint (Fig. 3.9). Note that you are now receiving proprioceptive impulse from your palpating hand at the radiohumeral joint, as well as from your hand as it passively introduces, through the subject's hand and wrist, the pronation and supination effort (Fig. 3.10). Again look for total range of movement, the quality of movement during the range, and the end feel. In supination and pronation, which has the greatest range? Which has the tighter or looser end feel? How does this compare with the active movement? Now let us take it one step further. While passively introducing pronation and supination, you should notice that tension increases the closer you get to the end points of the range. As you move in the opposite direction, it appears to be easier or more free. See if you can, by decreasing increments of pronation and supination, find the point between the two extremes of movement wherein the joint feel is the most free.

Even though pronation and supination is not a symmetrical range of movement at this joint, it is possible to find a point within the range that is the most free and could be described as the physiological neutral point.

We now have another concept of joint motion, the concept of "ease" and "bind" (Fig. 3.11). The more one moves in the direction of the neutral point, whether it be a midline neutral point in a normal range of motion or a pathological neutral point somewhere within the range of altered motion, it becomes more free, or there is more ease. Conversely, as one moves away from the neutral free point, one begins to sense a certain amount of bind or increase in resistance to the induced movement. Understanding this concept of ease and bind and the ability to sense this phenomenon are essential to mastering the functional (indirect) techniques (see Chapter 10). In the elbow exercise just accomplished, the hand palpating over the proximal radiohumeral joint

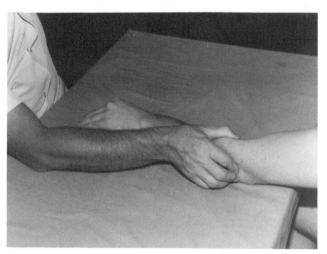

Figure 3.7.
Palpate radiohumeral joint.

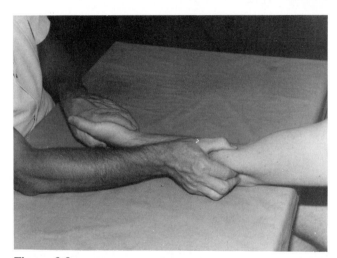

Figure 3.9.
Passive pronation-supination.

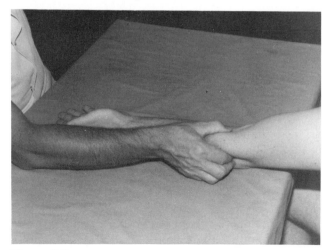

Figure 3.8.
Active pronation-supination.

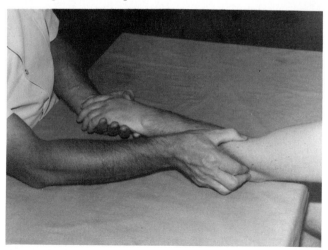

Figure 3.10.
Sensing hand of pronation-supination.

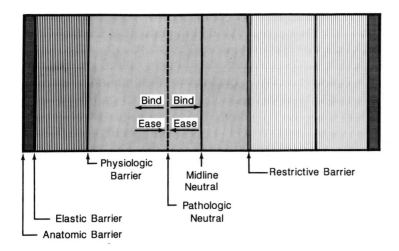

Physiologic
Barrier

Midline
Neutral

Restrictive Barrier

Pathologic
Neutral

Elastic Barrier

Anatomic Barrier

Figure 3.11.
Neutral ease-bind point.

was the "sensing hand" and your other hand, which introduced passive supination and pronation at the subject's hand, was the "motor hand."

RESTRICTIVE BARRIERS

The restrictive barriers limit movement within the normal range of motion and have different palpatory characteristics than the normal physiological, elastic, and anatomical barriers. The restrictive barrier can be within the following tissues:

Skin;
Fascia;
Muscle, long and short;
Ligament;
Joint capsule and surfaces.

Restrictive barriers can be found within one or more of these tissues, and the number and type contribute to the palpable characteristics at the restrictive barrier. Different pathological changes within these tissues can give quite different end feel sensations. For example, congestion and edema within the tissues will give a diffuse, boggy sensation quite like a sponge filled with water. Chronic fibrosis within these tissues will give a harder, more unyielding, rapidly ascending end feel when compared with the more boggy, edematous sensation. A restrictive barrier due to altered muscle physiology, whether it be spasm, hypertonus, or contracture, will give a more jerky and tightening type of end feel than one due to edema or fibrosis. Do not forget that pain can be a restrictive barrier as well. If a movement is painful, it will result in restriction as the body attempts to compensate for relief of pain by reduction of movement. When examining ranges of movement, and particularly when looking for normal and abnormal barriers to movement, one should constantly keep in mind the potential for hypermobility. The classical feel of a hypermobile range of motion is one of looseness for a greater extent of the range than would be antic-

ipated and with a rapidly escalating hard end feel when one approaches the elastic and anatomical barriers.

Restrictive barriers may also be long or short. They may involve a single joint or spinal segment or cross over more than one joint or series of spinal segments. It is important to identify the tissue or tissues involved in the restrictive barrier, their extent, and the functional pathology found within the tissues. Some types of manual medicine intervention are more appropriate for certain restrictive barriers than others.

In structural diagnosis, alteration of range of movement is an essential criterion for a diagnosis of somatic dysfunction. It is necessary to evaluate the total range of movement, the quality of movement available during the range, and the feel at the end point of movement to make an accurate diagnosis of the restrictive barrier. Therapeutic intervention by manipulative means can be described as an approach to these pathological barriers. Multiple methods are available and different activating forces can be used toward the goal of restoring maximal physiological movement available within the anatomy of the joint(s) and tissue(s).

DEFINITIONS

1. *Active motion:* movement of an articulation between the physiological barriers limited to the range produced voluntarily by the patient.

2. *Anatomical barrier:* the bone contour and/or soft tissues, especially ligaments, that serve as the final limit to motion in an articulation beyond which tissue damage occurs.

3. *Barrier:* an obstruction; a factor that tends to restrict free movement.

4. *Elastic barrier:* the resistance felt at the end of passive range of motion when the slack has been taken out.

5. *Motion:* movement, act, process, or instance of changing places.

6. *Paraphysiological space:* that sensation of a sudden "give" beyond the elastic barrier of resistance, usually accompanied by a "cracking" sound with a slight amount of movement beyond the usual physiological limit but within the anatomical barrier.

7. *Passive motion:* movement induced in an articulation by the operator. This includes the range of active motion as well as the movement between the physiological and anatomical barriers permitted by soft tissue resiliency that the patient cannot do voluntarily.

8. *Physiological barrier:* the soft tissue tension accumulation that limits the voluntary motion of an articulation. Further motion toward the anatomical barrier can be induced passively.

9. *Restrictive barrier:* an impediment or obstacle to movement within the physiological limits of an articulation that reduces the active motion range.

4

In the practice of medicine, it is essential that an accurate diagnosis be made before the institution of either curative or palliative therapy. When a therapeutic intervention is deemed to be indicated, particularly when using pharmacotherapeutic agents, a specific and accurate prescription needs to be written. No self-respecting physician would make a diagnosis of throat infection and write a prescription for antibiotic.

DX—Throat infection
RX—Antibiotic

The physician would seek to identify the infectious agent, either bacterial or viral, causing the throat infection. When a specific infectious agent was identified and was responsive to antibiotic therapy, a specific prescription would be written for the antibiotic agent. A prescription would identify the antibiotic to be used, the strength of each dose, the number of doses per day, and the duration of therapy.

In manual medicine it is common for practitioners to be lax in their specificity for the structural diagnosis and prescription of the manual medicine intervention to be applied. Too often a diagnosis is made of somatic dysfunction and manual medicine is the prescription.

DX—Somatic dysfunction
RX—Manipulative treatment

In manual medicine it is just as important to know the location, nature, and type of somatic dysfunction before a specific manual medicine therapeutic intervention is prescribed. The same elements are needed for a manual medicine prescription as for a pharmaceutical agent. One wants to be specific about the type of manual medicine, the intensity, the frequency, and the total length of the treatment plan. Therefore, the manipulative prescription requires an accurate diagnosis of the somatic dysfunction to be treated, a specific description of the type of manipulative procedure, the intensity, and the frequency.

Manipulative therapeutic procedures are indicated for the diagnostic entity somatic dysfunction or the manipulable lesion.

SOMATIC DYSFUNCTION

Somatic dysfunction is impaired or altered function of related components of the somatic (body framework) system; skeletal, arthrodial, and myofascial structures; and the related vascular, lymphatic, and neural elements.

MANIPULABLE LESION SYNONYMS

Joint blockage;
Joint lock;
Chiropractic subluxation;
Osteopathic lesion;
Loss of joint play;
Minor intervertebral derangements.

DIAGNOSTIC TRIAD

In defining somatic dysfunction, one uses three elements:

A Asymmetry of form or function of related parts of the musculoskeletal system;
R Range of motion, primarily alteration of motion, looking at range, quality of motion during the range, and the "end feel" at the limit of movement;
T Tissue texture abnormality with alteration in the feel of the soft tissues, mainly muscle hypertonicity, and in skin and connective tissues, described as hot-cold, soft-hard, boggy, doughy, and so on. Most of the tissue texture abnormalities result from altered nervous system function with increased α motor neuron activity maintaining muscle hypertonicity, and altered sympathetic autonomic nervous system function to the skin viscera, vasomotor, sudomotor, and pilomotor activity.

CLINICAL GOALS FOR MANIPULATIVE TREATMENT

As previously stated, the goal of manipulation is the use of the hands in a patient-management process using instructions and maneuvers to achieve maximal, painless, movement of the musculoskeletal (motor) system in postural balance. In achieving this goal, different types of therapeutic effects on the patient can be sought. They can be classified as follows:

1. Circulatory effects
   A. Move body fluids
   B. Provide tonic effect
2. Neurological effect: modify reflexes
   A. Somato-somatic
   B. Somato-visceral
   C. Viscero-somatic
   D. Viscero-visceral
   E. Viscero-somato-visceral
   F. Somato-viscero-somatic
3. Maintenance therapy for irreversible conditions

Depending on the desired outcome, the therapeutic application will use different models of manual medicine.

MODELS AND MECHANISMS OF MANUAL MEDICINE INTERVENTION

Several different conceptual models can be used in determining the manual medicine approach to a patient. Five such models are described, but it should be evident that when a manual medicine procedure is provided, it has multiple effects and is mediated through a number of different mechanisms.

Postural Structural or Biomechanical Model

The postural structural model is probably the one most familiar to practitioners of manual medicine. In this model the patient is approached from a biomechanical orientation toward the musculoskeletal system. The osseous skeleton is viewed as a series of building blocks piled one on top of the other, starting with the bones of the foot and ending with the skull. The ligamentous and fascial structures are the tissues that connect the osseous framework, and the muscles are the prime movers of the bones of the skeleton, working across single and multiple joint structures. Alteration of the patient's musculoskeletal system is viewed from the alignment of the bones and joints, the balance of muscles as movers and stabilizers of the skeleton, the symmetry of tone of the ligaments, and the integrity of the continuous bands of fascia throughout. Alteration in joint apposition and alteration in muscle function either because of hypertonicity or weakness, tightness or laxity of ligament(s), and shortening or lengthening of fascia are considered when approaching a patient from this perspective. The manual medicine treatment would be directed toward restoring maximal motion to all joints, symmetry of length and strength to all muscles and ligaments, and symmetry of tension within fascial elements throughout the body. The goal is to restore maximal function of this musculoskeletal system in postural balance, and the patient can be approached

either starting at the feet and ending with the head or vice versa.

The most important element of the postural structural model in this author's experience has been the restoration of maximum pelvic mechanics in the walking cycle. The pelvis becomes the cornerstone of the postural structural model. Influences from below or above must be considered to achieve symmetrical movement of the osseous pelvis during walking.

This model is most useful in approaching patients with pain from either single instances of trauma or microtrauma over time due to postural imbalance from such entities as anatomical shortening of one leg, unilateral fallen arch, and so on. This conceptual model includes much of the current biomechanical engineering research in the areas of joint mechanics; properties of ligaments, tendons, and fascia; and kinetics and kinematics.

Neurological Model

The neurological model concerns influencing neural mechanisms through manual medicine intervention. One mechanism of action is through the autonomic nervous system. There is a large body of basic research into the influence of the somatic (motor) system on the function of the autonomic nervous system, primarily the sympathetic division. This basic research is consistent with clinical observations, but additional clinical research is needed into the influence of alteration in function of the musculoskeletal system on total body function mediated through the sympathetic division of the autonomic nervous system.

Autonomic Nervous System Model. The concept is based on the organization of the sympathetic nervous system. The preganglionic fibers take their origin from the spinal cord from T1 to L3. The lateral chain ganglia are paired and overlie the posterior thoracic and abdominal wall where synaptic junction occurs with postganglionic fibers. The lateral chain ganglia in the thoracic region are tightly bound by the fascia to the posterior chest wall and overlie the heads of the ribs. It is hypothesized that altered mechanics of the costovertebral articulations could mechanically influence the lateral chain ganglia. There are peripheral ganglia through which the sympathetic nervous system synapses with postganglionic fibers that are relatively adjacent to the organs being innervated.

The sympathetic nervous system is the sole source of autonomic nervous system activity to the musculoskeletal system. There is no parasympathetic innervation to the somatic tissues. The sympathetic nervous system has wide influence on visceral function, endocrine organs, reticuloendothelial system, circulatory system, peripheral nervous system, central nervous system, and muscle. Korr has worked extensively on the function of the sympathetic nervous system and points out the wide diversity of influence that sympathetic hyperactivity has on target end organs. Many factors can affect sympathetic hypertonia, one of which is afferent impulses from segmentally related areas of soma. It would seem reasonable, therefore, to attempt to reduce aberrant afferent stimulus to hyperirritable sections of the sympathetic nervous system to reduce the hyperactivity on target end organs.

Because the sympathetic nervous system is organized segmentally, it can be used in a maplike fashion to look for both alterations of afferent stimulus and areas that might be influenced through manual medicine intervention. All of the viscera and soma above the diaphragm receive their preganglionic sympathetic nervous system fibers from above cord level T4. All visceral and soma below the diaphragm receive preganglionic sympathetic nervous system fibers from T5 and below. Understanding this anatomy helps in relating identified somatic dysfunction to the patient's problem and can lead the physician to give appropriate manual medicine treatment to those areas of somatic dysfunction thought to contribute increased somatic afferent stimuli to cord levels with manifestations of increased sympathetic nervous system activity.

The parasympathetic nervous system takes its origin from the brain, brainstem, and sacral segments of the cord. Its organization differs from the segmental aspects of the sympathetic division, but its segmentation relates to the origin of the cranial nerves in the brainstem and the segmentation of the sacral cord. The cranial nerves, including those with parasympathetic activity, exit from the skull through numerous foramina and penetrate the dura. These nerves are at risk for entrapment with alteration of cranial mechanics and dural tension. Many times the clinical goal of craniosacral technique is to improve the function of cranial nerves as they exit the skull and sacrum. The autonomic nervous system neurological model leads the therapist toward a patient approach based on the anatomy or physiology of the two divisions of the autonomic nervous system and how best to affect them through manual medicine means.

Pain Model. A second neurological model focuses more on the interrelationships of the peripheral and central nervous systems, their reflex patterns, and their multiple pathways. This model is particularly useful in managing patients with pain syndromes, such as back pain. Although controversy remains about the origin of back pain, much is known about the location and type of nociceptors and mechanoreceptors within the musculoskeletal system. The pain stimulus can originate in a number of tissues and can be transmitted by peripheral afferent neurons to the spinal cord for integration and organization. Different neurons end in different laminae of the dorsal horn and synapse with interneurons that transmit information up and down the spinal cord, affecting other neuronal pools through propriospinal pathways. Transmission up the cord to higher centers can be either through the fast or slow pain pathways. Pain is perceived in the brain, and stimulatory or inhibitory activities can enhance or reduce the pain perception. These processes are programmed through the brainstem and back down the cord to modulate activity at cord segmental level.

An understanding of the anatomy and physiology of the musculoskeletal system and nervous systems, particularly the spine and paraspinal tissues, is necessary to develop a therapeutic plan to manage the patient's pain syndrome. A clear distinction must be made between acute and chronic pain. Acute pain is that which is best known to the clinician. It results from tissue damage, is well localized, has clear objective evidence of injury, and has a sharp pricking quality. There may be some lingering burning and aching. Acute pain responds well to treatment and abates when the tissue damage has resolved. Chronic pain persists despite the lack of ongoing tissue damage. It is poorly localized with no objective evidence present. It has a burning aching quality with a strong associated affective component. Changes have occurred in the central pathways and central endogenous control. It is unclear as to when chronic pain begins, but it is generally accepted that ongoing pain beyond 3 months results in central pathway changes. Acute and chronic pain respond differently to therapeutic interventions. Manual medicine has a role in the treatment of both acute and chronic musculoskeletal pain syndromes. In the acute condition, manual medicine attempts to reduce the ongoing afferent stimulation of the nociceptive process. If it is determined that muscle contraction and hypertonicity are primary factors, then muscle energy procedures might be most beneficial. If it is believed that altered mechanoreceptive behavior in the articular and periarticular structure of the zygapophysial joint, a mobilizing procedure with or without impulse might be more appropriate. The goal of manual medicine in the chronic patient is to restore the maximum functional capacity of the musculoskeletal system that is possible to achieve so that exercises and increased activities of daily living can occur. It is difficult for a chronic pain patient to undergo exercise therapy and reconditioning rehabilitative processes in the presence of restricted mobility of the musculoskeletal system.

Neuroendocrine Model. The third concept within the neurological model is that of neuroendocrine control. Since the late 1970s, there has been a rapidly expanding body of knowledge about the role of endorphins, enkephalins, and other neural peptides. These substances are not only active in the nervous system but also profoundly affect the immune system. There appears to be ample evidence that alteration in musculoskeletal activity influences their liberation and activity. It has been hypothesized that some of the beneficial effects of manipulative treatment might result from the release of endorphins and enkephalins with subsequent reduction in the perception of pain. Because of the influence of the substances in areas other than the central nervous system, other systemic effects may result from manual medicine procedures. This neuroendocrine mechanism might explain some of the general body tonic effects.

All of these neurological mechanisms are highly complex and have been only superficially dealt with here. They can be used, however, as conceptual models to approach a patient with a myriad of problems.

Respiratory Circulatory Model

The respiratory circulatory model looks at a different dimension of the activity of the musculoskeletal system. In this model the patient is viewed from the perspective of blood and lymph flow. Skeletal muscles and the diaphragm are the pumps of the venous and lymphatic systems. The goal is restoring the functional capacity of the musculoskeletal system to assist return circulation and the work of respiration. The function of the diaphragm to modify the relative negative intrathoracic pressure to assist in inhalation and exhalation requires that the torso, including the thoracic cage and the abdomen, have the capacity to respond to these pressure gradient changes. Thus, the thoracic spine and the rib cage must be functionally flexible, particularly the lower six ribs where the diaphragm attaches. The lumbar spine must be flexible enough to change its anterior curvature for breathing. The abdominal musculature should have symmetrical tone and length and the pelvic diaphragm should be balanced and nonrestrictive.

The respiratory circulatory model looks at somatic dysfunction(s) and its influence on fluid movement and ease of respiration rather than on neural entrapment or biomechanical alteration. Thus, some of the techniques applied are less segmentally specific and are more concerned with tissue tension that might impede fluid flow. The guiding principle of this model is the progression from central to distal. The beginning point is usually in the thoracic cage, primarily at the thoracic inlet, so that the tissues of the thoracic cage are able to respond to respiratory effort and the pumping action of the diaphragm to receive the fluids trapped in the peripheral tissues. Attention to the thoracic inlet also aids in the drainage of fluid from the head, neck, and upper extremities. Recall that all of the lymph ultimately drains into the venous system at the thoracic inlet behind the anterior extremity of the first rib and the medial end of the clavicle. When the thoracic cage is functioning at maximal capacity, one progresses to the lumbar spine, pelvis, and lower extremities, attempting to remove any potential obstruction to fluid flow that occurs in these tissues. The therapeutic goals of the respiratory circulatory model are to reduce the work of breathing and to enhance the pumping action of the diaphragm and extremity muscles to assist lymphatic and venous flow.

Bioenergy Model

The bioenergy model is somewhat more ethereal than the preceding and focuses on the inherent energy flow within the body. Some clinicians are skilled at both observing and feeling energy transmission, or the absence of same, from patients. We are all familiar with the phenomena of Kirlian photography, which enables us to visualize radiant energy outside the anatomical limits of the body. This may be but one example of perceptible energy that emanates from the human organism. The bioenergy model focuses on the maximization of normal energy flow within the human body and its response to its environment. Many clinicians have reported sensations of release of energy during manual medicine procedure that appear to emanate from the patient.

There is also the element of the transfer of energy from the therapeutic touch of the physician. Many of the ancient, oriental forms of healing have focused on elements of "life force," "energy field," and so on, and it is within this domain that a manual medicine practitioner can apply this conceptual model. The craniosacral manual medicine approach is one in which one of the major goals of treatment is to restore the normal inherent force of the central nervous system, including the brain, spinal cord, meninges, and cerebral spinal fluid, to maximize a symmetrical, smooth, normal rhythmic cranial rhythmic impulse.

Psychobehavioral Model

The psychobehavioral model views the patient from the perspective of enhancing the capacity to relate to both the internal and external environment. There are many racial, social, and economic factors that influence the patient's perception of such things as pain, health, illness, disease, disability, and death. The patient's ability or inability to cope with all the stresses of life may well manifest itself in a wide variety of symptoms and physical signs. The physician's ability to understand the patient's response to stress and coping mechanisms and methods to assist the patient with this process are important components of this conceptual model. "Therapeutic touch" is an integral part of the doctor-patient interaction in this model. The influence of manual medicine may be less a biomechanical, neurological, or circulatory effect than just an important caring function. Awareness of this model is also important in understanding the difficulty in clinical research within manual medicine because of the "placebo" effect of the "laying on of hands."

It is beyond the scope of this volume to do anything but highlight the various models that are available for consideration when using a manual medicine intervention. It should be obvious that more than one model can be operative at the same intervention. It is strongly recommended, however, that the physician use some conceptual model before a manual medicine intervention. I support the contention of F.L. Mitchell, Jr. (personal communication) that manual medicine therapy is more than "a search and destroy mission of somatic dysfunction."

MANUAL MEDICINE ARMAMENTARIUM

Manual medicine procedures are classified and described below.

Soft Tissue Procedures

The soft tissue procedures are those in which manual application of force is directed toward influencing specific tissue(s) of the musculoskeletal system or, by peripheral stimulation, enhancing some form of reflex mechanism that alters biological function. The direct procedures include massage, effleurage, kneading, stretching, and friction rub, to name a few. These procedures can prepare the tissues for additional specific joint mobilization, or they can be a therapeutic end in themselves. The therapeutic goals are to overcome congestion, reduce muscle spasm, improve tissue mobility, enhance circulation, and to "tonify" the tissue. These procedures are some of the first learned and practiced by manual medicine physicians and can be used effectively in a variety of patient conditions.

A number of reflex mechanisms have been described that stimulate the peripheral tissues of the musculoskeletal system. These include acupuncture, reflex therapy, Chapman's reflexes, and Travell's trigger points. etc. Some manual, mechanical, or electrical stimulus is applied to certain areas of the body to enhance a therapeutic response. Some of these systems have been postulated on neurological models, lymphatic models, neuroendocrine models, and, in some instances, without any explanation for the observable clinical phenomena. Suffice it to say that many of these peripheral stimulating therapeutic points are consistent across patients, observable by multiple examiners, and provide a predictable response.

Articulatory Procedures

The articulatory procedures (mobilization without impulse) are used extensively in physiotherapy. They consist primarily of putting the elements of the musculoskeletal system, particularly the articulations, through ranges of motion in some graded fashion, with the goal of enhancement of the quantity and quality of motion. These procedures are therapeutic extensions of the diagnostic process of evaluating range of motion. If there appears to be a restriction of motion in one direction, with some alteration in sense of ease of movement in that direction, a series of gentle, rhythmic, operator-directed efforts in the direction of motion restriction can be found therapeutically effective. These articulatory procedures are especially useful for their tonic and/or circulatory effect.

Specific Joint Mobilization

The specific joint mobilization procedures all have two common elements: method, which is the method of approaching the restricted barrier, and activating force, which is the intrinsic or extrinsic force(s) exerted.

Methods. The specific joint mobilization methods are as follows.

1. Direct method. All direct procedures engage the restrictive barrier and by application of some force attempt to move the restrictive barrier closer to the normal physiological barrier to active movement.

2. Exaggeration method. This therapeutic effort applies a force against the normal physiological barrier in the direction opposite the motion loss. The force is usually a high-velocity low-amplitude thrust and has been found to be quite successful. There are systems of manual medicine that only provide therapeutic force in the direction of pain-free movement, and it is within this exaggeration method that such therapy seems to be operative.

3. Indirect method. In these procedures the operator moves the segment away from the restrictive barrier into the range of "freedom" or "ease" of movement to a point of balanced tension ("floating" of the segment[s]). The segment can then be held in that position for 5–90 seconds to relax the tension in the tissues around the articulations so that enhanced mobility occurs. Procedures using this method are termed functional technique, balance-and-hold technique, and release-by-positioning technique.

4. Combined method. Sometimes it is useful to use combinations of direct, exaggeration, and indirect methods in sequence to assist in the ultimate therapeutic outcome. Frequently, a combined method series of procedures is more effective than multiple applications of the same method.

5. Physiological response method. These procedures apply patient positioning and movement in response to position direction to obtain a therapeutic result. A series of body positions may use nonneutral mechanics to restore neutral mechanics to the musculoskeletal system. Another example of a physiological method is the use of respiratory effort to affect mobility of vertebral segments within spinal curvatures. Inhalation effort enhances straightening of the curves and hence backward bending movement in the thoracic spine and forward bending in the cervical and lumbar spines; exhalation effort causes just the reverse.

Activating Forces. The activating forces can be categorized into extrinsic and intrinsic. The extrinsic forces are those that are applied from outside the patient's body directly to the patient. These can include

1. Operator effort, such as guiding, springing, and thrust;
2. Adjunctive, such as straps, pads, traction, and so on;
3. Gravity, which is the weight of the body part and the patient position.

The intrinsic group are those forces that occur from within the patient's body and are used for their therapeutic effectiveness. They are classified as

1. Inherent force, or nature's tendency toward balance and homeostasis
2. Respiratory force
   a. Inhalation, which straightens curves in vertebral column and externally rotates extremities
   b. Exhalation, which enhances curves in vertebral column and internally rotates extremities
3. Muscle force of the patient
   a. Muscle cooperation
   b. Muscle energy, especially isometrics
4. Reflex activity
   a. Eye movement
   b. Muscle activation

Afferent Reduction Procedures

The afferent reduction procedures appear to work on a model of reducing aberrant afferent activity from the various mechanoreceptors found within the various tissues of the musculoskeletal system. The working hypothesis is that altered behavior of the musculoskeletal system provides aberrant stimulation to the central nervous system that alters the programing of musculoskeletal function. Identifying various positions and maneuvers that reduce the afferent bombardment of multiple reflexes at cord and central levels can provide an opportunity to restore more normal behavior. It is thought that many of the indirect approaches, including the dynamic functional techniques, balance and hold techniques, and release by positioning techniques, work through this mechanism.

MANIPULATION UNDER ANESTHESIA

Manipulation under anesthesia has had a long history in manual medicine. It is used for dysfunction within the spinal complex, particularly the lumbosacral and cervical regions, as well as peripheral joints. The procedures performed are mobilization with impulse (high velocity, low amplitude thrust technique) with the patient under general anesthesia. Its use requires skilled anesthesia and a high level of competence of the manipulating practitioner. The indications are acute or chronic vertebral dysfunctions that cannot be managed by nonoperative conservative means. Muscle spasm and irritability may preclude a successful manual medicine procedure without anesthesia. In chronic myofibrositis, manipulation under anesthesia may enhance the response unobtainable by more conservative measures. The indications are not high. Morey reported only 3% of patients hospitalized with musculoskeletal disorders in a 3-year period required manipulation under anesthesia. Complications are rare, but the procedure is contraindicated in patients who cannot tolerate the anesthetic and those in which manual medicine is not viewed as appropriate.

It is possible to design multiple variations of method and activating force to achieve the desired clinical goal. All of the procedures in manual medicine can be viewed as having a common goal, which is to reprogram the behavior of the central nervous system. Using the analogy of the computer, manual medicine deals with the "hardware" of the musculoskeletal system and modulates the behavior of the "software" in the central nervous system. The more optimal the behavior of the central nervous system, the better the function of the musculoskeletal system. The anatomy (hardware) may be altered by developmental variant; trauma, both single and repetitive; and surgery. Despite the changes in the anatomy, the goal of manual medicine is to restore the maximum functional capacity that the anatomy will allow. The more skilled one becomes in using different methods and activating forces, the more successful one becomes as a manual medicine therapist.

FACTORS INFLUENCING TYPE OF MANIPULATIVE PROCEDURES

In addition to a wide variety of types and styles of manual medicine procedures available and a number of different clinical goals, there are other factors that influence the type of manual medicine procedure instituted.

1. Age of patient;
2. Acuteness or chronicity of problem;
3. General physical condition of patient;
4. Operator size and ability;
5. Location (office, home, hospital);
6. Effectiveness of previous and/or present therapy.

If one were prescribing a pharmaceutical agent, the dosage would be adjusted to the age of the patient, so too in the use of manual medicine. Clearly, one approaches an infant differently than a young adult. In an elderly debilitated patient, one is much more careful and judicious in the use of some of the more forceful direct action types of technique. Osteoporosis in the female is not necessarily a contraindication to manual medicine, but indirect procedures with intrinsic activating forces would be more appropriate.

The type of manual medicine procedure is also modified by the acuteness or chronicity of the problem. In acute conditions, inflammatory swelling and acute muscle spasm are frequently encountered. The physician might use the respiratory circulatory model to relieve the inflammatory congestion and perhaps some soft tissue procedure to reduce the amount of acute muscle spasm. In more chronic conditions with long-standing fibrosis in the ligaments, muscles, and fascia, a more direct action myofascial release or direct action high-velocity thrust procedure might be more appropriate. In the patient who is acutely ill, with reduced capacity to withstand aggressive and intensive therapy, a more conservative approach, such as indirect technique, might be more appropriate. Also remember that manual medicine procedures, particularly those using intrinsic activating forces, result in energy expenditure by the patient. Keep the therapeutic application within the physical capacity of the acutely ill patient. In chronic conditions do not expect to overcome all of the difficulty with a single manual medicine intervention.

The operator's size, strength, and technical ability will also influence the type of procedure used. Although strength is not necessarily the primary determinant of a successful procedure, the proper application of leverage usually is. Understanding of and ability in a number of manual medicine procedures makes a more effective clinician. With only one antibiotic available, the ability to treat infectious disease is clearly hampered. Likewise, with only one form of manual medicine treatment, one is clearly hampered as an effective manual medicine practitioner.

The physician should have the capacity to provide an effective manual medicine treatment irrespective of the location of the patient. Although there are some procedures that are more effective in the office setting with specific therapeutic tables, stools, and other equipment, one should be able to devise an effective procedure anywhere. In a hospital bed or at home on a soft mattress, the capacity to use a high velocity, low amplitude thrust is compromised. Muscle energy activating forces and other intrinsic force techniques are more appropriate in such locations.

Past therapy is also highly important in determining the type of procedure to be used. You must know whether there has been a previous surgical intervention, manual medicine intervention, or pharmacotherapeutic treatment. If surgery has changed the anatomy, you might wish to modify the therapeutic procedure to meet the altered anatomy. Lack of response to previous manual medicine is not necessarily a reason not to use a different form of manual medicine treatment. Previous medication, particularly muscle relaxants, tranquilizers, and antiinflammatory agents, might modify the type of procedure to be used. With long-standing steroid therapy, be aware of the potential for laxity of ligaments and softening of cancellous bone.

These are but a few of the factors that affect the choice of a manual medicine procedure. In addition there are three cardinal rules for any effective manual medicine procedure: control, balance, and localization.

Control includes the physician's control of body position in relationship to the patient, control of the patient in a comfortable position, control of intrinsic or extrinsic forces, and control of the type of therapeutic intervention being applied. Balance of both patient and operator ensures adequate patient relaxation and the ability of the operator to engage the restrictive barrier in comfort. Localization refers to adequate engagement of a restrictive barrier in a direct action procedure, localization on the point of maximum ease in a balance-and-hold indirect procedure, and localization of a most pain-free position in a release by positioning procedure.

CONTRAINDICATIONS TO MANUAL MEDICINE PROCEDURES

Much has been written about absolute and relative contraindications to manual medicine procedures. This author holds the view that there are none if (and it is a big if) there is an accurate diagnosis of somatic dysfunction that requires treatment to effect the overall management of the patient and the manual medicine procedure is appropriate for that diagnosis and the physical condition of the patient. However, there are a number of conditions that require special precautions. Some of these are as follows:

1. The vertebral artery in the cervical spine;
2. Primary joint disease (e.g., rheumatoid arthritis, infectious arthritis);
3. Metabolic bone disease (e.g., osteoporosis);
4. Primary or metastatic malignant bone disease;
5. Genetic disorders (e.g., Down's syndrome), particularly in the cervical spine;
6. Hypermobility in the involved segments. This should clearly be avoided. One should look for restricted mobility elsewhere in the presence of hypermobility.

Following these principles, a specific and appropriate manual medicine therapeutic prescription can be written for a diagnosis much as with traditional therapeutic interventions. Returning to our original example, the thinking physician identifies the infectious agent in a throat infection before deciding on a therapeutic intervention. If, for example, the throat infection was due to a streptococcus, the physician might select ampicillin as the antibiotic of choice. With the specific infectious agent identified and an appropriate antibiotic chosen, then adequate dosage on an appropriate schedule for a sufficient length of time would be ordered.

DX—Throat infection (streptoccocal)
RX—Ampicillin 250 mg every 6 hours for 10 days

With an appropriate diagnosis of somatic dysfunction, an accurate manual medicine prescription can be written based on the principles addressed above. One would choose the type of procedure and specify the method, activating force, dosage, length of treatment time, and frequency of treatments.

DX—Somatic dysfunction, T6, extended, rotated, and sidebent, right (ERS_{right}).
RX—Manual medicine, direct action muscle energy type to flexion, left rotation, and left sidebending. Reexamine in 48 hours.

The specific somatic dysfunction has been identified with its position and subsequent motion restriction. A direct procedure and an intrinsic activating force was chosen. It was anticipated that the effectiveness of the procedure would last 48 hours and therefore reexamination at that time was indicated.

COMPLICATIONS

It is difficult to have an accurate estimation of the incidence of complications of manual medicine procedures. Some authors have defined the rate at one to two per million procedures. A well-controlled study (Dvorak and Orelli, Manuelle Medizine, 1982) identified symptom exaggeration as one in 40,000 and a significant complication as one in 400,000. Most of the complications involve vascular and neural structures. Obvious complications occur when a procedure is contraindicated. Many of the complications occur from manipulation in the cervical spine, resulting in insult to the vertebral-basilar artery system. Fractures and dislocations have been identified as well as spinal cord injury. Complications of exaggeration of disc herniation with progressive radiculopathy after manipulation are controversial. Some authors view mobilization with impulse as being contraindicated in the presence of disc herniation, whereas others believe that it is indicated in certain conditions if appropriately applied. Postmanipulation injury to the vertebral basilar artery system occurs in the 30- to 45-year-old age group, with a slight preponderance in the female population. Death rates approach 22% and significant disability in 75–80%. Complete recovery is available to only a small number. The avoidance of complications requires the practitioner to be knowledgeable about the patient's diagnosis, appreciate their own level of skill and experience, and to be able to deal with complications if they occur. Although the incidence is low, they are to be avoided if possible.

As manual medicine practitioners, we should all prescribe our therapy as precisely as we prescribe any other therapeutic agent. It is hoped that these principles will assist in the appropriate use of manual medicine.

5

NORMAL VERTEBRAL MOTION

The vertebral column consists of 26 segments. There are usually 7 cervical segments, 12 thoracic segments, and 5 lumbar segments. Anomalous development occurs in the spine and is most common in the lumbar region where four or six segments are occasionally found. The lumbar region is also the site of the greatest number of developmental changes, particularly in the shape of the transverse processes and zygapophysial joints. The first and second cervical segments are uniquely atypical. The vertebral motion segment consists of two adjacent vertebrae and the intervening ligamentous structures (Fig. 5.1). The typical vertebra consists of two parts: the body and the posterior arch. The vertebral body articulates with the intervertebral disk above and below at the vertebral end plate. The posterior arch consists of the two pedicles, two superior and two inferior zygapophysial joints, two laminae, two transverse processes, and a single spinous process. Two adjacent vertebra are connected ventrodorsad by the anterior longitudinal ligament, the intervertebral disk with its central nucleus and surrounding annulus, the posterior longitudinal ligament, the articular capsules of the zygapophysial joints, the ligamentum flavum, the interspinous ligament, and the supraspinous ligament.

CERVICAL REGION

Atlas

In the cervical region, we find the atypical atlas (C1) and axis (C2). The atlas (Fig. 5.2) does not have a vertebral body and consists primarily of a bony ring with two lateral masses. On the posterior aspect of the anterior arch is a small joint structure for articulation with the anterior aspect of the odontoid process of the axis. Each lateral mass consists primarily of the articular pillars. The shape of the superior zygapophysial joints is concave ventrodorsad and laterally. The long axis of each superior zygapophysial joint projects from the lateral to medial dorsoventrad. This results in an anterior wedging of the long axis of these joints. They articulate with the condyles of the occiput, and their shape is a major determinant of the amount and type of motion available between the occiput and the atlas. The inferior zygapophysial joints are quite flat but when the articular cartilage is attached become convex ventrodorsad and laterally. These inferior zygapophysial joints articulate with the superior zygapophysial joints of the axis. The transverse processes are quite long and are easily palpable in the space between the tip of the mastoid process of the temporal bone and the angle of the mandible.

Axis

The axis (C2) (Fig. 5.3) has atypical characteristics in its superior portion and more typical characteristics in its inferior portion. The vertebral body is surmounted by the odontoid process, developmentally the residuum of the body of the atlas. On the anterior aspect of the odontoid process is an articular facet for the posterior aspect of the anterior arch of the atlas; the posterior aspect has an articular facet

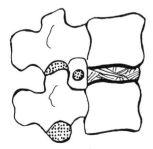

Figure 5.1.
Vertebral motion segment.

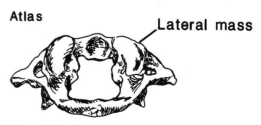

Figure 5.2.
Atlas (C1).

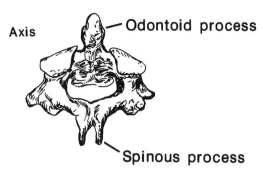

Figure 5.3.
Axis (C2).

for the transverse atlas ligament. The superior zyga-pophysial joints are convex ventrodorsad and later-ally. They are higher on the medial than lateral as-pect and their contour resembles a pair of shoulders. The spinous process of C2 is quite long and is one of the more easily palpable spinous processes in the cervical region.

Typical Cervical Vertebrae

The typical cervical vertebrae, from the inferior sur-face of C2 down to the cervical thoracic junction, have the following characteristics (Fig. 5.4). The ver-tebral body is relatively small in relation to the poste-rior arch. The superior surface is convex ventrodor-sad and concave laterally, whereas the inferior surface is concave ventrodorsad and convex laterally. When two typical vertebral bodies are joined by the intervertebral disk, the shape is similar to a universal joint. At the posterolateral corner of each vertebral body is found a small synovial joint called the unco-vertebral joint of Luschka. These joints are found only in the cervical region and are subject to degen-erative change that occasionally encroaches on the intervertebral canal posteriorly. The pedicles are quite short and serve as the roof and floor of the related intervertebral canal. The articular pillars are relatively large and are easily palpable on the pos-terolateral aspect of the neck. The zygapophysial joints are relatively flat and face backward and up-ward at an approximate 45° angle. The shape and direction of the zygapophysial joints and the univer-sal joint characteristics between the vertebral bodies largely determine the type of movement available in the typical cervical spinal segments. The laminae are flat, and the spinous processes are usually bifid with the exception on C7. The transverse processes are unique in this region, having on each side the inter-transverse foramen for the passage of the vertebral artery. The tips of the transverse processes are bifid and serve as attachments for the deep cervical mus-cles. They are quite tender to palpation and are not easily used in structural diagnosis of the cervical

spine. The intervertebral canals on each side are ovoid in shape and are limited by the inferior margin of the pedicle above, the posterior aspect of the in-tervertebral disk and Luschka's joints in front, the superior aspect of the pedicle of the vertebral below, and by the anterior aspect of the zygapophysial joints behind. The vertebral canal is relatively large and provides the space necessary for the large area of the spinal cord in the cervical region.

Thoracic Vertebrae

In the thoracic region (Fig. 5.5), the vertebral bodies become somewhat larger as they descend and have unique characteristics for articulation with the heads of the ribs. T1 has a unifacet found posterolaterally for the articulation of the head of rib one bilaterally. From the inferior surface of T1 down are found de-mifacets, which together with the intervertebral disk provide an articular fossa for the head of each rib. The zygapophysial joints are vertical in orientation and the superior facets project backward and later-ally. Theoretically, this should provide a great deal of freedom of movement in multiple directions, but the attachment of the ribs to the thoracic vertebra mark-edly restricts the available motion. The transverse processes have an articular facet on their anterior as-pect for articulation with the tubercle of the rib. This forms the costotransverse articulation bilaterally. The transverse processes become progressively narrower in descent, with those at T1 being widest at their tips

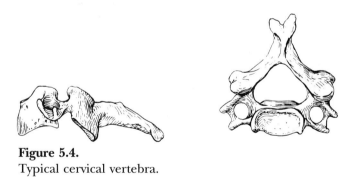

Figure 5.4.
Typical cervical vertebra.

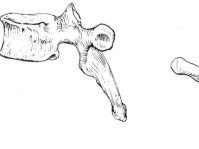
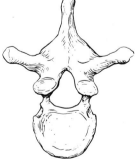

Figure 5.5.
Thoracic vertebra.

and at T12 the narrowest. The laminae are shingled and continue to the spinous processes that are also shingled from above downward. The spinous processes are quite long and overlap each other, particularly in the middle to lower region. The relation of the palpable tips of the spinous processes to the thoracic vertebral bodies is spoken of as "the rule of 3s" (Fig. 5.6). The spinous processes of T4–6 project one-half vertebra below that to which they are attached. The spinous processes of T7–9 are located a full vertebra lower than the vertebra to which they are attached. The spinous processes of T10–12 return to being palpable at the same level as the vertebral body to which they are attached.

Lumbar Vertebrae

In the lumbar region the vertebral bodies (Fig. 5.7) become even more massive and support a great deal of weight. The spinous processes project posteriorly in relation to the vertebral body to which they are attached and are broad, rounded, and easily palpable. The transverse processes project laterally with those attached to L3 being the broadest in range. The zygapophysial joints have a concave-convex relationship between the superior and inferior zygapophysial joints of adjacent vertebra that greatly restricts the amount of sidebending and rotation available. The plane of zygapophysial joints is usually considered a sagittal *(yz)* plane with the lumbosacral zygapophysial joints considered closer to the coronal *(xy)* plane. However, in the lumbar region asymmetrical facing of the zygapophysial joints is not uncommon.

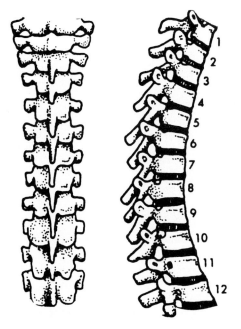

Figure 5.6.
Thoracic spine rule of 3s.

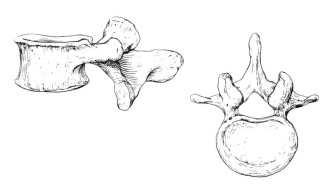

Figure 5.7.
Lumbar vertebra.

Vertebral Column Muscles

The muscles overlying the vertebral column are many and layered. They can be described as follows:

> Layer one: the trapezius, latissimus dorsi, and lumbodorsal fascia;
> Layer two: the levator scapulae, the major and minor rhomboids;
> Layer three: the erector spinae mass, including the spinalis, semispinalis, longissimus, and iliocostalis;
> Layer four: multifidi, rotatores, and intertransversarii.

The anteroposterior curves of the vertebral column develop over time. The primary curve at birth is convex posteriorly. The first secondary curve to develop is in the cervical region that becomes convex anteriorly when the infant begins to raise its head. The second curve develops in the lumbar region on assuming the biped stance. This is convex anteriorly. Appropriate alignment of the three curves of the vertebral axis is an essential component of good posture (Fig. 5.8).

LAYER PALPATION

The palpation of these structures is an essential component of structural diagnosis. The following exercise in palpation might be useful in gaining familiarity with some of them for further use both diagnostically and therapeutically.

1. Place the palms and palmer surfaces of the fingers over the shawl area of the cervicothoracic junction (Fig. 5.9). Palpate the skin for thickness, smoothness, and temperature.

2. Move the skin on the subcutaneous fascia overlying the deep structures in a synchronous and alternating fashion anteroposteriorly and from medial to lateral (Fig. 5.10). Note that in one direction

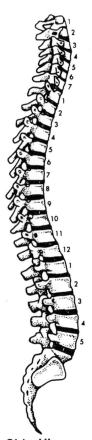

Side View
Figure 5.8.
Normal vertebral curves.

it will be more free and the other somewhat tighter. This tight-loose characteristic is a sensation of great significance when using myofascial release technique.

3. Using the thumb and index finger on each hand, pick up the skin and subcutaneous fascia and gently roll the skin over your thumbs by the action of your index fingers coming from below upward (Fig. 5.11). Repeat starting medially and going laterally. Perform this procedure symmetrically on each side looking for differences in thickness and pliability of the skin and ascertaining whether this procedure produces patient pain. Skin rolling that identifies tightness and tenderness is a valuable tool in identifying levels of somatic dysfunction.

4. Place the palm of your hand over each acromion process with the long finger extending to the anterior aspect of the shoulder girdle with the finger pad palpating the tip of the coracoid process (Fig. 5.12). Be gentle as this location is quite tender in all subjects. Palpate for the sensation of the resilience of bone. Move your finger pad slightly inferiorly to palpate a rounded, smooth, firm tendon of the short head of the biceps brachii. Return to the tip of the coracoid process and proceed medially and palpate

the broader but still smooth and firm tendon of the pectoralis minor muscle.

5. Place the palms of the fingers of both hands overlying the upper thoracic region just medial to the spinous process of the scapula (Fig. 5.13). Palpate through skin, subcutaneous fascia, and the deeper fascia overlying the first layer muscle, the midportion of the trapezius. Move your fingers from side to side as well as superiorly to inferiorly sensing for muscle fiber direction. This is somewhat easier by having the patient retract the scapulae actively. Note that it appears more smooth to move your hands from side to side and more rough when you move your hands from above to below. That smoothness

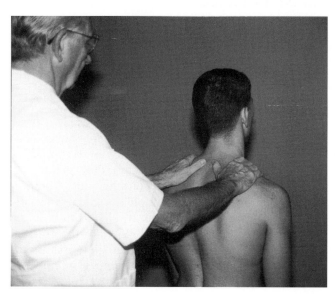

Figure 5.9.
Layer palpation of shawl area.

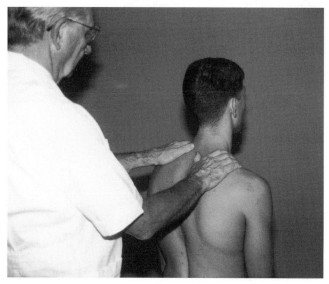

Figure 5.10.
Skin motion on subcutaneous fascia.

versus roughness characteristic is typical of muscle fiber direction.

6. Place your left hand where your right hand was in the last example and grasp the elbow with your right hand (Fig. 5.14). Palpate through the tissues, including the horizontal portion of the trapezius, and concentrate on the next layer of muscle below the rhomboids. The rhomboid can be more easily palpable if you resist the patient's effort to push the elbow toward the table. Note that the muscle has a different fiber direction than the trapezius at the same level. It is oblique from medial to lateral and from above downward. The inferior margin is easily palpable to give you the fiber direction.

7. Palpate the midline overlying the spinous processes (Fig. 5.15). As you move from above downward, note that the skin is very tightly attached at the midline. As you course from above downward you note a bump and hollow characteristic with the bumps being the bony spinous processes and the hollow being the interspinous space. Note the tension of the interspinous space reflecting the tension of the supraspinous and intraspinous ligaments.

8. Place three fingers in the interspinous spaces of the middle to upper thoracic spine. Introduce flexion through the head, sensing for opening of the interspinous spaces (Fig. 5.16). Reverse the process by taking the head and neck into extension and note

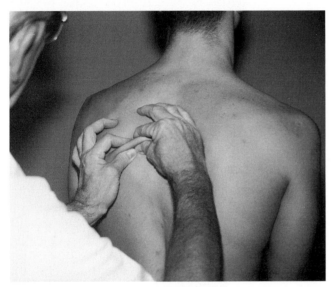

Figure 5.11.
Skin rolling.

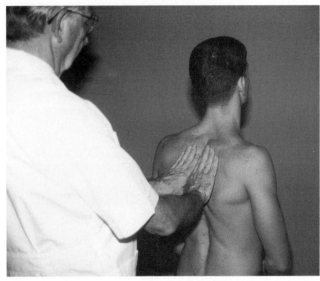

Figure 5.13.
Layer palpation of trapezius muscle.

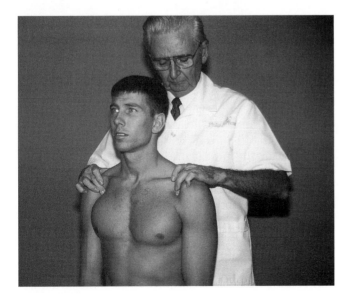

Figure 5.12
Palpation of shoulder girdle and corocoid process.

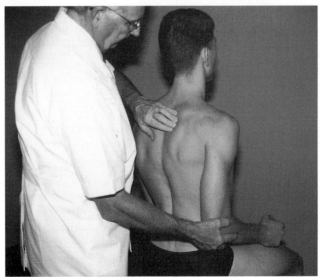

Figure 5.14.
Layer palpation of rhomboid muscle.

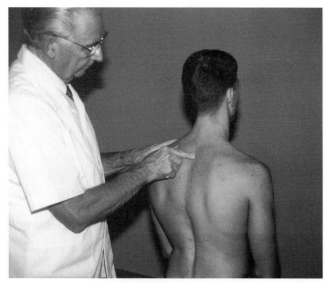

Figure 5.15.
Layer palpation of spinous processes.

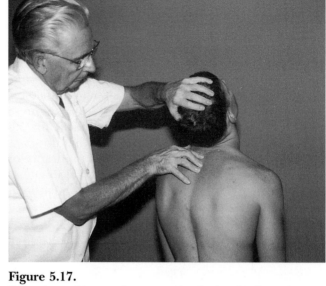

Figure 5.17.
Palpation of interspinous spaces during backward bending.

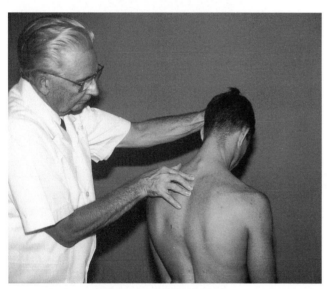

Figure 5.16.
Palpation of interspinous spaces during forward bending.

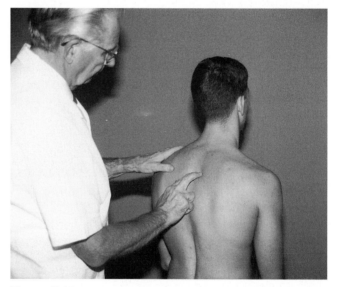

Figure 5.18.
Palpation in medial groove erector spinae muscles.

that the interspinous spaces narrow (Fig. 5.17). Repeat this process several times, noting how the interspinous spaces open and close. Attempt to move the head and neck such that you can localize the opening of the interspinous space beneath the middle finger during flexion, but not the finger below, and repeat the same process in extension so that you can close the interspinous space under the middle finger but not the one below. This is an important exercise in identifying your capacity to localize to a single vertebral segment.

9. Place your index finger on one side of the spi-
nous process and your middle finger on the other and palpate the fascial groove between the spinous process and the third layer of muscle, the erector spinae mass (Fig. 5.18). Actually, the fascial plane is between the spinalis muscle, which is intimately attached to the lateral aspect of the spinous processes, and the medial side of the longissimus, the easily palpable "rope" of the erector spinae mass. As you move from cephalward to caudad in this groove, you should feel symmetry and no palpable structure. Should you palpate anything in this medial groove, it is a reflection of hypertonicity of the deeper fourth

layer muscle primarily at the multifidus layer. Fourth layer hypertonic muscle is rounded and tense and is about the size of a small piece of a tootsie roll candy. They are usually quite sensitive to the patient and found unilaterally. Occasionally, a bilateral fourth layer muscle hypertonic area can be palpated in the presence of bilateral flexion or extension restrictions of a vertebral segment. Palpable fourth layer hypertonic muscle (the "tootsie roll sign") is one of the cardinal diagnostic findings in vertebral segmental somatic dysfunction.

10. Move laterally from the medial groove over the rounded mass of the longissimus and note there is a lateral deep fascial groove separating the lateral aspect of the longissimus from the medial aspect of the iliocostalis muscle. Place your thumbs on the lateral aspect of the longissimus in the lateral groove in a symmetrical fashion (Fig. 5.19). Move your thumbs symmetrically in an anteromedial direction until you feel a deep resistance (Fig. 5.20). Note there has been elevation of the belly of the longissimus muscle. While maintaining your palpation at this deeper level, move your thumbs in a cephalic to caudad direction, sensing for a bump and hollow contour similar to that identified over the spinous processes in the midline. At the level you are now palpating, you are overlying the transverse processes of the thoracic vertebra that are the bumps. The intertransverse space is the hollow. Try to palpate one pair of transverse processes in a symmetrical fashion and ask the patient to actively flex and extend their head and neck while you attempt to maintain contact with the transverse processes. Note that it is easier to feel the transverse process during the extension movement than during flexion. Acquisition of the skill of follow-ing transverse processes in three-dimensional space is most valuable in making a diagnosis of vertebral somatic dysfunction.

11. Move your hands more laterally overlying the most posterior aspect of the thoracic cage (Fig. 5.21). You are palpating over the rib angles and the associated attachment of the iliocostalis muscle. Move from cephalward to caudad and note that the rib angles diverge from medial to lateral. Each rib angle should participate in the posterior convexity of the thoracic cage. If one rib angle is more or less prominent than those above and below, it is a significant finding in the diagnosis of rib somatic dysfunction. Any palpable hypertonicity of muscle at the rib angle is indicative of hypertonic iliocostalis that is only found in the

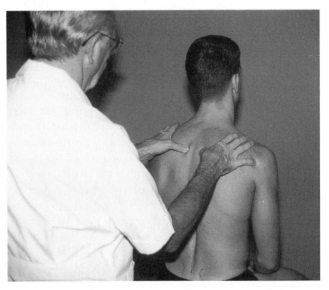

Figure 5.20.
Palpation of transverse processes.

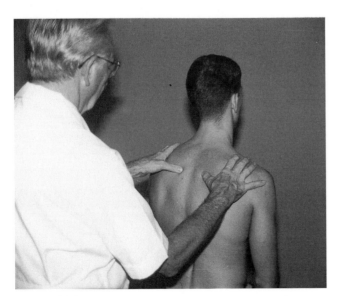

Figure 5.19.
Palpation in lateral groove erector spinae muscles.

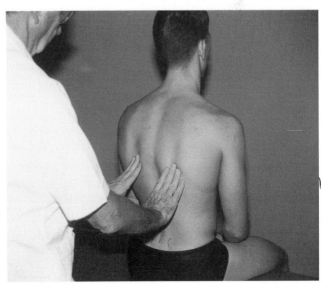

Figure 5.21.
Palpation of rib angles and iliocostalis muscle.

presence of rib dysfunction. Again, hypertonic iliocostalis at a rib angle is frequently tender to the patient.

12. Place your thumb overlying the rib angle of the most posterior aspect of the thoracic cage, usually the seventh rib (Fig. 5.22). Move your thumb over the rib shaft at the angle, noting the posterior convexity. Move to the superior and inferior aspect of the rib, noting the rib edge. Most commonly the inferior edge is somewhat more easily palpable than the superior. Of importance is the contour of the rib in comparison to the one above and below, as well as on the contralateral side. Prominence of the superior or inferior rib edge is significant in the diagnosis of rib somatic dysfunction. Palpate the interspace above and below the rib and compare it with the opposite side. Is one more narrow or wide than the other? Palpate the intercostal muscle to see whether it is hypertonic and tender. Abnormal width above and below a rib and intercostal hypertonicity are both significant findings in certain rib somatic dysfunctions.

13. From the rib angle continue to monitor rib shaft and move medially with the palm of your thumb on the rib shaft until the tip of your thumb runs into an obstruction (Fig. 5.23). The tip of your thumb has now struck the lateral aspect of the transverse process. The portion of bone from the rib angle to the tip of the transverse process is an important component of the rib that is used in some of the subsequently described techniques for rib somatic dysfunction. Again note that the longissimus muscle becomes more prominent as you have moved from lateral to medial along the rib shaft.

This layer palpation exercise of the back will provide you with the ability to palpate anatomical structures necessary for the accurate diagnosis of vertebral axis and costal cage somatic dysfunction. Particularly important is the ability to follow paired transverse processes through a range of motion and the ability to identify tender tense hypertonic muscle of the fourth layer. Practice this exercise on a regular basis until it becomes habitual.

VERTEBRAL MOTION

Certain conventions are used in describing all vertebral motion. The vertebral motion segment consists of the superior and inferior adjacent vertebra and the intervening disc and ligamentous structures. By convention, motion of the superior vertebra is described in relation to the inferior. Motion is further defined as the movement of the superior or anterior surface of the vertebral body. In describing rotation, the anterior surface is used rather than the elements of the posterior arch. For example, in rotation of T3 to the right in relation to T4, the anterior surface of T3 turns to the right and the spinous process deviates to the left. Therefore, remember that descriptions relate to the anterior or superior surfaces of the vertebral body. In addition to describing characteristics of a vertebral motion segment, we also speak of movement of groups of vertebrae (three or more).

Vertebral motion is also described in relation to the anatomically oriented cardinal planes of the body using the right orthogonal coordinate system. Most of the clinical literature relates to the anatomically described cardinal planes and axes, whereas the biomechanical research literature uses the coordinate system extensively. Motion can be described as rotation around an axis and translation along an axis with the body moving within one of the cardinal

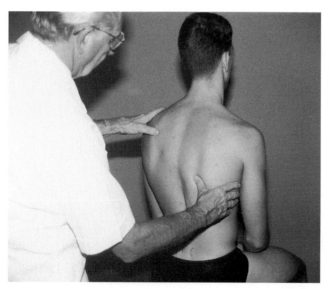

Figure 5.22.
Palpation of rib angle contour.

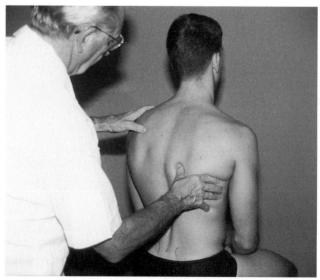

Figure 5.23.
Palpation of rib shaft to tip of transverse process.

planes. By convention, the horizontal axis is the *x* axis, the vertical axis is the *y* axis, and the anteroposterior axis is the *z* axis. The coronal plane is the *xy* plane, the sagittal plane is the *yz* plane, and the horizontal plane is the *xz* plane. The ability to rotate around an axis and to translate along an axis results in 6 df for each vertebra. Vertebral motion can then be described as overturning moment (rotation around an axis) and translatory movement (translation along an axis).

TERMINOLOGY

At the present time, convention in clinical practice describes vertebral motion in the following terms: forward-bending; backward-bending; sidebending, right and left; and rotation, right and left.

Forward-bending

A superior vertebra rotates anteriorly around the *x* axis and translates somewhat forward along the *z* axis. In forward-bending (Fig. 5.24), the anterior longitudinal ligament becomes somewhat more lax, posterior pressure is placed on the intervertebral disc, and the posterior longitudinal ligament becomes more tense as do the ligamentum flavum, the interspinous and supraspinous ligaments. The inferior zygapophysial facet of the superior vertebra moves superiorly in relation to the superior zygapophysial facet of the inferior vertebra. This has been described as "opening" or "flexing" of the facet.

Backward-Bending

In backward-bending the vertebra rotates backward around the *x* axis and moves posteriorly along the *z* axis (Fig. 5.25). The anterior longitudinal ligament becomes more tense. There is less tension on the posterior longitudinal ligament, the ligamentum flavum, and the interspinous and supraspinous ligaments. The inferior zygapophysial facet of the superior segment slides inferiorly in relation to the superior zygapophysial facet of the inferior vertebra. The facets are spoken of as having "closed" or "extended." Forward-bending and backward-bending result in an accordiontype movement of the opening and closing of the zygapophysial joints. If something interferes with the capacity of a facet joint to open or close, restriction of motion of either forward-bending or backward-bending will result.

Sidebending

In sidebending there is rotation around the anteroposterior *z* axis and translation along the horizontal *x* axis. Sidebending is seldom a pure movement and is usually coupled with rotation. In sidebending to the right, the right zygapophysial joint "closes" and the left zygapophysial joint "opens." Interference with a facet's capacity to open or close can interfere with sidebending and the coupled rotatory movement.

Rotation

Rotation of a vertebra is described as rotation around the *y* axis with the translatory movement being dependent on the vertebral segment involved. Rotation is always coupled with sidebending with the exception of the atlantoaxial joint.

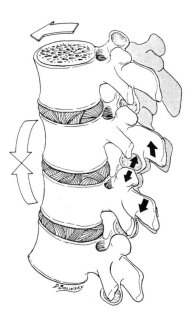

Figure 5.24.
Vertebral forward-bending.

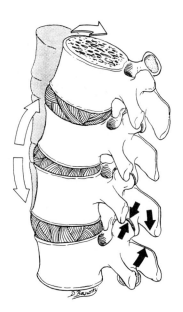

Figure 5.25.
Vertebral backward-bending.

COUPLED MOVEMENTS

Sidebending and rotation are coupled movements and do not occur individually. In some instances rotation is coupled in the same direction as sidebending (e.g., sidebending right, rotation right) and at other times at opposite directions (e.g., sidebending right, rotation left). Coupled movements change in response to the anteroposterior curves of the vertebral axis.

NEUTRAL MECHANICS

Neutral mechanics, or its synonym, type I, result in coupled movement of sidebending and rotation to opposite sides. Neutral mechanics occur when the patient is in the erect position with normal anteroposterior curves. For example, in the lumbar spine, with a normal lumbar lordosis present, sidebending of the trunk to the left results in rotation of lumbar vertebra to the right (Fig. 5.26). You can demonstrate this on yourself by standing erect and placing four fingers of your hand over the posterior aspect of the transverse processes of the lumbar spine. Now sidebend to the left and feel the tissues under your right hand become more full. This fullness is interpreted as posterior movement of the right transverse processes of the lumbar vertebra as they rotate right in response to sidebending left.

NONNEUTRAL MECHANICS

A nonneutral mechanical coupling, or its synonym, type II, results in sidebending and rotation of a vertebra to the same side. This occurs when there is alteration in the anteroposterior curve into forward-bending or backward-bending. To demonstrate, stand and forwardbend at the waist and place both fingers overlying the posterior aspect of the transverse processes of the lumbar spine. Introduce sidebending to the right. You will feel fullness occur under the fingers of your right hand, interpreted as resulting from posterior orientation of the right transverse processes during a right rotational response to the right sidebending coupled movement (Fig. 5.27). Return to the midline before returning to the erect posture. Nonneutral mechanics occur in the lumbar spine when it is forwardbent. In backward-bending, the lumbar spine demonstrates neutral coupling.

In the thoracic spine there is the capability of both neutral and nonneutral coupling. The type of coupling appears to be a function of where you are in the thoracic curve, above or below the apex, and whether you introduce sidebending or rotation first. In general, if sidebending is introduced first, then rotation will occur to the opposite side. If rotation is introduced first, then sidebending couples to the same side.

Nonneutral (type II) mechanics include the coupling of all three arcs of vertebral motion and all 6 df. Nonneutral coupling results in significant reduction in freedom of motion. It is for this reason that the vertebral column appears to be at risk for dysfunction when nonneutral mechanics are operative. Particularly in the lumbar region with the trunk forwardbent, sidebent, and rotated to the same side, any

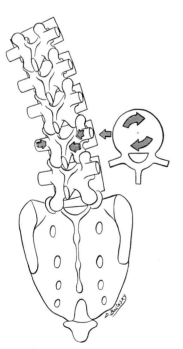

Figure 5.26.
Neutral (type I) vertebral motion.

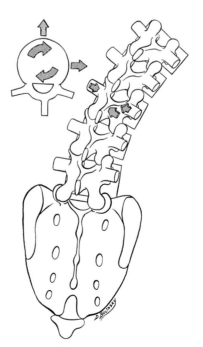

Figure 5.27.
Nonneutral (type II) vertebral motion.

additional movement places the lumbar spine at risk for muscle strain, zygapophysial joint dysfunction, annular tear of the intervertebral disc, or posterolateral protrusion of nuclear material in a previously compromised disc annulus.

TYPE III MECHANICS

Type III refers to the observation that when motion is introduced in the vertebral column in one direction, motion in all other directions is reduced. To demonstrate this phenomena, have your patient sit erect on an examining couch and passively introduce rotation of the trunk to the right and left. Ascertain the range and quality of movement. Now have the patient slump on the table with a posterior thoracolumbar convexity and again introduce trunk rotation to the right and left. Note the reduction in range and the restricted quality of movement during the range with the patient in this slumped position. The phenomena of type III vertebral motion is therapeutically applied during localization to dysfunctional segments. Introduction of motion above and below a dysfunctional vertebral segment can be accurately localized to a single vertebral motion segment that will then be treated by introduction of some activating force.

Table 5.1
Vertebral Motion

Segment(s)	Type(s)
C0–C1 (occipitoatlantal)	(neutral) I (always)
C1–C2 (atlantoaxial)	(rotation)
C2–C7 (typical cervical)	(nonneutral) II
C7–L5 (typical thoracic and lumbar)	(neutral) I and (nonneutral) II

TYPES OF MOTION AVAILABLE

The type of coupled movement available in the vertebral column varies from region to region and posture to posture. In the areas of the vertebral column that have both neutral and nonneutral movement capability, their vertebral segments can become dysfunctional with either type of motion characteristic (Table 5.1).

An understanding of the anatomy of the vertebral column, the ability to palpate the tissues therein, and an understanding of the concepts of vertebral motion are essential to understand and diagnose vertebral dysfunctions.

6

VERTEBRAL MOTION DYSFUNCTION

In the application of manual medicine procedures to the vertebral column, it is essential to make appropriate, accurate diagnosis of vertebral somatic dysfunction.

Somatic dysfunction is defined as impaired or altered function of related components of the somatic (body framework) system; skeletal, arthrodial, and myofascial structures; and related vascular, lymphatic, and neural elements. (Hospital Adaption of the International Classification of Disease, ed 2. 1973.)

This term is codable under current classification systems, International Classification of Diseases, 9th Revision, Clinical Modification (ICD-9-CM) codes 739.0–739.9. Somatic dysfunction replaces old terms such as osteopathic lesion, chiropractic subluxation, 'joint blockage, joint lock, loss of joint play, or minor vertebral derangement. Concern for the function of the musculoskeletal system requires a method of evaluating motion within the vertebral complex to determine whether it is normal, increased, or decreased. The motion spectrum advances from ankylosis to hypomobility, to normal motion, to hypermobility, to instability. Manual medicine procedures are most appropriate for segments with hypomobility that retain the capacity to move.

THEORIES OF VERTEBRAL MOTION DYSFUNCTION

Many theories have been proposed to explain the clinically observed phenomena of hypomobility. One theory proposes entrapment of synovial material or a synovial meniscoid between the two opposing joint surfaces. There is some anatomical evidence that meniscoids do occur, but whether they actually cause joint restriction has not been demonstrated. The joint meniscoid has innervation by C fibers that suggest nociception function.

A second theory suggests a lack of congruence in the point-to-point contact of the opposing joint surfaces. This theory postulates alteration in the normal tracking mechanism between the joint surfaces and that the role of manual medicine is to restore the joint to the "right track."

A third theory suggests an alteration in the physical and chemical properties of the synovial fluid and synovial surfaces. In essence, the smooth gliding capacity has been lost because the opposing surfaces have become "sticky." After a high velocity, low amplitude thrusting procedure (mobilization with impulse), in both vertebral and extremity joints in which separation of the joint surfaces has occurred, the "cavitation" phenomena has been demonstrated. In addition to the audible popping sound, a negative density within the joint on x-ray has also been observed. This "vacuum phenomena" appears to have the density of nitrogen, and the gaseous shadow is present for a variable period of time before it is no longer observable, suggesting a change from liquid to gaseous state as a result of the thrusting procedure.

A fourth theory regards the restriction of motion as a result of altered length and tone of muscle. Muscles can become hypertonic and shortened in position, whereas others become lengthened and weaker. Of greatest significance is the loss of muscle control. Control of muscle physiologically is highly complex and includes the behavior of mechanoreceptors in joints and related soft tissue, muscle spindle and golgi tendon apparatus, cord level and propriospinal pathway reflexes, pathways to the motor cortex, corticobulbar and corticospinal pathways modulated by the cerebellum, and the final common pathway of the α motor neuron to muscle fiber. Any alteration in afferent stimulus to this complex mechanism, or alteration of function within the system, can result in dysfunctional muscle activity and ultimately affect joint mechanics. Any alteration in muscle tone then restricts normal motion and serves as a perpetuating factor in altered joint movement. Whether the abnormal muscle activity is primary or secondary to the vertebral dysfunction is purely conjectural. However, altered muscle component of a vertebral dysfunction should always be dealt with in some fashion by the treatment provided. Using the analogy of a computer, the nervous system can be viewed as the software and the musculoskeletal system as the hardware. Altered function of the nervous system (the software) does not allow the musculoskeletal system (hardware) to function appropriately. Some manual medicine practitioners view the effectiveness of manual medicine treatment as being the reprograming of the software through the alteration of mechanoreceptor behavior at the joint and soft tissue levels.

A fifth theory considers changes in the biomechanical and biochemical properties of the myofascial elements of the musculoskeletal system, the capsule, the ligamentous structures, and fascia. When these structures are altered through traumatic, inflammatory, degenerative, or other changes, reduction of normal vertebral mobility can result.

Regardless of the theory to which one might subscribe, the clinical phenomenon of restricted vertebral motion can be viewed as the influence on the paired zygapophysial joints of the segment. We speak of the capacity of facets to open and close and refer primarily to the accordion-type movement and not the separation-type movement. In forward-bending the facets should normally open and in backward-bending they should close. If something interferes with the capacity of both facets to open, forward-bending restriction will occur. Conversely, if something interferes with both facets' capacity to close, backward-bending restriction will occur. It is also possible for one facet to move normally and the other to become restricted. If, for example, the right facet does not open but the left functions normally, right sidebending is possible but left sidebending is restricted. Because sidebending and rotation are coupled movements in the typical vertebral segments, rotation can also be affected by alteration in facet joint movement.

DIAGNOSIS OF VERTEBRAL MOTION DYSFUNCTION

Dysfunctions in the vertebral column can be described as single-segment dysfunctions involving one vertebral motion segment and group dysfunctions involving three or more vertebrae. After one completes a screening-and-scanning examination and fine tunes the diagnostic process to segmental definition, one is particularly interested in the motion(s) lost by the vertebra(e) involved. There are many methods to accomplish the process. The most commonly used is palpating the same bony prominence of two or more vertebrae (e.g., spinous processes or transverse processes) and actively or passively putting the segment(s) through successive ranges of movement into forward-bending, backward-bending, sidebending right, sidebending left, rotation right, and rotation left, comparing the motion of one segment with another. These procedures are most frequently done passively, and the operator attempts to define restriction and quality of restriction of movement in one or more directions. Although this method is frequently

effective, it does have two serious drawbacks. First, every time multiple-plane motion is introduced in a dysfunctional segment diagnostically, a therapeutic effect occurs because an articulatory (mobilization without impulse) procedure is accomplished. This results in constant change. A second disadvantage is the difficulty in making an assessment after a treatment procedure, that is, knowing whether the amount of range present before the procedure was modified. It is difficult to accurately remember all of the nuances of motion restriction that were present before the therapeutic intervention.

A second method, preferred by this author, is to follow a pair of transverse processes through an arc of forward-bending and backward-bending and interpret the findings based on the phenomena of facet opening and closing. Regardless of the method used, one can describe vertebral motion from the perspective of the motion available, the position in which the segment is restricted, or the motion of the segment that is restricted. In Table 6.1 a suffix is used in each term, either a static suffix, which represents the position of the segment, or a motion suffix, which describes the motion available or the motion lost. The current convention of describing vertebral dysfunction is either the position of the restricted segment or the motion that is lost in the restricted segment. Therefore, a segment that is backward bent (extended), right rotated, and right sidebent has forward-bending (flexion), left sidebending, and left rotation restriction. A plea is made for the use of appropriate terminology either to describe position or motion restriction. One should learn to translate between the two systems of positional and motion restriction diagnosis, but clearly a statement of terms is necessary for accurate communication between examiners.

DYSFUNCTIONS OF SINGLE VERTEBRAL MOTION SEGMENT

Single vertebral motion segment dysfunctions can be easily identified by the finding of hypertonicity of

Table 6.1
Factors that Describe Vertebral Motion

Position	Motion Restriction	Motion Available
T$_3$ on T$_4$		
Flexed	Extension	Flexion
Left rotated	Right rotation	Left rotation
Left sidebent	Right sidebending	Left sidebending
Extended	Flexion	Extension
Right rotated	Left rotation	Right rotation
Right sidebent	Left sidebending	Right sidebending

fourth-layer vertebral muscle in the medial grove adjacent to the spinous processes. Palpable fourth-layer muscle hypertonicity is not present in normal vertebral motion segments. When palpable at a vertebral level, the practitioner should identify the motion characteristics of that vertebra in relation to the one above and below. A second clue to the possibility of a single vertebral motion segment dysfunction is the scanning examination finding of prominence overlying one transverse process, suggesting the possibility of rotation of the vertebra to that side (Fig. 6.1). The segmental definition diagnostic process is performed by placing the thumbs over the posterior aspect of the transverse process of a segment that is suspected of being dysfunctional. The patient then is put through a forward-bending to backward-bending movement arc either actively or passively. In the upper thoracic spine the active movement of the head on the trunk is frequently used, whereas in the lower thoracic and lumbar region, the patient is examined in three different positions: prone neutral on the table, fully backward bent (prone prop position), and fully forward bent (Figs. 6.2–6.4). For the purpose of description, assume that something interferes with opening of the right zygapophysial joint. In the neutral position the right transverse process appears to be somewhat more posterior than the left. As the patient increases the amount of forward-bending, the right transverse process becomes more prominent than the left. The restricted right zygapophysial joint holds the right half of the posterior arch of that vertebra in a posterior position, whereas the free-moving zygapophysial joint on the left side allows the left half of the posterior arch to move forward and superior with the left transverse process, seeming to become less prominent. In backward-bending both transverse processes appear to become more symmetric because the right transverse process is already held posterior by the restricted right zygapophysial joint, whereas the left zygapophysial joint closes in backward-bending, allowing the left transverse process to move posteriorly and inferiorly, becoming more symmetric in appearance.

Now let us assume that something interferes with the left zygapophysial joint's ability to close. In this instance we usually find the right transverse process a little more prominent in the neutral position. In asking the patient to move into backward-bending the right transverse process appears to become more prominent. This is the result of normal closure of the right zygapophysial joint that allows the transverse process to move posteriorly, whereas the left zygapophysial joint is restricted in its capacity to close and holds the left transverse process in a more anterior position. Upon forward-bending, both transverse processes become more symmetrical. The left transverse process is already held in an anterior position by the restricted left zygapophysial joint, and the motion of the right zygapophysial moving into an open position carries the right transverse process more anteriorly.

These single vertebral motor unit dysfunctions are also described as nonneutral dysfunctions because the restricted coupled movement is sidebending and rotation to the same side. Historically, they have been described as type II dysfunctions. The characteristics are as follows:

1. Single vertebral motion unit involved;
2. Includes either flexion or extension restriction component;
3. Motion restriction of sidebending and rotation to the same side.

We have described the phenomenon that occurs if one or the other zygapophysial joint loses the capacity to open or close. If there is a single vertebral motion segment involved in which both zygapophysial joints are restricted, the transverse processes remain in the same relative position throughout forward-bending and backward-bending movement. One can determine the case of bilateral zygapophysial joints being closed or bilaterally being open by monitoring the interspace between the spinous process during forward-bending and backward-bending. If the z joints are able to open, the interspinous distance will increase during forward-bending. If the z joints are able to close in a bilaterally symmetrical fashion, the interspinous distance becomes smaller during backward-bending.

There are several reasons why this method of vertebral motion testing is recommended. First, this method remains consistent and reproducible over time. The challenge to the motion segment is in only one plane of movement. No multiaxial changes in movement characteristics are introduced, as in the procedure described earlier. This method does not put the segment through an articulatory procedure

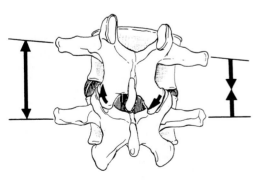

Figure 6.1.
Single segment right prominent transverse process.

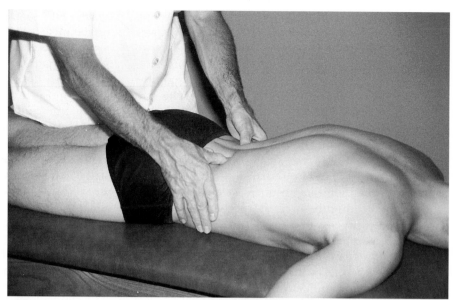

Figure 6.2.
Vertebral motion testing prone
neutral.

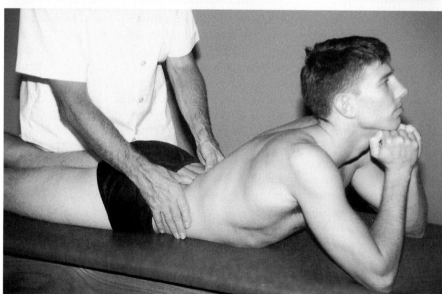

Figure 6.3.
Vertebral motion testing backward bent.

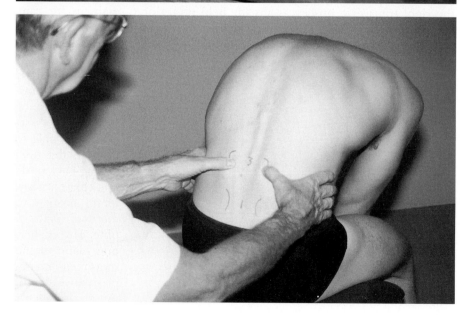

Figure 6.4.
Vertebral motion testing forward bent.

and thus is not changing the vertebral mechanics to any appreciable amount. This makes it possible for the examiner to be more confident in the posttreatment evaluation of a segment that, in fact, some change has occurred in the motion present before and after treatment.

Second, this procedure is easier for multiple examiners to apply because of the nontreatment aspect of the method. This allows more consistent student teaching and evaluation of vertebral diagnostic procedures. If five separate examiners tested a given segment by putting it through multiple ranges of movement, by the time the fifth examiner described the findings, the first examiner would believe it was a different patient. Using this single-plane movement challenge, the findings remain much more consistent across examiners and across time.

A third reason to recommend this process is the examiner's capacity to differentiate between structural and functional asymmetry of a vertebral segment. Structural asymmetries do occur fairly frequently, and palpation of a posterior transverse process cannot distinguish asymmetrical development from actual dysfunction of a rotational nature. If the prominent transverse process is because of nonneutral (type II) single vertebral motion segment dysfunction, the prominence of the transverse process will change during a forward-bending and backward-bending arc. In one position it will become worse, and in the other position it will become more symmetrical. If the transverse process is prominent because of asymmetrical development and the segment is basically functional, the transverse process will retain the same amount of prominence throughout the forward-bending and backward-bending movement arc. There is a third possibility for the finding of a transverse process being more prominent on one side than the other. This can occur when one zygapophysial joint does not open and the other does not close. This bilateral restriction retains the same amount of prominence of the posterior transverse process throughout the movement arc. One can distinguish this bilateral restriction from a structural asymmetry by evaluating the forward-bending and backward-bending capacity while monitoring at the interspinous space.

Figure 6.5 shows an example of the findings in the presence of nonneutral dysfunctions identified within the lumbar spine. A fundamental principle of the use of the diagnostic process is the importance of relating the behavior of the superior vertebra on the one below. The inferior segment is the plane of orientation against which the superior segment is related. The base reference plane is the coronal plane. If the inferior segment is rotated to the left and the superior is level against the coronal plane, then the superior vertebra in relation to the inferior segment is rotated to the right. Remember, always relate the behavior of the superior segment to the inferior. In this example the sacrum is level against the coronal plane in all three positions of forward-bending, neutral, and backward-bending. At L5 the left transverse process becomes more prominent during forward-bending, whereas it is symmetrical against the coronal plane in neutral and backward-bending. This finding results from something interfering with the capacity of the left zygapophysial joint to open during forward-bending. In both neutral and backward-bending, the transverse processes are symmetric, indicating the capacity of the zygapophysial joints to close symmetrically in backward-bending. The amount of restriction is not great because it is not evident by rotation to the left in neutral. The diagnosis would be L5 is extended, rotated, and sidebent, left (ERS$_{\text{left}}$) with motion restriction of forward-bending, right sidebending, and right rotation. Also note that in forward-bending the left transverse processes of L1–4 are also more prominent on the left. This finding is a result of the fact that L5 has rotated left during forward-bending and the other four lumbar vertebra have followed in a normal fashion with symmetrical opening of their zygapophysial joint during forward-bending.

At L4 we have a different observation. At this level in backward-bending, the right transverse process becomes more prominent in relation to the symmetric transverse processes at L5. In both neutral and forward-bending, L4 follows the behavior of L5. In backward-bending it does not. In backward-bending something has interfered with the capacity of the left zygapophysial joint to close. During backward-bending the normal closure of the right zygapophysial joint carries the vertebra into right rotation, right sidebending, and backward-bending on the right side. The diagnosis is L4 is flexed, rotated, and sidebent, right (FRS$_{\text{right}}$) with motion restriction of backward-bending, left sidebending, and left rotation. Again note that the transverse processes of L1–3 are also posterior on the right in backward-bending. This is a normal finding as they follow the right rotation of L4. Their zygapophysial joints have the capacity to close symmetrically and follow the right rotation at L4.

NEUTRAL (GROUP) DYSFUNCTION

The characteristics of a neutral group dysfunction are

1. A group of segments (three or more);
2. Minimal flexion or extension component of restriction;

3. Restriction of the group to sidebending in one direction and rotation in the opposite (Fig. 6.6).

With three or more vertebral segments involved in motion restriction, a lateral curvature results to one side. There is prominence on the side of convexity of the group of segments because of rotation of the vertebra to that side. On palpatory examination one finds a fullness overlying the transverse processes of three or more adjacent vertebra. This finding is frequently misdiagnosed as muscle hypertonicity or spasm because the muscle overlying the posterior transverse processes is more prominent and the impression is that the muscle is spastic or is hypertonic or tight. It is true that the muscle is more prominent, but it is the result of the rotation of the vertebra that the transverse process is taking the muscle mass posteriorly.

During the diagnostic process of trunk, neutral, forward-bending, and backward-bending, the palpable fullness over the transverse processes on one side is maintained. It may get a little better or a little worse in its deformity during the movement arc, but there is no position in which the transverse processes on each side become symmetrical. The motion restriction found in this group of segments will be minimal forward-bending or backward-bending restriction but major restriction of sidebending to the side of convexity and rotation to the side of concavity.

Neutral group dysfunctions are also called type I restrictions with a restricted coupled movement being sidebending to one side and rotation to the opposite. These dysfunctions are present in compensatory scoliotic mechanisms and are frequently found above or below a single vertebral motion segment dysfunction. They are frequently secondary to change elsewhere, but because they involve a large number of vertebral segments, they receive a lot of diagnostic attention. Because these dysfunctions are secondary to other findings, their treatment should follow appropriate treatment to the cause of the dysfunction, either a nonneutral dysfunction or unleveling of the sacral base.

Figure 6.7 portrays the findings in a group dysfunction. Again note that L5 shows a nonneutral single segment dysfunction that is ERS_{left} as in Figure 6.5. In this example the left transverse processes are prominent from L1–4 in forward-bending, neutral, and backward-bending. No matter what position the patient assumes, there is rotation of L1–4 to the left. This dysfunction is a neutral group dysfunction of L1–4 with the positional diagnosis being neutral, sidebent right, and rotated left. Another diagnostic description for this group dysfunction is L1–4 EN (easy normal) left (indicating left convexity).

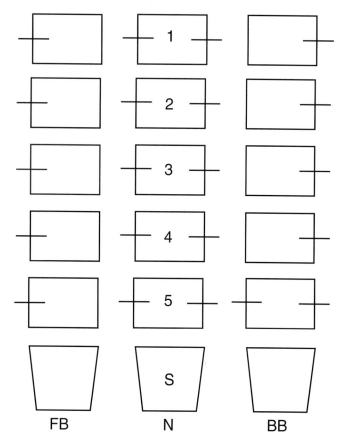

Figure 6.5.
Single segment nonneutral vertebral dysfunction example.

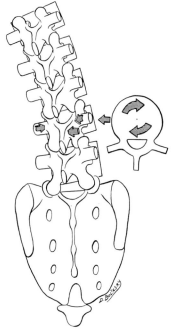

Figure 6.6.
Neutral group vertebral dysfunction.

In the therapeutic process the practitioner identifies and treats all nonneutral dysfunctions first, and if any group dysfunctions remain, they are addressed separately.

HYPERMOBILITY

Manual medicine procedures are appropriate for restriction of articular structures (hypomobility), but if used on hypermobile segments they could be detrimental, enhancing the hypermobility. In structural diagnosis we are concerned with three types of hypermobility: *(a)* hypermobility due to disease such as Ehlers-Danlos syndrome, Marfan's syndrome, the Marfanoid hypermobility syndrome, and others even more rare; *(b)* physiological hypermobility seen in certain body types (ectomorphic) and frequently observed in gymnasts, ballet dancers, and other athletic types; and *(c)* compensatory hypermobility due to hypomobility elsewhere in the musculoskeletal system.

The pathological hypermobilities are a group of conditions in which there is alteration in the histology and biochemistry of the connective tissues. In Ehlers-Danlos syndrome there is articular hypermobility, dermal extensibility, and frequent cutaneous scarring. This condition has been noted in circus performers who are classified as "elastic people." The classic Marfan syndrome demonstrates long slender (Lincolnesque) limbs, ectopic lentis, dilation of the ascending aorta, and mitral valve prolapse. Although the severity of each of the components of the Marfan syndrome vary from patient to patient, all exhibit joint hypermobility. After joint injury the hypermobility is increased, and it is very difficult to manage patients with this condition who have somatic dysfunction superimposed on their musculoskeletal anatomy. The Marfanoid hypermobility syndrome has the same musculoskeletal system findings but seems not to demonstrate either the eye or the vascular changes.

In the physiological hypermobility group there is hypermobility of fingers, thumbs, elbows, knees, and trunk forward-bending. A nine-point scale has been devised for the paired fingers, thumbs, elbows, and knees with one point being assigned to trunk forward-bending. Patients with this trait find it easy to become gymnasts and ballet dancers, and increased mobility can result from training and exercise. In normal individuals joint mobility reduces rapidly during childhood and then more slowly during adulthood. Patients with increased physiological hypermobility are at risk for increased musculoskeletal system symptoms and diseases, particularly osteoarthritis.

It is in the secondary hypermobility states that the manual medicine practitioner becomes more involved. Compensatory hypermobility appears to develop in areas of the vertebral column as a secondary reaction to hypomobility within the complex. The segments of compensatory hypermobility can be either adjacent to or some distance from the area(s) of major joint hypomobility. Clinically, there also appears to be relative hypermobility on the opposite side of a segment that is restricted. The major difficulty encountered with these areas of secondary compensatory hypermobility is that they are frequently the ones that are symptomatic. Because they attempt to compensate for restricted motion elsewhere, they receive excess stimulation from increased mobility and frequently become painful and tender. As the painful areas, they receive a great deal of attention from the manual medicine practitioner, who can become trapped into treating the hypermobile segment because it is symptomatic and not realizing that the symptom is secondary to restricted mobility elsewhere. In most instances of compensatory hypermobility, the condition requires little or no direct treatment but responds nicely to appropriate treatment of hypomobility elsewhere in the vertebral column. Many practitioners of musculoskeletal medicine use sclerosant-type injection into the ligaments of a hypermobile segment as part of treatment. This system was used empirically for many years, but recently

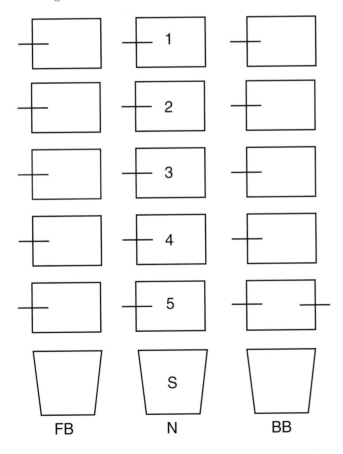

Figure 6.7.
Neutral group dysfunction example.

there have been both clinical and animal studies that support the observation that proliferent therapy does enhance joint stability and reduce nociception. In this author's experience, most areas of secondary compensatory hypermobility are self-correcting once the hypomobility areas are adequately treated and the total musculoskeletal system is restored to functional balance.

One cannot discuss hypermobility without referring to instability. Instability occurs when the damage is sufficient and the opposing joint structures lose their anatomical integrity. The dividing line between extensive hypermobility and instability is very hard to define. In actual instability the appropriate treatment is either a stabilizing surgical procedure or a restraining orthopedic device.

Diagnosing Hypermobility

The diagnosis of hypermobility in the Ehlers-Danlos and Marfan syndrome groups is not difficult as long as the index of suspicion is present and the other physical findings are identified. The nine-point scale previously mentioned helps give an overall assessment of relative hypermobility. It is in the evaluation of local compensatory hypermobility that the difficulty exists. The diagnostic procedures are variations on regional segmental motion testing. In these procedures, one attempts to hold one segment and move the other in relation to it, comparing it with the perceived normals of the segments above and below the one suspected of hypermobility. Translatory motion challenges have been found to be the most effective. With the lumbar spine, the patient can be in the lateral recumbent position while the operator monitors each vertebral segment. By grasping two spinous processes with the thumb and index finger, a to-and-fro lateral translatory movement can be introduced and compared above and below (Fig. 6.8). Using the same lateral recumbent position with the knees and hips flexed, the operator can monitor a given segment holding the superior one and then introducing an anteroposterior translatory movement by movement of the operator's thigh against the patient's knees (Fig. 6.9). Combined sidebending and rotation challenge can occur in the same position with the operator grasping the feet and ankles and lifting the extremities off the table (Fig. 6.10), and dropping them down below the table (Fig. 6.11) while monitoring the posterior elements of the lumbar vertebrae. Another hypermobility test builds on the fact that in backward-bending, as the zygapophysial joints symmetrically close, there is reduction in available lateral translatory movement. With the patient in the prone prop backward-bent position on the table (Fig. 6.12), the operator places thumbs on each side of the spinous process overlying the transverse processes of the vertebra and translates from left to right (Fig. 6.13) and from right to left. Comparing the translatory mobility from segment to segment gives the operator an impression of whether one is more mobile than the other. Testing for hypermobility requires a great deal of practice, and the judgment is highly individualistic. If one suspects significant segmental hypermobility, stress x-ray procedures in the flexion-extension and right and left sidebending modes should be used to assist in the diagnosis.

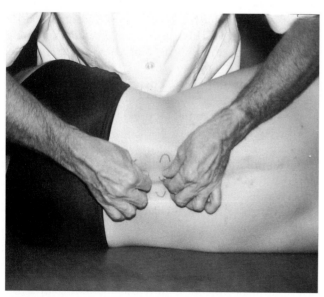

Figure 6.8.
Hypermobility testing lateral translation.

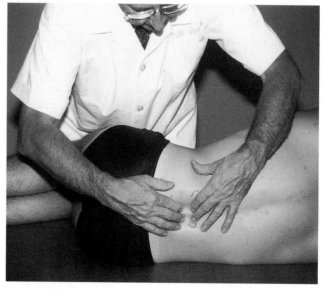

Figure 6.9.
Hypermobility testing anteroposterior translation.

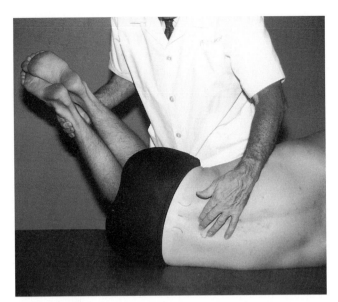

Figure 6.10.
Hypermobility testing sidebending rotation.

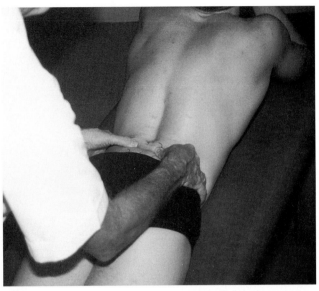

Figure 6.12.
Hypermobility testing beginning with thumb contact of spinous and transverse processes while backward bent.

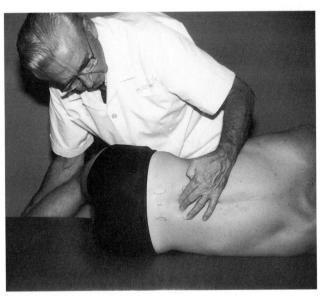

Figure 6.11.
Hypermobility testing sidebending rotation.

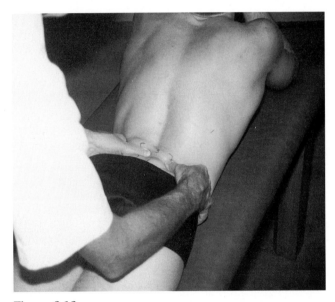

Figure 6.13.
Hypermobility testing translation from left to right while backward bent.

CONCLUSION

Although there is still a need for more research into the biomechanics of vertebral segmental motion and pathologies that might restrict vertebral motion, the concepts and methodologies described here will pro-vide the practicing manual medicine clinician with sufficient accurate diagnostic information for treatment purposes, for accurate records, and for communicating with a colleague. The hallmark of structural diagnosis of restricted vertebral function is practice and experience.

7

SOFT TISSUE AND MOBILIZATION WITHOUT IMPULSE (ARTICULATORY) TECHNIQUE

There are a great number of "hands-on" approaches to the body. They can all be classified as peripheral stimulation therapies. Chapter 4 mentioned soft tissue therapy procedures, including Travell trigger points, Chapman's reflexes, acupuncture, and others. This chapter describes soft tissue procedures with long acceptance and use in the field of manual medicine. Many of the procedures are the same as, or similar to, those found in traditional massage.

DEFINITION

Soft tissue technique is defined as a "procedure directed towards tissues other than the skeleton while monitoring response and motion changes using diagnostic palpation. It usually involves lateral stretching, linear stretching, deep pressure, traction, and/or separation of muscle origin and insertion" (Glossary of Osteopathic Terminology. *J Am Osteopath Assoc* 80:552–567, 1981).

PURPOSE OF SOFT TISSUE TECHNIQUE

Soft tissue procedures are widely used in a combined diagnostic and therapeutic mode. They are frequently a prelude to other more definitive manual medicine procedures to the underlying articular structures. They prepare the soft tissues for other technique procedures. They are also used as the only manual medicine intervention to achieve a specific therapeutic goal.

Mechanisms

These procedures have mechanical, circulatory, and neurological effects and are useful in both acute and chronic conditions. Soft tissue procedures can mechanically stretch the skin, fascia, and muscle tissues of the body to enhance their motion and pliability. These procedures are useful in encouraging circulation of fluid in and around the soft tissues of the musculoskeletal system, enhancing venous and lymphatic return and decongesting parts of the body compromised by injury or a disease process. These

same procedures can have a neurological effect, particularly modifying muscle physiology to overcome hypertonicity and spasm. These neurological effects can be stimulatory or inhibitory depending on how the procedure was applied. Another neurological effect is the relief of musculoskeletal pain after their use. This may result from the release of endogenous opioids and other neurohumoral substances. Another possible mechanism is the modulation of spinal reflex pathways by the stimulation of mechanoreceptors, proprioceptors, and nociceptors in the soft tissues.

Tonic Effect

Soft tissue procedures are also useful for their general "tonic" effect on patients, particularly those who have been bedridden for any period of time because of illness or injury. They seem to enhance general physical tone and level of well-being. Because many of these procedures seem general in application and result in various outcomes, the manual medicine practitioner must have a specific therapeutic goal in mind before instituting any soft tissue procedure. Once the objective is clear, the procedure can be adapted to fit the patient condition, patient location, and operator's strength and ability.

TYPES OF SOFT TISSUE PROCEDURES

Soft tissue procedures are oriented toward the direction of a force being applied to the underlying muscle(s) (Fig. 7.1). A force at right angles to the long axis of the muscle is called lateral stretch. The force applied in the direction of the long axis of the muscle is called linear or longitudinal stretch. By applying a force in both directions along the long axis of a muscle, we achieve separation of origin and insertion. If steady deep pressure is applied to a muscle close to its attachment to the bone, the procedure is called deep pressure. Although these procedures are described in relation to muscle and its fiber direction, remember that application of external force

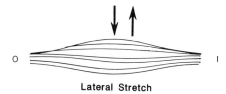

Lateral Stretch

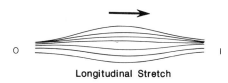

Longitudinal Stretch

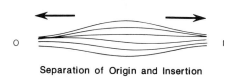

Separation of Origin and Insertion

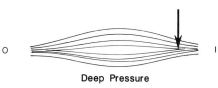

Deep Pressure

Figure 7.1.
Soft tissue procedures.

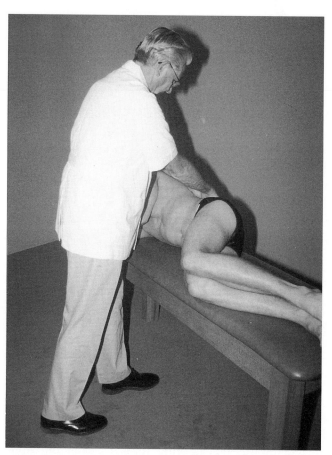

Figure 7.2.
Operator's stance.

to the muscle area also involves skin, subcutaneous fascia, and the deep fascia surrounding muscle. All of these tissues are affected by soft tissue procedures.

THERAPEUTIC PRINCIPLES OF SOFT TISSUE TECHNIQUE

As in all appropriate manual medicine procedures, the operator's body should be held in a posture that is comfortable and balanced to avoid undue strain or fatigue. The treatment table or bed should be at the appropriate height so that the operator need not bend forward unnecessarily (Fig. 7.2). The operator's stance should be relaxed with one foot slightly in front of the other so that the to-and-fro rocking of the operator's body mass provides the force, not operator muscle activity.

The patient should be in a comfortable and relaxed position. If the prone position is used, the head should be turned toward the operator so that lateral force does not put undue strain on the cervicothoracic junction. If a lateral recumbent position is used, an appropriate pillow height should maintain the head and neck in the long axis of the trunk. It is useful to have the patient's feet and knees together

with the knees and hips slightly flexed. This provides both comfort and stability to the patient. It is most important that the relationship of the patient and the operator be relaxed and synergistic.

The placement and use of the hands in soft tissue procedures becomes most important. These procedures use mainly the fingerpads, the thenar eminence of the hand, and the palmer aspect of the thumb. When the operator uses the fingerpads to engage the tissues, the distal interphalangeal joint flexion that occurs is a function of the flexor digitorum profundus (Fig. 7.3). Beginners in manual medicine have to practice strengthening the profundus tendon flexor action to maintain appropriate application of force to soft tissues. The thenar eminence and palmer surface of the thumb can be laid along the long axis of muscle and used singly (Fig. 7.4), paired (Fig. 7.5), or with one hand reinforcing the other (Fig. 7.6). It is very important that the soft tissues be adequately and accurately engaged at the appropriate layer. In treating the erector spinae mass, there are two common errors to be avoided. The first is pressure toward the spinous processes, instead of away from the spinous processes, on the side being treated. This causes painful compression of the

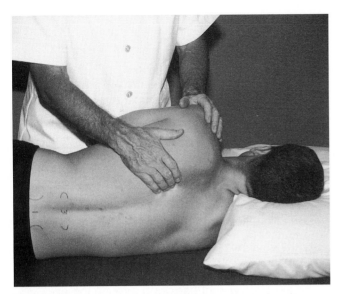

Figure 7.3.
Soft tissue, flexed finger pad contact.

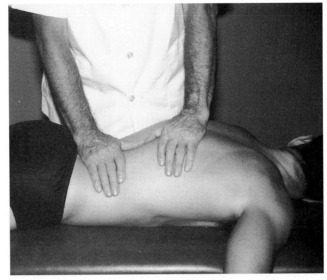

Figure 7.5.
Soft tissue, paired thenar eminence and thumb contact.

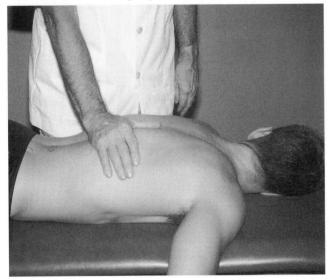

Figure 7.4.
Soft tissue, single thenar eminence contact.

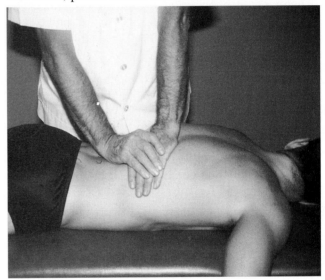

Figure 7.6.
Soft tissue, reinforced two hand contact.

erector spinae mass against the lateral side of the spinous process and is counterproductive. The second error is allowing the therapeutic hand to "snap over" an area of hypertonic muscle through failure of control at the muscle layer. Hand placement and control become most important.

The dosage of soft tissue procedures is modified by the rate, rhythm, and length of time of application and, most importantly, by the constant feedback from the tissues of the response obtained. Constant reassessment of the response is the hallmark of soft tissue procedures. The operator should continue until the desired response is obtained and stop as soon as it has been achieved. If the tissue response is not as anticipated, the procedure should be stopped and reassessment of the diagnosis and status of the patient should be made. Slow and steady soft tissue procedures appear to have inhibitory effects on the tissues. More rapid and vigorous applications of force appear to be stimulatory. The application of force is modified by the goal to be achieved and the response of the tissues. The operator must also be aware of other reactions within the patient in addition to those of the tissue being treated. Sometimes patients become quite agitated; other times they become very relaxed and almost euphoric. It must be remembered that although these procedures are passive, they are still fatiguing, and the length of treatment might well be modified by the response of the patient.

Soft Tissue Techniques

Cervical Spine

Procedure: Unilateral lateral stretch

1. Patient supine on table with operator on side of the table facing the patient (example left side) (Fig. 7.7).
2. Operator's right hand stabilizes patient's forehead.
3. Operator's left hand grasps the patient's right cervical paravertebral musculature with fingertips medial to the muscle mass and just lateral to the spinous processes.
4. Lateral stretch is placed on the cervical musculature by the operator's left hand pulling laterally and somewhat anteriorly with the operator's right hand maintaining the stability of the patient's head.
5. Lateral stretch is applied and released rhythmically throughout the cervical musculature with particular reference to areas of increased muscle tone and soft tissue congestion.
6. The procedure can be varied to allow the patient's head to rotate toward the left during the application of force by the operator's left hand and a counter force can be applied by the operator's right hand in a "push-pull" manner.
7. The procedure can be repeated on the opposite side by having the operator now stand on the patient's right.

Soft Tissue Techniques

Cervical Spine

Procedure: Bilateral-lateral stretch

1. Patient supine on table with operator standing at head of table (Fig. 7.8).
2. Operator's fingerpads bilaterally contact the medial side of the cervical paravertebral musculature.
3. The operator puts simultaneous lateral stretch on both sides of the cervical musculature, moving from above downward or below upward, and focusing on side of greater tissue reaction and muscle hypertonicity.
4. The operator may also apply some long axis extension in combination with the lateral stretch by leaning the body weight backward through the extended arms.

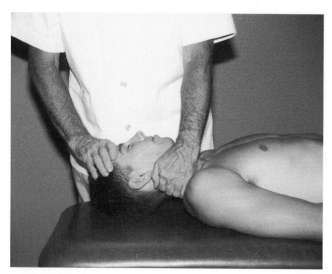

Figure 7.7.

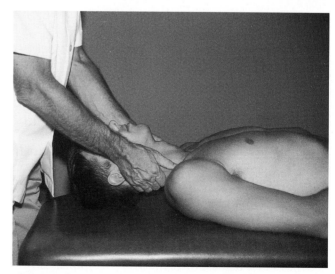

Figure 7.8.

Soft Tissue Techniques

Cervical Spine

Procedure: Long axis longitudinal stretch

1. Patient supine with operator sitting at head of table.
2. Operator's one hand cradles the skull with the index finger and thumb in contact with the insertion of the cervical musculature into the occiput and the chin held by the other hand (Fig. 7.9).
3. By the use of body weight, the operator puts long axis extension (traction) in a cephalic direction and then releases.
4. Repeat as necessary.

Caution: Too much traction is frequently counterproductive.

Soft Tissue Techniques

Cervical Spine

Procedure: Suboccipital muscle deep pressure

1. Patient supine with operator sitting at head of table.
2. Operator's fingertips of each hand contact the bony attachment of the deep cervical musculature at the suboccipital region.
3. By flexing the distal interphalangeal joints, the operator puts sustained deep pressure over the muscular attachment to the occipital bone (Fig. 7.10).
4. Pressure is applied on each side to achieve balance in tension and tone.
5. Pressure is released when bilateral relaxation occurs.

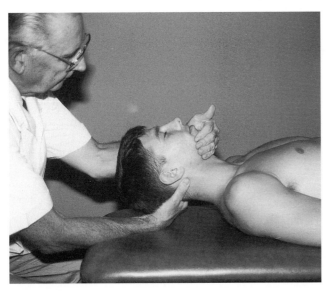

Figure 7.9.

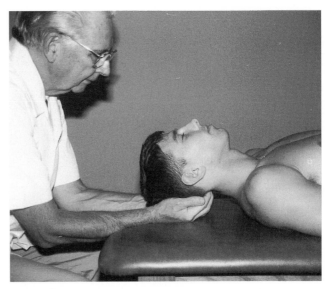

Figure 7.10.

Soft Tissue Techniques

Cervical Spine

Procedure: Separation origin and insertion (example: right upper trapezius)

1. Patient supine with operator sitting or standing at head of table.
2. Operator's left hand is placed over the patient's occiput and controls head and neck position.
3. Operator's right hand is placed over the patient's right acromium process (Fig. 7.11).
4. Operator's left hand sidebends the head and neck to the left with some left rotation while right hand puts counterforce on the acromial process, separating the origin and insertion of the upper fibers of the trapezius.
5. By reversal of hand position, the opposite side can be treated with the goal of symmetry of length and tone of each trapezius.

Soft Tissue Techniques

Thoracic Spine

Procedure: Lateral stretch

1. Patient is in lateral recumbent position lying with involved side uppermost with operator standing and facing patient.
2. For upper thoracic region, patient's left arm is draped over operator's right arm and fingerpads contact medial side of paravertebral musculature (Fig. 7.12).

3. Operator pulls thoracic paravertebral musculature laterally and releases in a rhythmical fashion.
4. A counterforce can be applied by the operator's left hand against the patient's left shoulder for additional leverage.
5. For rhomboid stretch the same body position as for upper thoracic spine but operator's fingers contact the vertebral border of the scapula (Fig. 7.13). The scapula is swept anterolaterally around the chest wall with stretch in the direction of the fibers of the rhomboid muscle.
6. Repeat as necessary.

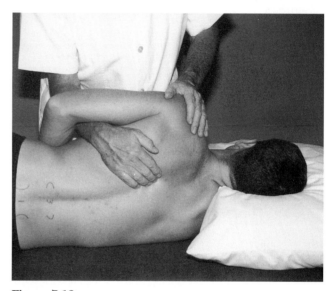

Figure 7.12.

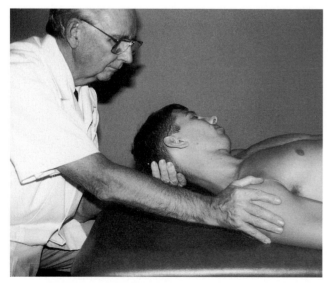

Figure 7.11.

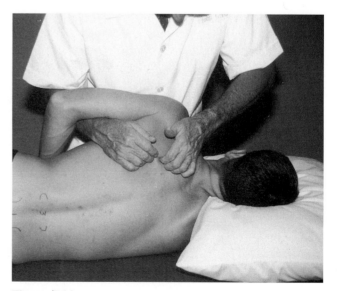

Figure 7.13.

Soft Tissue Techniques

Thoracolumbar Spine

Procedure: Lateral stretch

1. Patient lies in lateral recumbent position with involved side uppermost. Operator faces patient.

2. Operator's right hand grasps the thoracolumbar paravertebral muscle mass on the involved side with the left hand stabilizing the patient's left shoulder (Fig. 7.14).

3. An alternate hand position is with the operator's left hand grasping the thoracolumbar paravertebral muscle mass and with the right hand stabilizing the patient's pelvis over the left ilium (Fig. 7.15).

4. Operator's hand in contact with the paravertebral musculature stretches laterally against the counterforce applied either at the pelvis or at the shoulder girdle.

5. Repeat as necessary throughout the thoracolumbar muscle region.

6. Variation sometimes allows patient's right arm to be flexed at the elbow and the operator's right hand to be threaded through before application to paravertebral musculature.

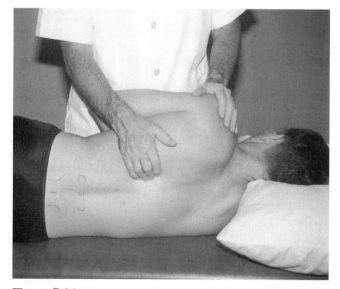

Figure 7.14.

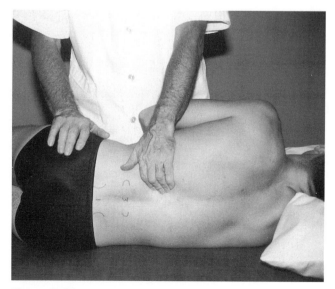

Figure 7.15.

Soft Tissue Techniques

Thoracolumbar Spine

Procedure: Lateral and longitudinal stretch

1. Patient in lateral recumbent position with involved side uppermost. Operator faces patient.

2. Operator's left forearm is threaded through the patient's left axilla with the left hand in contact with the left paravertebral muscle mass.

3. Operator's right forearm is on the superior aspect of the patient's left ilium with fingerpads in contact with the left paravertebral musculature.

4. Fingerpad contact of both hands stretches paravertebral musculature laterally (Fig. 7.16).

5. Simultaneously with lateral stretch, the operator's forearm or arms are separated with the right arm going caudally and the left cephalically applying a longitudinal stretch (Fig. 7.17).

6. Repeat as necessary throughout the lumbar and thoracic paravertebral musculature.

Soft Tissue Techniques

Thoracolumbar Spine

Procedure: Prone lateral stretch

1. Patient lies prone on table with arms at side and face turned toward operator.

2. Operator stands at side of table.

3. Operator's thumbs and thenar eminences are placed on medial side of involved paravertebral

musculature. Lateral stretch is applied rhythmically throughout the involved areas (Fig. 7.5).

4. A variation is applying lateral stretch using one hand on top of the other as reinforcement (Fig. 7.6).

5. Another variation is for the operator's right hand to grasp the patient's right anterior superior iliac spine while the left thumb and thenar eminence puts lateral stretch on the involved paravertebral musculature (Fig. 7.18). Lifting the patient's right ilium provides a counterforce.

6. Repeat as necessary.

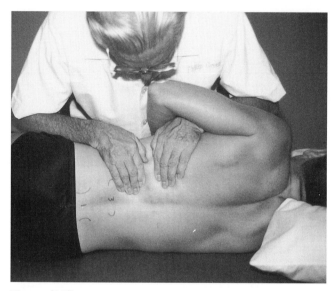

Figure 7.17.

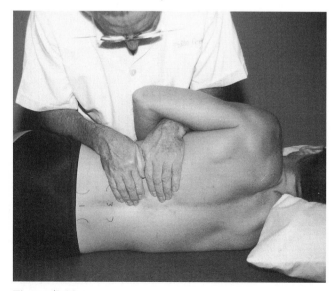

Figure 7.16.

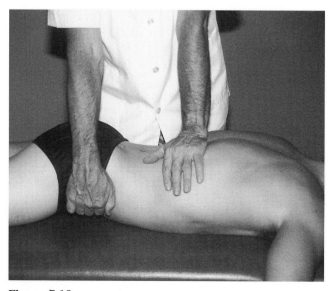

Figure 7.18.

Soft Tissue Techniques

Thoracolumbar Spine

Procedure: Deep pressure

1. Patient is prone on table.
2. Operator places thumbs, or thumb reinforced by hand, over area of hypertonic muscle (Fig. 7.19). This is most effective in the medial groove between the spinous process and the longissimus and overlying the hypertonic fourth-layer vertebral muscle.

3. Steady pressure is applied in a ventral direction and sustained until tissue release is felt.
4. A variation is the placement of the operator's olecranon process of the elbow overlying the hypertonic muscle. Body weight can be used to provide ventral compressive force against hypertonic muscle (Fig. 7.20).
5. Repeat as necessary.

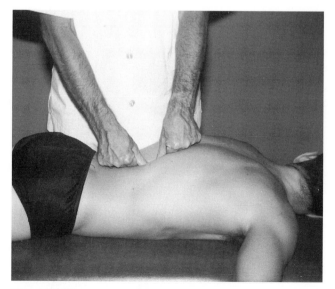

Figure 7.19.

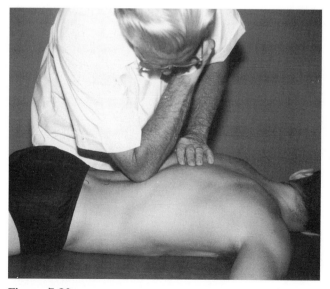

Figure 7.20.

Soft Tissue Techniques

Gluteal Region

Procedure: Deep pressure

1. Patient is in the prone or lateral recumbent position with involved side uppermost.

2. Operator can stand at the side or in front of the patient.

3. Reinforced thumbs are placed over the hypertonic areas of gluteal musculature either near origin on the ilium, within the belly, or at insertion in greater trochanter (Fig. 7.21).

4. Deep pressure is maintained until relaxation is felt.

5. A variant in application of force is the use of the olecranon process of the elbow as the contact point with the body weight being applied against the hypertonic muscle (Fig. 7.22).

6. Repeat as necessary.

Soft Tissue Techniques

Lymphatic Pump

Lymphatic pump treatment procedures apply the principle of the respiratory circulatory model of manual medicine. The therapeutic goal is to enhance venous and lymphatic flow throughout the body and to enhance respiratory exchange. These procedures apply force to the extremities, as well as to the thoracic cage, in a "pumping" fashion. Although the goal is to enhance fluid flow and respiratory exchange, the forces applied mobilize articular structures and the fascias of the body from superficial to deep. These techniques are of great value in patients with acute and chronic pulmonary disease, particularly bronchitis and pneumonia, and in both the obstructive and restrictive components of chronic obstructive pulmonary disease. The techniques are potent in mobilizing peripheral edema. Appropriate dosage should be applied so that cardiac function is not compromised. These techniques can be applied in patients with acute musculoskeletal injuries to enhance the drainage of the soft tissue swelling associated with acute trauma to the peripheral joints. Always remember the principle of working from central to distal when applying the respiratory circulatory model in the patient's care.

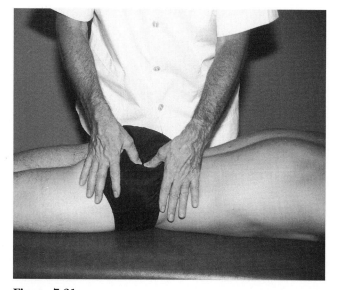

Figure 7.21.

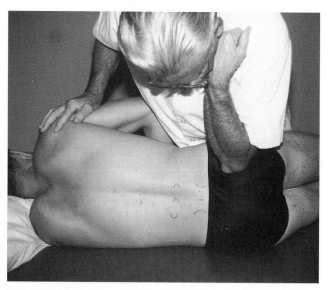

Figure 7.22.

Soft Tissue Techniques

Lymphatic Pump

Procedure: Thoracic lymphatic pump

1. Patient supine with operator at head of table.
2. Operator places both hands in contact with anterior aspect of the thoracic cage with heel of hand just below the clavicle (Fig. 7.23).
3. Patient is instructed to inhale deeply and then exhale.
4. During exhalation phase, the operator puts oscillatory compression on chest cage.
5. At end of exhalation patient is instructed to breathe in while operator holds chest wall in exhalation position for a momentary period of time.
6. Operator rapidly releases compression of chest during patient's inhalation effort.
7. Repeat steps 2 through 6 several times.

Soft Tissue Techniques

Lymphatic Pump

Procedure: Unilateral thoracic lymphatic pump

1. Patient supine with operator at side of table.
2. Operator's left arm grasps the patient's right upper extremity.
3. Operator's right hand contacts the patient's right thoracic cage (Fig. 7.24).
4. During patient's inhalation, operator applies traction on patient's right upper extremity.

5. During exhalation phase, traction of upper extremity is released, and operator applies oscillatory force against thoracic cage during exhalation.
6. Operator's right hand maintains compression on chest wall during initial phase of inhalation and then rapidly releases pressure while simultaneously lifting patient's right upper extremity in a cephalic direction.
7. Repeat steps 2 through 6 several times.
8. A lateral recumbent variation has the patient with the treated side uppermost. The operator's left hand grasps the patient's right upper extremity while the operator's right hand is applied to the patient's right thoracic cage (Fig. 7.25). Repeat steps 2 through 6 several times.

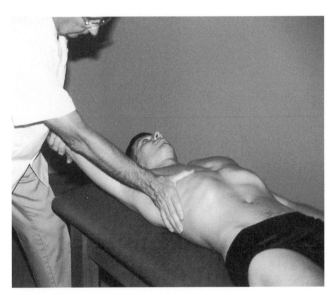

Figure 7.24.

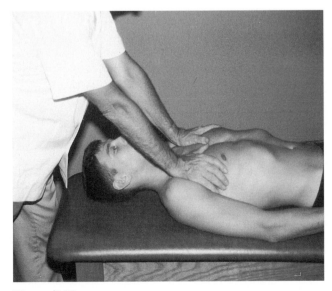

Figure 7.23.

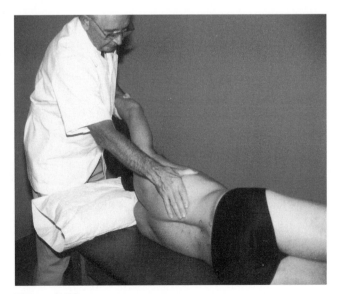

Figure 7.25.

Soft Tissue Techniques

Lymphatic Pump

Procedure: Lymphatic pump lower extremity

1. Patient supine with operator at end of table.
2. Operator grasps dorsum of both feet with each hand and introduces plantar flexion (Fig. 7.26).
3. Operator applies oscillatory movement in a pedad direction noting oscillatory wave of lower extremities up to the trunk.

4. Operator grasps toes and ball of patient's foot and introduces dorsi flexion (Fig. 7.27).
5. Cephalic oscillatory movement is applied to the dorsi flexed feet.
6. Repeat in both the dorsi and plantar flexed directions several times.

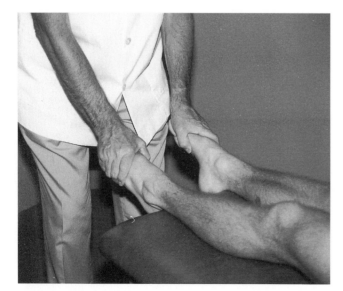

Figure 7.26.

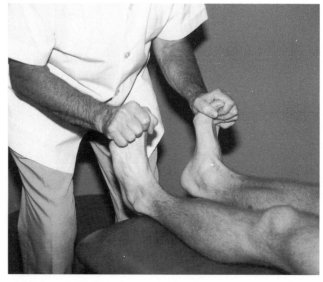

Figure 7.27.

Soft Tissue Techniques

Lymphatic Pump

Procedure: Lymphatic pump upper extremity

1. Patient supine with operator at head of table.
2. Patient raises both hands above head and operator grasps each wrist (Fig. 7.28).
3. Operator applies intermittent cephalic oscillatory traction on patient's upper extremities noting response in the thoracic cage.
4. Repeat as necessary.

Soft Tissue Techniques

Miscellaneous Soft Tissue Techniques

Procedure: Pectoral release

1. Patient supine with operator at head of table.
2. Operator's two hands, particularly using the middle fingers, grasp patient's inferior border of pectoral muscles (Fig. 7.29).
3. Operator applies bilateral cephalic traction on the inferior aspect of the pectoral muscles.
4. The response elicited is release of muscle tension.
5. Observe thorax and abdomen for change from thoracic to abdominal breathing.

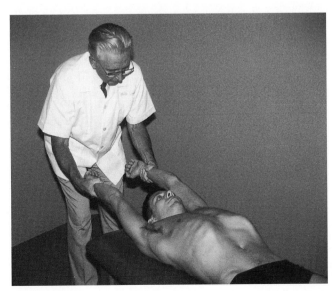

Figure 7.28.

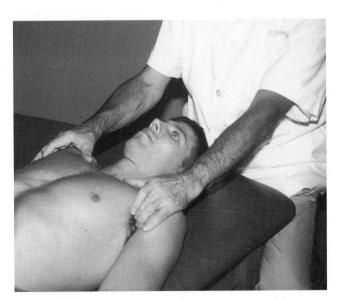

Figure 7.29.

Soft Tissue Techniques

Miscellaneous Soft Tissue Techniques

Procedure: Diaphragmatic release sitting technique

1. Patient sits on edge of table with operator behind.

2. Operator's fingerpads bilaterally contact the inferior surface of the diaphragm below the costal arch (Fig. 7.30).

3. Patient slumps against operator by forward-bending the trunk (Fig. 7.31).

4. Operator maintains cephalic compression on the inferior aspect of the diaphragm.

5. Operator maintains compression on diaphragm during patient's inhalation effort.

6. Several applications may be necessary with fine tuning of operator's fingers on specific areas of diaphragmatic tension.

7. A variation finds the operator sitting in front of the patient with the thumbs in contact with the inferior surface of the diaphragm below the costal arch (Fig. 7.32). Patient slumps forward on operator's thumbs. Exhalation effort is followed by upward pressure by operator against points of diaphragmatic tension. Repeat until diaphragmatic release is obtained (Fig. 7.33).

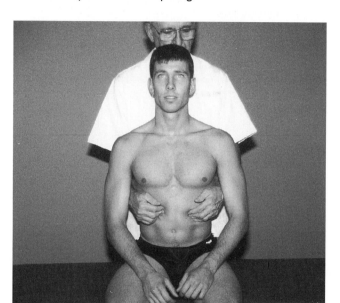

Figure 7.30.

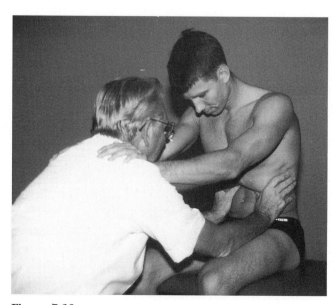

Figure 7.32.

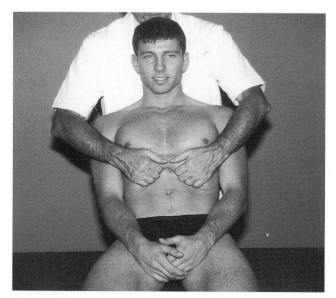

Figure 7.31.

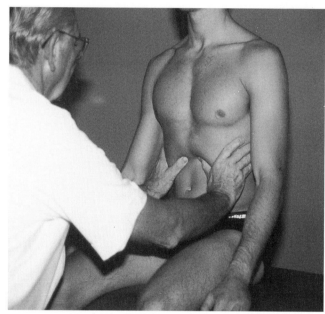

Figure 7.33.

Soft Tissue Techniques

Miscellaneous Soft Tissue Techniques

Procedure: Diaphragmatic release patient supine

1. Patient supine on table with operator standing at side.
2. Operator's fingerpads make contact along inferior surface of diaphragm just below costal arch on each side (Fig. 7.34).
3. Operator maintains cephalic pressure on the inferior aspect of diaphragm. Exhalation effort is encouraged and maintained by fingertip compression until diaphragm is released.

Soft Tissue Techniques

Miscellaneous Soft Tissue Techniques

Procedure: Pelvic diaphragm

1. Patient in lateral recumbent position with hips and knees flexed, involved side uppermost.
2. Operator stands in front of patient with extended fingers of right hand placed on medial side of left ischial tuberosity (Fig. 7.35).
3. Fingers slowly move along the ischium to the lateral aspect of the ischiorectal fossa until fingertips contact pelvic diaphragm.
4. During patient exhalation, operator's fingers move cephalward and hold against pelvic diaphragm as patient performs deep inhalation.
5. With release of diaphragmatic tension, the palpating fingers observe the diaphragm to move freely into fingers during inhalation and away during exhalation.
6. Repeat on both sides as necessary.

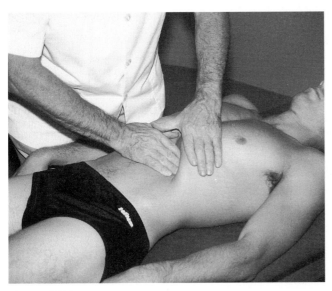

Figure 7.34.

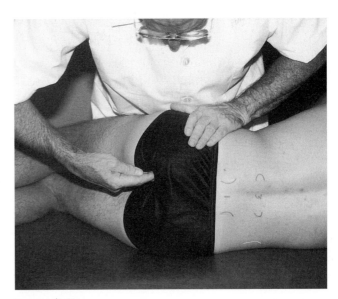

Figure 7.35.

Soft Tissue Techniques

Miscellaneous Soft Tissue Techniques

Procedure: Supine mesenteric release

1. Patient supine on table with operator standing at side.
2. Operator places both hands on each side of the anterior abdomen (Fig. 7.36).
3. Operator applies clockwise and counterclockwise rotation to the anterior abdominal wall with slight abdominal compression.
4. The endpoint is sensation of release of underlying abdominal contents.

Soft Tissue Techniques

Miscellaneous Soft Tissue Techniques

Procedure: Mesenteric release prone position

1. Patient prone on table in knee-chest position.
2. Operator stands at side or head of table.
3. Operator places both hands over lower abdomen above the pubis (Fig. 7.37).
4. Operator lifts abdominal contents in slow oscillatory and rotary fashion until release is felt.

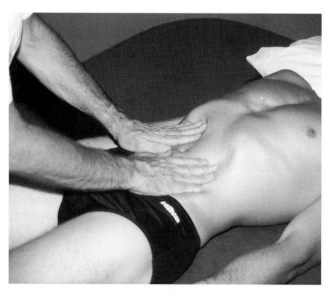

Figure 7.36.

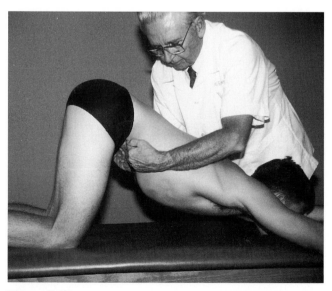

Figure 7.37.

MOBILIZATION WITHOUT IMPULSE

Mobilization without impulse, or articulatory, procedures are an extension of motion testing. Like soft tissue procedures, they are repetitively applied and modified by the response of the tissues. In mobilization without impulse one's goal is to increase the range of motion in an articulation with hypomobility. Repetitive, oscillatory efforts are applied by the operator against the resistant barrier in the arc or plane of restricted articular movement. These procedures require good visualization of the articular anatomy and the range and arc of restricted movement. The operator constantly monitors the end feel of the motion introduced, with the goal being restoration of a "normal" end feel. A graded series of mobilizing efforts from 1 to 4 can be made depending on the amount of motion introduced (1 being limited and 4 being maximum) and with increasing degrees of arc of movement. During these procedures, one is interested in the range of movement, the quality of movement during the range, and the end feel. The goal is a smooth symmetrical range of movement in all of the planes of motion available within the articulation. These procedures can be regionally applied to a group of segments or individually to a single articulation.

The purpose of mobilization without impulse is to restore range of motion and stretch the connective tissue surrounding the restricted articulation. One anticipates modulation of neural activity to relieve pain and restore normal reflex activity in the related spinal cord segments. The same admonitions for soft tissue technique apply to mobilization without impulse, namely the relaxation of the patient, the relaxation and control by the operator, and the localization of the procedure to the appropriate area. These techniques are direct action (force against the restrictive barrier) with an extrinsice activating force (the operator in an oscillatory and rhythmic mode).

CONCLUSION

Soft tissue and mobilization without impulse (articulatory) procedures are useful in a wide variety of acute to chronic patient conditions. They are applicable to all regions of the body. They are useful as independent procedures or can be combined with other manual medicine procedures. Experience in palpating the tissue response to both soft tissue and mobilization without impulse is necessary to properly use them for the appropriate diagnosis.

8

MUSCLE ENERGY TECHNIQUE

In the evolution of manual medicine, a great deal of emphasis has been placed on the osseous skeleton and its articulations. The heritage of the "bonesetters" gave all practitioners of manipulation the aura of "putting a bone back in place." The muscle component of the musculoskeletal system did not receive as much attention by manual medicine practitioners. Early techniques did speak of muscle relaxation with soft tissue procedures, but specific manipulative approaches to muscle appear to be a 20th century phenomena. In osteopathic medicine, Dr. T.J. Ruddy developed techniques that he described as resistive duction. A series of muscle contractions against resistance were accomplished by the patient with a tempo approximating the pulse rate. He used these techniques in the cervical spine and around the orbit in his practice as an ophthalmologist-otorhinolaryngologist.

Dr. Fred L. Mitchell, Sr., is acknowledged as the father of the system we now call muscle energy technique. He took many of Dr. Ruddy's principles and incorporated them in a system of manual medicine procedures that could be applicable to any region of the body or any particular articulation. Dr. Mitchell was a great student of anatomy and gifted osteopathic physician. He was a skilled practitioner and an excellent teacher who gave much time and effort to the educational programs of the American Academy of Osteopathy. Early in his career, he lectured and demonstrated to large audiences, but it was later in small group tutorials that some of his most effective teaching occurred.

WHAT IS MUSCLE ENERGY TECHNIQUE?

Muscle energy technique is a manual medicine treatment procedure that involves the voluntary contraction of patient muscle in a precisely controlled direction, at varying levels of intensity, against a distinctly executed counterforce applied by the operator. Muscle energy procedures have wide application and are classified as active techniques in which the patient contributes the corrective force. The activating force is classified as intrinsic. The patient is responsible for the dosage applied.

Muscle energy technique has many clinical uses. It can be used to lengthen a shortened, contractured, or spastic muscle; to strengthen a physiologically weakened muscle or group of muscles; to reduce localized edema and relieve passive congestion (the muscles are the pump of the lymphatic and venous systems); and to mobilize an articulation with restricted mobility. The function of any articulation in the body that can be moved by voluntary muscle action, either directly or indirectly, can be influenced by muscle energy procedures. The amount of patient effort may vary from a minimal muscle twitch to a maximal muscle contraction. The duration of the effort may vary from a fraction of a second to a sustained effort lasting several seconds.

TYPES OF MUSCULAR CONTRACTION

There are four different types of muscle contraction in muscle energy technique: isometric, concentric isotonic, eccentric isotonic, and "isolytic." With an isometric contraction, the distance between the origin and the insertion of the muscle is maintained at a constant length. A fixed tension develops in the muscle as the patient contracts the muscle against an equal counterforce applied by the operator, preventing shortening of the muscle from the origin to the insertion. A concentric isotonic contraction occurs when the muscle tension causes the origin and insertion to approximate. An eccentric isotonic contraction is one in which there is muscle tension that allows the origin and insertion to separate. In fact, the muscle actually lengthens. An "isolytic" contraction is a nonphysiological event in which the contraction of the patient attempts to be concentric with approximation of the origin and insertion but an external force applied by the operator occurs in the opposite direction.

With the elbow as an example, let us see how each of these contractions operates. With the patient's elbow flexed, the operator holds the distal forearm and shoulder. The patient is instructed to bring the wrist to the shoulder while the operator holds the wrist and shoulder in the same relative position. The force inserted by the patient's contracting biceps has an equal counterforce applied by the operator. This results in isometric contraction of the biceps brachii muscle. Muscle tone increases, but the origin and insertion do not approximate.

A concentric isotonic contraction occurs during the process of holding a weight in the hand and bringing it to the shoulder by increasing the flexion at the elbow. The concentric isotonic contraction of the biceps brachii increases muscle tone, and the origin and insertion are approximated.

An eccentric isotonic contraction occurs when the weight that had been brought to the shoulder is now returned to the starting position by increasing the amount of elbow extension. There is tone within the biceps brachii, allowing the origin and insertion to separate in a smooth and easy fashion as the elbow extends and the weight is taken away from the shoulder.

An "isolytic" contraction occurs when the elbow is flexed at 90° and the patient attempts to increase the flexion of the elbow by bringing the hand to the shoulder while the operator holds the shoulder and wrist, forcefully extending the elbow against the effort of the patient to concentrically contract the biceps brachii. An "isolytic" procedure must be used cautiously to lengthen a severely contractured or hypertonic muscle because rupture of musculotendinous junction, insertion of tendon into bone, or muscle fibers themselves can occur.

MUSCLE PHYSIOLOGY AND PRINCIPLES

Muscle energy technique uses the highly complex principles of muscle physiology and motor control. It is beyond the scope of this volume to describe all of the elements, and the reader is referred to a physiology text for details.

Muscles are composed of extrafusal and intrafusal fibers. The extrafusal fibers are innervated by α motor neurons. In normal resting tone, some extrafusal fibers are contracting while others are in a relaxed state so that all fibers are not contracting at the same time. The intrafusal fibers, or spindles, lie in series with the extrafusal fibers, and their role is to monitor the length and tone of the muscle. The spindle is innervated by γ fibers that set the length and tone of the spindle. When the spindle is stimulated by stretch or muscle contraction, afferent type II fibers project information to the spinal cord. The spindle is sensitive both in change in length and rate of change. Through complex central control systems, the spindle is preset for the anticipated action of the muscle. If the muscle action and the spindle set are not congruent, abnormal muscle tone might well result. This has been one of the hypothetical constructs of somatic dysfunction, namely muscle imbalance of hypertonic muscle tone. The golgi tendon apparatus lies in series with the extrafusal fibers and is sensitive to muscle tension. As the muscle contracts or is put on passive stretch, tension builds up on the golgi tendon apparatus, which provides information through IB fibers, resulting in inhibition of α motor neuron output.

The control of muscle tone is highly complex and includes afferent information coming from mechanoreceptors of the articulations, periarticular structures, and from the muscle spindle and golgi tendon apparatus. This information is processed at the cord level with many muscle functions being preprogramed in the cord through local reflexes and propriospinal tracts. The cord has the capacity to learn both normal and abnormal muscle programs. Persistent abnormal afferent stimulation from the periphery can change cord level programing and result in aberrant muscle behavior. There are complex ascending and descending spinal pathways for motor control that integrate both conscious and subconscious motor behavior. These pathways are altered by many disease processes, but of more importance to the manual medicine practitioner is alteration in functional behavior.

Muscle fibers are of two types: fast twitch fibers, which contract and relax rapidly, and slow twitch fibers, which relax slowly. All muscles have combinations of both fast and slow twitch muscle fibers, and the composition of the muscle is important for its postural and phasic function. Muscles can be classified as postural or tonic muscles and those that are primarily phasic. The postural muscles frequently become hypertonic, short, and tight, whereas the phasic muscles become weak and inhibited. The postural muscles of major significance in vertebral somatic dysfunction are the short fourth-layer muscles, the multifidi, rotatories, intertransversarii. These muscles are very dense in spindles and function more as proprioceptors than prime movers. When they become dysfunctional, they maintain altered joint mechanics through their local effect and alter the behavior of the larger muscles of the erector spinae mass.

USES OF MUSCLE CONTRACTION IN MUSCLE ENERGY TECHNIQUE

The muscle contractions used most frequently in muscle energy technique are isometric and concentric isotonic. Isometric technique is used primarily in the vertebral axis to overcome short, hypertonic muscle that functions as a biomechanical tether, preventing motion, and through the law of reciprocal innervation, inhibits its antagonist. Through complex neurological mechanisms, including the spindle, golgi tendon apparatus, and spinal cord and cortical reflexes, the following phenomena occurs. After an isometric contraction, a hypertonic, shortened muscle can be stretched to a new resting length. When this hypertonic agonist is relaxed, it no longer contributes inhibition to its antagonists, resulting in more equal muscle tone and balance. Isotonic contractions are more frequently used in the extremities. In the presence of an inhibited, weakened muscle group, a series of concentric isotonic contractions can be made against progressively increasing resistance, resulting in increased tone and strength of the muscle. Concurrently, increasing strength of repetitive actions of a muscle throughout its range concentrically will also inhibit its antagonist, resulting in more symmetrical muscle tone. Occasionally, a concentric isotonic contraction is used to mobilize a joint directly against its motion barrier. This is less commonly used to address joint motion restriction because the concentric isotonic contraction against the resisted barrier is frequently painful for the patient and does not result in a good outcome.

MUSCLE MOBILIZING TECHNIQUE

Isometric and concentric isotonic contraction can be used in three different ways to overcome a joint restrictor. Let us take a simple example of restriction of a segment to right rotation. The left rotator muscle will be hypertonic, short, and tight, whereas the right rotator muscle will be more weak. One approach would be to engage the resisted barrier of right rotation and ask the left rotator muscle to contract isometrically. After a series of these isometric contractions, the hypertonic left rotator muscle can be stretched to a new resting length, enhancing the segments capacity to move in right rotation. A second approach would be to ask the right rotator muscle to contract with concentric isotonic action, resulting in a pull of the joint through its range of right rotation. Although this might be effective, it is frequently too painful for the patient to perform and too difficult for the operator to control. A third option would be to engage the right rotational barrier and ask the right rotator muscles to isometrically contract. No motion occurs, but a sustained isometric contraction

of the right rotator muscle will inhibit the hypertonic shortened left rotator muscle so that after the contraction, some lengthening of the tight left rotator muscle can occur, enhancing right rotation (Figs. 8.1 and 8.2).

All of these muscle contractions influence the surrounding fascia, connective tissue ground substance, and interstitial fluids and alter muscle physiology by reflex mechanisms. Fascial length and tone is altered by muscle contraction. Alteration in fascia influences not only its biomechanical function but also the biochemical and immunological functions. The patient's muscle effort requires energy and the metabolic process of muscle contraction results in carbon dioxide, lactic acid, and other metabolic waste products that must be transported and metabolized. It is for this reason that the patient will frequently experience some increase in muscle soreness within the first 12–36 hours after a muscle energy technique treatment. Muscle energy procedures provide safety for the patient because the activating force is intrinsic and the dosage can be easily controlled by the patient, but it must be remembered that this effort comes at a price. It is easy for the inexperienced practitioner to overdo these procedures and, in essence, overdose the patient.

ELEMENTS OF MUSCLE ENERGY PROCEDURES

The following five elements are essential for any successful muscle energy procedure:

1. Patient-active muscle contraction;
2. Controlled joint position;
3. Muscle contraction in a specific direction;
4. Operator-applied distinct counterforce; and
5. Controlled contraction intensity.

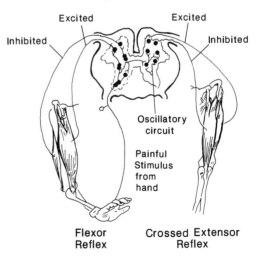

Figure 8.2.
Reciprocal inhibition reflex arc.

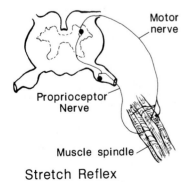

Stretch Reflex

Figure 8.1.
Muscle spindle reflexes.

The patient is told to contract a muscle while the operator holds an articulation or portion of the musculoskeletal system in a specific position. The patient is instructed to contract in a certain direction with a specified amount of force, either in ounces or pounds. The operator applies a counterforce: one that prevents any approximation of the origin and insertion (making the procedure isometric), one to allow yielding (for a concentric isotonic contraction), or one that overpowers the muscle effort (resulting in an "isolytic" procedure).

The common errors patients make during muscle energy procedures are that they contract too hard, contract in the wrong direction, sustain the contraction for too short a time, or do not relax appropriately following the muscle contraction. The most common operator errors are not accurately controlling the joint position in relation to the barrier to movement, not providing the counterforce in the correct direction, not giving the patient accurate instructions, and moving to a new joint position too soon after the patient stops contracting. The operator must wait for the refractory period after an isometric contraction before the muscle can be stretched to a new resting length.

Clinical experience has shown that three to five repetitions of muscle effort for 3–7 seconds each are effective in accomplishing the therapeutic goal. Experience will tell the operator when longer contraction or more repetitions are needed. The isometric contraction need not be too hard (Table 8.1). It is important that it be sustained and that the muscle length be maintained as nearly isometric as possible. After the sustained but light contraction, a momentary pause should occur before the operator stretches the shortened and contracted muscle to a new resting length. Isotonic procedures require forceful contraction by the patient because the operator wants to recruit the firing of muscle fibers and make them work as hard as possible, resulting in relaxation of the antagonist. The muscle should contract over its total range. After any muscle energy procedure, the patient should relax before repositioning against a new resistant barrier.

MUSCLE ENERGY TECHNIQUES

In succeeding chapters muscle energy techniques are described for specific regions. Here we shall use the elbow as an example. Assume there is restriction of elbow movement into full extension, that is, the elbow is flexed. One etiology for restricted elbow extension is hypertonicity and shortening of the biceps brachii muscle. The operator might choose an isometric muscle energy technique to treat this condition as follows:

1. Patient sits comfortably on the treatment table with the operator standing in front.
2. Operator grasps patient's elbow with one hand and distal forearm with the other (Fig. 8.3).
3. Operator extends the elbow until the first extension barrier is felt.
4. Operator instructs the patient to attempt to bring the forearm to the shoulder by using a few ounces of force in a sustained manner.
5. Operator provides equal counterforce to the patient's effort.
6. After 3–7 seconds of contraction, the patient is instructed to stop contracting and relax.
7. Operator waits until the patient is completely relaxed after the contracting effort and extends the elbow to a new resistant barrier (Fig. 8.4).
8. Steps 2 through 7 are repeated three to five times until full elbow extension is restored.

Table 8.1.
Comparison of Isometric and Isotonic Procedures

Isometric	Isotonic
1. Careful positioning	1. Careful positioning
2. Light to moderate contraction	2. Hard to maximal contraction
3. Unyielding counterforce	3. Counterforce permits controlled motion
4. Relaxation after contraction	4. Relaxation after contraction
5. Repositioning	5. Repositioning

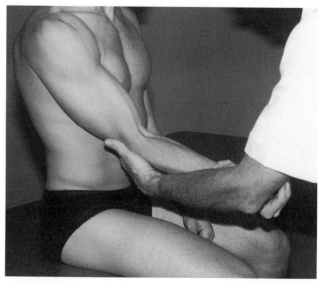

Figure 8.3.
Restricted elbow extension. Isometric contraction of biceps brachii.

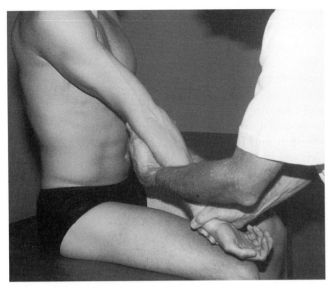

Figure 8.4.
New extension resistant barrier engaged after postisometric relaxation.

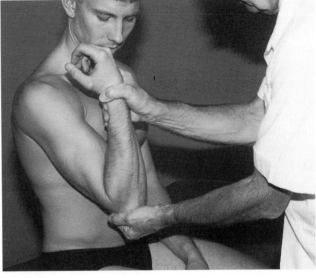

Figure 8.5.
Restricted elbow extension. Concentric isotonic contraction of triceps beginning at full flexion.

The restriction of elbow extension might also be the result of length and strength imbalance between the biceps muscle as the elbow flexor and the triceps muscle as the elbow extender. A weak triceps could prevent full elbow extension. The operator might choose an isotonic muscle energy technique to treat this condition as follows:

1. Patient sitting on table with operator in front.
2. Operator grasps shoulder and distal forearm and takes elbow into full flexion (Fig. 8.5).
3. Patient is instructed to extend the elbow with as much effort as possible, perhaps several pounds.
4. The operator provides a yielding counterforce that allows the elbow to slowly but steadily extend throughout its maximal range (Fig. 8.6).
5. Operator returns elbow to full flexion and the patient repeats the contraction of the triceps to extend the elbow, but this time the operator provides increasing resistance to elbow extension.
6. Several repetitive efforts are accomplished with the operator providing increasing resistance each time and with the patient endeavoring to take the elbow through full extension with each effort.
7. Approximately three to five repetitions are usually necessary to achieve full elbow extension.

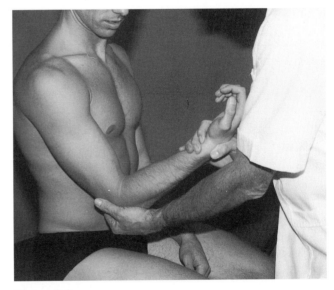

Figure 8.6.
Operator resists triceps contraction through full range of elbow extension.

In any of these muscle energy procedures, it is important to accurately assess the resistant barrier. With an isometric technique, the first barrier sensed must be the point where the careful joint position is held by the operator. If the operator "crashes into" the muscle resistant barrier in positioning the joint, an increase in the muscle hypertonicity will result, just the opposite of the desired therapeutic effort. Second, when using these procedures in a joint with multiple planes of movement available, each motion barrier must be engaged in the same fashion. In the vertebral column with motion restriction around and along three different axes, precision in the engagement of the restrictive barrier is essential for therapeutic effectiveness.

Successful muscle energy technique can be ensured if the operator will constantly keep in mind the following three words: control, balance, and localization. Both the operator and patient must be balanced, and the operator must be in control of the localization against the resistant barrier. There must be continued control of the muscle effort by the patient and the yielding or unyielding counterforce by the operator. Each element is essential with each effort during the procedure.

CONCLUSION

In this author's opinion, muscle energy is one of the most valuable forms of manual medicine therapy because many therapeutic effects result from a single procedure and the procedures are physiologically and anatomically quite safe. It is possible to achieve increased joint movement, normalization of muscle strength and length, stretch of shortened fascia, and removal of passive congestion, all during a single procedure. Not only has muscle effort been used to move a joint, but more normal physiology has been restored to the muscle.

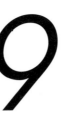

9 MOBILIZATION WITH IMPULSE (HIGH VELOCITY, LOW AMPLITUDE THRUST) TECHNIQUE

The scientific advisory committee of the International Federation of Manual Medicine in the 1980s recommended the term "mobilization with impulse" to replace the terms "high velocity, low amplitude thrust" and "manipulation." Before that time, the term manipulation was used to designate mobilization techniques with an operator-applied extrinsic thrusting force. Currently, the use of the term manipulation is better applied to the "therapeutic use of the hands." This technique is one of the oldest and most widely used forms of manual medicine and has long been deemed the treatment of choice for the "manipulable lesion." These techniques emphasize alteration in articular function and the periarticular structures. Some of the older terms for somatic dysfunction, including "joint lock," "joint blockage," and "chiropractic subluxation," show the emphasis on the joint and its mechanics. The use of an extrinsic-applied thrusting force was found useful in overcoming restricted articular movement.

Despite recent developments in manual medicine procedures with the introduction of muscle energy technique, functional indirect technique, myofascial release technique, and craniosacral technique, mobilization with impulse (high velocity, low amplitude thrust) remains one of the most frequently used forms of manual medicine. Inappropriate use yields poor or no therapeutic results and risks complications. These procedures should be applied only after arriving at an appropriate diagnosis and being performed in a proper manner.

JOINT PLAY

Mennell is credited with contributing the concept of joint play to manual medicine. He defines joint play as movement within a synovial joint that is independent of, and cannot be introduced by, voluntary muscle contraction. The movements are small (less than 1/8″ in any plane), with a precise range that depends on the contour of the opposing joint surfaces. These joint-play movements are deemed essential for the normal, pain-free, nonrestricted movement of the particular articulation. If these movements are ab-

sent, normal voluntary movements are restricted and frequently painful. Mennell defines joint dysfunction as loss of joint-play movement that cannot be recovered by the action of voluntary muscle, that is, joint dysfunction is loss of joint play. These principles apply to all synovial joints and are applicable in both the spine and the extremities. Mennell's diagnostic system tests for normal joint play movements in each articulation and introduces therapeutic joint manipulation to restore movement and function. Mennell's 10 rules of therapeutic manipulation are as follows:

1. Patient must be relaxed.
2. Therapist must be relaxed. Therapeutic grasp must be painless, firm, and protective.
3. One joint is mobilized at a time.
4. One movement in a joint is restored at a time.
5. In performance of movement, one aspect of joint is moved upon the other, which is stabilized.
6. Extent of movement is not greater than that assessed in the same joint on opposite unaffected limb.
7. No forceful or abnormal movement must ever be used.
8. The manipulative movement is a sharp thrust, with velocity, to result in approximately 1/8″ gapping at the joint.
9. Therapeutic movement occurs when all of the "slack" in the joint has been taken up.
10. No therapeutic maneuver is done in the presence of joint or bone inflammation or disease (heat, redness, swelling, and so on).

These 10 rules are applicable to all procedures described as high velocity, low amplitude thrust techniques or mobilization with impulse.

THEORIES OF JOINT DYSFUNCTION

Many theories have been proposed to explain joint dysfunction and the therapeutic effect of mobilization with impulse. They include alteration in the relationship of opposing joint surfaces, the articular capsules and associated meniscoids, and upon neural mechanisms from the articular mechanoreceptors and nociceptors, and the resultant effect on segmentally related muscle function. These theories should be considered as working hypotheses at this time with a need for more research being evident. Theories involving joint surfaces include "lack of tracking" of opposing joint surfaces and "hitching within the joint." It has been suggested that a change in the thixotropic property of the synovial fluid might make it more "sticky." It has been postulated that a fringe of synovium from the articular capsule might become caught between the two opposing joint surfaces. It has been demonstrated that meniscoids are present in the zygapophysial joints of the spine and contain innervation by C fibers. It seems reasonable that they might become entrapped between the opposing joint surfaces, and gapping of the joint might release the entrapped meniscoid resulting in enhanced function. This theory remains controversial and to date has not been demonstrated in a research study. More recently, it has been postulated that stress on the capsule of the involved joint alters the afferent nerve traffic from the type I mechanoreceptors so that central control of motion cannot determine the joint's spatial relationship. This alteration in neural control is postulated to affect the length and tone of the segmentally related muscles, further restricting normal joint movement.

CAVITATION PHENOMENON

Research into the mechanisms of a mobilization with impulse (high velocity, low amplitude thrust) has demonstrated the cavitation phenomenon. Cavitation occurs at the time of the audible joint pop. A radiographic negative shadow appears within the joint with the density of nitrogen. This gaseous density remains present for a variable period of time, usually less than 20 minutes. The cavitation phenomenon suggests that the synovial fluid changes from a liquid to a gaseous state. The exact effect on the synovial fluid is unknown at this time.

An additional observation that occurs in a spinal zygapophysial joint undergoing a mobilization with impulse procedure involves the segmentally related musculature. After the thrust there is temporary electrical silence of the segmentally related muscles, with a refractory period before normal electrical activity returns. It is hypothesized that the segmentally related muscle returns to more normal function after the thrusting procedure and contributes to the positive therapeutic response. Much more research is needed, but clinical experience shows that joint dysfunction (somatic dysfunction) responds positively to

the application of mobilization with impulse technique.

INDICATIONS FOR THE USE OF MOBILIZATION WITH IMPULSE

These procedures appear to be most effective in somatic dysfunction when the restriction is in and closely around the joint itself, the so-called "short restrictors." They are usually applied as precisely as possible to a single joint level and for specific joint motion loss. Although Mennell states that a therapeutic procedure should occur in only one plane, it is possible to influence all three planes of vertebral movement simultaneously by specific localization and leverage application. These procedures appear to be much more effective in subacute and chronic conditions than in acute somatic dysfunction. Although most are designed for a single joint and its motion loss, some of the procedures can be applied in a regional fashion. The procedures advocated by Zink, for use with his respiratory-circulatory model, are designed to mobilize regions of the body to enhance fluid circulation and not to overcome a specific joint restriction. The difference between specific and nonspecific mobilization with impulse lies with the principle of localization and locking described below.

High velocity, low amplitude thrusting procedures are used in direct and exaggeration methods. The most common usage is direct, with engagement of the restrictive barrier and thrusting through the barrier to achieve more normal joint motion. Some authors advocate the exaggeration method (also called "rebound thrust") in which the thrust is against the normal physiological barrier in the direction opposite the motion loss. This author uses only the direct method and would use something other than an exaggeration thrust if a direct action thrust was not possible. The activating force is extrinsic, a thrusting procedure by the operator. Other assisting forces are gravity (patient seated or standing versus recumbency) and patient respiratory efforts, both for relaxation and for influence on joint position desired.

PRINCIPLES OF TECHNIQUE APPLICATION

Joint Gapping

All thrusting procedures result in gapping of the joint, requiring that the operator know the anatomical contour and the movement possible at that articulation. Joint gapping can be in the plane of the joint, at right angles to the plane, or with joint distraction. Any successful mobilization with impulse procedure contains an element of joint distraction and gapping. The audible joint pop or click appears to coincide with joint gapping. It must be remembered that the production of joint noise is not the therapeutic goal. In fact, Kimberly states that the goal of successful thrusting procedures is "painless and noiseless restoration of maximum joint function."

Localization

Localization limits this thrusting procedure to the joint needing treatment, but other joints do receive the mobilizing impulse. This relates to Mennell's principle of holding one bone of the articulation and moving the other bone in relation to it.

One localization principle that is most useful is the introduction of convexities in two different planes precisely to the segment under treatment. The first convexity introduced is into the forward-bending and backward-bending arc of movement. The objective is to engage the forward-bending (flexion) or backward-bending (extension) component of the nonneutral vertebral somatic dysfunction. The goal is to place the segment under treatment at the apex of the convexity introduced either through a forward-bending and backward-bending movement or an anteroposterior or posteroanterior translatory movement. For example, if L1 has forward-bending restriction on L2, forward-bending of the trunk is introduced from above downward through the thoracic spine to L1. Flexion of the lower extremities, pelvis, and lumbar spine from below upward is introduced to L2. The L1–2 interspace becomes the apex of the forward-bending curve introduced and is localized against the forward-bending (flexion) barrier. This localization can also be performed by translatory movement from anterior to posterior localized at the L1–2 level. The second convexity introduced is that of sidebending, creating a convexity right or left. Introduction of sidebending while forward bent (flexed) or backward bent (extended) couples the rotation to the same side (nonneutral vertebral mechanics). If in our example of L1–2 the sidebending and rotation restrictions are to the right, sidebending to the right establishes a convexity of the thoracolumbar spine to the left with the apex at the L1–2 interspace. This left convexity can be established by a right to left translatory movement as well as right sidebending from above and below. The introduction of two convexities, one from front to back and the other through sidebending, with the apex of each convexity at the segment to be treated is the principle used for nonneutral (type II) vertebral dysfunctions in which there is either a forward-bending or backward-bending restriction, together with sidebending and rotation restriction to the same side.

In the neutral, group (type I) vertebral dysfunctions localization is accomplished by the introduction of sidebending and rotation to opposite sides from above downward and from below upward to the segment requiring treatment. Forward-bending and backward-bending is introduced only to place the joint under treatment at its point of maximum ease in the forward-bending and backward-bending arc that is "neutral" at that level. This is best demonstrated when using the lateral recumbent (lumbar roll) technique. With the patient in the left lateral recumbent position, the apex of the group curve is placed in the neutral position of the forward-bending and backward-bending arc. With L1–2 as our example, forward-bending and backward-bending is introduced until L1–2 is in its neutral position in the anteroposterior curve. The operator pulls the patient's left upper extremity anteriorly and caudally, introducing left sidebending and right rotation of the vertebral column down to the L1 level. With the other hand the operator rolls the patient's pelvis anteriorly introducing rotation to the left from below upward until L2 is reached. This results in a neutral group localization at L1–2 and any thrusting force summates at that level. The goal is to localize so that the segment under treatment is maintained in the coronal *(xy)* plane. The lower the lumbar spine localization is desired, the more movement is introduced from above downward and less from below upward. Higher in the lumbar spine and into the lower thoracic spine, less movement is introduced from above downward and more from below upward.

Levers

Levers are classified as short or long. A short lever is one in which a portion of one vertebra (spinous process) is firmly held while force is applied to a bony prominence of the adjacent vertebra (spinous process, transverse process, mammillary process) and the resultant applied force is sufficient to move one segment on the other. Long levers are established by using one of the extremities, or multiple segments within the vertebral column, in a "locking" maneuver. Long levers have the advantage of reducing the force required and increasing the distance the force travels. Long-lever technique requires precise localization and limitation of force. A vertebral column long lever involves the principle of ligamentous or bony lock. A ligamentous lock occurs when the spine is sufficiently forward bent to place maximum tension on the posterior ligamentous structures surrounding the zygapophysial joints. A joint lock occurs when the spine is backward bent with engagement of the posterior zygapophysial joints. Both of these maneuvers reduce joint mobility. Levers can also be established after concept three of vertebral motion in which introduction of motion in one direction reduces vertebral motion in all others. The introduction of a neutral (type I) vertebral movement (sidebending and rotation to opposite sides) limits the movement of the vertebra involved and can include as many segments of the vertebral column as desired. Long levers are used to establish localization at any specific vertebral segmental level. Segments above and below the dysfunctional vertebral segment are "locked" in a long lever while the segment to be treated is "free" to receive the activating force to be applied. It is not uncommon for the neophyte practitioner to use excessive force to a joint that is inappropriately locked through poor localization.

Fulcrum

A fulcrum is used in many mobilization with impulse techniques, particularly in the cervical and thoracic spine. Some practitioners use firm rubber blocks of varying sizes and shapes. This author prefers to use hand positions to establish a fulcrum. The advantage of using fingers or hand combinations for a fulcrum is the ability to sense localization at the segment under treatment. In the cervical area, a fingerpad pressure against a zygapophysial joint line serves as fulcrum around which the vertebra can be moved to overcome restriction of the opposite zygapophysial joint. In the thoracic spine, various hand positions can be used to block the lower segment of the vertebral motion segment under treatment, allowing the operator to move the superior segment in any direction necessary to engage the restrictive barrier. In rib dysfunctions, the thenar eminence above or below a dysfunctional rib can serve as an appropriate fulcrum against which an activating force can be localized.

Velocity

Velocity means speed of application not force. In mobilization with impulse technique, the velocity is high. The maneuver should have quickness. The common mistake is that the maneuver is a "push" rather than a "quick thrust." The thrusting maneuver should be applied only when all of the "slack" within the joint is removed. One must engage the restriction at its elastic barrier so that the thrusting procedure reestablishes the residual joint play available until one reaches the firm anatomical barrier. Remember that additional force does not make up for poor localization and poor velocity. The neophyte practitioner frequently "backs off" from the barrier in an attempt to get a "running start" against the barrier. This must be avoided by careful localization against the elastic barrier of the restriction and moving with velocity from that point in the direction of motion loss.

Amplitude

Mobilization with impulse technique attempts to create movement of 1/8″ at the joint under treatment. The thrusting force should be applied quickly and for a short distance. With short-lever technique, the amplitude of the thrust to achieve a 1/8″ gapping at the joint is considerably less than with a long-lever technique. When two long levers are used, a great deal of movement is introduced by the operator to the patient. What must be remembered is that the summation of all of the movement results in a thrust amplitude at the joint under treatment of 1/8″.

Balance and Control

As in any successful manual medicine procedure, the operator and patient must be in body positions that are comfortable, easily controlled, and balanced. The patient can be completely relaxed so the operator can apply the thrust with maximum efficiency. The table must be at the appropriate height for the patient and operator size. If the table is too high, the operator's ability to control the patient is compromised. The patient should be appropriately placed on the table, not too far away, not too close to the operator, so that localization can be accurate and the patient not fear falling. The thrust is most appropriately provided by a weight transfer of the operator's body rather than by a specific muscle action. In performing the lateral recumbent lumbar and sacroiliac mobilization with impulse procedures, many operators attempt to introduce the thrust by an adduction movement of the arm placed on the pelvis rather than by a total body movement. It is difficult to provide appropriate velocity and amplitude by an adductor muscle contraction of the operator's upper extremity. It is easier to apply the appropriate thrust by the dropping of the operator's body weight in the correct direction.

Therapeutic Goals of Mobilization with Impulse Technique

These procedures are useful in increasing range of movement of an articulation that has dysfunction (loss of joint play). Although the motion loss seemed to be only in one direction, a successful thrust procedure will increase range of movement in all possible directions. While moving the joint, one might attempt to realign the skeletal parts in their normal anatomical relationship, intending to restore normal joint receptor activity at that level. An additional outcome is reduction of muscle hypertonicity and/or spasm in an attempt to restore balance to the segmentally related musculature. Another therapeutic outcome might be the stretching of shortened connective tissues surrounding the articulation. The fascial connective tissues may be shortened and tightened as the result of the altered position of the articulation, the healing of the inflammatory process after injury. As suggested earlier, the therapeutic goal might be the movement of fluid, both intravascular and extravascular, by "wringing out" the tissues. One or more of these therapeutic goals might be the objective of a procedure, but many of the others would be operative simultaneously. These procedures seem most effective for subacute and chronic dysfunctions that appear to be due to short restrictors.

Contraindications

As in all forms of manual medicine, accurate diagnosis is essential and precision and accuracy of therapeutic intervention is required. When these criteria are met for mobilization with impulse, the contraindications become fewer. However, these procedures have more contraindications, both absolute and relative, than others. Absolute contraindications for mobilization with impulse are hypermobility and instability of an articulation and the presence of inflammatory joint disease.

There are many relative contraindications and authors classify them differently. In the cervical spine there is a major concern regarding the vertebral artery. The vertebral artery is anatomically at risk at the craniocervical junction. Movements of extension and rotation will narrow the normal vertebral arteries. Techniques then should avoid extensive extension and rotation. In the presence of vertebral artery disease, these movements become potentially more dangerous. The need for precision of diagnosis and technique application becomes crucial in the presence of vertebral artery disease. The cervical spine is also the site of developmental and congenital conditions that might contraindicate a thrusting procedure. These include agenesis of the odontoid process and the Down's syndrome. Throughout the vertebral column, there is concern for metabolic and systemic bone disease, particularly osteoporosis and metastatic carcinoma. With careful and precise localization and the appropriate amount of force, mobilization with impulse technique can restore loss of joint play despite the alteration in osseous architecture. Degenerative joint disease of the zygapophysial and uncovertebral

joints of Luschka are also a relative contraindication. Degenerative joint disease alters the capacity of the zygapophysial joints to function and an inappropriate mobilization with impulse technique could damage these joints. However, somatic dysfunction of these joints can complicate the degenerative joint process. The joint dysfunction can be successfully treated by mobilization with impulse procedures if the aforementioned principles are applied properly. The thrusting impulse is appropriately placed against the elastic barrier of the joint dysfunction even in the presence of altered anatomical barrier because of the degenerative joint disease.

Of major concern is the use of mobilization with impulse procedures in the presence of intervertebral disc disease, particularly in the acute phase. Some authors believe that it is the treatment of choice, whereas others believe that it is contraindicated. The concern is the possibility of exacerbating the disc pathology into increased herniation and sequestration with entrapment of neural elements. This author has used mobilization with impulse procedures in the presence of known disc herniation demonstrated by appropriate imaging with successful therapeutic results. It is interesting to note that little change has occurred in the imaging of the disc by the procedure. It has been reported that an acute cauda equina syndrome has followed the use of mobilization with impulse technique in the presence of lumbar disc disease. This potential danger should always be considered.

CONCLUSION

Mobilization with impulse (high velocity, low amplitude thrusting techniques) are valuable in the armamentarium of the manual medicine practitioner. They require an accurate diagnosis and precision of the therapeutic intervention. Appropriate application of velocity rather than force is a skill to be mastered when using these techniques.

10

FUNCTIONAL (INDIRECT) TECHNIQUE

Functional (indirect) technique is not as well known as many others in the field of manual medicine. These procedures are viewed by many as being highly complex, although the principles are relatively simple and straightforward. These procedures focus more on the functional aspect than the structural in the structure-function interface.

HISTORY

Functional (indirect) techniques developed within the American osteopathic profession in the 1940s and 1950s. Several groups of osteopathic physicians in different areas of the country simultaneously worked on the development of the system. One group in the pacific northwest worked with both Drs. Hoover, whereas members of the New England Academy of Osteopathy on the east coast, particularly Drs. Bowles and Johnston, developed a study group. Dr. George Andrew Laughlin of Kirksville, Missouri developed his variation of this technique by building on the balanced membranous tension concepts of Dr. W.G. Sutherland, the founder of the craniosacral concept. These techniques have gained in popularity and now are included in many manual medicine practitioners armamentarium.

STRUCTURE-FUNCTION INTERFACE

The interrelationship of structure and function in the body and the body's tendency to self-regulation are well-recognized basic principles. Functional (indirect) techniques build on these principles, particularly from the perspective of function. In viewing a dysfunctional vertebral segment, the thought is not that the bone is out of place but that it has abnormal behavior in relation to the rest of the organism. The classic structural approach would attempt to "put the bone back in place," whereas the functional approach would attempt to restore coordinated activity with other segments of the vertebral column and the related soft tissues. A helpful analogy is to imagine a rank of soldiers marching in a parade. One soldier in the rank is out of step. The soldier is in line in the rank, he is not out of place, but he is highly visible because he is "out of step." He does not function in a coordinated manner with his fellow soldiers. The soldier's commanding officer would not take the soldier out of the rank and put him elsewhere but would change his stride so that it matched the remaining soldiers in the rank. The practitioner using functional technique focuses on restoring coordinated activity in an involved vertebral dysfunction in a similar fashion to the change in behavior in the soldier who is out of step in the rank.

BARRIER CONCEPTS

Chapter 3 described normal and restrictive barriers. In the absence of dysfunction, there is a midrange neutral point of maximum ease or freedom within the total range of motion. In the presence of somatic dysfunction, the neutral point is no longer in midline but is found as the point of maximum ease or freedom between the restrictive barrier in one direction and the normal physiological and anatomical barriers in the opposite direction. Direct action techniques, such as muscle energy and mobilization without impulse and mobilization with impulse, are interested in engaging the restrictive barrier and applying an activating force in the direction of motion loss. Functional technique is more interested in the behavior of the motion present than in its specific relationship to the barrier. The practitioner is more interested in the quality of motion, rather than the quantity, and how the dysfunctional segment behaves when motion is introduced. Functional diagnosis looks for the normal and reasonably expected coordination of movement and the quality and ease of movement in any given area or segment.

NEUROLOGICAL HYPOTHESIS

The working hypothesis for functional technique is the premise that dysfunction results in altered neural activity. The abnormal dysfunction stimulates aberrant afferent impulses from mechanoreceptors and nociceptors. These impulses are transmitted to the spinal cord for processing, locally at the cord level and centrally through ascending and descending neural pathways. This abnormal neural traffic results in abnormal efferent signals to the final common pathway of the α motor neuron to muscle. Hypothetically, restoration of more normal afferent signals to the central nervous system returns the neural traffic at the spinal cord to more normal levels, resulting in restoration of more normal neural activity to the muscle. Functional techniques can be described as afferent reduction procedures. The functional diagnostic process is extensive in that it searches for alteration in behavior of all segments within the musculoskeletal system, attempts to restore more normal behavior, and requires that each dysfunctional segment is given appropriate attention.

FUNCTIONAL DIAGNOSIS

Functional diagnosis begins by identifying areas of tissue tension and/or the areas of most restriction. One diagnostic process has the operator percussing with fingertips over vertebral motion segments and their adnexal tissues. Loss of tissue resilience is identified in areas of significant dysfunction. A second diagnostic method finds the operator passively introducing ranges of motion throughout the vertebral axis in a symmetrical fashion, seeking areas of resistance to the induced motion. A third process is to identify vertebral somatic dysfunction by the biomechanical method described in Chapter 6 and then assess the functional characteristics of the dysfunction.

EASE-BIND CONCEPT

In functional technique the practitioner searches for the quality of movement rather than range. Is the movement easy and free (ease) or is the movement restricted and difficult (bind)? The spectrum runs from maximum ease to maximum bind with many gradations between. Functional diagnosis searches for the ease-bind interface.

The procedure to identify ease and bind is as follows. A palpating hand is placed over the suspected segmental dysfunction and is called the "listening hand." Contact is maintained in a quiet and noninvasive fashion, focusing on changes that occur at the dysfunctional segment and its adnexal tissues. The listening hand seldom introduces movement or energy. It is a "receiver" of information. The operator's other hand contacts some area of the musculoskeletal system distant from the dysfunctional segment and either introduces motion or monitors the motion the patient performs under verbal cues. This hand is

called the "motor hand." It introduces the movement that the listening hand monitors, responding either as ease or bind. The process requires a motion demand and a response. The motion hand initiates the demand, and the listening hand monitors the response.

Functional technique has a constant diagnostic and treatment interaction. The motor hand introduces diagnostic and therapeutic motions and the listening hand monitors the response, giving constant feedback as the outcome. The diagnosis-treatment can be viewed as a cybernetic loop of continuous input and output with feedback assessment throughout the process. Because of the dynamic process involved in functional technique, the practitioners may look as though they are performing many different things with little standardization. In fact, the processes are quite standard in that there is motion introduced by one hand and constantly monitored by the other.

THERAPEUTIC USE

Acute Conditions

Functional technique is particularly useful in acute conditions because it is nontraumatic and can be performed repeatedly and frequently. Functional technique does not seek a major structural change but a tissue response. Reprograming of aberrant afferent stimulation is important in acute conditions as well as in chronic. Acute conditions appear to respond quite favorably and rapidly to functional technique. Special equipment is not necessary and it can be performed in any location even in an intensive care unit.

Chronic Conditions

Functional technique is also effective in chronic conditions because it overcomes the abnormally programed neural response and not just alter position. Restoring the position of a dysfunctional vertebral segment is of little value without restoring the neuromuscular mechanisms that control its function. The diagnostic component of functional technique is useful in chronic conditions as it monitors tissue response and behavior irrespective of the therapeutic intervention.

Prognostic Value

Functional diagnostic technique is of prognostic value. It assesses the therapeutic response of a dysfunctional level irrespective of the therapeutic intervention. For example, lift therapy for an anatomically short lower extremity and pelvic tilt mechanism (a structural intervention) will change the functional capacity of the entire musculoskeletal system. Functional diagnosis helps determine whether the structural intervention of the lift has accomplished improvement in musculoskeletal function both locally and distantly.

TYPES OF FUNCTIONAL TECHNIQUE

All functional techniques can be classified as afferent reduction procedures. Most functional technique can be placed in one of three categories: balance and hold, dynamic functional procedures, and release by positioning.

Balance and Hold

These procedures are performed in any body position: standing, sitting, supine, prone, or lateral recumbent. The listening hand monitors at the dysfunctional segment as the motor hand introduces motion passively or the patient assumes body positions under the practitioner's verbal commands. Motion is sequentially introduced in six different directions, seeking the balance point of maximum ease within each range. Each is then held in that position while stacking one on top of the other. The stacking sequence makes little difference. The ranges introduced are forward-bending–backward-bending; side-bending right–sidebending left; rotation right–rotation left; translation anterior–posterior; translation laterally, both right and left; translation cephalic-caudad.

The last movement introduced is respiratory. Once each of the ranges within the dysfunctional segment has been "stacked" at the point of maximum ease, inhalation and exhalation effort is introduced. The phase of respiration found to be the most free is then held as long as comfortably possible. This is usually for 5–30 seconds. At the end of the comfortable holding of the breath, the patient is instructed to breath normally and naturally. A new balance point is sought for each of the motion directions. The respiratory effort is repeated. The entire process is repeated until release of restriction is felt and increased mobility is obtained. The usual operator sense is that the neutral point is returning more and more toward normal and that range is increasing.

Dynamic Functional Procedures

The second category of functional technique is described as dynamic functional. The focus is on the restoration of normality to the apparently abnormal tracking of the dysfunction. The process follows the inherent tissue motion. Inherent tissue motion is a function of many physiological phenomena, particularly the cranial rhythmic impulse, contraction relaxation of muscle tone, and dynamic effects of respiration and circulation. In dynamic functional technique, the listening hand monitors the response to motion introduced by the motor hand and directs the motion demand along the path of increasing ease. The goal is to restore more normal movement patterns, and the operator attempts to "ride out" the dysfunction. The operator continually seeks ease and avoids bind. These techniques look quite varied because of the dynamic motion patterns introduced. They can be standardized by the formula C-C-T-E-T.

C (1)—contact over the adnexal tissue of the dysfunctional segment;
C (2)—control of the induced motion by the motor hand;
T (1)—test the adnexal tissue response;
E—evaluate the compliance of the segment as normal or abnormal;
T (2)—treatment by constantly monitoring the bind-ease point of the dysfunctional segment.

Release by Positioning

The third category of functional technique is release by positioning. This system was originated and developed by Lawrence Jones, D.O., F.A.A.O., and is described as counterstrain. There are two cardinal features of this system. The first is the identification and monitoring of palpable tender points in various locations throughout the musculoskeletal system. Many of these tender points coincide with similar locations reported by other authors (Travell myofascial trigger points, Chapman's reflex points, and acupuncture points). The release by positioning system uses these tender points diagnostically and to monitor the therapeutic intervention. The second element is the assumption of a body position in which the patient has the least pain and is the most comfortable. A number of different body positions are used and include combined sitting and recumbent positions. When a tender point is identified, a body position is assumed that reduces both the patient's pain and the tenderness and tissue tension felt by the operator. The position is then held for 90 seconds. At the end of this time, the patient is slowly returned to a more normal body posture and reevaluated. These procedures are supported by specific exercise programs. A study of the manual "Strain and CounterStrain" (Jones LH, Colorado Springs, 1981, American Academy of Osteopathy) is recommended before attempting the use of this technique.

FUNCTIONAL PALPATION EXERCISE

The following exercise is useful in learning the principles of functional diagnosis and treatment.

1. Patient sits on examining table in an erect position with arms folded across the chest, each hand holding the opposite shoulder.

2. Operator stands behind and to the side of the patient, placing fingertips of the listening hand over the upper thoracic region. The listening hand should be as quiet as possible.

3. Operator's other hand becomes the motor hand and is placed on top of the head. This hand leads the patient through certain movements in the fashion of the use of the reins on the bridle of a horse. The motor hand introduces passive movement and also monitors the response of a patient movement from operator verbal commands.

4. Operator introduces forward-bending in a slow and smooth fashion, attempting to identify (with the listening hand) changes in ease and bind from maximum ease to maximum bind. Operator reverses the procedure into backward-bending. Several repetitions are made, constantly evaluating the range of ease to bind motion in both directions.

5. With the patient in the neutral starting position, the motor hand introduces sidebending to the right and rotation to the left of the head and neck on the trunk. This introduces neutral (type I) vertebral motion. Operator monitors the range of this coupled movement through the ease and bind phenomena. Reverse the movement to sidebending left and rotation right. Is there symmetry to the ease and bind? As you modulate sidebending and rotation, is there difference in the ease and bind of each component of the motion?

6. Beginning at the neutral position, operator introduces a small amount of forward-bending, right sidebending, and right rotation of the head and neck on the trunk. This introduces nonneutral (type II) coupled movement. The listening hand monitors for ease and bind of this motion. Repeat to the left side. Are they symmetrical in the quality of ease and bind and in each component of the motion?

This exercise can be repeated throughout the vertebral axis in a number of positions. Diagnostically, the operator is attempting to classify each segment as normal, marginally dysfunctional, or significantly dysfunctional. The normal segment has a wide range of minimal signaling throughout the procedure. A significantly dysfunctional segment has a narrow range of rapid signaling in the ease-bind range. It is not uncommon to find a segment that is marginally dysfunctional, and it is important to decide how significant it is within the total musculoskeletal complex. This decision can only be achieved through experience, which is the only and best teacher.

FUNCTIONAL TECHNIQUES

The following techniques demonstrate the system of functional technique attributed to George Andrew Laughlin, D.O., of Kirksville, Missouri. These techniques have been refined and standardized by Edward Stiles, D.O., F.A.A.O., who had the opportunity to study extensively with Dr. Laughlin. This is but one of the many systems of functional (indirect) technique but show examples of both the balance and hold and the dynamic functional principles. The diagnosis attributed to these techniques follows the postural structural model for terminology purposes, but to successfully use these techniques, the principles identified previously need to be implemented.

Functional Technique

Lumbar Spine
Sitting
Diagnosis: Nonneutral dysfunctions: extended, rotated, sidebent (ERS) and flexed, rotated, sidebent (FRS)

1. Patient sitting on table.

2. Operator sits behind patient.

3. Operator's listening hand is placed over dysfunctional segment with index finger on superior and thumb on inferior vertebra (Fig. 10.1).

4. Operator's motion hand placed on patient's shoulder to control sidebending and rotation from above (Fig. 10.2).

5. Operator places head at the patient's thoracolumbar region to control flexion and extension through anteroposterior translation (Fig. 10.3).

6. Operator introduces sidebending and rotation through the motion hand and flexion-extension through anteroposterior translation to the balance point of ease in all 6 degrees of freedom (Fig. 10.4).

7. Inhalation-exhalation efforts are used to find point of maximum ease and held until release occurs (Balance and Hold).

8. A dynamic indirect approach can be implemented by applying a load from the motion hand to the listening hand at step 6 and following the unwinding inherent motion in the tissues as they seek balance.

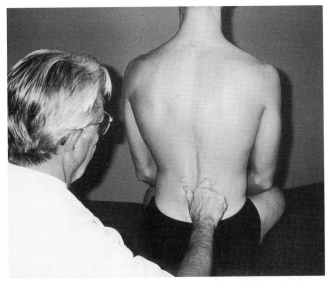

Figure 10.1.

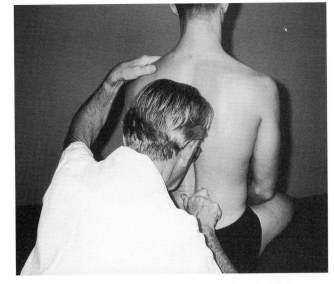

Figure 10.3.

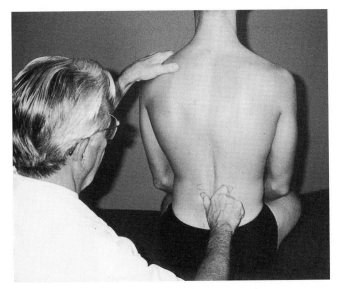

Figure 10.2.

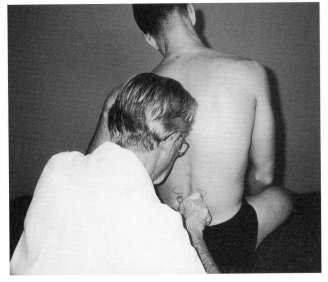

Figure 10.4.

Functional Technique

Pubes
Supine
Diagnosis: Superior or inferior pube

1. Patient supine, knees flexed, and dropped into abduction with the soles of feet together.

2. Operator stands at side of table and palpates right and left side of the pubic symphysis with index fingers above and thumbs below (Fig. 10.5).

3. Operator introduces cephalic to caudad motion to point of maximum ease (Fig. 10.6).

4. Balance and hold approach uses respiratory force assist until balance of symmetrical position and motion occurs.

5. A dynamic approach introduces motion in the direction of ease and follows inherent motion until balance of function is achieved.

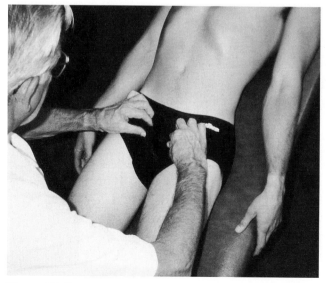

Figure 10.5.

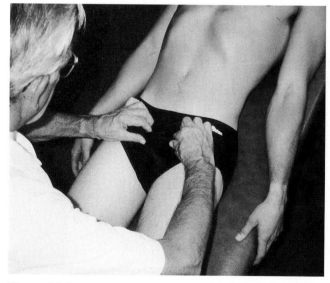

Figure 10.6.

Functional Technique

Sitting
Sacroiliac
Diagnosis: Left on left torsion

1. Patient sitting on table.

2. Operator sits behind patient with the right hand over the right sacral base as the listening hand (Fig. 10.7) and the left hand on the left shoulder as the motion hand (Fig. 10.8).

3. Operator's head is placed in the thoracolumbar region to control flexion-extension by anteroposterior translation (Fig. 10.9).

4. Operator's right thumb is over the sacral base while the right index finger exerts lateral distraction on the medial side of the posterior superior iliac spine, sensing for ease at the upper pole of the right sacroiliac joint.

5. Operator's head introduces anteroposterior translation and flexion-extension to ease at the listening hand.

6. Operator's (left) motion hand introduces left side-bending and right rotation of the patient's trunk to ease at the listening hand (Fig. 10.10).

7. The balance and hold approach fine tunes ease at the listening hand and then introduces respiratory effort to achieve release of tension and return of function. Several repetitions may be necessary with fine tuning after each respiratory assist.

8. The dynamic indirect approach initiates motion in the direction of ease and follows the inherent tissue response as the tissues "unwind." The thumb of the right hand may be moved to the left inferior lateral angle to initiate and assist the process.

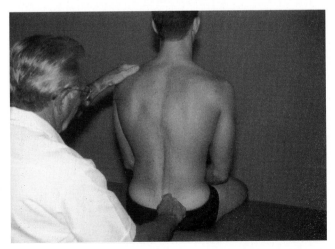

Figure 10.7.

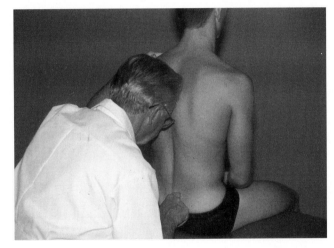

Figure 10.9.

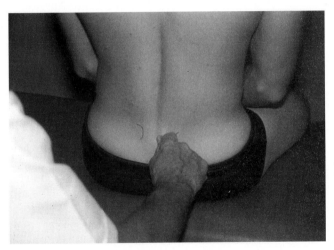

Figure 10.8.

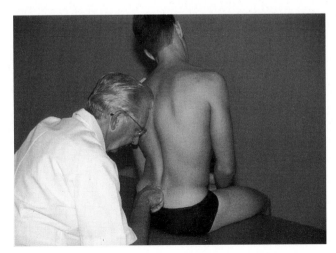

Figure 10.10.

Functional Technique

Sacroiliac
Sitting
Diagnosis: Left sacrum flexed

1. Patient sitting on table.

2. Operator sits behind patient with the left hand over the left sacral base as the listening hand with the thumb over the sacrum and the index finger medial to the left posterior superior iliac spine (Fig. 10.11).

3. Operator's right hand is placed on the patient's right shoulder as the motion hand (Fig. 10.12).

4. Operator's head is placed at the thoracolumbar junction.

5. Operator introduces flexion-extension, anteroposterior translatory motion through the head until ease is felt at the listening hand (Fig. 10.13).

6. Operator motion hand introduces right sidebending and left rotation until ease is felt at the listening hand (Fig. 10.14).

7. The balance and hold approach maintains the point of ease and uses respiratory action to achieve release of restriction in the tissues.

8. The dynamic indirect approach initiates motion in the direction of ease through the motion hand and follows the inherent tissue motion as it seeks ease and balance of tension. The operator's left thumb can be moved to the left inferior lateral angle to assist in release. The motion hand controls the trunk as ease is sought in all dimensions.

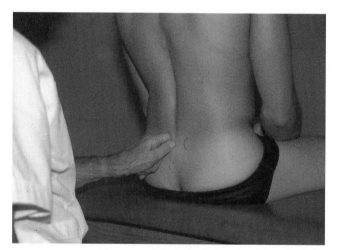

Figure 10.11.

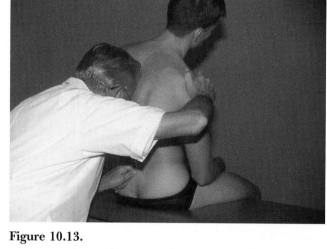

Figure 10.13.

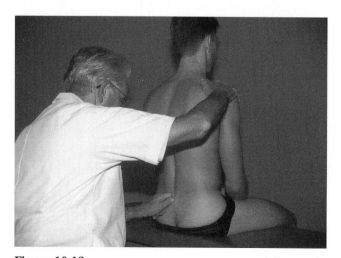

Figure 10.12.

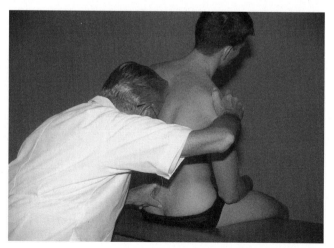

Figure 10.14.

Functional Technique

Sacroiliac
Sitting
Diagnosis: Right sacrum extended

1. Patient sitting on table.
2. Operator sitting behind patient with the right hand over the upper pole of the right sacroiliac joint as the listening hand. The thumb is over the right sacral base and the right index finger provides lateral distraction on the right posterior superior iliac spine.
3. Operator's left hand is on patient's left shoulder as the motion hand (Fig. 10.15).
4. Operator's head is at the thoracolumbar junction.
5. Operator introduces a little flexion, posterior translation and right sidebending-rotation until ease is felt at the listening hand. The patient's weight is shifted to the right ischial tuberosity (Fig. 10.16).
6. The balance and hold approach maintains the point of maximum ease at the right sacral base by fine tuning and then using respiratory effort to achieve balance of tissue tension.
7. The dynamic indirect approach initiates motion at the right sacral base through the motion hand and follows the balance point until tissue release occurs and function restored.

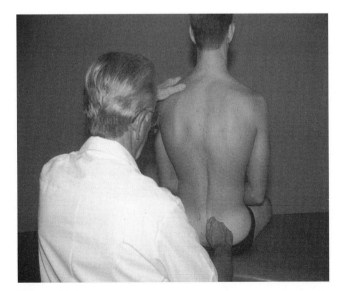

Figure 10.15.

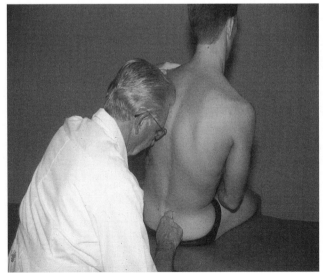

Figure 10.16.

Functional Technique

    Sacroiliac
    Sitting
Diagnosis: Left on right torsion

1. Patient is sitting on the table.
2. Operator sitting behind patient with the left hand over the upper pole of the left sacroiliac joint as the listening hand. The thumb is on the sacral base and the index finger gives lateral distraction on the left posterior superior iliac spine.
3. Operator's right hand is placed on the patient's right shoulder as the motion hand (Fig. 10.17).
4. Operator's head is placed at the thoracolumbar junction.

5. Operator introduces flexion and posterior translation to localize to the listening hand.
6. Operator's motion hand introduces sidebending and rotation to the left to balance at the left sacral base. The patient's weight is usually on the left ischial tuberosity (Fig. 10.18).
7. The balance and hold approach localizes ease in all dimensions at the left sacral base and initiates respiratory action to achieve tissue balance.
8. The dynamic indirect approach initiates motion through the motion hand in the direction of ease at the listening hand and follows the inherent tissue motion in the direction of ease to tissue balance.

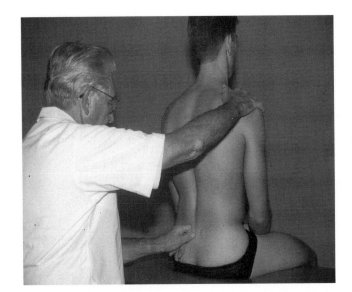

Figure 10.17.

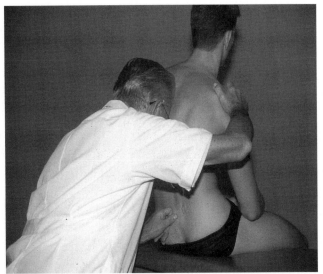

Figure 10.18.

Functional Technique

Iliosacral
Sitting
Diagnosis: Right anterior ilium

1. Patient is sitting on the table.
2. Operator sitting behind the patient.
3. Operator's right hand lies over the right iliac crest with the thumb over the sacrum at the lower pole of the sacroiliac joint as the listening hand.
4. Operator's left hand contacts the patient's left shoulder as the motion hand (Fig. 10.19).
5. Operator's head is placed at the thoracolumbar junction.

6. Operator introduces anteroposterior translation until the right ilium starts to move forward and then left sidebending and rotation until ease is felt over the upper pole of the right sacroiliac joint. The patient's weight is usually on the left ischial tuberosity (Fig. 10.20).
7. The balance and hold approach seeks ease in all dimensions, adds respiratory effort, and fine tunes until balance of tissue tension occurs.
8. The dynamic indirect approach is initiated by loading through the motion hand in the direction of the listening hand and following the inherent tissue motion until tissue balance is achieved.

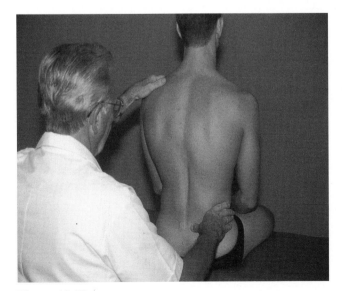

Figure 10.19.

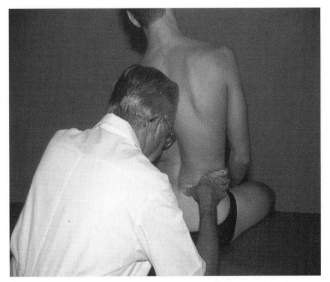

Figure 10.20.

Functional Technique

Iliosacral
Sitting
Diagnosis: Left posterior ilium

1. Patient sitting on the table.
2. Operator sitting behind patient.
3. Operator's left hand contacts the left iliac crest with the thumb over the sacrum at the lower pole of the left sacroiliac joint as the listening hand.
4. Operator's right hand contacts the patient's right shoulder as the motion hand (Fig. 10.21).
5. Operator's head is at the thoracolumbar junction.

6. Operator introduces anteroposterior translation to localize to the lower pole left sacroiliac joint (Fig. 10.22) and then introduces left sidebending until the left ilium moves to ease in posterior rotation (Fig. 10.23).
7. The balance and hold approach seeks ease in all dimensions and adds respiratory effort to achieve balanced tissue tension.
8. The dynamic indirect approach introduces motion through the motion hand toward the left sacroiliac joint and follows inherent tissue motion until balanced tissue tension is achieved.

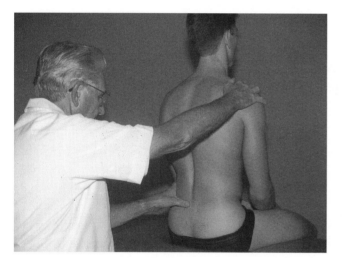

Figure 10.21.

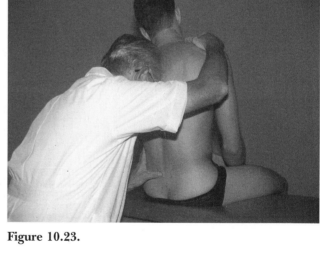

Figure 10.23.

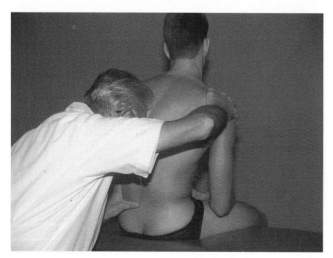

Figure 10.22.

Functional Technique

Pelvis
Sitting
Diagnosis: Pelvic compression

1. Patient sitting on table.

2. Operator sitting behind patient.

3. Operator's two hands grasp the ilia with the thumbs over the sacral base and the fingers along the iliac crests (Fig. 10.24).

4. Operator's head contacts the thoracolumbar junction.

5. Operator introduces anteroposterior translatory motion until ease is felt at the two sacroiliac joints (Fig. 10.25).

6. Operator's two hands compress the pelvis and rotate anteriorly and posteriorly on each side to the point of ease (Fig. 10.26).

7. The balance and hold approach holds the two ilia at the point of maximum ease and using respiratory effort seeks release and balance of tissue tension.

8. The dynamic indirect approach introduces motion through both hands and follows inherent tissue motion until balance in three dimensions is achieved.

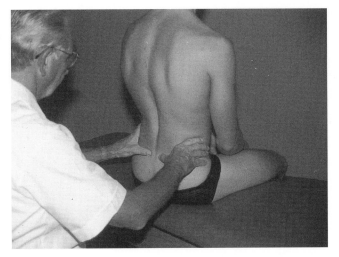

Figure 10.24.

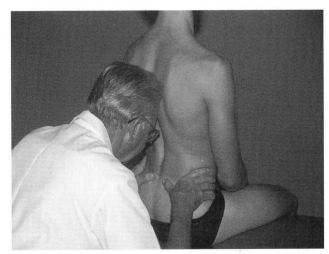

Figure 10.26.

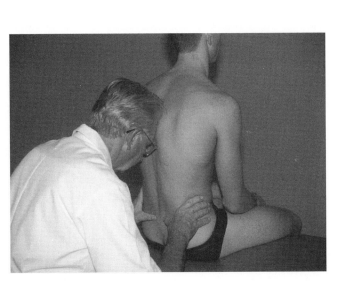

Figure 10.25.

Functional Technique

Thoracolumbar Spine
Sitting
Diagnosis: Vertebral dysfunction either ERS or FRS

1. Patient sitting on the table with arms folded across chest.

2. Operator sitting behind patient.

3. Operator's right hand contacts the thoracolumbar spine as the listening hand.

4. Operator's left hand grasps patient's left elbow as the motion hand (Fig. 10.27).

5. Operator's listening hand introduces flexion and extension through anteroposterior translation and then adds cephalic distraction to the point of ease.

6. Operator's motion hand introduces sidebending and rotation of the trunk, plus cephalic distraction, to the point of maximum ease (Fig. 10.28).

7. The balance and hold approach introduces motion to maximum ease in all dimensions and adds respiratory effort until balance in tissue tension is achieved.

8. The dynamic indirect approach introduces motion through the motion hand in the direction of ease and follows inherent tissue motion until balance of tissue tension is achieved.

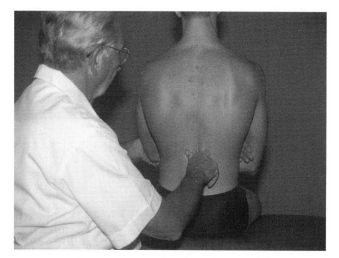

Figure 10.27.

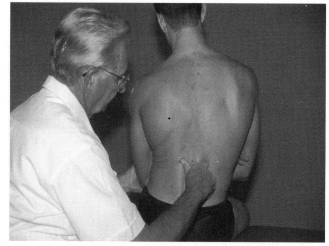

Figure 10.28.

Functional Technique

Upper Thoracic Spine
Sitting
Diagnosis: Vertebral dysfunction either ERS or FRS

1. Patient sitting on the table.

2. Operator standing behind patient with the patient's trunk against the operator for control.

3. Operator's left hand contacts the dysfunctional segment as the listening hand with fingers on each vertebra.

4. Operator's right hand contacts the top of the patient's head as the motion hand (Fig. 10.29).

5. Operator introduces flexion (Fig. 10.30) and extension (Fig. 10.31) through anteroposterior translation to maximum ease at the listening hand.

6. Operator's motion hand introduces sidebending and rotation to the dysfunctional segment, seeking maximum ease at the listening hand (Fig. 10.32).

7. The balance and hold approach seeks balance in all dimensions and then adds respiratory effort until tissue tension balance is achieved.

8. The dynamic indirect approach introduces motion through the motion hand in the direction of the listening hand and follows inherent tissue motion until tissue tension balance is achieved.

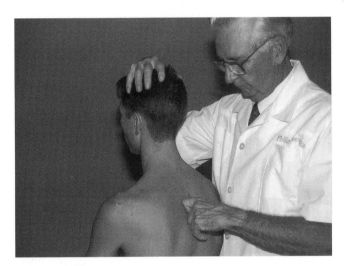

Figure 10.29.

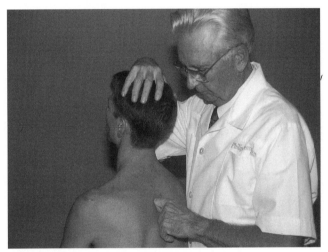

Figure 10.31.

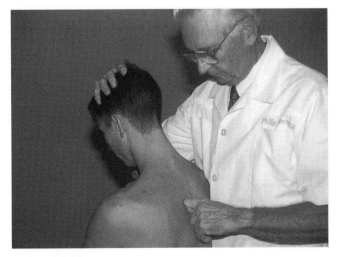

Figure 10.30.

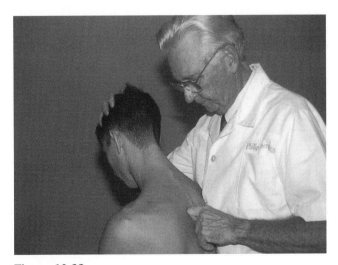

Figure 10.32.

Functional Technique

Middle and Lower Thoracic Spine
Sitting
Diagnosis: Vertebral dysfunction either ERS or FRS

1. Patient sitting on the table.

2. Operator stands behind patient with the patient trunk against the operator's torso for control.

3. Operator's left hand contacts the dysfunctional segment with a finger contact on each of the two vertebra as the listening hand.

4. Operator's right hand lies over the patient's right shoulder with the hand behind the patient's neck as the motion hand (Fig. 10.33).

5. Operator introduces flexion (Fig. 10.34) or extension (Fig. 10.35) through anteroposterior translation to ease at the listening hand.

6. Operator's motion hand introduces sidebending and rotation to ease at the listening hand (Fig. 10.36).

7. The balance and hold approach seeks ease in all dimensions and adds respiratory effort until balance of tissue tension is achieved.

8. The dynamic indirect approach initiates motion through the motion hand in the direction of ease at the listening hand and follows inherent tissue motion until balance of tissue tension is achieved.

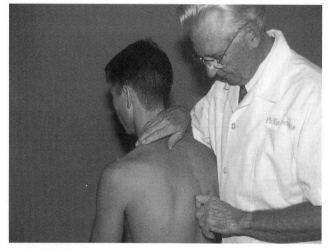

Figure 10.33.

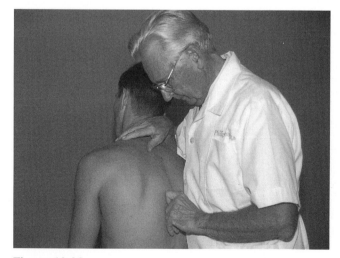

Figure 10.35.

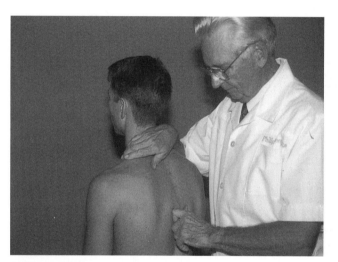

Figure 10.34.

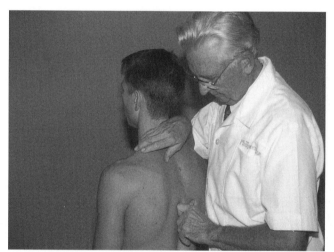

Figure 10.36.

Functional Technique

  Thoracic Spine and Ribs
  Sitting
Diagnosis: Combined vertebral and rib dysfunction

1. Patient sitting on the table with the left hand on the back of the neck.

2. Operator stands behind patient with the left hand grasping patient's left elbow as the motor hand (Fig. 10.37).

3. Operator's right hand is placed in the medial groove adjacent to the spinous processes over the restricted segments and serves as the listening hand. The thumb lies over the zygapophysial joints and the palm over the costotransverse articulation of the rib (Fig. 10.38).

4. Operator introduces flexion (Fig. 10.39) and extension (Fig. 10.40) through anteroposterior translation to ease at the listening hand.

5. Operator introduces sidebending and rotation to ease at the listening hand.

6. The balance and hold approach seeks ease in all dimensions and adds respiratory effort until balance in tissue tension is achieved.

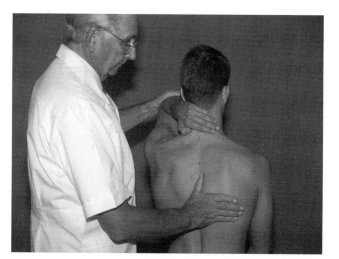

Figure 10.37.

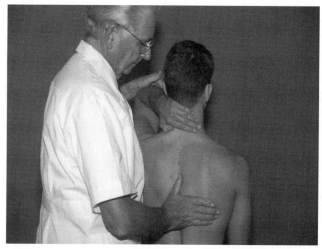

Figure 10.39.

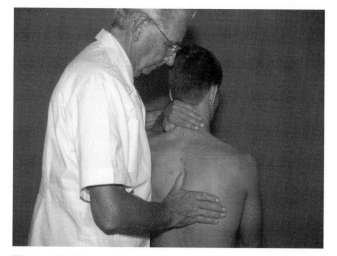

Figure 10.38.

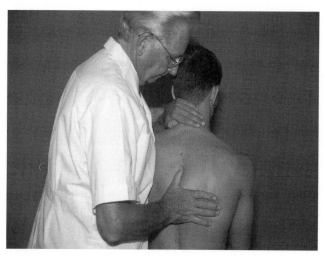

Figure 10.40.

7. The dynamic indirect approach initiates motion through the motion hand to ease at the listening hand and follows inherent tissue motion until three-dimensional tissue tension balance is achieved.

8. A variant of this technique has the patient's left hand grasping the right shoulder and the operator's left hand becoming the listening hand over the thoracic vertebra and ribs and right hand grasping the patient's left elbow as the motion hand (Fig. 10.41). The rest of the procedure follows as above. This variant allows for different combinations of flexion-extension and sidebending-rotation to the listening hand (Fig. 10.42).

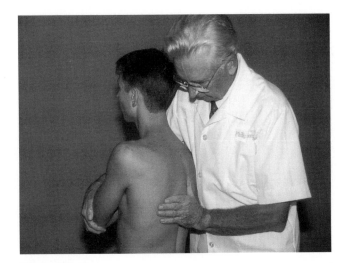

Figure 10.41.

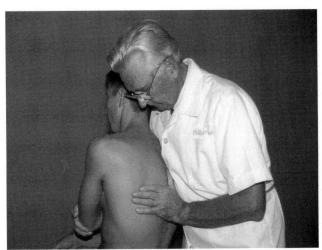

Figure 10.42.

Functional Technique

Middle and Lower Ribs
Sitting
Diagnosis: Structural or respiratory rib dysfunction

1. Patient sitting on the table.
2. Operator stands behind patient with the trunk supporting the patient's torso.
3. Operator's right hand is placed over the medial side of the rib angle with the fingers along the rib shafts of the dysfunctional rib(s) as the listening hand (Fig. 10.43).
4. Operator's left arm reaches across the patient's upper trunk and grasps the right shoulder as the motion hand.

5. Flexion-extension is introduced through anteroposterior translation to ease at the listening hand.
6. Operator's motion hand introduces sidebending and rotation to ease at the listening hand (Fig. 10.44).
7. The balance and hold approach localizes ease in all dimensions at the listening hand and uses respiratory effort until balance of tissue tension is achieved.
8. The dynamic indirect approach introduces movement through the motion hand in the direction of ease at the listening hand and follows inherent tissue motion until balance in tissue tension is achieved. Occasionally, compression is useful in initiating the inherent tissue motion.

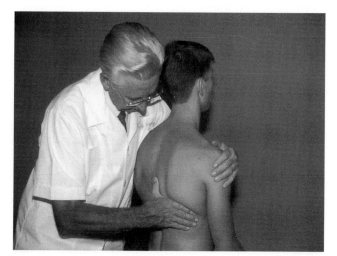

Figure 10.43.

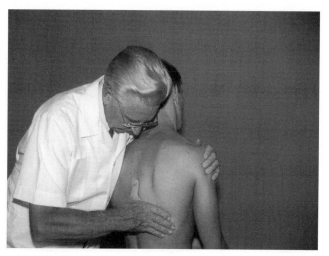

Figure 10.44.

Functional Technique

First Rib
Sitting
Diagnosis: Respiratory dysfunction first rib

1. Patient sitting on the table with right hand grasping back of neck.

2. Operator stands behind patient with the listening left hand palpating the patient's right first rib with the thumb on the posterior and the fingers on the anterior aspect (Fig. 10.45).

3. Operator's motion right hand grasps the patient's right elbow.

4. Operator introduces anteroposterior trunk translation and internal-external rotation of the patient's right arm, localizing ease at the listening hand (Fig. 10.46).

5. The balance and hold approach localizes ease in all directions and adds respiratory effort until balance of tissue tension occurs.

6. The dynamic indirect approach initiates a compressive action in the direction of ease through the motion hand and follows inherent tissue motion until tissue tension is relieved and motion reestablished.

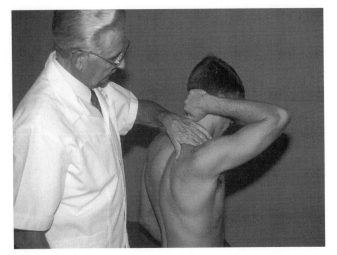

Figure 10.45.

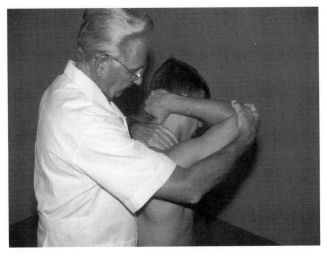

Figure 10.46.

Functional Technique

Upper Ribs
Sitting
Diagnosis: Respiratory rib dysfunction

1. Patient sitting with left hand grasping the right shoulder.
2. Operator stands behind patient with thorax supporting the patient's torso.
3. Operator's left listening hand contacts the upper left ribs (Fig. 10.47) with the thumb behind and the fingers over the anterior aspect.
4. Operator's right motion hand controls the patient's left upper extremity through the elbow.

5. Operator's body introduces anteroposterior translation and the motion hand introduces flexion, adduction, and abduction of the patient's upper arm to maximum ease at the listening hand (Fig. 10.48).
6. Additional ease may be obtained by the patient sidebending and rotating the head to the right.
7. The balance and hold approach maintains ease in all dimensions and adds respiratory effort until tissue balance and motion is restored.
8. The dynamic indirect approach initiates motion through the motion hand in the direction of ease at the listening hand and follows the inherent tissue motion until tissue tension is relieved and motion restored.

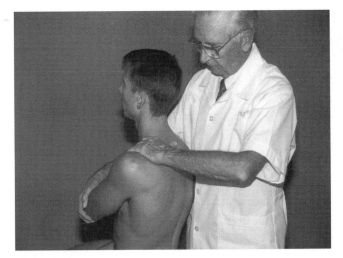

Figure 10.47.

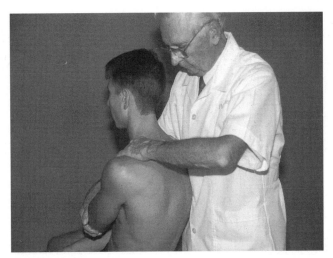

Figure 10.48.

Functional Technique

Single Rib (Variation 1)
Sitting
Diagnosis: Respiratory or structural rib dysfunction

1. Patient sitting on table.
2. Operator stands or sits at side of patient and identifies dysfunctional rib (Fig. 10.49).
3. Operator places both thumbs at the midaxillary line of the dysfunctional rib with the middle fingers span-

ning and holding the rib shaft anteriorly and posteriorly (Fig. 10.50).
4. Patient is instructed to lean toward the operator's hands and gently sidebend and rotate the trunk away (Fig. 10.51).
5. Operator translates the patient until the rib appears to "float" and then initiates respiratory effort until release of tissue tension and restoration of motion occurs.

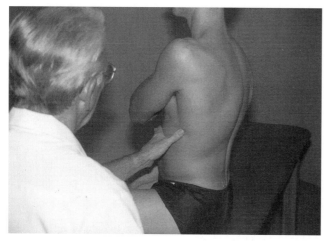

Figure 10.49.

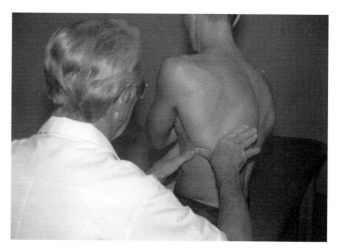

Figure 10.51.

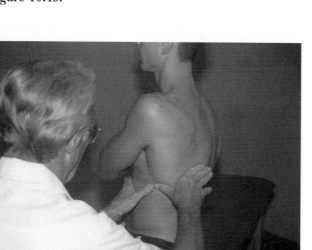

Figure 10.50.

Functional Technique

Single Rib (Variation 2)
Sitting
Diagnosis: Respiratory or structural rib dysfunction

1. Patient sitting on table.
2. Operator stands behind patient with thorax supporting the patient's torso.
3. Operator's listening hand is placed over the posterior aspect of the dysfunctional rib with the thumb near the costotransverse articulation and the fingers along the rib shaft.
4. Operator's motion hand reaches across anterior upper thorax of the patient and grasps the shoulder on the side of dysfunction (Fig. 10.52).
5. Operator introduces translation of the patient's body and moves the shoulder through elevation, depression, anterior, and posterior rotation until ease is felt at the listening hand (Fig. 10.53).
6. The balance and hold approach seeks ease in all dimensions and adds respiratory effort until release of tissue tension and restoration of motion is achieved.
7. The dynamic indirect approach initiates motion in the direction of ease and follows the inherent tissue motion until tissue tension is released and motion restored.

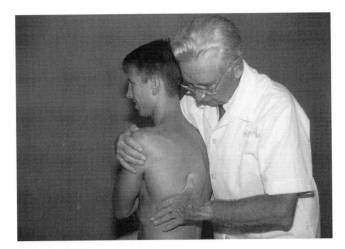

Figure 10.52.

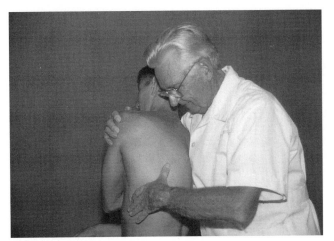

Figure 10.53.

Functional Technique

Single Typical Rib Dysfunction
Supine
Diagnosis: Respiratory or structural rib dysfunction

1. Patient supine on the table.
2. Operator sits at side of dysfunction. (Hand position shown with patient sitting, Figure 10.54).
3. Operator's posterior hand slides under patient and contacts the posterior shaft while the anterior hand contacts the anterior shaft of the dysfunctional rib (Fig. 10.55).

4. Operator introduces anteroposterior compression and seeks point of maximum ease.
5. Balance and hold approach adds respiratory effort to achieve tissue tension balance and restored function.
6. The dynamic indirect approach initiates motion through both hands in the direction of ease and follows inherent tissue motion until tissue tension is relieved and motion restored.

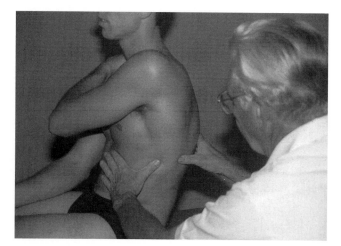

Figure 10.54.

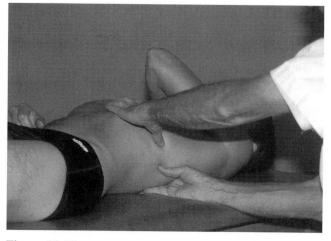

Figure 10.55.

Functional Technique

Sternum
Supine
Diagnosis: Manubrioglodiolar sternal dysfunction

1. Patient supine on the table.
2. Operator stands at side of the patient.
3. Operator places one hand over the sternum (Fig. 10.56) with the other hand overlying the first and pointed in the opposite direction (Fig. 10.57). A variant of the hand position has one hand over the body of the sternum pointed vertically and the other horizontally across the manubrium with the two hands adjacent to the angle of Louis (Fig. 10.58).
4. Operator introduces slight compression followed by cephalic-caudad, clockwise (Fig. 10.59) and counterclockwise (Fig. 10.60), shifting side to side, and anteroposterior rocking movements seeking point of maximum ease.
5. The balance and hold approach seeks the point of maximum ease and introduces respiratory effort until balanced motion is achieved.

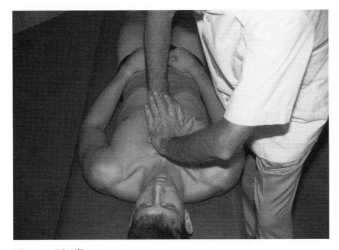

Figure 10.56.

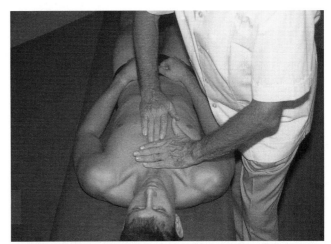

Figure 10.58.

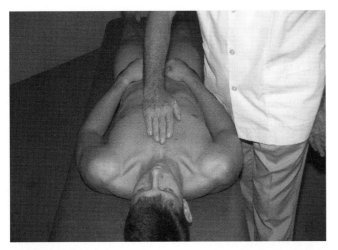

Figure 10.57.

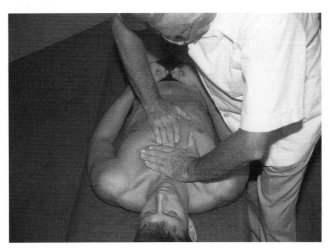

Figure 10.59.

6. The dynamic indirect approach initiates motion by added compression and follows the inherent tissue motion until tissue tension is relieved and motion restored.

Functional Technique

Occipitoatlantal Junction (C0–1)
Sitting
Diagnosis: Flexion-extension C0–1 dysfunction

1. Patient sitting on table.

2. Operator stands behind patient with chest wall and abdomen supporting the patient posterior torso.

3. Operator's two hands grasp the skull with the thumbs along the occipital protuberance (Fig. 10.61).

4. Operator's arms contact the patient's shoulders, and a cephalic lift to the head is applied until ease is felt.

5. Operator fine tunes ease with head flexion-extension, rotation, and sidebending to maximum (Fig. 10.62).

6. The balance and hold approach holds ease in all dimensions and adds respiratory effort until tissue tension is relieved and motion restored.

7. The dynamic indirect approach initiates motion in the direction of ease and follows inherent tissue motion until release is felt and motion established.

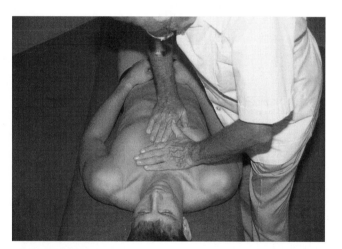

Figure 10.60.

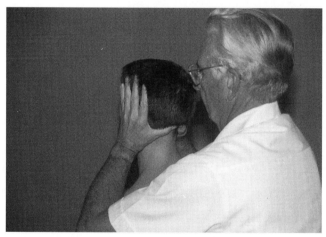

Figure 10.62.

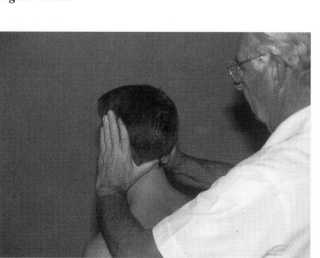

Figure 10.61.

Functional Technique

> Upper Cervical Spine (C1–2)
> Sitting

Diagnosis: Dysfunction at C1–2

1. Patient sitting on table.

2. Operator stands behind patient with chest wall and abdomen supporting the patient's posterior torso.

3. Operator's left hand is placed over the front of the skull and the right under the occiput with the thumb and index fingers in contact with the atlas-axis region (Fig. 10.63).

4. Operator introduces cephalic distraction followed by flexion-extension and sidebending-rotation, seeking the point of maximum ease.

5. The balance and hold approach would hold the point of maximum ease and apply respiratory effort until tissue tension is released and motion restored.

6. The dynamic indirect approach initiates motion in the direction of ease through combined motion of both hands and follows the inherent tissue motion until tissue tension is released and motion restored.

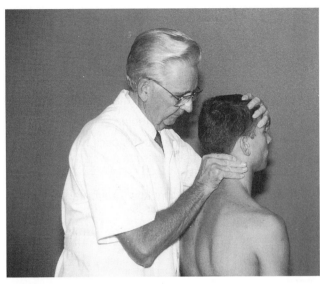

Figure 10.63.

Functional Technique

    Occipitoatlantal Junction (C0–1)
    Supine
Diagnosis: Flexion-extension dysfunction

1. Patient supine on the table, arms at sides.

2. Operator sitting at head of table.

3. Operator's left hand cradles the occiput with the thumb and index finger in contact with the posterior arch of the atlas (Fig. 10.64).

4. Operator's right hand contacts the frontal area (Fig. 10.65).

5. Operator introduces small anterior-posterior nodding movements of the skull until the atlas is at maximum ease.

6. Operator applies compression-distraction through the occiput and right-left translation through the atlas to the point of maximum ease (Fig. 10.66).

7. The balance and hold approach holds the point of maximum ease and applies respiratory effort until tissue tension releases and motion restored.

8. The dynamic indirect approach initiates motion in the direction of ease through both hands and follows inherent tissue motion until tissue tension releases and motion restored.

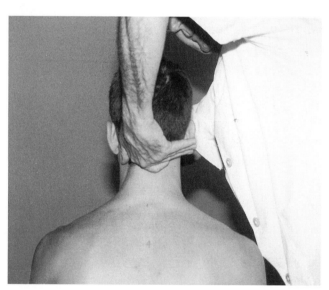

Figure 10.64.

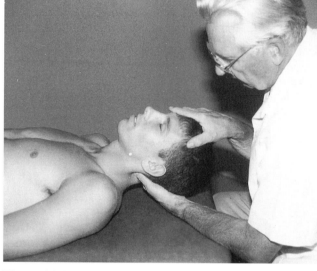

Figure 10.66.

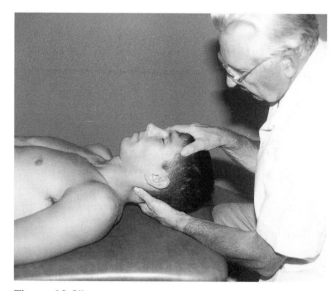

Figure 10.65.

Functional Technique

Typical Cervical Spine
Sitting

1. Patient sitting on table.

2. Operator standing behind patient with chest and abdomen supporting patient's posterior torso.

3. Operator's listening left hand is placed over the dysfunctional segment of the lower cervical spine. The thumb and index finger span either the posterior pillars or transverse processes (Fig. 10.67).

4. The motion right hand is placed on the patient's forehead.

5. Operator introduces flexion-extension, sidebending, and rotation through the motion hand to maximum ease at the listening hand (Fig. 10.68). Anterior-posterior translatory movement can be introduced through the operator's trunk. Cephalic to caudad translation can be introduced through combined movement of both hands.

6. The balance and hold approach maintains the point of maximum ease and applies respiratory effort until tissue tension releases and motion is restored (Fig. 10.69).

7. The dynamic indirect approach introduces motion through the right hand in the direction of ease and follows inherent tissue motion until tissue tension releases and motion restored.

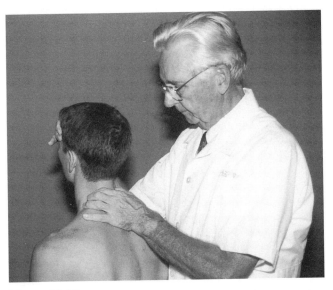

Figure 10.67.

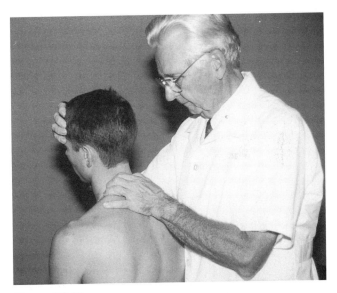

Figure 10.69.

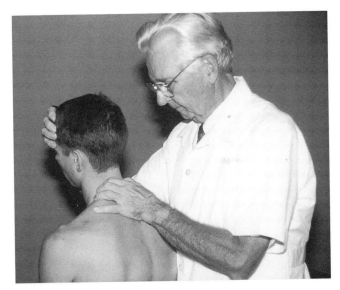

Figure 10.68.

Functional Technique

Typical Cervical Spine
Supine

1. Patient supine on the table.

2. Operator sitting at head of table.

3. Operator hands support patient's head and upper cervical spine with the index and middle fingers over the articular pillar of the dysfunctional segment (Fig. 10.70).

4. Operator introduces flexion-extension, anterior-posterior translation, sidebending, and rotation through combined movement of both hands, seeking point of maximum ease under finger tips (Fig. 10.71).

5. The balance and hold approach maintains the point of maximum ease and applies respiratory effort until tissue tension is released and motion restored (Fig. 10.72).

6. The dynamic indirect approach initiates motion in the direction of ease and follows the inherent tissue motion until tissue tension releases and motion is restored.

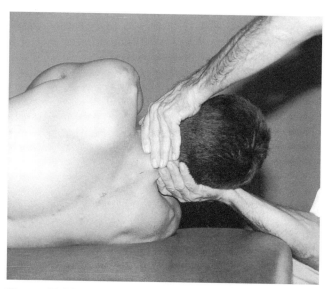

Figure 10.70.

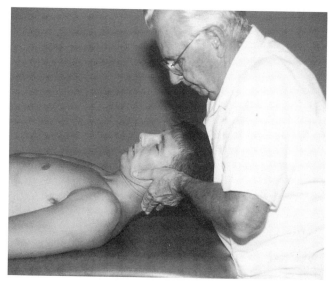

Figure 10.72.

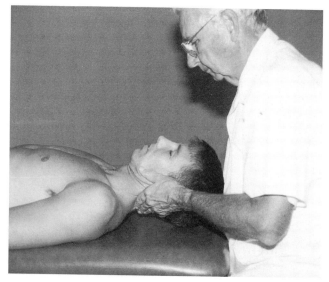

Figure 10.71.

Functional Technique

Shoulder Girdle
Step 1

1. Patient supine on the table.

2. Operator sits at the side of the shoulder to be treated.

3. Operator's listening hand is placed over the patient's clavicle with the little finger along the shaft and the fourth and fifth fingerpads over the sternoclavicular joint. The heel of the hand is over the acromioclavicular joint (Fig. 10.73).

4. Operator's motion hand grasps the patient's arm either above or below the elbow and abducts to about 90° (Fig. 10.74).

5. Operator's motion hand introduces adduction-abduction, internal-external rotation, and compression-distraction along the humerus to ease at the listening hand.

6. The balance and hold approach maintains the point of ease and adds respiratory effort until release of tissue tension occurs.

7. The dynamic indirect approach introduces motion in the direction of ease and follows the inherent tissue motion until tissue tension is relieved.

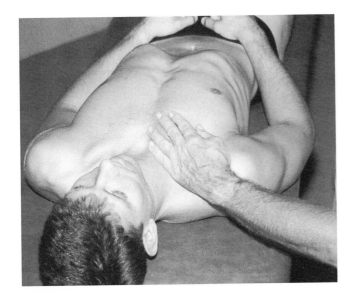

Figure 10.73.

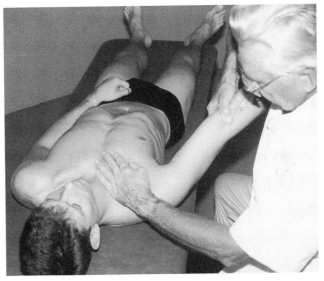

Figure 10.74.

Functional Technique

Shoulder Girdle
Step 2

1. Operator and patient position as in step one.

2. Operator's listening hand is placed over the gleno-humeral joint with the thumb behind and the fingers in front (Fig. 10.75).

3. Operator's motion hand grasps the patient's arm in the same fashion as step 1 and introduces abduction to 80–90° and then fine tunes through the lis-tening hand by internal-external rotation and compression-decompression until maximum ease is obtained (Fig. 10.76).

4. The balance and hold approach maintains ease and adds respiratory effort until release of tissue tension is achieved.

5. The dynamic indirect approach initiates motion in the direction of ease through the motion hand and follows inherent tissue motion until tissue tension is released and motion restored.

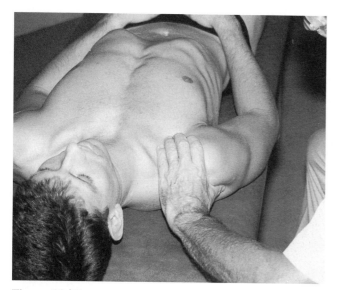

Figure 10.75.

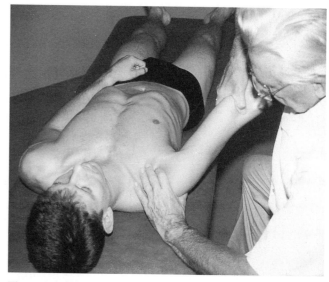

Figure 10.76.

Functional Technique

Shoulder Girdle
Step 3

1. Operator and patient position as in steps 1 and 2.

2. Operator switches hands with the listening hand over the pectoral region in the direction of the fibers of the pectoralis minor. The motion hand controls the arm and introduces abduction so that the arm is in the direction of the pectoral muscle fibers (Fig. 10.77).

3. Operator's motion hand introduces compression-decompression, internal-external rotation, and adduction-abduction until the point of maximum ease is felt at the listening hand.

4. The tissues are balanced between the two hands.

5. The balance and hold approach maintains the point of maximum ease and adds respiratory effort until tissue tension is relieved and motion returned.

6. The dynamic indirect approach initiates motion in the direction of ease and follows inherent tissue motion until tissue tension is relieved and motion restored.

Functional Technique

Acromioclavicular and Glenohumeral Joints
Sitting

1. Patient sitting on table.

2. Operator stands behind patient and supports patient's trunk against operator's body.

3. Operator's foot is placed on table on side being treated and drapes patient's relaxed arm over knee with medial hand placed over the patient's acromioclavicular and glenohumeral area (Fig. 10.78).

4. Operator's lateral hand grasps the patient's elbow.

5. Operator introduces anteroposterior and medial-lateral translation and rotation of the patient to ease at both the shoulder and the elbow (Fig. 10.79).

6. The balance and hold approach identifies the point of maximum ease and adds respiratory effort until tissue tension is relieved and motion restored.

7. The dynamic indirect approach introduces motion in the direction of ease, frequently with a compression-decompression maneuver in the long axis of the arm, and follows the inherent tissue motion until tissue tension is relieved and motion restored.

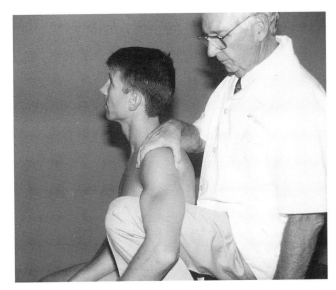

Figure 10.78.

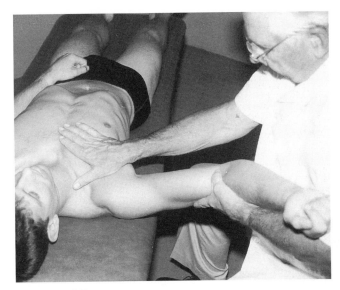

Figure 10.77.

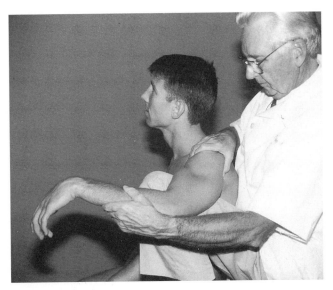

Figure 10.79.

Functional Technique

Radial Head
Sitting

1. Patient sitting.

2. Operator stands in front of patient with listening hand over the dysfunctional elbow with the thumb over the anterior and the index finger over the posterior aspects of the radial head (Fig. 10.80).

3. Operator's motion hand grasps the patient's distal forearm and introduces flexion-extension, internal-external rotation, adduction-abduction, and compression-decompression to the point of maximum ease (Fig. 10.81).

4. The balance and hold approach maintains the point of maximum ease and introduces respiratory effort until tissue tension is relieved and motion restored.

5. The dynamic indirect approach introduces motion in the direction of ease and follows inherent tissue motion until tissue tension is relieved and motion restored.

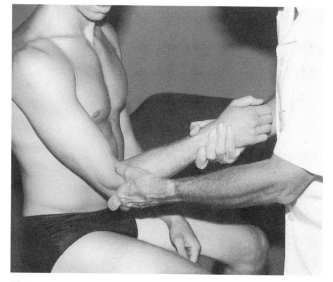

Figure 10.80.

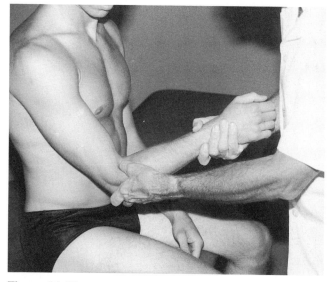

Figure 10.81.

Functional Technique

Wrist and Hand
Sitting

1. Patient sitting on table.
2. Operator stands in front of patient grasping the dysfunctional wrist and hand with the proximal hand over the distal forearm (Fig. 10.82).
3. Operator's distal hand grasps the patient's hand either with a handshake hold (Fig. 10.83) or the fingers interdigitating (Fig. 10.84).
4. Operator's distal hand introduces flexion-extension, internal-external rotation, adduction-abduction, and compression-decompression to the point of maximum ease (Fig. 10.85).
5. Balance and hold technique maintains the point of ease and adds respiratory effort until tissue tension is relieved and motion restored.
6. The dynamic indirect approach introduces motion in the direction of ease and follows inherent tissue motion until tissue tension is relieved and motion restored.

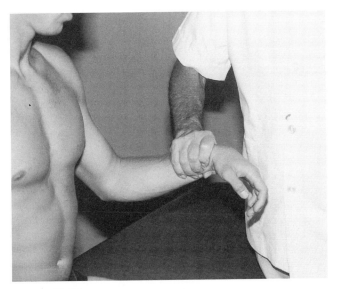

Figure 10.82.

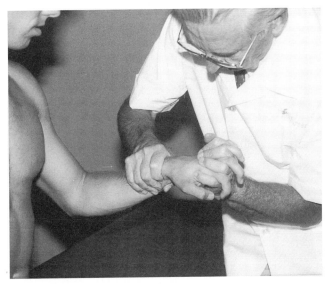

Figure 10.84.

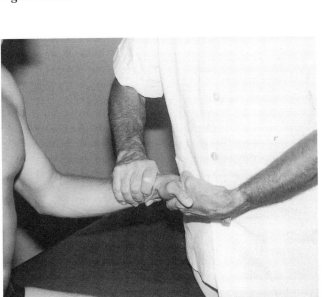

Figure 10.83.

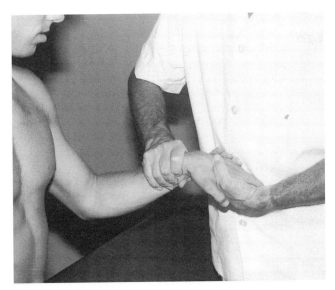

Figure 10.85.

Functional Technique

Hip and Leg
Supine

1. Patient supine on table.

2. Operator stands at side of table on side of dysfunctional leg and one foot on the table.

3. Operator flexes patient's leg to about 90° of hip and knee flexion with the leg draped over the operator's thigh.

4. Operator's proximal hand is on the patient's knee with the distal hand holding the patient's foot (Fig. 10.86).

5. Operator introduces compression-decompression through the thigh and/or leg until ease is obtained. Fine tuning is done by medial-lateral rotation, adduction-abduction, and flexion-extension of the hip and knee (Fig. 10.87).

6. The balance and hold approach maintains the point of maximum ease and adds respiratory effort until tissue tension is relieved and motion restored.

7. The dynamic indirect approach initiates motion in the direction of ease and follows the inherent tissue motion until tissue tension is relieved and motion restored.

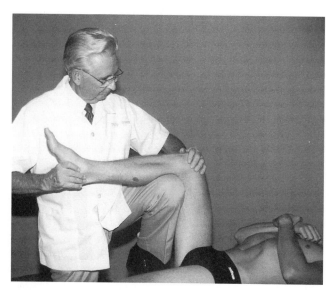

Figure 10.86.

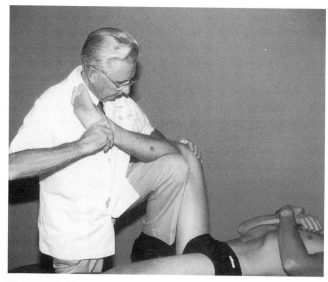

Figure 10.87.

Functional Technique

Knee and Fibular Head
Sitting

1. Patient is sitting on the table with legs dangling.

2. The operator sits in front of the patient.

3. Operator's listening hand palpates the knee with the thumb over the medial meniscus and the fingers on the fibular head (Fig. 10.88).

4. Operator's motion hand holds the foot and ankle and introduces compression-decompression to loose pack the tibia on the femur.

5. Operator fine tunes ease at the listening hand by introducing abduction-adduction, internal-external rotation, and flexion-extension (Fig. 10.89).

6. The balance and hold approach maintains maximum ease and adds respiratory effort until tissue tension is relieved and motion restored.

7. The dynamic indirect approach initiates motion in the direction of ease and follows inherent tissue motion until tissue tension is relieved and motion restored.

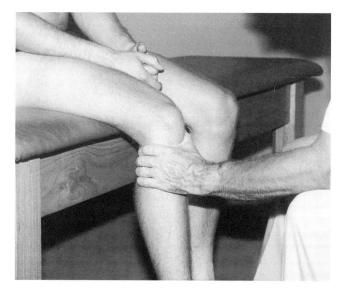

Figure 10.88.

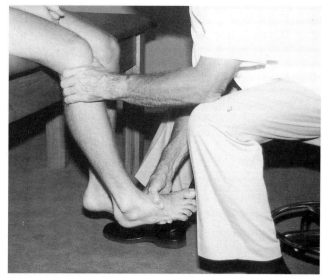

Figure 10.89.

Functional Technique

Foot and Ankle

1. Patient sitting or supine on table.

2. Operator's listening hand grasps the heel of the patient (Fig. 10.90).

3. Operator's motion hand grasps the forefoot and initiates motion through compression (Fig. 10.91).

4. Operator fines tunes maximum ease through the introduction of dorsi and plantar flexion, inversion-eversion, and adduction-abduction (Fig. 10.92).

5. The balance and hold approach maintains maximum ease and uses respiratory effort until tissue tension is relieved and motion restored.

6. The dynamic indirect approach initiates motion primarily through compression-distraction and follows inherent tissue motion until tissue tension is relieved and motion restored.

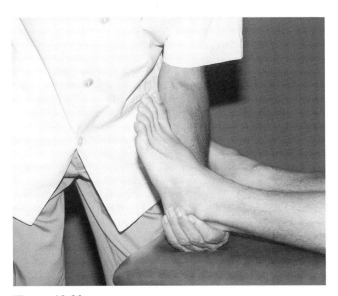

Figure 10.90.

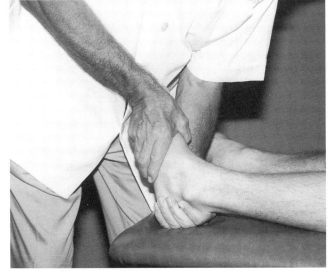

Figure 10.92.

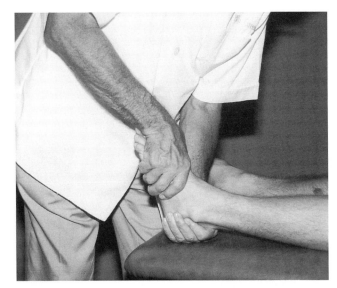

Figure 10.91.

CONCLUSION

Functional (indirect) techniques are based on a common neurological model in which reducing the flow of abnormal afferent impulses into the central nervous system reprograms the "central computer" to a more normal function. These procedures focus on the quality of movement, particularly the quality on the initiation of motion, rather than the amount of range or the feel of its end point. They are primarily nontraumatic and easily used in a variety of patient conditions and health care settings. They require considerable practice to educate the senses to the ease and bind phenomena and to the point of maximum pain-free position for the tissues of the musculoskeletal system. The value of these procedures in patient care warrants the expenditure of time and effort needed for the student to acquire proficiency.

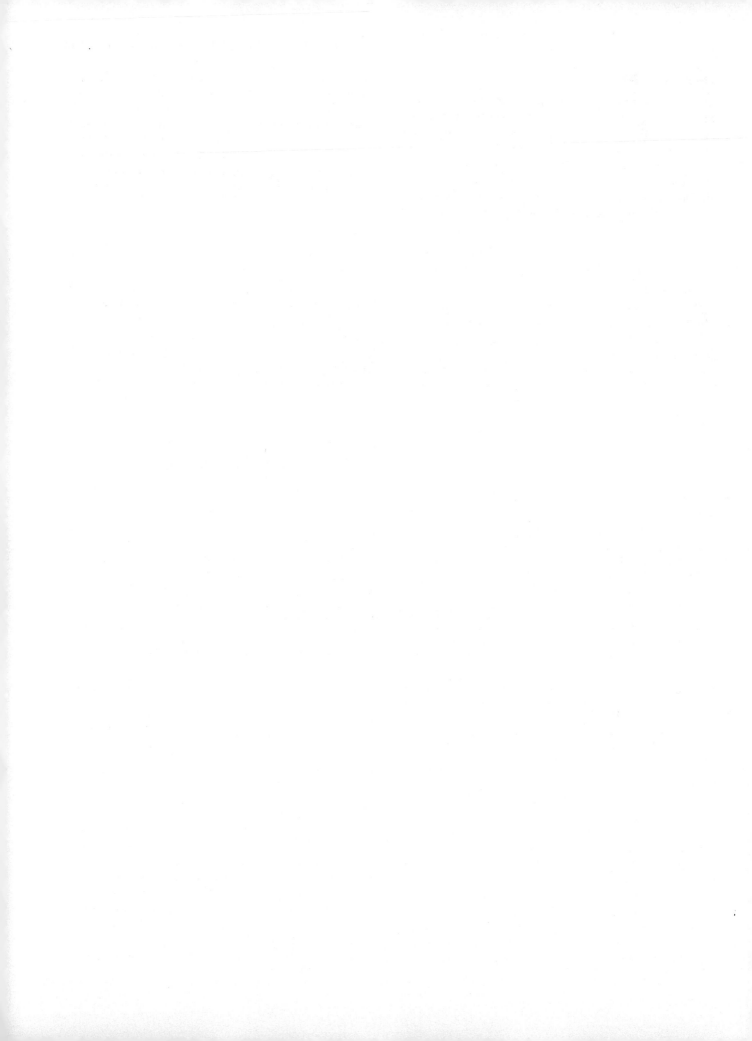

11

MYOFASCIAL RELEASE TECHNIQUE

Myofascial release technique is one of the newer additions to the field of manual medicine. Ward described myofascial release technique as a "bridging" technique spanning the spectrum of manual medicine procedures. It combines many of the principles of soft tissue technique, muscle energy technique, indirect technique, and inherent force craniosacral technique. There are multiple authors and teachers of myofascial release technique with many similarities and differences.

Fascia has received the attention of many individuals, including the osteopathic physician Neidner, who used twisting forces on the extremities to restore fascial balance and symmetry. Ida Rolf was famous for deep pressure and stretching of the fascia from the top of the head to the tips of the toes. Rolfing requires extensive investment in time and energy, both by the patient and operator, and the process is not always comfortable.

Myofascial release technique described here can be classified as either direct or indirect and frequently is used in a combined fashion. It applies the principles of biomechanical loading of soft tissue and the neural reflex modifications by stimulation of mechanoreceptors in the fascia. The resistant barrier may be engaged directly with tissue stretching, or loading can occur in the direction away from the resistant barrier in an indirect fashion. These are frequently called direct and indirect barriers. Frequently, the barriers are addressed in a combined fashion in each direction.

Myofascial release technique builds on inherent tissue motion. Living tissues have an inherent motion that continues at various rates and amplitudes. The inherent tissue motion of the musculoskeletal system is thought to be the result of rhythmic change in tone of muscle, pulsile forces of arterial circulation, the effects of respiration, and the inherent force of the cranial rhythmic impulse.

Activating forces in myofascial release technique are both intrinsic and extrinsic. The intrinsic forces include inherent tissue motion, inherent body rhythms, respiration, muscle contraction, and eye movement. Extrinsic activating forces applied by the operator include the application of loads, primarily of compression, traction, and twisting, to apply the appropriate tension in the soft tissues to affect biomechanical and reflex change. This technique is used for regional and local dysfunctions. It shares the common goal of all manual medicine procedures to achieve symmetrical pain-free motion of the musculoskeletal system in postural balance.

FASCIA

The clinician using myofascial release technique must have a thorough working knowledge of the continuity and integration of fascia. The fascia of the body is continuous from region to region and totally invests all other elements of the body. Various portions of fascia carry individual names, but all fascia is continuous.

Fascia can be described as consisting of three layers. The superficial fascia is attached to the undersurface of the skin and is loosely knit, fibroelastic, areolar tissue. Within the superficial fascia are found fat, vascular structures (including capillary networks and lymphatic channels) and nervous tissues, particularly the pacinian corpuscles referred to as skin receptors. The skin can be moved in many directions over the deeper structures because of the loosely knit nature of superficial fascia. Within the superficial fascia is potential space for the accumulation of fluid and metabolites. Many of the palpatory changes of tissue texture abnormalities are the result of changes within the superficial fascia.

Deep fascia is tough, tight, and compact. It compartmentalizes the body. It envelops and separates muscles, surrounds and separates internal visceral organs, and contributes greatly to the contour and function of the body. The peritoneum, the pericardium, and the pleura are specialized elements of the deep fascia. The tough, resistant, and confining characteristics of deep fascia can create problems such as the compartment syndromes. Trauma with hemorrhage in the anterior compartment of the lower leg can cause swelling that is detrimental to the sensitive nerve structures within the compartment. Frequently, surgical fasciectomy is necessary to relieve the compression on neural elements.

Subserous fascia is the loose areolar tissue that covers the internal visceral organs. The many small circulatory channels and fluid within this fascia lubricate the surfaces of the internal viscera.

Function of Fascia

Fascia provides support for vessels and nerves throughout the body. It enables adjacent tissues to move upon each other while providing stability and contour. It provides lubricating fluid between structures for movement and nutrition. The pacinian corpuscles in the superficial fascia provide afferent information for many complex reflexes involving the neuromuscular system. The fascia described is continuous with specialized elements such as ligaments and tendons. These tissues have unique characteristics but share with the general fascia collagen fibers, elastic fibers, cellular elements, and ground substance. Specialized mechanoreceptors and proprioceptors are found within these specialized elements of fascia that report information to the spinal cord and brain on body position and movement, both normal and abnormal. Within the ground substance of the fascia are many of the substances that contribute to immune mechanisms within the body.

Biomechanics of Fascia

Fascia's intimate connection with muscle provides the opportunity for contraction and relaxation. Fascia has elasticity that allows it to both retain its shape and respond to deformation. Elastic deformation is the capacity of fascia to recover its original shape when the load is removed. If the load is great and applied for a longer period of time, fascia may not be able to recover its original size and shape; this results in plastic deformation. When subjected to an extension load and held constant, fascia has the capacity to "creep." The relaxation of the tissue that accompanies creep allows less resistance to a second application of load. This phenomenon has clinical significance when the clinician observes the effects of acute and repetitive injury, and long-term stress, on connective tissues. Fascia has the capacity to change when subjected to stress and lose energy. This phenomenon, called hysteresis, is used therapeutically in myofascial release technique.

Fascial Injury

Fascia responds to acute injury, or chronic recurrent microtrauma (such as postural imbalance due to anatomical short leg), in a variety of ways. The first is the inflammatory process of injury, spanning the spectrum from acute to chronic change. Inflammatory fluid can be easily contained and absorbed in the superficial fascia, but when within the tight compartments of deep fascia, it becomes quite detrimental. These fascial changes are palpable by the trained hand and are contributors to the tissue texture abnormalities characteristic and diagnostic of somatic dysfunction.

Fascia under stress responds biomechanically. Depending on the amount and type of load, deformation may be temporary or permanent. The number and type of collagen and elastic fibers within the connective tissue, and the type of load applied, determine the fascial change that occurs under biomechanical stress. The biomechanical stress of fascial injury causes the receptors to send afferent information to the central nervous system for processing. The ability, or inability, of these receptors to adapt, and the facility of the central nervous system to adjust, determines the short-term or long-term effect on neural integration resulting from the connective tissue injury.

Biochemical and immunological changes occur within the ground substance of the fascia and have general systemic effects that seem quite far removed from the injury to the soft tissues. Scarring during the healing process frequently interferes with the functions of support, movement, and lubrication. Many detrimental symptoms result that are difficult to objectify. Soft tissue changes lead to persistent symptoms long after healing of the acute tissue injury. Victims of flexion extension cervical injuries (whiplash injury) from motor vehicle and other accidents frequently have persistent symptoms that are difficult to explain. Recent research identified fatty replacement of deep cervical muscles in some of these people, which may indicate the effects of "soft tissue injury" accompanying the trauma (see Chapter 21).

MUSCLE

Muscle is the second main focus of myofascial release technique. Muscles can be classified as those that maintain posture, the so-called static muscles, and those that provide movement, the so-called phasic muscles. Muscles can perform both functions, but usually one will predominate. Clinically, the muscles that have postural function respond by facilitation, hypertonicity, and shortening. In the lower half of the body, these include the iliopsoas, rectus femoris, tensor fascia lata, quadratus lumborum, adductors, piriformis, hamstrings, and lumbar erector spinae. In the upper half of the body, the postural muscles that respond by facilitation, hypertonicity, and shortening are the levator scapulae, upper trapezius, sternocleidomastoid, pectorals, scalenes, latissimus dorsi, subscapularis, and flexors of the upper extremity. Dynamic phasic muscles respond by inhibition, hypotonicity, and weakness. In the lower half of the body, these include the gluteus maximus, medius and minimis, rectus abdominous, internal and external abdominal obliques, peroneals, vasti of the thigh, and tibialis anterior. In the upper half of the body, these include the middle and lower trapezius, serratus anterior, rhomboids, supra and infraspinatus, deltoid, deep neck flexors, and extensors of the upper extremity.

Each muscle action has an equal and opposite muscle reaction, the agonist-antagonist principle. Sherrington's law of reciprocal innervation and inhibition balances the tone and function of agonist and antagonist muscles both on the ipsilateral and contralateral side. Sophisticated neuromuscular reflexes constantly maintain body posture and prepare for, initiate, and continue movement patterns.

Function of muscle in the musculoskeletal system is an integrated and highly complex process: motor control through the central nervous system from the premotor cortex through the brainstem, cerebellum, spinal cord, and finally to the final common pathway, the α motor neuron to skeletal muscle. This control system for muscle function is highly complex and has both voluntary and involuntary components. This complex motor programing is altered by afferent impulses coming from the mechanoreceptors within the articular and fascial symptoms. When this central control system is working efficiently, movement patterns are symmetrical, coordinated, and free. When altered, inefficient and uncoordinated movement results. One need only contrast the performance of an olympic-level runner and a patient with advanced Parkinson's disease. Between these two extremes are gradations of hypertonicity, hypotonicity, and altered integrative coordination, particularly noted in patients with minimal brain dysfunction.

Muscle injury interferes with its anatomy and function. Acute trauma results in muscle tears, disturbances at the myotendinous junction, and alterations of insertion of tendon into bone. These injuries undergo fibrosis as part of the healing process similar to other injuries of soft tissues. Functional loss can result. Injury not only alters the anatomy of the muscle but interferes with its neuroreflexive response to motor control and contributes to persistent long-term symptoms.

CONCEPTS IN MYOFASCIAL RELEASE TECHNIQUE

The first concept is *tight-loose*. Within the myofascial system, tightness creates and weakness permits asymmetry. There are biomechanical and neural reflexive elements to the tight-loose concept. Increased stimulation causes an agonist muscle to become tight, and the tighter it becomes, the looser its antagonist becomes of reciprocal inhibition. The fascia surrounding a hypertonic contracted muscle shortens and requires loosening of the fascia in the opposite direction for accommodation. One cannot step a mast on a boat by pulling on the forestay if the backstay is not sufficiently loose to permit movement. In acute conditions, the cycle can be described as continuing spasm-pain-spasm. The result is tightness that progresses from the acute condition of muscle contraction to muscle contracture leading to chronicity. In chronic conditions, the cycle is described as pain-looseness-pain. Manual medicine practitioners are familiar with the painful symptoms of hypermobility. The practitioners using myofascial release procedures apply the fundamental tight-loose concept on a continuing basis.

The second concept is the use of *palpation* in myofascial pain syndromes. Many diagnostic and therapeutic systems build on peripheral stimulation and include acupuncture, acupressure, Chapman's reflexes, Travell's trigger points, and Jones' tender points. Skilled palpation of myofascial elements frequently identifies locations of myofascial pain that can be therapeutically addressed by the hands. Frequently noted is the occurrence of myofascial pain in areas of soft tissue looseness. Sensitivity of the myofascial elements, particularly in the chronic state, frequently have a burning quality. Recall that the sympathetic division of the autonomic nervous system is the only division that innervates the musculoskeletal system. Many symptoms found in myofascial pain syndromes are probably mediated by sympathetic nervous system reflexes.

The third concept is *neuroreflexive change* occurring with the application of manual force on the musculoskeletal system. Hands-on application of force to the musculoskeletal system results in afferent stimulation through mechanoreceptors that require central processing at the spinal cord, brainstem, and cortical levels. Afferent stimulation frequently results in efferent inhibition. When afferent stimulation of a stretch is applied during a myofascial release procedure, the operator waits for relaxation in the tight tissues by efferent inhibition. The neuroreflexive response is highly variable and modified by the amount of pain, the patient's pain behavior, the level of wellness, the nutritional status, stress response, and basic life-style of the individual, including the use and abuse of alcohol, tobacco, and drugs, including prescription medications.

The fourth concept is the *release* phenomenon. The sensation of release is found in other forms of manual medicine, particularly in craniosacral technique and the ease-bind of functional-indirect technique. When using myofascial release technique, appropriate application of stress on tissue results in tissue relaxation both in the fascia and in muscle. Tightness "gives way" or "melts" under the application of load. Release of tightness is sought to achieve improvement in symmetry of form and function. The release phenomena is both an enabling and terminal objective when applying a myofascial release procedure. Release can occur in several directions and through different levels of tissue during a myofascial release procedure. The release phenomena is one that guides the practitioner through the treatment process.

PRINCIPLES OF MYOFASCIAL RELEASE EVALUATION

Ward has expanded his mnemonic M A I (N)4 to B E M A I (N)4. *B* stands for behavior, particularly as to the patient response to stress. Behavioral response to stress is modified by many factors, including race, education, family, financial status, religion, among others. Patients respond differently to the stress of their injuries as well as to the hands-on process of the patient-provider interaction. Behavioral issues, particularly in patients with chronic pain, are significant in any therapeutic outcome.

E stands for endocrine status. The endocrine system influences all of the other systems of the human organism. It has major influence on the musculoskeletal system and responds to stress within the musculoskeletal system. Alteration in thyroid function and carbohydrate metabolism in diabetes alters the response of the musculoskeletal system to stress and injury and alters its response to treatment interventions. Assessment of the musculoskeletal system by palpation identifies tissue texture abnormalities that may be associated with disturbances of the endocrine system. Therapeutic interventions used within the myofascial release technique system will alter the stimulation to the endocrine system and its close linkage with the nervous system.

M stands for mechanical analysis of the musculoskeletal system for its symmetry-asymmetry, looseness-tightness, and its response to postural balance or imbalance. Mechanical loading is important in the injury process and is also involved in the therapeutic process.

A stands for anatomy and the overall functional capacity of the body. Assessment is made in a three-dimensional sense of all of the anatomy of the body with particular reference to muscle function, joint mechanics, and nervous system control. The practitioner should have a working knowledge of the integration of all elements of the musculoskeletal system, particularly the integrating aspects of fascia and the motor control of the musculoskeletal system. The examiner assesses both symmetry or asymmetry of form and function, recognizing that asymmetry is the rule, whereas symmetrical function is the goal of any treatment outcome.

I stands for the immune system and the response of the patient to stress. The patient's immune system is highly complex and responds to many factors beginning with the general health status of the patient and the response to stressors in the internal and external environment. Altered immune function, particularly associated with rheumatological conditions, strongly influence the musculoskeletal system and its response to stress and to treatment interventions.

N stands for altered neurological function. The central nervous system is highly complex and is subject to both functional and pathological change. Assessment of the patient's nervous system function by traditional neurological examination assists in differentiating functional from organic pathologies of the central nervous system. There are many other neurological considerations, including the assessment of autonomic nervous system function. Are there palpable changes in the musculoskeletal system that may reflect alteration in autonomic nervous system balance and tone? Nervous system responses are influenced by the patient's life-style and psychological status. As part of neurological response, the examiner is interested in the nociceptive behavior of the patient. A patient's response to pain, pain behavior, and life-style will influence the patient's response to a nociceptive episode. The patient's nutritional status strongly affects the nervous system. Poor nutrition, particularly of the inadequacy of B-complex vitamins, results in abnormal nervous system function. Nutritional status, along with alcohol and tobacco use or abuse and prescribed medications and street drug use, strongly influences response of the patient's nervous system.

The assessment of the patient using the myofascial release system must be viewed from a total integrative perspective. All of these behavioral, anatomical, and physiological factors must be kept in mind when assessing the patient and when providing the therapeutic intervention.

MYOFASCIAL RELEASE TREATMENT CONCEPTS

Ward has coined another mnemonic to describe the principles of myofascial release treatment, P O E (T)². P O E stands for *point of entry* into the musculoskeletal system. Entry may be made from anywhere in the musculoskeletal system, including the lower extremity, the upper extremity, the thoracic cage, the abdomen, and the vertebral complex from the cranial cervical junction to the pelvis. (T)² stands for *traction and twist*. Traction and twist are but two of the applications of load that are of assistance in the diagnostic and treatment process. Traction produces stretch along the long axis of myofascial elements that are short and tight. Stretch should always be applied in the long axis rather than transversely across myofascial elements. Twisting force provides the opportunity to localize the traction, not only at the point of contact with the patient but also at points some distance away. Compressive and shear forces are also used to localize to different levels of the myofascial system and to provide different loads. The practitioner should develop the ability to sense change both locally at the point of contact as well as at some distance away. For example, when grasping the lower extremity near the ankle, the operator should attempt to feel through the extremity to the knee, thigh, hip, sacroiliac joint, and into the vertebral column, sensing changes that occur at each level. This is all perceived through the contact point at the ankle. This skill requires concentration, practice, and an appreciation for the three-dimensional aspects of the musculoskeletal system.

The treatment process includes assessment of tightness and looseness throughout the system and the application of loads, both into the direct and indirect barriers, seeking the release phenomena. Tightness and looseness can be different between the superficial and deep layers of the musculoskeletal system. Frequently, tightness in the superficial layers is found overlying the looseness in the deeper structures surrounding the articular elements. This may well be compensatory in nature, but the superficial tightness and the deep-level looseness should both be approached appropriately so that the result is more symmetric function throughout the system.

Patient activity during the treatment process can assist in the achievement of the therapeutic goal. These *enhancers* include muscle contraction, joint motion of both the upper and lower extremities, respiration, and eye movement. Any activity that increases the central nervous system processing seems to enhance the effectiveness of the practitioner-applied loading forces. One or more enhancers may be used throughout the treatment process.

After treatment by these techniques, patients are given specific exercises that are individualized for their problem. Stretching exercise maintains the added length of the tight tissues, and strengthening exercise restores the functional capacity of the weaker inhibited muscles. In treatment of muscle imbalance, first stretch the short tight muscle groups and follow with strengthening exercise for the weaker loose muscle groups. Exercise programs should also enhance the integrative function of muscle balance. Such exercises as cross-pattern pep walking, swimming, square dancing, rebounding, and so on can be used. The goal is to increase mobility and strength but also to enhance muscular coordination.

These procedures are more than biomechanical and neuroreflexive. They address the total patient. General health issues such as life-style, coping mechanisms, appropriate use of alcohol and other medications, discontinuance of tobacco, adequate and appropriate nutrition, and weight control are all issues that need to be addressed concurrently with the myofascial release treatment program.

EXERCISES IN PALPATION

Myofascial release procedures require skill at palpating the musculoskeletal system for something other than one bone moving on the other. One must learn to "read the tissues" for their tightness-looseness and their inherent mobility, in addition to the usual soft tissue texture abnormalities of hard-soft, cool-warm, smooth-rough, and so on referred to in Chapter 2. One needs to develop increased sensitivity to the patient's tissues both at point of contact and at some distance. There are many exercises in palpation that can be useful, and the following exercises are but a few.

Place the fingertips of all five fingers together without contact with the rest of the hand. Introduce force from one hand to the other and then reverse. Sense what goes on with the hand generating the force and the one receiving the force. Are they different from side to side? Now take one hand and stroke with the fingerpads down the volar surface of the fingers and palms, first with light stroking and then with increased pressure. Repeat using the other hand as the motor hand. Sense the difference in the sensitivity of the hand being stroked, as well as the sensation of touch by the fingerpads of the motor hand. To properly sense what goes on in the patient, you must have an awareness of your own palpatory skills and sensations and your own self-body awareness.

Fold your hands together interlacing all your fingers. You will find that either the right or the left second metacarpophalangeal joint is on top. Now reverse the position so that the other metacarpophalangeal joint is on top. Sense the difference, with one appearing to be more comfortable than the other and with the less comfortable one feeling tighter.

Stretch your arms out ahead of you, crossing them at the wrist and pronating both hands until the palmar surfaces meet. Interlace your fingers and raise the extended arms over your head. As you reach toward the ceiling, feel the difference in tension between the right and left sides of your body. Return to the starting position, reverse the way in which your wrists are crossed, and repeat the procedure. Again, note the difference in tension from side to side and the difference introduced by alternate crossing of the wrists.

Working with a patient partner, return to the forearm described in Chapter 2. This time start with your palpating hand some distance from the forearm and slowly move toward the forearm until you begin to feel radiant energy from the patient. This is usually sensed as heat. Repeat the procedure several times with your eyes closed to see whether you can repeatedly stop at the point where you first feel the sensation and whether the distance from your palpating hand to the forearm is consistent. Continue to approach the forearm until you are palpating just the superficial hair and course up and down over the forearm, attempting to sense what is going on under your hand. See whether you can identify differences in the proximal forearm, distal forearm, wrist, and hand. Place your hand in contact with the skin and concentrate, applying no motion of your own, but attempt to sense the inherent movement of the patient's tissues under your hand. It takes several seconds to several minutes to begin to sense an inherent oscillatory movement within the forearm.

When you have mastered the ability to apply pressure but not movement and the ability to sense inherent movement within your patient, place the palm of your hand in contact with the bony sacrum. This should be done both in the supine and prone posi-

tion. The contour of the sacrum fits nicely in the palm of your hand. In the prone position, it is sometimes necessary to use a slight compressive force to begin to feel the inherent motion of the sacrum. In a supine position, the patient's body weight on your hand is sufficient to initiate inherent sacral movement. Try to follow the sacrum in the directions in which it wishes to move. Do not attempt to direct it. What is the rhythm, amplitude, and direction of the sacrum moving in space? When you have been able to identify inherent soft tissue and bony movement, you are well on your way to being able to use myofascial release technique.

EXAMPLES OF MYOFASCIAL RELEASE TECHNIQUE

There are a wide variety of myofascial release techniques in use by many practitioners. They are highly individualized to the skill of the practitioner and to the needs of the patient at the treatment visit. The following examples are those taught by Ward but have been found most effective in this author's hands. They provide the reader with only a small sample of the total system.

Myofascial Release Technique

Lumbosacral Spine One

Prone with longitudinal traction

1. Patient prone with arms off side of table, feet over the end, with head turned to the most comfortable side.

2. Operator stands at side of patient facing foot of table, if right handed, on patient's left, if left handed, on patient's right.

3. Operator places distal hand over sacrum with heel of hand at lumbosacral junction. Operator's proximal hand is placed in the midline over the thoracolumbar junction with fingers pointing caudally (Fig. 11.1).

4. Operator introduces compression and separates both hands in a longitudinal fashion sensing for symmetry or asymmetry (Fig. 11.2).

5. Operator follows inherent tissue motion, sensing direct and indirect barriers, constantly searching for balance of tightness and looseness.

6. Operator applies twisting and torsional loads as necessary to achieve balance while the patient uses enhancing maneuvers.

7. After release(s) is achieved, reassess for enhanced motion and balance.

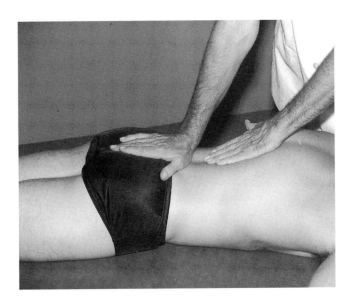

Figure 11.1.

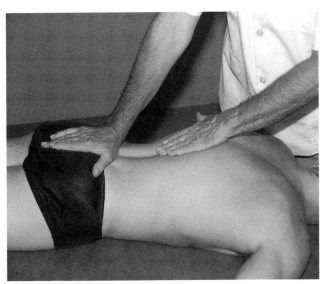

Figure 11.2.

Myofascial Release Technique

Lumbosacral Spine

Prone with transverse traction

1. Patient prone on table with arms at side and feet off end and with head turned to most comfortable position.

2. Operator stands at side of table with cephalic hand transversely across the thoracolumbar junction and the caudal hand transversely across the lumbosacral junction and sacral base (Fig. 11.3).

3. Operator applies compression and introduces transverse shear in opposite directions sensing for tightness and looseness (Fig. 11.4).

4. Operator may apply a twisting force as barriers are engaged (Fig. 11.5).

5. Operator follows inherent tissue motion sensing for balance of tightness and looseness while patient performs enhancing maneuvers.

6. After release(s) are achieved, reassess for enhanced motion and balance.

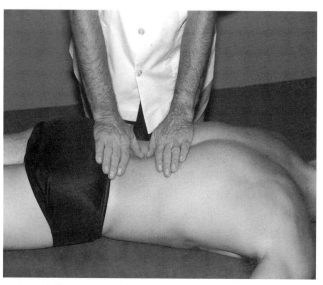

Figure 11.3.

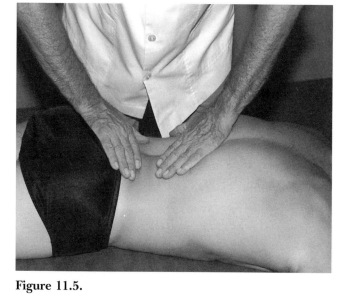

Figure 11.5.

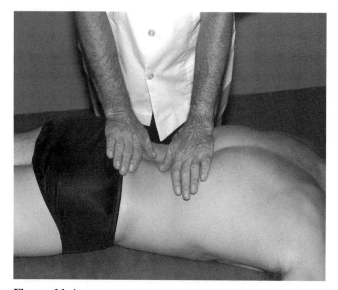

Figure 11.4.

Myofascial Release Technique

Thoracolumbar Junction and Posterior Diaphragm

Prone

1. Patient prone with arms off side of table and feet off the end and with head turned to the most comfortable side.
2. Operator stands at side of patient facing toward the head.
3. Operator's hands are placed on each side of the thoracolumbar junction with the thumbs vertical along the spinous processes and the remainder of the hand along the lower ribs overlying the posterior diaphragm (Fig. 11.6).
4. Operator's whole hand introduces compressive load and the left moves clockwise while the right moves counterclockwise in a lateral and superior direction (Fig. 11.7).
5. Operator assesses direct and indirect barriers from superficial to deep sensing for tissue balance while patient performs enhancing maneuvers.
6. Redness of the skin is frequently seen after this technique and is described as the "blush" phenomenon.
7. After release(s) is achieved, reassess for enhanced motion and balance.

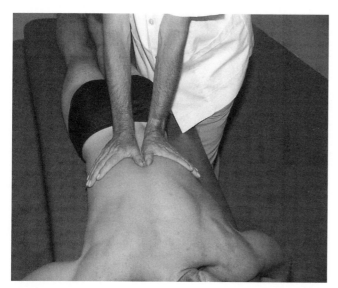

Figure 11.6.

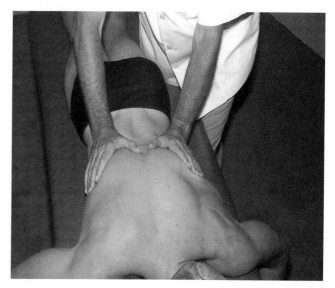

Figure 11.7.

Myofascial Release Technique

Prone

Sacral release
1. Patient prone with arms off side and feet off end of table with head turned to the most comfortable side.
2. Operator places hand over sacrum with heel over base and fingers over the apex, including the inferior lateral angles (Fig. 11.8).
3. Operator's other hand is placed on top (Fig. 11.9).

4. Operator's hand pressure is anterior and inferior with a rocking motion from side to side, forward and backward, and across the oblique axes.
5. Operator follows the inherent sacral motion sensing for indirect barriers (looseness) and direct barriers (tightness) until release(s) occurs.
6. Patient performs enhancing maneuvers to assist in treatment procedure.
7. Treatment goal is balance of the sacrum between the innominates.

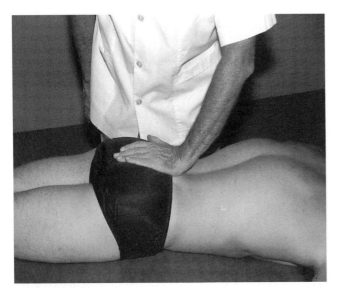

Figure 11.8.

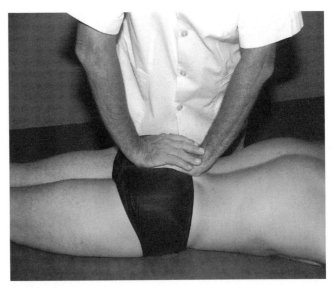

Figure 11.9.

Myofascial Release Technique

Prone

Sacrotuberous ligament and urogenital diaphragm release

1. Patient prone with arms off side and feet off end of table with head turned to the most comfortable side.

2. Operator at side of table facing cephalward places hands over buttock area with the thigh in contact with the sacrotuberous attachments at the inferior lateral angles of the sacrum (Fig. 11.10).

3. Tension in the sacrotuberous ligaments is tested for symmetrical balance.

4. Operator's hands twist in a clockwise and counter-clockwise direction sensing for tightness and looseness (Fig. 11.11).

5. Operator applies load to balance tension in the sacrotuberous ligament while the patient performs enhancing maneuvers.

6. Treatment goal is balance of the sacrotuberous ligaments and urogenital diaphragm.

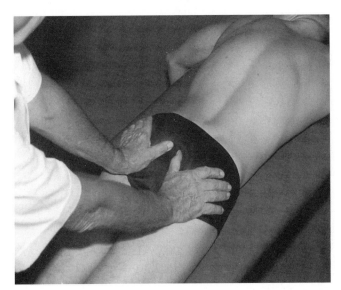

Figure 11.10.

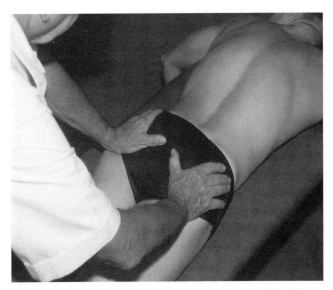

Figure 11.11.

Myofascial Release Technique

Supine or Sitting

Thoracic inlet (necklace) technique

1. Patient sitting on table with operator standing behind with both hands encircling the thoracic inlet (Fig. 11.12) with the thumbs on each side of the spinous process of T1 (Fig. 11.13).

2. Patient supine on table with operator sitting at head of table and hands placed on thoracic inlet as above (Fig. 11.14).

3. Operator's hands in contact with thoracic inlet with palms over trapezius and fingers contacting the medial end of the clavicle and upper sternum introducing compression followed by twisting and traction load seeking direct and indirect barriers (Figs. 11.15 and 11.16).

4. Operator using a steering wheel action rotates the thoracic inlet to symmetry of anteroposterior and rotary balance.

5. Various arm positions of the patient are used to enhance load application. Patient performs enhancing maneuvers to increase release(s).

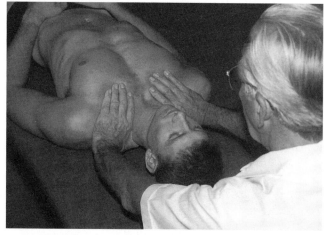

Figure 11.14.

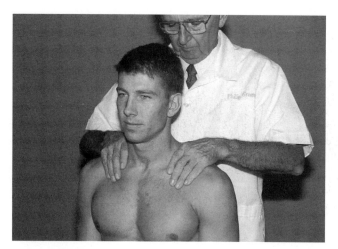

Figure 11.12.

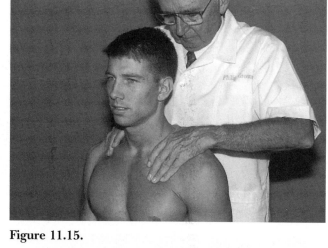

Figure 11.15.

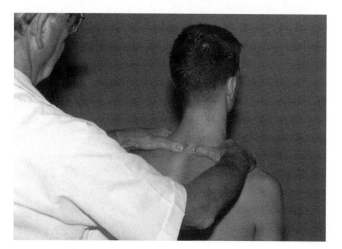

Figure 11.13.

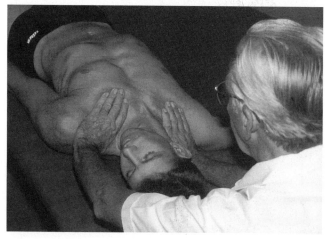

Figure 11.16.

Myofascial Release Technique

Sitting

Thoracic Spine

1. Patient sitting on table with operator sitting facing away from the patient with the trunk against the patient for stability.

2. Operator's anterior hand is vertically placed over the sternum with the fingertips covering the manubriosternal junction (Fig. 11.17).

3. Operator's posterior hand is placed vertically over the spinous processes of the lower to midthoracic spine (Fig. 11.18).

4. For the upper thoracic spine, the operator's left hand is transversely placed across the sternum, upper ribs, and medial end of the clavicles (Fig. 11.19).

5. Operator's posterior hand is transversely placed across the upper thoracic spine (Fig. 11.20).

6. Operator's hands apply compression, cephalic to caudad shear, transverse shear, and clockwise and counterclockwise twisting loads seeking direct and indirect barriers.

7. Patient performs enhancing maneuvers to assist in the enhancement of release(s).

These are but a few examples of myofascial release technique. They can be used as the primary manual medicine intervention or as a terminal technique to assess the success of other manual medicine interventions to ensure that myofascial balance has been achieved. Some practitioners find these techniques to be fatiguing and time consuming, whereas others find them easy.

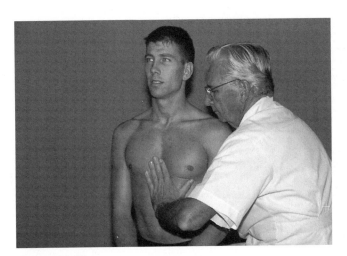

Figure 11.17.

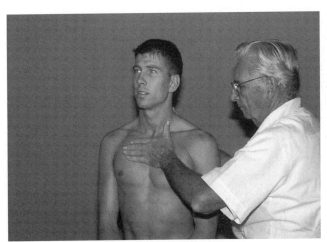

Figure 11.19.

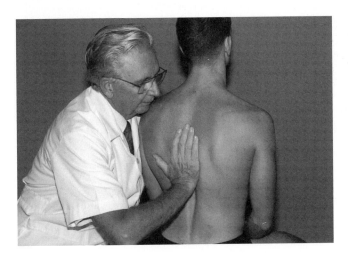

Figure 11.18.

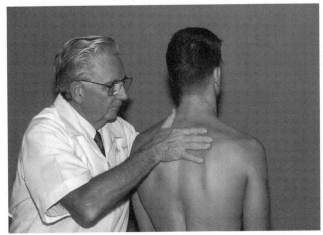

Figure 11.20.

CONCLUSION

Myofascial release techniques use both direct and indirect action with activating forces that are both extrinsic and intrinsic. They influence the biomechanics of the musculoskeletal system and the reflexes that direct, integrate, and modify movement. The goal is restoring functional balance to all of the integrative tissues in the musculoskeletal system, and the techniques are useful in acute, subacute, and chronic conditions, with simple and complex problems. The techniques can be used in multiple patient positions.

They usually consist of symmetrical placement of the operator's hands, introducing some twisting force to engage the tissues and then following directly or indirectly along fascial planes to sense areas of tightness and looseness. Traction is placed on the tight area awaiting the sensation of release. Release is hypothesized as following reflex neural efferent inhibition and biomechanical hysteresis within the tissues. The techniques are highly individualized to the patient's need and the operator's training and experience.

12

William G. Sutherland, D.O., is credited with extending the osteopathic concept and osteopathic manipulative treatment above the craniocervical junction. After many years of study, research, and self-manipulation, Sutherland began to teach the principles of craniosacral technique in the mid-1940s. Craniosacral technique procedures were not readily received in the professional community but have become increasingly popular through the work of Sutherland and his many students.

Sutherland extended the principle of Andrew Taylor Still to the articulations of the skull. He reasoned that the sutures functioned as joints between the bones of the skull and were intricately fashioned for the maintenance of motion. The sutures are present throughout life and consistently have similar areas of bevel change. Skulls can be disarticulated by "explosion" (filling with beans through the foramen magnum and then immersing in water), and the bones consistently separate at the sutures. The bone does not fracture; the sutures separate. Sutherland reasoned that the skull would have normal mobility during health and show restrictions in response to trauma or systemic disease. Clinical observations were consistent with his hypothesis. Since Sutherland's time, an increasing body of clinical evidence and research support some of the basic premises of his concept. Craniosacral technique requires the practitioner to make an intense study of the osseous cranium, sutures, and meninges and finely tune the palpatory sense necessary to perceive inherent mobility within the craniosacral mechanism. Application of manual medicine procedures to the cranium and sacrum require precision and dexterity.

ANATOMY

The skull can be divided into three elements: (a) the vault, consisting of portions of the frontal bone, the two parietal bones, the occipital squama, and the temporal squama which develop from membrane; (b) the base, consisting of the body of the sphenoid, the petrous and mastoid portions of the temporals, and the basilar and condylar portions of the occiput that form in cartilage; and (c) the facial bones. The bones of the skull can be further divided into those that are paired and unpaired. The unpaired midline bones are the occiput, sphenoid, ethmoid, and vomer. The paired bones include the parietals, temporals, maxillae, zygoma, palatines, nasals, and the frontal. The frontal is viewed as a paired bone because of the functional characteristics it provides and the fact that the metopic suture frequently remains open during life. The mandible has both paired and unpaired characteristics. It is bilaterally related to the temporal bones, but when the teeth are present and approximated, they serve as a long suture between the mandible and the two maxillae.

MOTION

The motion of the midline bones is primarily flexion and extension with an overturning moment around a transverse (x) axis. The flexion-extension movement is described as occurring at the sphenobasilar junction, a synchondrosis. During this movement, the sphenoid and occiput rotate in opposite directions. During sphenobasilar flexion, the sphenoid rotates anteriorly with the basisphenoid being elevated and the pterygoid processes moving inferiorly. Concurrently, the occiput rotates posteriorly with the basiocciput being elevated and the squama portion and condylar parts being depressed caudally. During sphenobasilar flexion, the ethmoid rotates in the opposite direction to the sphenoid and in the same direction as the occiput. During sphenobasilar flexion, the vomer is carried caudad as the anterior portion of the sphenoid moves in that direction. During sphenobasilar extension, all of the motions are reversed. The paired bones move into internal and external rotation as they accompany sphenobasilar flexion and extension. During sphenobasilar flexion, there is external rotation of the paired bones, and during extension, there is internal rotation.

The combination of flexion and extension of the midline unpaired bones and the internal-external rotation of the paired bones causes observable change in cranial contour. With flexion, the transverse diameter of the skull increases, the anteroposterior diameter decreases, and the vertex flattens. With sphenobasilar extension, the transverse diameter decreases, the anteroposterior diameter increases, and the vertex becomes more prominent. The facial bones can be viewed as being suspended from the frontal bone.

The paired bones consist of the parietal, temporal, frontal, zygoma, maxilla, palatine and nasal bones. Their motion is described as internal and external rotation and is normally synchronous with sphenobasilar flexion and extension. During sphenobasilar flexion, there is external rotation of the paired bones, and during extension, there is internal rotation. The sphenoid determines the motion characteristics of the paired facial bones. Dysfunction of the front half of the cranium, particularly the facial bones, is related to altered function of the sphenoid. Dysfunction of the posterior half of the cranium relates to dysfunction of the occipital bone.

MENINGES

The dura is attached at the foramen magnum and continues down the spinal canal with attachment to the upper two or three cervical vertebra and continues freely until attachment at the second segment of the sacrum. This membrane attachment appears to link the sacral component of the craniosacral mechanism. As one of many movements, the sacrum has an involuntary nutation-counternutation movement that is synchronous with flexion-extension at the sphenobasilar junction. During sphenobasilar flexion, the foramen magnum is elevated and the tension on the dura causes the base of the sacrum to move posteriorly and the apex anteriorly. This counternutational movement is described as craniosacral flexion. During sphenobasilar extension, the foramen magnum moves inferiorly, reducing tension on the dura and resulting in the sacral base moving anteriorly and the apex posteriorly. This nutational movement is called craniosacral extension. The terms flexion and extension are the reverse of that used in a postural-structural model for sacral mechanics. Despite the terminology confusion, the concept to be understood is the relationship of the movement of the occiput and the sacrum that normally occurs in synchronous directions.

SUTURES

The sutures are joints that join the bones of the skull. There are many different types of sutures that are designed to permit and direct specific types of movement between opposing cranial bones. The sutures contain extensions of the dura and other connective tissue, primarily Sharpey's fibers. Anatomical and histological study of the sutures shows that the fiber direction is not haphazard and random but specific at each sutural level. The sutures contain blood vessels with accompanying nerves for vasomotor control. Free nerve endings with unmyelinated C fibers are found within the sutures, suggesting the possibility of pain perception and transmission. A detailed description of the cranial sutures is beyond the scope of this text. The reader is strongly urged to study not only the classical anatomical work but the sutures found on each bone of a disarticulated skull.

SUTURE PALPATION EXERCISE

The following palpation exercise identifies palpable sutures in a living subject and the location of anatomical parts used in diagnosis and treatment of cranial dysfunctions:

1. Palpate the depression at the base of the nose and between each orbit (Fig. 12.1). This is the junction of the two nasal bones and the frontal bone and is called nasion.
2. Proceed laterally over the upper margin of the orbit and follow it laterally and inferiorly to the upper-outer portion and feel the frontozygomatic suture.
3. Continuing inferiorly along the lateral aspect of the orbit and beginning to move medially, one feels the zygomaticomaxillary suture.
4. Continuing medially along the inferior aspect of the orbit and up its medial way, palpate the suture of the maxillonasal junction and the maxillofrontal suture.
5. Returning to the nasion, move upward between the two supra orbital ridges of the frontal bone, the midline of which is a point called glabella. Moving superiorly from glabella along the midline, the palpator may feel the remnant of the metopic suture either as a depression or a ridge.
6. Continuing toward the vertex of the skull in the midline, one strikes a depression approximately one-third of the way posteriorly on the vertex. This depression is the junction of the sagittal and coronal sutures and is the remnant of the anterior fontanelle and is called bregma.
7. Moving posteriorly from bregma along the midline, the sagittal suture is palpable, and by moving the fingerpads from side to side, one can feel the serrated sutural contour.
8. Starting from bregma, palpate bilaterally along the coronal suture, feeling the junction of the frontal and the parietal bone on each side (Fig. 12.2). At the lower extremity of the coronal suture, the palpating finger moves somewhat deeper and palpates the

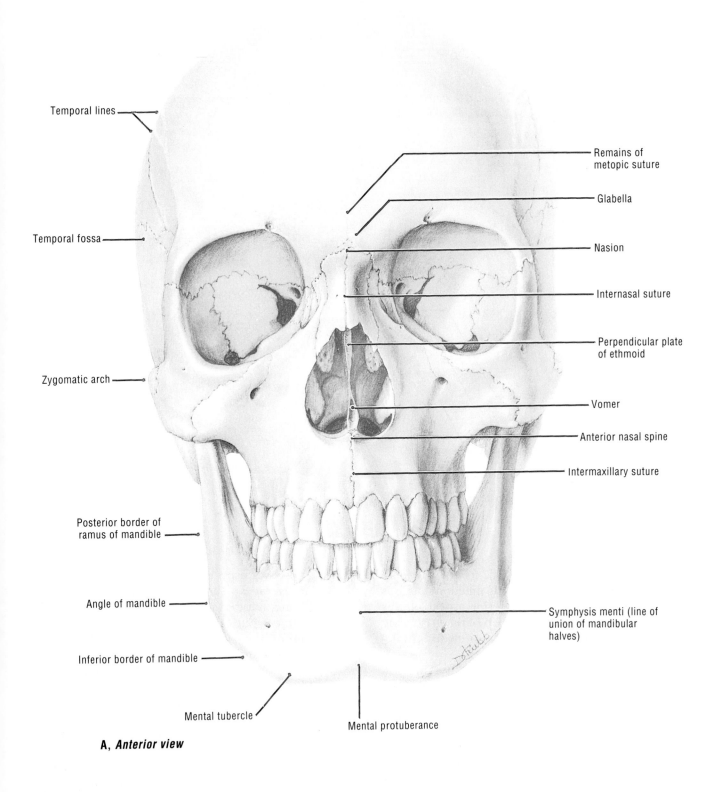

Temporal lines

Temporal fossa

Zygomatic arch

Posterior border of
ramus of mandible

Angle of mandible

Inferior border of mandible

Mental tubercle

Remains of
metopic suture

Glabella

Nasion

Internasal suture

Perpendicular plate
of ethmoid

Vomer

Anterior nasal spine

Intermaxillary suture

Symphysis menti (line of
union of mandibular
halves)

Mental protuberance

A, *Anterior view*

Figure 12.1.
Skull, frontal view.

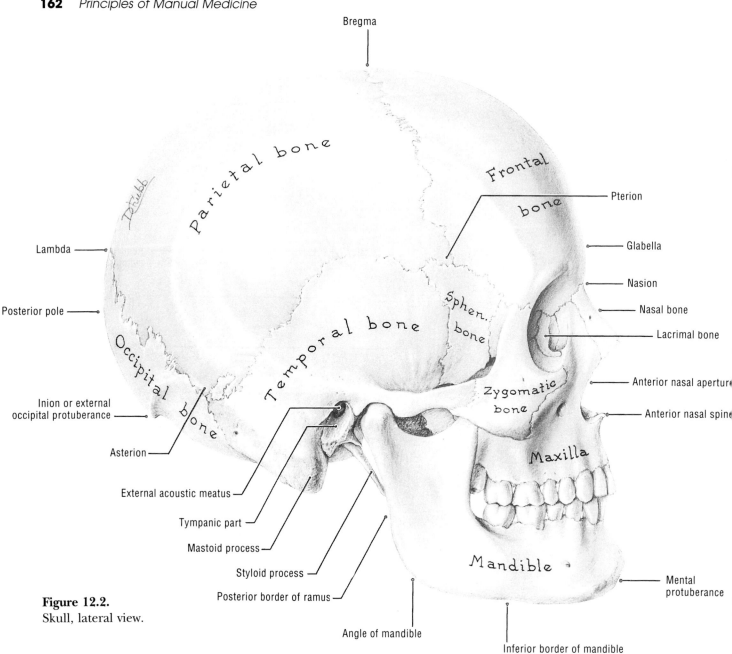

Figure 12.2.
Skull, lateral view.

junction of the sphenoid, frontal, parietal, and temporal bones. This junctional area is called pterion. The inferior aspect of this junction is the palpable tip of the great wing of the sphenoid used extensively for craniosacral diagnosis and treatment.

9. From the pterion, follow the suture line posteriorly along the junction of the parietal and temporal squama. This suture courses over the top of the ear in a circular fashion and ends just posterior to the ear.

10. Moving straight posteriorly from the posterior inferior aspect of the suture between the parietal and the temporal squama is a short suture between the parietal bone and the mastoid portion of the temporal. At the

posterior aspect of this suture is a slight depression at the junction of the parietal bone, mastoid portion of the temporal, and the occiput called the asterion.

11. From the asterion, move inferiorly along the posterior aspect of the mastoid process, following the occipital mastoid suture. The lower portion of this suture is lost in the soft tissues of the muscular attachment of the head to the neck.

12. From the asterion on each side, course medially and superiorly along the lambdoidal suture separating the parietal bone from the occipital squama, and where the two sutures join with the sagittal suture is found the point called lambda (Fig. 12.3). The

lambdoidal sutures are frequently asymmetric and occasionally contain extra bony structures called wormian bones.

This exercise should be repeated on multiple patients until the examiner is confident of the ability to palpate the sutures of the skull and identify landmarks used to control the bones of the skull during the examination and the treatment process. The pterion and asterion are the two most frequently used in the craniosacral technique system.

CRANIAL MENINGES

The meninges are divided into three layers: the pia, arachnoid, and dura (Fig. 12.4). The external layer of the dura is continuous with the periosteum and the cranium. The internal layer has several duplications that separate segments of the brain and encircle the venous sinuses.

There are three duplications of the dura with intricate fiber directions in each and are named the falx cerebri, tentorium cerebelli, and falx cerebelli.

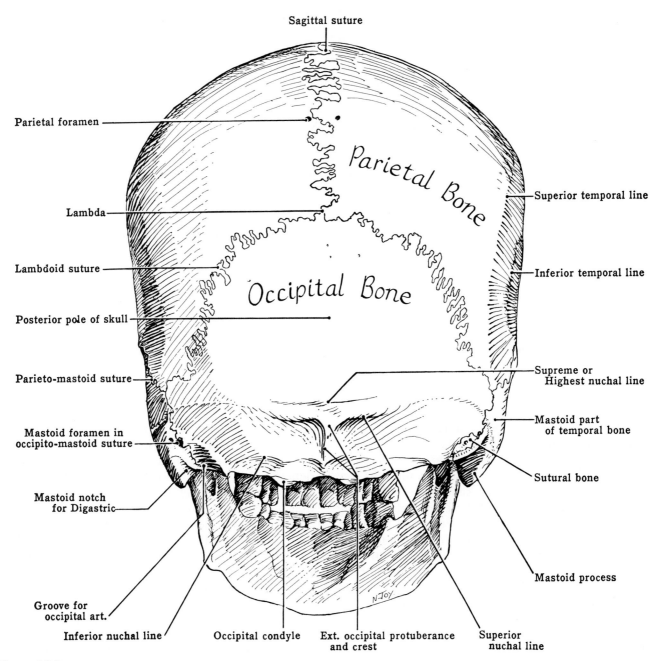

Figure 12.3.
Skull, posterior view.

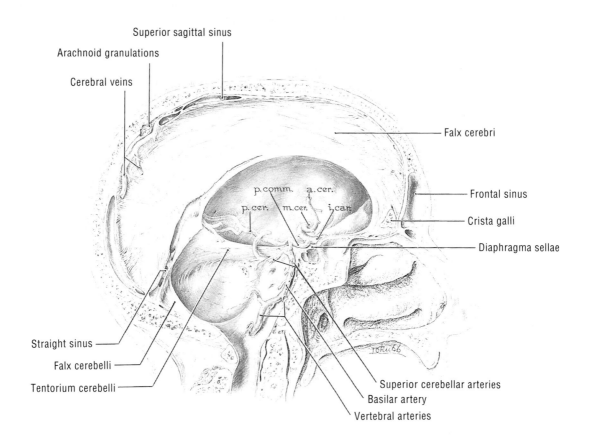

Superior sagittal sinus

Arachnoid granulations

Cerebral veins

Falx cerebri

p.comm. a.cer.

p.cer. m.cer. i.car.

Frontal sinus

Crista galli

Diaphragma sellae

Straight sinus

Falx cerebelli

Tentorium cerebelli

Superior cerebellar arteries

Basilar artery

Vertebral arteries

Figure 12.4.
Cranial meninges.

The falx cerebri is attached anteriorly to the crista galli of the ethmoid, the frontal bone, both parietal bones, and the occipital squama. It encloses the superior sagittal sinus at its osseous attachment. At its free border is found the inferior sagittal sinus. The falx cerebri separates the two cerebral hemispheres. The tentorium cerebelli separates the cerebrum and cerebellum and attaches to the sphenoid, occiput, both parietals, and temporal bones. It attaches to the petrous ridges of the temporal bones and along the occipital squama where it encloses the transverse sinus. It is attached to the posterior inferior corner of each parietal bone where the transverse sinus starts into the sigmoid sinus. At the junction of the falx cerebri and the tentorium cerebelli is found the straight sinus. This junction is of significance as the location of the reciprocal tension membrane, called the "Suther-

land fulcrum." The falx cerebelli separates the two hemispheres of the cerebellum. The diaphragm sellae covers the sella turcica of the sphenoid and is penetrated by the stalk of the pituitary. These dural membranes are under constant dynamic tension so that increased tension in one requires relaxation in another and vice versa. During sphenobasilar flexion, there is shortening of the falx cerebri from before backward because of the overturning of the sphenoid and occiput in opposite directions. This is accompanied by flattening of the tentorium cerebelli, resulting from external rotation of the two temporal bones. During sphenobasilar extension, the reverse occurs with the lengthening of the anteroposterior diameter of the skull by rotation of the sphenoid and the occiput and elevation of the tentorium cerebelli because of internal rotation of the temporal bones.

Craniosacral motion combines articular mobility and change in tension within the membranes. The membranous attachment at the foramen magnum of the occiput and at S2 of the sacrum determines the synchronous movement of the cranium and the sacrum. This dural attachment allows the examiner to influence the cranium through the sacrum and the sacrum through the cranium.

RESPIRATION AND THE THREE DIAPHRAGMS

Sphenobasilar flexion and extension is related to and influenced by voluntary respiratory activity. Inhalation enhances sphenobasilar flexion and exhalation enhances sphenobasilar extension. The tentorium cerebelli can be viewed as the diaphragm of the craniosacral mechanism. It descends and flattens during inhalation similar to the thoracoabdominal diaphragm. The pelvic diaphragm is intimately related to the sacrum within the osseous pelvis. The pelvic diaphragm also descends during inhalation. One can then view the body from the perspective of the three diaphragms: the tentorium cerebelli, the thoracoabdominal diaphragm, and the pelvic diaphragm. In health, these diaphragms should function in a synchronous fashion. If dysfunction interferes with the capacity of any of the three, it is reasonable to assume that the other two will be altered as well. This observation has been made in clinical practice.

PRIMARY RESPIRATORY MECHANISM

By placing both hands over the superior and lateral aspects of the skull like a wet towel, waiting for a sufficient period of time, the examiner experiences the palpatory sensation of widening and narrowing of the skull. This motion sensation occurs at a normal rate of 10–14 times per minute and is of a relatively low amplitude. This sensation, called the cranial rhythmic impulse, is interpreted as the result of the primary respiratory mechanism. Sutherland postulated the existence of the primary respiratory mechanism as consisting of the following five components.

1. Inherent mobility of brain and spinal cord. The living tissue of the brain appears to have an inherent mobility observable during a craniotomy procedure. The motion has been described as that of coiling and uncoiling of the cerebral hemispheres. During the uncoiling process, the cerebral hemispheres appear to swing upward and the unpaired bones move into flexion while the paired bones move into external rotation. During the coiling process, the cerebral hemispheres descend and the unpaired midline bones move into extension motion while the paired bones move into internal rotation. The cause of this inherent bone motility is unknown at this time but is one of the biological rhythms that cannot be artificially restored if lost.

2. Fluctuation of the cerebral spinal fluid (CSF). The CSF is formed in the vesicles in the lateral ventricles and flows through the third and fourth ventricles, into the cisterns of the skull, and throughout the spinal canal. Obstruction to the flow of CSF leads to pathological conditions such as hydrocephalus. The site of exit of the CSF from the system is not well known, but CSF follows dural attachments to the spinal nerves and to the spinal nerves themselves. The coiling of the brain seems to increase the volume of the cerebral ventricles, whereas uncoiling seems to compress them. This may explain some of the mechanisms for the circulation of CSF fluid.

3. Motility of intracranial and intraspinal membranes. The falx cerebri, falx cerebelli, and tentorium cerebelli are all duplications of the intracranial dura. The membranes within these structures have an intimate and intricate pattern suggestive of stress bands. The intracranial membranes are continuously under dynamic tension so that a change in one requires adaptive change in another. During sphenobasilar flexion, the tent descends and flattens and the falx cerebri shortens from before backward. In sphenobasilar extension, the reverse occurs. The intracranial membranes connect with the intraspinal membranes through continuity from the firm attachment at the foramen magnum down the spinal canal to the upper two or three cervical vertebra and then to the attachment to the second sacral segment. Movement of the foramen magnum alters tension on the anterior and posterior aspects of the spinal dura, resulting in motion of the sacrum between the two innominates.

4. Articular mobility of cranial bones. The sutures appear to be developed to permit and guide certain types of movement between cranial bones. The cranial bones and sutures are intimately attached to the dura and contain vascular and nervous system elements. Sharpey's fibers within the sutures have a consistent direction between anatomical specimens. These fibers appear to permit and yield to motion in certain directions. Sutural obliteration does not appear to occur normally during the aging process. Patent sutures in humans have been identified into the ninth decade. The amount of motion across any individual suture is quite small, but when aggregated throughout the multiple bones of the skull with multiple sutures, there appears to be sufficient motion to be easily palpable clinically.

5. The involuntary mobility of the sacrum between the ilia. The sacrum is suspended between the two ilia by the ligaments of the sacroiliac joints. The posterior sacroiliac ligaments are thick and strong with multiple fiber directions. They can be viewed as analogous to the ropes of a child's swing. The anterior sacroiliac ligaments are inferior as well as ante-

rior and appear to support the sacrum from below like the seat of a child's swing. The sacrum can be cupped in an examiner's hand in either the prone or supine position. With light palpatory compression, the examiner normally feels a to-and-fro oscillating movement of the base and apex of the sacrum synchronous with the flexion and extension motion palpated in the cranium.

The primary respiratory mechanism and its related cranial rhythmical impulse (CRI) responds to trauma, disease processes, psychological stress, exercise, and respiration and can be influenced by the skilled application of craniosacral manual medicine procedures. The normal rate of the CRI is 10–14 per minute, quite close to the patient's respiratory rate. A patient can voluntarily control diaphragmatic respiration but cannot directly influence the primary respiratory mechanism. Voluntary inhalation and exhalation can influence the CRI and the inherent mobility of the osseous and membranous cranium.

CRANIOSACRAL DIAGNOSIS

The diagnostic process begins with observation and palpation in a screening examination. The examiner looks for skull symmetry from the anterior, posterior, superior, and both lateral views. Observation is made for symmetry of the frontal bosses, orbits, nose, zygoma, maxillae, mandible, level of the ears, and overall cranial contour. The screening examination proceeds by palpation of skull contour in all dimensions and particularly palpating the sutures as described. Palpation of the sutures looks for widening, narrowing, tension, and tenderness. The skull is assessed by palpation for resiliency to see whether it is more hard and less resilient than normal. Normal bone has a pliability that is lost in the presence of motion restriction. Palpation over the parietotemporal region by the "wet towel" application of the two hands ascertains the rate, rhythm, and amplitude of the CRI.

Another screening examination of assistance in determining whether there is asymmetric loss of cranial motion is the temporal lift (Fig. 12.5). The examiner grasps each temporal bone with the middle finger in the external auditory meatus, the thumb and index fingers on the superior and inferior aspect of the zygomatic process, and the mastoid process between the ring and little finger. With the patient supine on the table, the examiner pulls both temporal bones in a direction toward the vertex. Each temporal bone is then allowed to settle back to its neutral position. The examiner assesses the symmetry or asymmetry of the small amount of joint play motion available in each temporal bone. The horizontal portion of the sphenosquamous suture and the horizontal portion of the occipital mastoid suture are beveled such that the temporal bone sits on top of

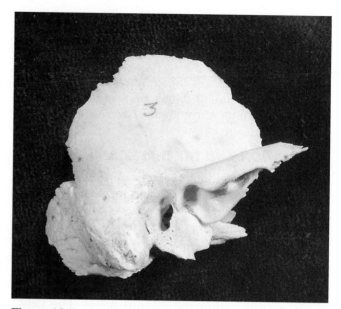

Figure 12.5.
Temporal bone, lateral view.

the sphenoid and occiput. The temporal lift procedure assesses the presence or absence of mobility of the temporal bones on each side.

The sacrum is screened for its anterior and posterior nutational movement between the two ilia in either prone or supine position. The examiner cradles the sacrum in the palm of the hand and assesses the sacral movement and its relation to the cranial rhythmic impulse palpated at the skull. A finding of exaggerated, depressed, or irregular movements instead of the normal anterior and posterior nodding movement requires additional diagnostic assessment. If the screening examination provides evidence of craniosacral dysfunction, additional scanning and segmental definition examinations are necessary.

ASSESSMENT OF SPHENOBASILAR MOTION

Evaluation of sphenobasilar mechanics is accomplished by placing the hands and fingers over the skull in a position that is called the vault hold (Fig. 12.6). There are several variations of the vault hold, but with each there is control of the great wings of the sphenoid at the pterion and with the occiput at the asterion. The classic vault hold has the index finger on the sphenoid at the pterion and the little finger at the asterion and with the ear between the middle and ring fingers. This four-point contact provides the examiner the opportunity to evaluate sphenobasilar mechanics. A second vault hold uses the thumbs on the sphenoid at the pterion with the little finger on the occiput at the asterion and with ear between the index and middle finger. A third vault hold finds the examiner cradling the occiput in the palm of one hand holding posterior to the occipito-mastoid suture and the other hand spanning the front of the skull with the thumb on one great wing of the sphenoid and the long finger on the opposite great wing. Each of these vault holds have their uses. The beginning student should use the vault hold first described.

With sphenobasilar flexion, the index and little fingers separate as they move in a caudad direction. With sphenobasilar extension, the fingers on each side move closer together as the hands move cephalically. With sphenobasilar sidebending-rotation to the right, the fingers of the right hand separate and move in a caudad direction while the fingertips on the left side narrow and move cephalically, resulting in the right side of the skull appearing to become more convex. Sphenobasilar left sidebending-rotation results in similar findings on the opposite side. Sphenobasilar torsional movement is introduced through the four-point contact by alternately turning one hand forward while the other turns backward.

The hand moving anteriorly carries the sphenoid caudad and elevates the occiput on that side. The hand that rotates posteriorly carries the sphenoid high and the occiput low on the same side. This torsional movement should be bilaterally symmetric, but if restricted, the dysfunction is named for the side in which the sphenoid is held in a cephalic (high) position.

Sphenobasilar flexion-extension, sidebending-rotation, and torsion are all present physiologically. Other altered movements of the sphenobasilar junction that usually results from trauma include lateral strain, vertical strain, and sphenobasilar compression. Traumatic episodes can include birth trauma, childhood falls, sports injuries, motor vehicle accidents, industrial accidents, altered muscle balance from chronic postural deficit, abnormal chewing from poor dental hygiene, and many others. Injury to the skull from before backward and behind forward can easily result in sphenobasilar compression that, if present, restricts the midline sphenobasilar move-

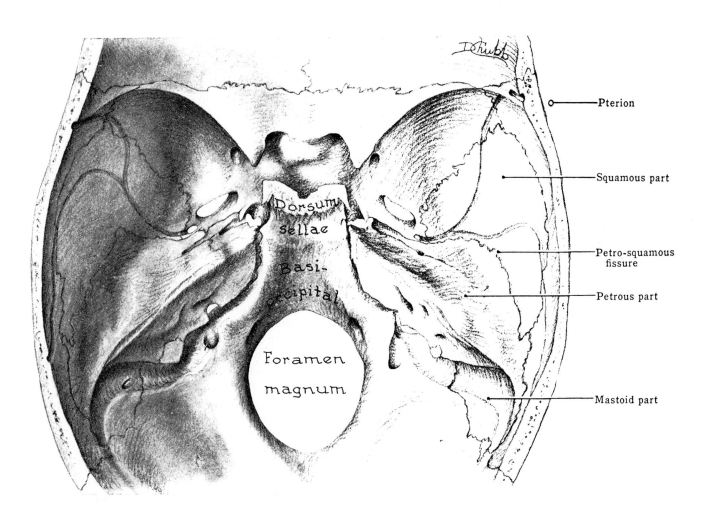

Figure 12.6.
Sphenobasilar junction from above.

ment patterns. The skull usually compensates for this restriction by increased internal and external rotation of the paired lateral bones. Lateral compression can occur with trauma from right to left or left to right, resulting on impaction of the temporal bone on that side. Trauma from left to right or right to left in front of or behind the sphenobasilar junction alters the relation of the sphenoid and occiput in the horizontal plane. Trauma from above downward or below upward on either the sphenoid or occiput can alter the relation of the sphenobasilar junction in the sagittal plane. Both of these strain mechanisms alter the central axis through the sphenobasilar junction. Traumatic lateral and vertical strains, and compressions, significantly alter the craniosacral mechanism.

To test for a lateral strain with the patient supine using the vault hold, one hand lifts one side of the head toward the ceiling and reverses it on the opposite side. This introduces side-to-side translatory movement. If this motion test is asymmetric, it is described as a lateral strain to the side in which the basisphenoid moves freely. To test for vertical strain, both hands of the vault hold move in a rotary fashion forward and then backward symmetrically, introducing a cephalic to caudad translatory movement. If asymmetric, the vertical strain dysfunction is named for the direction in which the basisphenoid moves more freely in a cephalic (superior vertical strain) or caudad (inferior vertical strain) direction. Sphenobasilar compression is identified by loss of overall cranial mobility, particularly at the sphenobasilar junction, and the inability of separation of the four-point contact of the vault hold in the anteroposterior direction.

After evaluation of sphenobasilar mechanics, a specific motion test of each suture can be evaluated. Specific sutural motion testing is beyond the scope of this volume, and the reader is referred to standard texts in the field. Specific motion tests are available for the bones of the vault and of the face.

PRINCIPLES OF CRANIOSACRAL TREATMENT

The goals of craniosacral technique are to improve motion in articular restrictions, reduce membranous tension restrictions, improve circulation (particularly of the venous system), reduce potential neural entrapment from exit foramen at the base of the skull, and increase the vitality of the cranial rhythmic impulse. These techniques have local effects within the head and neck region, distal effects throughout the body, and all are directed toward enhancing the level of wellness of the patient. All of these goals can be accomplished by the restoration of balanced membranous tension. Normal dynamic reciprocal tension of the falx cerebri and tentorium cerebelli is absent in the presence of restriction or alteration in rela-

tionship of cranial bones and their sutures. Alteration in membranous tension affects the venous sinuses within the skull, resulting in the reduction of venous drainage and overall intracranial congestion. The dura is intimately attached to the periosteum on the internal surface of the skull and at each exit foramen. Abnormal dural tension might contribute to neural entrapment and result in altered neural function. Restoring maximum mobility to the osseous cranium restores balanced membranous tension; enhances venous flow; reduces neural entrapment; and permits normal CRI rate, rhythm, and amplitude.

Treatment of the craniosacral system can begin at either the sacrum or the cranium or can be done concurrently. A sequence for treatment proven to be clinically effective begins by screening the cranium and identifying whether the skull is rigid or nonrigid. If rigid, the approach is to decongest the head by venous sinus release and enhance the CRI by CV4 procedures. After the reduction of rigidity within the skull, the sphenobasilar mechanics are assessed and appropriately treated. If sphenobasilar compression is identified, it should be addressed so that the remaining sphenobasilar motions can be more efficient. Treatment of sphenobasilar strain patterns may include approaches both from the cranial and sacral ends of the system. Temporal bone rotational capability is then assessed, and if asymmetric, appropriate sutural evaluation and treatment are performed to restore symmetry of internal and external temporal rotation. The facial component is then assessed and treated as appropriate. Successful craniosacral treatment restores functional balance to both the cranial and sacral limbs of the mechanism, enhances mobility of the cranial bones, balances membranous tension, and enhances the vitality of the cranial rhythmic impulse.

METHODS OF CRANIOSACRAL TECHNIQUE

Craniosacral technique shares with other forms of manual medicine the approach to barriers. In addition to the usual methods of direct action, indirect action, and exaggeration technique, there are two others, namely disengagement and molding. In the direct action method, the barrier is engaged and an activating force is applied in the direction of motion loss. The exaggeration method moves in the opposite direction to motion loss against the physiological barrier and applies an activating force. The indirect method finds the neutral point between the area of normal motion in one direction and restricted motion in the opposite and holds that position while activating forces are applied. The disengagement method applies an activating force to separate sutures, particularly at pivot areas. Molding technique modifies resiliency and contour of bone by the application of external force while waiting for intrinsic activating forces to alter the contour and resiliency of bone. The most commonly applied procedures in craniosacral technique are indirect balanced procedures and exaggeration. Direct action technique is used more commonly in infants and children before the full development of the sutural components to the cranial bones.

ACTIVATING FORCES

The primary activating force in craniosacral technique is the inherent primary respiratory mechanism. Fluctuation of cerebral spinal fluid is a potent intrinsic activating force that is easily directed from the exterior of the skull. The normal fluid fluctuation is in an anterior-to-posterior midline direction but can be altered for intrinsic activating force purposes by being directed with finger contact exactly opposite to the area of skull restriction. This principle is frequently used in V-spread technique. As an example, in the presence of restriction of the left occipitomastoid suture, the operator's index and middle fingers are placed on each side of the occipitomastoid suture on the posterior aspect of the mastoid process and over the anterior portion of the occiput posterior to the occipitomastoid suture. The index finger of the right hand is placed over the right frontal bone directly opposite the left occipitomastoid suture. After separation of the two fingers of the left hand, an attempt is made to direct the fluid from the right frontal to the left occipitomastoid region. Minimal compression on the right frontal area results in a sensation of surflike pounding against the restricted joint until release occurs. The same fluid fluctuation activating force is used in some of the molding method techniques.

Respiratory assistance is a second activating force. Voluntary inhalation enhances flexion movement of the craniosacral mechanism, and voluntary exhalation enhances extension movement. The use of forced inhalation or exhalation and holding respiration at the extreme of movement can be used as an activating force to enhance motion in any direction. A third activating force is enhancement of dural tension by application of effort at the sacrum and from the feet. Enhancement of flexion and extension movement can be made directly from the sacrum by the operator's hand in either direction as desired. Dorsiflexion and plantar flexion of the foot, either voluntarily by the patient or passively by an operator, enhances the intrinsic activating force. Dorsiflexion appears to enhance flexion at the sphenobasilar junction, whereas plantar flexion enhances extension. The principle of the longest diagonal is used by dorsiflexing or plantar flexing the right foot when working on the left side of the skull and by using the left foot when working on the right side.

The fourth activating force is the procedure called CV4. This procedure is performed by the operator cradling the skull in the hands with the thenar eminence against the occiput just medial to the occipitomastoid suture. During normal craniosacral flexion, this portion of the occipital bone appears to become fuller and wider and during exhalation less full and narrower. After tuning into the cranial rhythmic impulse, the operator resists the occiput during the flexion phase until a "still point" is reached. The sensation experienced is that no motion is felt. The operator holds the occiput in this position for several cycles awaiting the return of fluid fluctuation that is perceived by the inherent force pushing the hands away. The operator then allows restoration of the normal flexion and extension movement through the occipital bone. The outcome seems to be the enhancement of fluid movement, change in the rhythm of the diaphragms, and increased temperature in the suboccipital region. A still point can be achieved by a similar process of compression in places other than the occiput that results in a temporary period of reduced motion in the cranial rhythmic impulse.

CRANIOSACRAL TECHNIQUES

This section describes methods of enhancing activating forces in craniosacral techniques. The main activating force continues to be the inherent mobility of the brain, meninges, and CSF. This can be termed inherent force technique and is intrinsic in nature. Enhanced fluctuation of the CSF by respiratory assistance, sacral or extremity force applications, or by the CV4 maneuver all ultimately depend on the intrinsic inherent force reestablishing normal mobility.

Venous Sinus Technique

The goal of venous sinus technique is to enhance the flow of venous blood through the venous sinuses to exit from the skull through the jugular foramen. It is particularly useful when the initial palpatory screening examination reveals a hard rigid skull with loss of resiliency. Venous congestion is believed to contribute to this hard rigid sensation, and the operator attempts to enhance venous return to the central venous circulation.

The operator performs this procedure by initially placing fingertip contact with the middle fingers over the external occipital protuberance of the occipital bone. The weight of the head is carried on these fingerpads, and the operator awaits a softening sensation of bone and beginning of a sensation of freer mobility. The fingers are moved sequentially along the midline of the occiput in the direction of the foramen magnum, awaiting the same softening sensation. The examiner returns to the external occipital protuberance and applies firm pressure with the pads of all four fingers along the superior nuchal line with increasing pressure from medial to lateral until softening is felt. This reduces congestion within the transverse sinus. Returning to the external occipital protuberance, the examiner places a thumb on each side of the occiput, addressing the superior sagittal sinus while applying a pressure with the palmar surface of the thumb in a separation manner. The operator continues from posterior to anterior along the superior sagittal sinus working one thumb breadth at each application until reaching the bregma. From the bregma forward, the operator places the pads of four fingers on each side of the midline of the frontal bone and applies compression and lateral distraction waiting for the sensation of softening and release. Venous sinus technique is frequently used before approaching specific articular restrictions.

Condylar Decompression

The patient lies supine with the operator sitting at the head of the table cradling the skull in the palms of the hands. The middle finger pads are placed along the inferior aspect of the occiput beginning at the inion and sliding forward as far as possible. By flexing the distal interphalangeal joints of the middle fingers, the operator applies cephalic and posterior traction on the occiput. The operator's elbows are brought together, resulting in supination of both hands and separation of the middle fingers. The resultant force vector is cephalic and posterolateral on each side of the occiput posterior to the foramen magnum. This pressure is continued until release of tension is felt, particularly the sensation of equal softening on each side of the occipital bone.

CV4: Bulb Compression

This technique has been previously described under activating forces. It is used independently or in combination with other approaches to restore function to the craniosacral mechanism. CV4 technique is particularly valuable in the enhancement of the amplitude of the cranial rhythmic impulse.

Sphenobasilar Symphysis

Dysfunctions at the sphenobasilar symphysis, both physiological and traumatic, are addressed by one of the vault holds. The operator controls the greater wing of the sphenoid at the pterion and the occiput at the asterion and determines the sphenobasilar strain patterns present. Addressing the sphenobasilar strain pattern that appears to be the most restricted is frequently a valuable first approach. The operator addresses the dysfunction in either a direct, exaggeration, or indirect method. The most commonly used is the indirect method of balanced membranous tension. The operator finds the point of maximum ease within the range of the strain pattern and holds the mechanism at a balanced point until some release is achieved. Respiratory assistance and membranous enhancement from the sacrum and lower extremities is frequently concurrently used. Decompression of the sphenobasilar symphysis is accomplished by finding the balanced point of each of the strain patterns in a stacked fashion and applying a distraction force by separating the finger contact on the sphenoid and occiput in an anteroposterior direction.

Temporal Rocking

With the patient supine on the table and the operator sitting at the head, the skull is supported in the palms of the hand with each thumb behind the ear in front of the mastoid process. This thumb placement allows control of the temporal bones on each side. Pressure by the distal phalanx of the thumb in a posteromedial direction on the inferior aspect of the mastoid process introduces external rotation. Compression in a posteromedial direction with the base of the thumb on the mastoid portion of the temporal bone enhances internal rotation. Movement of the thumbs can rock the temporal bones into internal and external rotation, either synchronously (both temporals into internal rotation or external rotation) or nonsynchronously (one temporal moving into internal rotation and the other external rotation). Asynchronous rocking of the temporals through several cycles appears to change the fluid fluctuation from an anteroposterior to-and-fro movement to a side-to-side to-and-fro movement. Once asynchronous rocking is symmetrical on each side, synchronous rocking is reintroduced to restore the normal anteroposterior to-and-fro fluid fluctuation. The operator should never leave a patient with asynchronous motion of the temporals as an adverse reaction of dizziness and nausea can result. Enhancement of synchronous rocking of the two temporals appears to have a beneficial effect on membranous balance. It is also of value in the temporomandibular joint function because asymmetrical relationship of temporal movement interferes with symmetrical temporomandibular joint function.

V Spread

This procedure is useful to separate restricted and impacted sutures wherever present. The principle is to place two fingers on each side of the restricted suture with a distraction and separation and using fluid fluctuation as the activating force by applying pressure with the opposite hand at a point of greatest distance and opposite to the suture under treatment. The occipitomastoid suture is one frequently treated by means of V spread, but the principles can be applied to any suture within the skull or face.

Lift Technique

Frontal and parietal lift technique is commonly used to aid in the balance of membranous tension. To perform a frontal lift, the patient is supine on the table with the operator sitting at the head. The operator grasps the inferior and lateral corner of the frontal bone on each side with either one hand spanning the frontal bone or two hands interlaced with the pisiforms on the frontal bone. The hands apply a medial compression force to disengage the frontal bone and then it is lifted toward the ceiling, sensing for a release. A frontal lift puts longitudinal traction on the falx cerebri as it lifts the frontal bone from the sphenoid. When the frontal bone appears to be in the midline and has been released anteriorly, it is slowly allowed to settle back to its normal relationship. It is not uncommon during this procedure to have the sensation that the frontal bone is wobbling from side to side when being distracted.

A parietal lift is performed by a four finger contact on the two anterior inferior and posterior inferior corners of the parietal bones. Compressive force is applied through the tips of the four fingers and each parietal bone is lifted toward the vertex. The four-corner compression disengages the parietal bone, allowing for the lift that results in external rotation of the two parietal bones. The parietal lift places a transverse stress on the tentorium cerebelli, balancing its tension from right to left. As with the frontal lift, when balance is achieved, the operator reduces the lifting force and allows the parietals to settle back into the skull. Lift techniques distract one bone from the other and apply loads to the meninges to achieve membranous balance.

SEQUENCE OF TREATMENT

Sequence of treatment varies from practitioner to practitioner, from patient to patient, and from one treatment to the next. There are several general principles that can be useful and applied and adapted individually for the patient need. First and foremost, the craniosacral mechanism must be viewed within the context of the total musculoskeletal system. Craniosacral dysfunction may be primary, secondary, or of little significance in the overall patient status. Secondary cranial dysfunction resulting from altered functional capacity elsewhere in the system will not respond well until the primary dysfunction is identified and appropriately treated. Conversely, continued treatment to dysfunction of the musculoskeletal system elsewhere in the system, without addressing the craniosacral dysfunction, will lead to less than satisfactory results.

Treatment of the craniosacral mechanism can follow that identified in the preceding section on the principles of craniosacral treatment. The goal should be to reduce venous congestion, mobilize articular restrictions, balance the sphenobasilar symphysis, and enhance the rate and amplitude of the cranial rhythmic impulse.

Craniosacral treatment, like all manual medicine, needs to be prescribed in the dosage appropriate for the individual patient need. These procedures do not appear to be aggressive and forceful but are powerful and if inappropriately applied can result in a poor outcome by the patient.

COMPLICATIONS AND CONTRAINDICATIONS

Complications to craniosacral treatment are fortunately quite rare but do occur. The brainstem with its many control functions for the total body is intimately related to the sphenobasilar junction. Craniosacral treatment, particularly that which addresses sphenobasilar strain patterns, might lead to alteration in nervous system control of systemic function, resulting in symptom exacerbation. This may include alteration in heart rate, blood pressure, respiration, and gastrointestinal irritability with nausea, vomiting, and diarrhea. These exacerbated symptoms appear to result from alteration in autonomic nervous system control. A second area of potential symptom exacerbation and complications is in the area of the cervicocranial syndromes with headache, dizziness, and tinnitus. The vestibular system is highly sensitive to balance or imbalance of the temporal bones. Overly aggressive or improperly applied temporal rocking of the synchronous and asynchronous nature may exacerbate symptoms of dizziness, vertigo, nausea, and vomiting. Care must be exercised in using craniosacral technique in individuals with psychological and psychiatric problems. These procedures can cause significant emotional change in response to the patient environment. Neurological complications and symptom exacerbation can occur in patients with seizure states and dystonia of the central nervous system. Dystonia is related to the central nervous system. Traumatic brain injury is a common, but frequently unrecognized, patient problem. Great care must be used in applying craniosacral techniques to patients with traumatic brain injury as it is difficult to predict the outcome of craniosacral treatment in these patients. The practitioner must be aware of, and prepared to deal with, symptom exacerbation or onset of new symptoms when under craniosacral treatment.

Contraindications are few but include suspicion for acute intracranial bleed or increase in intracranial pressure. These should be evaluated by appropriate diagnostic testing before implementing craniosacral treatment. Skull trauma requires adequate investigation to rule out fractures of the cranial base or depressed fractures of the vault or subarachnoid hemorrhage. Seizure states are not an absolute contraindication but are relative depending on the control of the seizure status.

Although the complications and contraindications are few, the admonition of "primum non nocere" (first do not harm) applies when using craniosacral technique.

CONCLUSION

Craniosacral technique is a valuable addition to the armamentarium of the manual medicine prac-

titioner. Craniosacral technique requires extensive study and practice. It should be performed within the context of total patient evaluation because of its powerful systemic effects. It influences, and is influenced by, the rest of the musculoskeletal system. This chapter includes basic and preliminary information about the craniosacral system. The student is recommended to pursue additional study from the standard texts in the field and pursue structured courses of instruction.

Section **//** *TECHNIQUE PROCEDURES*

13

The cervical spine is an important region of the vertebral column in the field of manual medicine. It receives a great deal of attention by manual medicine practitioners. It functions as the support of the skull and biomechanically provides mobility for a number of activities of daily living. A myriad of head, neck, and upper extremity symptoms have been observed when the cervical spine is dysfunctional. Symptomatic conditions in the area can be categorized as cervicocephalic syndrome, cervical syndrome, and cervicobrachial syndrome. Cervicocephalic syndrome includes pain and restriction of motion of the upper cervical spine and associated superficial and deep pain in the head. This syndrome frequently demonstrates functional alteration in vision, vertigo, dizziness, and nystagmus. Cervical syndrome includes painful stiffness of the neck of varying severity from mild to acute spastic torticollis. Cervicobrachial syndrome couples painful stiffness of the cervical spine with symptoms in the shoulder girdle and upper extremity. The upper extremity symptoms result from alteration of the functional capacity in the brachial plexus or altered vascular function through the arterial, venous, and lymphatic systems. Associated dysfunction of the thoracic inlet, particularly the first and second ribs, contribute to the cervicobrachial syndrome.

The cervical spine is subjected to acute injuries, such as the flexion-extension "whiplash" injury, and chronic repetitive injury from improper posture and abnormal positions of the head and neck. It is seldom that the whiplash injury is a true flexion-extension injury. Most commonly, a rotary torque is included in the trauma, giving rise to a number of motion-restriction possibilities and different vectors of soft tissue injury. It is common in our society to have patients with a forward head carriage as a component to poor posture. Forward head posture results in an increase in the upper cervical lordosis and a flattening in the lower cervical spine. The balance of the head on the neck is altered, resulting in muscle imbalance and tightness of the neck extensors and weakness of the deep neck flexors.

The cervical spine is the area of the musculoskel-etal system in which most of the reported complications of manual medicine treatment have occurred. Traumatic insult to the vertebral-basilar artery system is a rare but catastrophic event. Congenital, inflammatory, and traumatic alteration in the upper cervical region place the cervical spinal cord at risk from improper diagnostic and manual medicine treatment methods. Down's syndrome, rheumatoid arthritis, agenesis of the odontoid process, and fracture of the odontoid base are but a few of these conditions. The student and practitioner must understand the anatomy, physiology, and biomechanics of the region to understand the therapeutic role of manual medicine and to avoid potential complications.

FUNCTIONAL ANATOMY AND BIOMECHANICS

The cervical spine can be divided into the atypical segments of the upper cervical complex and the typical cervical vertebra from C3 to C7. The upper cervical complex, consisting of the occipitoatlantal (C0–1), atlantoaxial (C1–2), and the superior aspect of C2, function as an integrated unit. The biomechanics of this region are complex and continue under intense research and study. Although the C0–3 region functions as an integrated unit, it is useful to assess each level individually to identify its contribution to the overall function of the complex.

Occipitoatlantal Articulation

The occipitoatlantal junction (C0–1) consists of two articulations formed by the occipital condyles and the superior articular facets of the atlas. The occipital condyles are convex from the front to the back and from side to side. The superior articular facets of the atlas are concave from the front to the back and from side to side. The two articulations are divergent from before backward. The primary movement is forward-bending and backward-bending. There is a small amount of coupled sidebending and rotation to opposite sides that becomes highly clinically significant when lost. During sidebending, one occipital condyle slides upward on one side of the atlas and downward on the other. This sidebending component is approximately 5° each direction. Rotation couples to the opposite side of sidebending and is in the range of 5° to each side. The coupling of rotation to the opposite side appears to be a function of the ligamentous attachments of the occiput to the atlas and axis, the relationship of the slope of the side of the superior facets of the atlas, and the divergence posteriorly.

Atlantoaxial Articulation

There are four articulations at the atlantoaxial junction (C1–2). The right and left zygapophysial joints are formed by the inferior facet of the atlas articulating with the convex superior facet of the axis. The inferior facet of the atlas is covered by an articular cartilage that is convex anteroposteriorly and from side to side. This results in a unique convex to convex apposition of joint surfaces. The superior articular facets of the axis are convex anteroposteriorly and from side to side and face superiorly and laterally, giving the appearance of a pair of shoulders. The other two articulations at the atlantoaxial junction involve the odontoid process. The anterior surface of the odontoid articulates with small facet on the posterior aspect of the anterior arch of the atlas. On the posterior aspect of the odontoid process is an articulation with the transaxial ligament. The integrated functions of these four articulations, modified by ligamentous and muscular attachment, result in a small amount of forward-bending, backward-bending, and sidebending, with the primary motion being rotation to the right and left. There is a small amount of cephalic to caudad translatory movement that accompanies rotation. This is a result of the unique convex to convex articular apposition of the zygapophysial joints. As the atlas turns right on the axis, the right facet of the atlas slides downward on the posterior aspect of the right facet of the axis and the left inferior facet of the atlas slides downward on the anterior aspect of the left facet of the axis, resulting in caudad translation. Upon returning to neutral, the inferior facets of the atlas ascend on the articular shoulders of the facets of the axis, resulting in a cephalic translatory movement.

C2 functions as a transitional segment with its atypical superior surface articulating with the atlas and to the occiput through ligamentous and muscular attachments. The inferior surface is the same as the remaining typical cervical segments below.

Typical Cervical Articulations

The typical cervical segments from C3 to C7 articulate at the vertebral bodies with an intervening intervertebral disc. The vertebral bodies superior surface is convex from before backward and concave from side to side, whereas the inferior surface is convex from side to side and concave from before backward.

This joint configuration with the intervening intervertebral disc allows it to move in all directions. The uncovertebral joint of Luschka is found at the posterolateral corner of the vertebral body and appears to function in the gliding movements during forward-bending and backward-bending. They also seem to protect the posterolateral aspect of the intervertebral disk from herniation in a posterolateral direction. These joints are subject to degenerative productive change resulting in lipping, which occasionally encroaches on the anterior aspect of the lateral intervertebral canal. The zygapophysial joints of the typical cervical vertebra face backward and upward at an angle of approximately 45°. Because of the facing of the zygapophysial joints and the characteristic of the vertebral bodies and intervening intervertebral disc, the motions available are forward-bending, backward-bending, and coupled sidebending and rotation movement to the same side. The result is that in the typical cervical segments, one only encounters nonneutral somatic dysfunction. There are no group dysfunctions in the typical cervical segments, although several segments can become dysfunctional one on top of the other.

Vertebral Artery

The course of the vertebral artery is of major significance in the field of manual medicine. The vertebral artery begins its relationship with the cervical spine at the level of C6–7, where it enters between the transverse processes, immediately turns cephalward, runs through the intertransverse foramen, and exits from the superior side of the transverse process of C1. Here it turns acutely posteriorly over the posterior arch of the atlas and penetrates the posterior occipitoatlantal membrane before entering the foramen magnum. It joins the vertebral artery of the opposite side to form the basilar artery. The vertebral artery is at risk at the acute angulation at C6–7, by productive change in and around the intertransverse foramen from C6 to C1, and at the occipitoatlantal junction. Normal vertebral arteries can narrow as much as 90% of there luminal size on the contralateral side to cervical rotation. This normal phenomenon is exacerbated when performed in backward-bending of the head on the neck. Congenital asymmetry, and even atresia, of the vertebral arteries is not uncommon, and they are subject to degenerative vessel disease. A commonly used provocative diagnostic test for the integrity of the vertebral artery is the hanging (De Kleyn) test. The examiner backward bends the head and neck over the end of the table and introduces rotation to the right and to the left, holding the head in each rotated position looking for the development of nystagmus. This author does not advocate this test because it unnecessarily puts normal vertebral arteries at risk. It also has a high false-positive rate. A less aggressive test that provides equally valid information is to have the sitting patient look up at the ceiling and then turn the head to both the left and to the right while the operator observes for the initiation of nystagmus and adverse symptoms such as dizziness. This is a hands-off test by the practitioner and asks only that the patient introduce normal ranges of active movement. Probably the best sign of impending cerebral anoxia is the symptom of acute anxiety and panic. If this occurs during a structural diagnostic or manual medicine procedure in the cervical spine, the operator should stop and immediately institute evaluation and treatment for potential vascular complications.

Mechanoreceptors and Nociceptors

The articular and periarticular structures of the cervical spine, particularly the upper cervical complex, are heavily invested by mechanoreceptors and nociceptors. Cervical spine dysfunction can result in altered afferent stimulation by these mechanoreceptors and nociceptors and influence the integrated function of the musculoskeletal system, as well as contribute to local and regional symptoms. The suboccipital cervical muscles have a large number of spindles per unit mass. The proprioceptive function of these muscles must have a high level of significance. Recent magnetic resonance imaging (MRI) research in this region demonstrated fatty replacement of the erectus capitis posterior major and minor muscle in patients with posttraumatic cervicocranial syndromes (see Chapter 21).

Autonomic Nervous System Relationships

Sympathetic autonomic nervous system control of cerebral blood flow emanates from the superior cervical ganglion. This structure is intimately related to the longus colli muscle and the anterior surface of C2 to which it is intimately bound by deep connective fascia. Somatic dysfunction of C2 is frequently found in cervicocephalic syndromes and in patients with internal visceral disease. A small branch of the second cervical nerve connects with the vagus as it descends through the trunk. Hypothetically, this neural connection may account for the clinical observation of somatic dysfunction of C2 in the presence of visceral disease.

STRUCTURAL DIAGNOSIS

The anatomy and biomechanics of the cervical spine result in basically five somatic dysfunctions. The typical cervical segments have nonneutral dysfunction with either forward-bending or backward-bending restriction together with coupled sidebending and rotation restriction to the same side. At the atlantoaxial junction (C1–2), the primary somatic dysfunction is that of restriction of rotation to one side or the other. Although there may be minor forward-bending, backward-bending, and sidebending components to the rotational restriction, adequate treatment to the rotational restriction restores the minor movement motion simultaneously. At the occipitoatlantal junction (C0–1), two dysfunctions are possible: either forward-bending or backward-bending restriction with coupled sidebending and rotation restriction to opposite sides.

The structural diagnostic process begins by identifying levels of palpable deep muscle hypertonicity. This identifies segments that need motion testing. The diagnostic and therapeutic process seems to be most satisfactory by beginning from below and moving cephalward.

The bony landmark of most value in the typical cervical segments is the articular pillar. They are palpated in the deep fascial grove between the semispinalis medially and the cervical longissimus laterally. The examiner's paired fingers can localize to the right and left articular pillars of any given cervical segment and introduce motion testing. The typical cervical segment articular pillar is the size of the examiner's fingerpad. The identification of the articular pillars begins by first identifying the spinous process of C2 and C7. C2 spinous process is the first bony prominence in the midline caudad to the external occipital protuberance (inion). The spinous process of C7 (vertebra prominens) is the spinous process that remains palpable during cervical backward-bending. The articular pillars of C2 and C7 are at the same level of the spinous processes. Placing the examiner's fingers between the pillars of C2 and C7 puts the fingerpads in contact with C3, C4, C5, and C6. This provides the ability to localize to any specific cervical segment. The structural diagnostic process can be performed in both the patient sitting and supine positions.

Cervical Spine Diagnosis

Typical Cervical Vertebra Sitting

1. Patient sitting on table or treatment stool.

2. Operator stands behind with thumb and index finger contacting zygapophysial joints bilaterally and with left hand on vertex of head to control motion (Fig. 13.1).

3. Operator's left hand introduces forward-bending, right sidebending, and right rotation with the left hand while monitoring left zygapophysial joint for opening movement (Fig. 13.2).

4. Operator introduces forward-bending, left sidebending, and left rotation palpating for opening of the right zygapophysial joint by the operator's right index finger (Fig. 13.3).

5. Operators left hand introduces backward-bending, right sidebending, and right rotation with the right index finger monitoring the right zygapophysial joints capacity to close (Fig. 13.4).

6. Operator introduces backward-bending, left sidebending, and left rotation with the left hand with the right thumb monitoring the left zygapophysial joints capacity to close (Fig. 13.5).

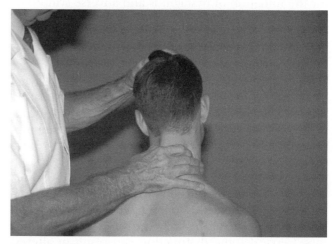

Figure 13.3.

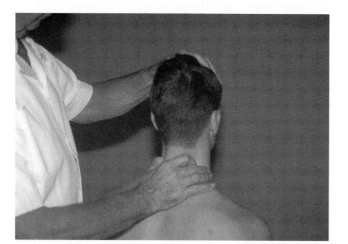

Figure 13.1.

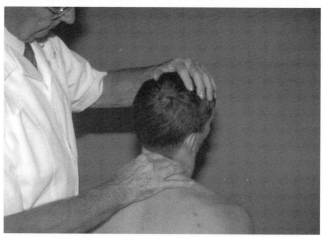

Figure 13.4.

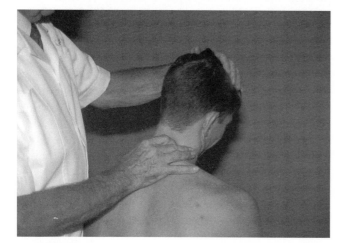

Figure 13.2.

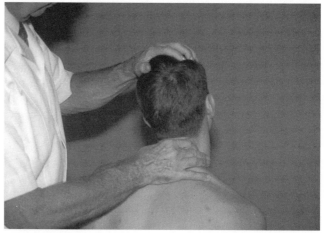

Figure 13.5.

Cervical Spine Diagnosis

Atlantoaxial (C1–2) Sitting

1. Patient sitting on table with operator behind.
2. Operator's two hands grasp the patient's head and introduce forward-bending (Fig. 13.6) to reduce rotation in lower typical cervical vertebra.
3. Operator introduces right rotation, sensing for resistance to movement (Fig. 13.7).
4. Operator introduces left rotation, sensing for resistance to left rotation (Fig. 13.8).

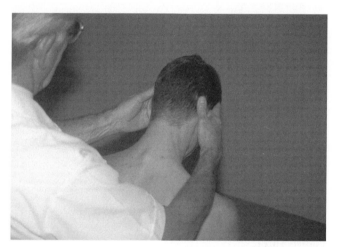

Figure 13.6.

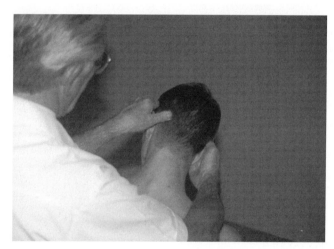

Figure 13.8.

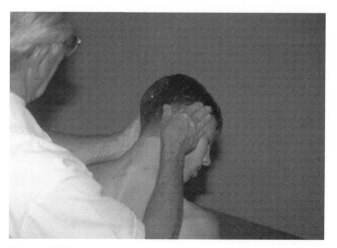

Figure 13.7.

Cervical Spine Diagnosis

Occipitoatlantal (C0–1) Sitting

1. Patient sitting on table.

2. Operator stands behind with thumb and index finger of the right hand grasping the posterior arch of the atlas and the left hand on top of the head to introduce movement.

3. Operator's left hand introduces backward-bending, left sidebending, and right rotation of the head, sensing for prominent fullness under the right thumb, indicating posterior rotation of the atlas on the left (Fig. 13.9).

4. Operator's left hand introduces backward-bending, right sidebending, left rotation of the head, and monitors for prominence of the right posterior arch of the atlas under the right index finger indicative of right rotation of the atlas (Fig. 13.10).

5. Operator introduces forward-bending, right sidebending, and left rotation with the left hand while monitoring for prominence of the right posterior arch of the atlas under the right index finger, indicating atlas right rotation (Fig. 13.11).

6. Operator introduces forward-bending, left sidebending, and right rotation of the head with the left hand while monitoring for prominence of the left posterior arch of the atlas under the right thumb, indicating left rotation of the atlas (Fig. 13.12).

Note: The right thumb and index finger assesses the rotation of the atlas in relation to the induced rotation of the occiput and not in relation to the coronal plane.

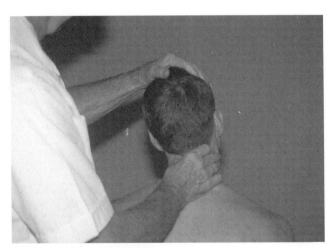

Figure 13.9.

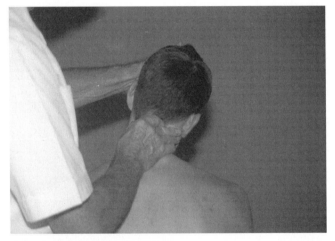

Figure 13.11.

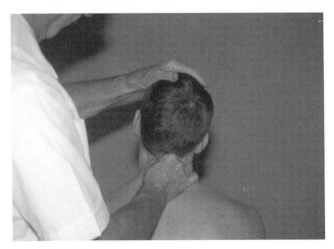

Figure 13.10.

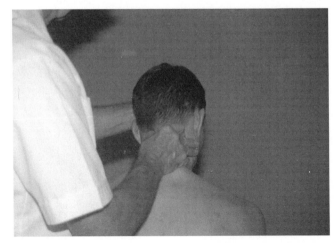

Figure 13.12.

Cervical Spine Diagnosis

Typical Cervical Segments (C3–7) Supine for Flexed, Rotated, Sidebent (FRS) Dysfunction

1. Patient supine on table with operator sitting at head of table.

2. Operator's index and middle fingers of each hand contact the pillar of the superior vertebra of the motion segment being tested (Fig. 13.13).

3. Operator's palms and thenar eminences control the patient's head and upper cervical spine (Fig. 13.14).

4. Operator's finger contacts translate the vertebra anteriorly to the backward-bending barrier (lift the fingers toward the ceiling) (Fig. 13.15).

5. The operator introduces translation from right to left, sensing for resistance to movement (Fig. 13.16). If resistance is encountered, the motion restriction is backward-bending, right sidebending, and right rotation (FRS$_{left}$). Something interfered with the capacity of the right facet to close.

6. Operator introduces translatory movement from left to right, sensing for resistance (Fig. 13.17). If resis-

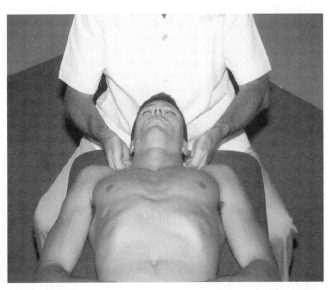

Figure 13.13.

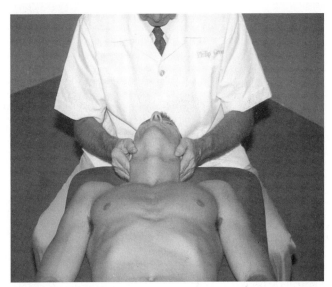

Figure 13.15.

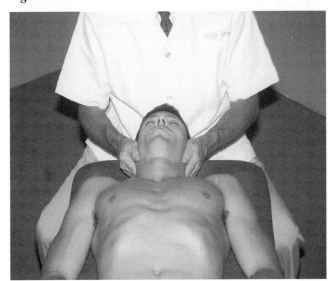

Figure 13.14.

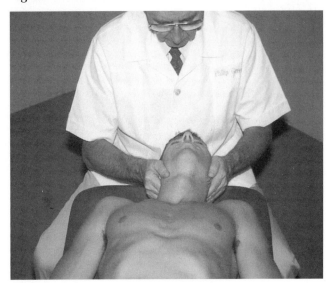

Figure 13.16.

tance is encountered, the motion restriction is backward-bending, left sidebending, and left rotation (FRS$_{right}$). Something interfered with the left facet to close.

Cervical Spine Diagnosis

Typical Cervical Segment (C3–7) Supine for Extended, Rotated, and Sidebent (ERS) Dysfunction

1. Patient supine on table with operator sitting at head of table.
2. Operator's index and middle fingers of each hand contact the pillar of the superior vertebra of the motion segment being tested (Fig. 13.13).
3. Operator's palms and thenar eminences control the patient's head and upper cervical spine (Fig. 13.14).
4. Operator flexes the head and neck down to the segment under examination (Fig. 13.18).
5. Operator introduces translation from right to left, sensing for resistance (Fig. 13.19). If resistance is felt, the motion restriction is forward-bending, right sidebending, and right rotation (ERS$_{left}$). Something has interfered with the capacity of the left facet to open.
6. Operator introduces translation from left to right, sensing for resistance (Fig. 13.20). If resistance is encountered, the motion restriction is forward-bending, left sidebending, and left rotation (ERS$_{right}$). Something interfered with the capacity of the right facet to open.

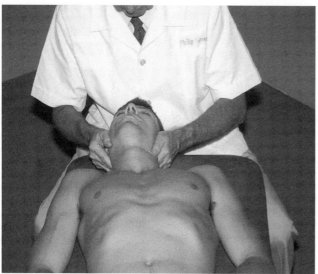

Figure 13.17.

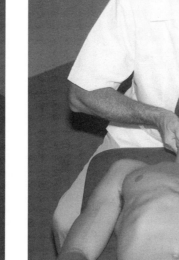

Figure 13.19.

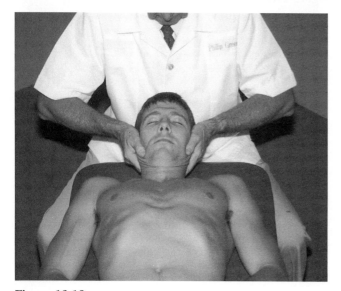

Figure 13.18.

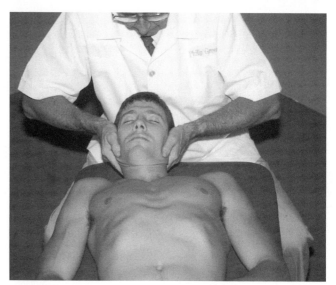

Figure 13.20.

Cervical Spine Diagnosis

Atlantoaxial (C1–2) Supine

1. Patient supine on table with operator standing (or sitting) at the head of the table.

2. Operator's two hands hold each side of the patient's head with index fingers monitoring the posterior arch of the atlas. Operator flexes the patient's head and neck to provide restriction of typical cervical segment rotation through ligamentous locking (Fig. 13.21).

3. Operator's hands introduce right rotation, sensing for resistance (Fig. 13.22). If resistance is encountered, the motion restriction is right rotation (atlas rotated left).

4. Operator rotates head to the left, sensing for resistance (Fig. 13.23). If resistance is encountered, the motion restriction is left rotation (atlas rotated right).

Note: Neck flexion must be maintained throughout the procedure. Do not allow the head and neck to go into backward-bending during the rotation effort.

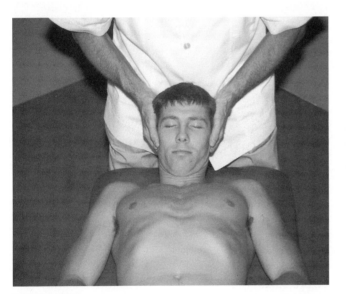

Figure 13.21.

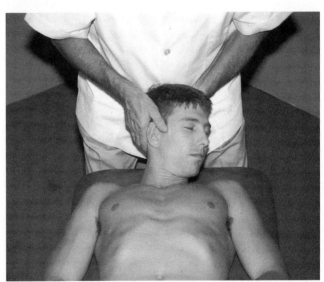

Figure 13.23.

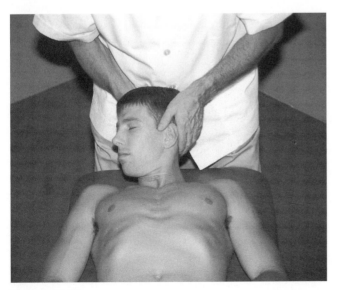

Figure 13.22.

Cervical Spine Diagnosis

Occipitoatlantal (C0–1) Supine Extension Restriction

1. Patient supine on table with operator sitting at the head of the table.

2. Operator's two hands grasp sides of patient's head with index fingers monitoring the posterior arch of the atlas.

3. Operator introduces backward-bending to the first barrier by rolling the head posteriorly around an axis of rotation through the external auditory meati (Fig. 13.24).

4. Operator introduces translation of the head from right to left while maintaining the eyes parallel to the head of the table, sensing for resistance (Fig. 13.25). If resistance is felt, motion restriction is backward-bending, right sidebending, and left rotation (FS_LR_R). Something interfered with the right condyle gliding forward.

5. Operator introduces translation from left to right, sensing for resistance (Fig. 13.26). If resistance is encountered, the motion restriction is backward-bending, left sidebending, and right rotation (FS_RR_L). Something interfered with the left condyle to glide forward.

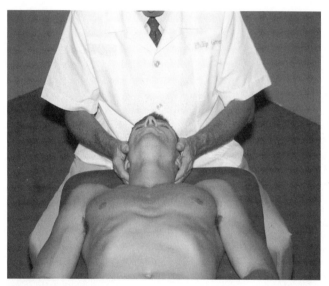

Figure 13.24.

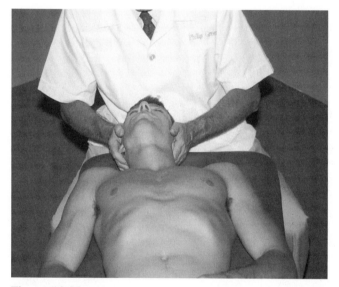

Figure 13.26.

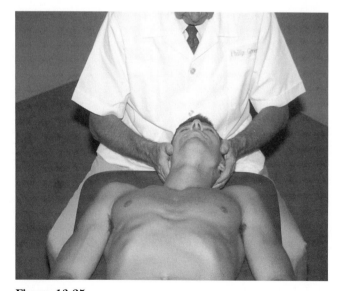

Figure 13.25.

Cervical Spine Diagnosis

Occipitoatlantal (C0–1) Supine for Flexion Restriction

1. Patient supine on table with operator sitting at head of table.

2. Operator's hands grasp the side of the patient's head with the index fingers monitoring the posterior arch of the atlas.

3. Operator forward bends the patient's head by rotation around an axis through the external auditory meati while monitoring for first movement of the atlas (Fig. 13.27).

4. Operator introduces translation from right to left, sensing for resistance (Fig. 13.28). If resistance is felt, the motion restriction is forward-bending, right sidebending, and left rotation ($ES_L R_R$). Something interfered with the left condyle to glide posteriorly.

5. Operator introduces translation from left to right, sensing for resistance (Fig. 13.29). If resistance is encountered, the motion restriction is forward-bending, left sidebending, and right rotation ($ES_R R_L$). Something interfered with the right condyle to glide posteriorly.

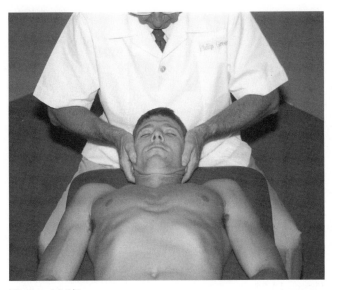

Figure 13.27.

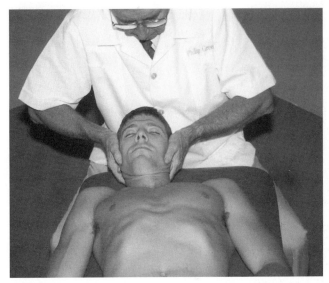

Figure 13.29.

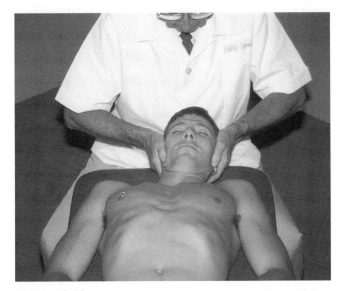

Figure 13.28.

Cervical Spinal Diagnosis

Occipitoatlantal (C0–1) Supine Condylar Glide

1. Patient supine on table with operator sitting at head of table.

2. Operator grasps the sides of the head with each hand and rotates the head 30° to the right (Fig. 13.30).

3. Operator introduces anterior translation by gliding the right condyle anteriorly, sensing for resistance (Fig. 13.31).

4. Operator translates the head posteriorly, requiring the right condyle to glide posteriorly (Fig. 13.32).

5. Operator rotates head 30° to the left (Fig. 13.33).

6. Operator introduces anterior translatory movement of the head, requiring the left condyle to glide forward (Fig. 13.34).

7. Operator introduces posterior translation of the head, requiring the left condyle to glide posteriorly, sensing for resistance to movement (Fig. 13.35).

Note: This tests the forward-bending and backward-bending capacity of each condyle. If resistance is encountered, the sidebending and rotational motion coupled to opposite sides will be restricted (the minor movements).

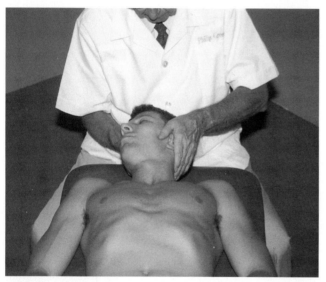

Figure 13.30.

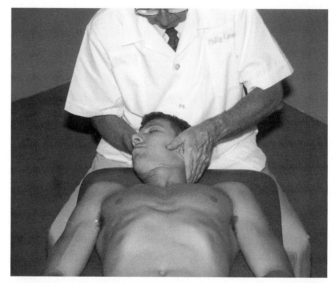

Figure 13.32.

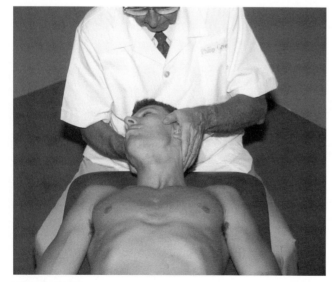

Figure 13.31.

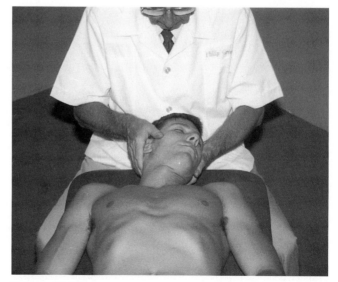

Figure 13.33.

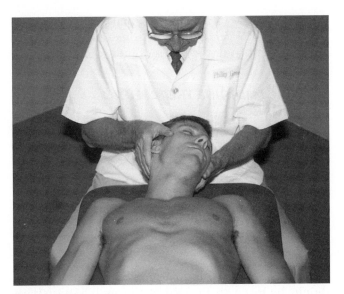

Figure 13.34.

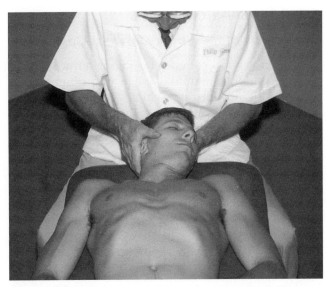

Figure 13.35.

CERVICAL SPINE DIAGNOSIS

Stress Tests of the Upper Cervical Complex

The upper cervical complex is subject to fracture, dislocation, and ligamentous damage after trauma. Fracture and dislocation are seldom a concern in the practice of manual medicine. Ligamentous damage may well be of concern to the manual medicine practitioner. The preceding diagnostic tests are most valuable for determining hypomobility as the result of somatic dysfunction. Early hypermobility is much more difficult to assess. Stress testing of the craniocervical junction is difficult to interpret. If the preceding diagnostic tests for the occipitoatlantal and atlantoaxial joints have full range and asymmetric loose end feel, the index of suspicion should go up for hypermobility due to ligamentous laxity.

This author uses two stress tests of the many available. The first is an anterior-posterior stress of upper cervical complex. In the supine position, the operator holds the occiput and anteriorly translates the atlas and axis, sensing for mobility. The thumbs are then placed on the anterior aspect of the transverse processes of the atlas and axis, and a posterior translatory force is applied. Abnormal anterior to posterior translatory movement may indicate some laxity of the transaxial ligament. The second test is to monitor the spinous process of C2 and introduce sidebending of the head on the neck. Right sidebending of the occiput should result in immediate right rotation of C2. Should this sidebending be asymmetric or delayed, the possibility of alar ligament damage should be suspected.

A major problem in motion testing for hypermobility in this region is that it may be compensatory to restricted motion in other areas of the upper cervical complex. Is the side of restriction hypomobile or is the hypermobility truly due to ligamentous damage?

If there is any question of significant ligamentous damage, it can be further evaluated by rotational stress films of the upper cervical complex using either computed tomography or MRI technology. Axial views in the right and left rotated positions provide the opportunity to assess segmental mobility and its symmetry. MRI technology is somewhat more valuable for identifying the status of individual ligaments.

MANUAL MEDICINE THERAPEUTIC PROCEDURES

The following procedures are all direct action because they directly engage the restrictive barrier. The two activating forces will be muscle energy technique, an intrinsic activating force, and mobilization with impulse technique, an extrinsic activating force. The muscle energy techniques are recommended to be performed initially because most of the somatic dysfunctions found within the cervical spine respond well. It is in those patients that muscle energy is not effective in maximizing motion that consideration should be given to the use of the mobilization with impulse technique. When the diagnostic process identifies what seems to be a deep articular or periarticular restriction, the mobilization with impulse techniques appear to be most effective.

It is recommended that the treatment sequence begin in the lower cervical spine and move upward toward the craniocervical junction; this provides easier and more accurate diagnosis of the superior segment on the inferior throughout the diagnostic process. It is not uncommon for several typical cervical segments to demonstrate stacked nonneutral dysfunction that need to be addressed individually. The goal of any manual medicine intervention is to balance the occiput on the vertebral column. This use of the biomechanical model would suggest that the craniooccipital junction be the last treated after balancing the system below. One major exception to this rule is to approach the most restricted segment first to influence the system to the maximum. However, if the most restricted area is also the most acute, the practitioner might wish to work around the acute area to remove related restrictors as well as to decongest the acute inflammatory process. In acute conditions of the cervical spine, functional (indirect) technique is the treatment of choice (see Chapter 10).

Cervical Spine Muscle Energy Technique

Typical Cervical Vertebra C5–6 Example

Diagnosis
Position: Flexed, rotated left, sidebend left
(FRS$_{left}$)
Motion restriction: Extension, right rotation, right
sidebending.

1. Patient supine on table with operator sitting at
   head.
2. Operator's fingertips of the right index and middle
   finger are placed on the right articular pillar of C6
   to hold the segment so that C5 can be moved
   upon it (Fig. 13.36).

3. The operator's left hand controls the left side of the
   patient's head and neck (Fig. 13.37).
4. The operator's right fingers translate the segment
   anteriorly, introducing motion to the backward-bending barrier (Fig. 13.38).
5. Operator's left hand introduces sidebending and rotation of the head and neck to the right, engaging
   the right rotation, right sidebending barrier (Fig.
   13.39).
6. The patient exerts a small isometric effort against
   the operator's resisting left hand into forward-bending, left sidebending, or left rotation.

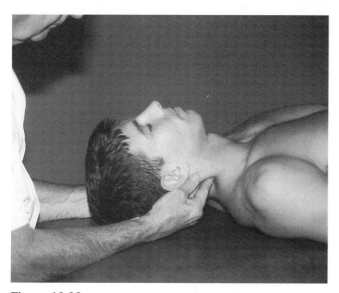

Figure 13.36.

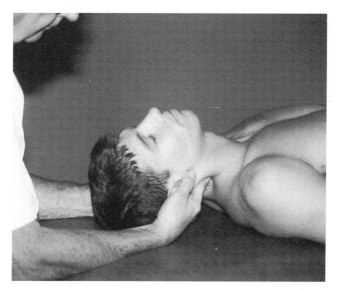

Figure 13.38.

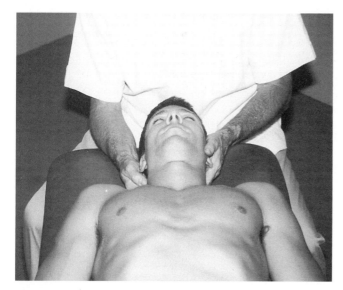

Figure 13.37.

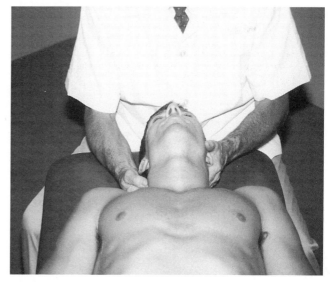

Figure 13.39.

7. After a 3- to 5-second muscle effort, the patient relaxes and the operator increases translatory movement in an anterior and a right to left direction engaging the backward-bending, right sidebending, and right rotation barrier (Fig. 13.40). The process is repeated three to five times.

8. Retest.

Note: An alternative activating force is eye movement. In this example of restriction of backward-bending, right sidebending, and right rotation, the patient's activating force is looking to the left or toward the feet against resistance. A new barrier is engaged during relaxation and the eye movement is repeated.

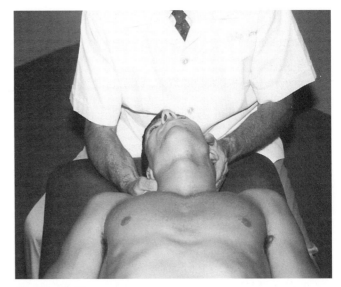

Figure 13.40.

Cervical Spine Muscle Energy Treatment

Typical Cervical Vertebra C2–3 Example

Diagnosis
Position: Extended, left sidebent, left rotated (ERS$_{left}$)
Motion restriction: Forward-bending, rotation right, sidebending right

1. Patient supine on table with operator sitting at head.

2. Operator's left hand supports the occiput with the left thumb over the left C2–3 zygapophysial joint and the left index finger blocking the right C2–3 zygapophysial joint (Fig. 13.41).

3. Operator's right hand is placed on the patient's right frontoparietal region to control head movement (Fig. 13.42).

4. Operator's two hands roll the head and upper neck into forward-bending as far as the C2–3 interspace (Fig. 13.43).

5. Operator introduces right sidebending and right rotation by right to left translation through the left index finger contact on the right zygapophysial joint of C2–3, engaging the flexion, right sidebending, right rotation restriction (Fig. 13.44).

6. The patient exerts a 3- to 5-second isometric contraction into backward-bending, or left sidebending, or left rotation. After relaxation, the operator engages the new flexion, right sidebending, and right rotational barrier and the isometric contraction is repeated three to five times.

7. Retest.

Note: Eye movement can be substituted for the activating force with the patient either looking up toward the eyebrows or to the left after each localization.

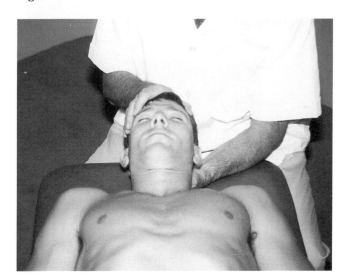

Figure 13.41.

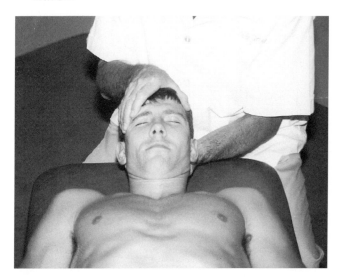

Figure 13.43.

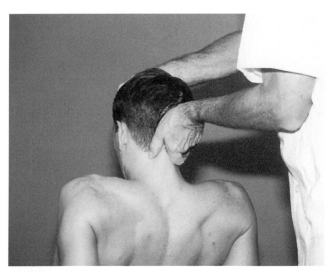

Figure 13.42.

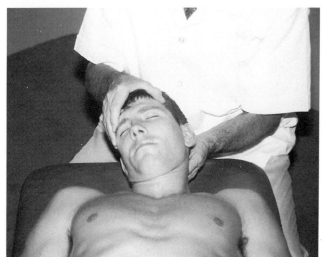

Figure 13.44.

Cervical Spine Muscle Energy Technique

Atlantoaxial (C1–2)

Diagnosis
Position: Atlas rotated right
Motion restriction: Atlas resists left rotation on axis

1. Patient supine on table with operator sitting or standing at head.

2. Operator grasps the head with the palms of the hands and flexes the head to approximately 30° (Fig. 13.45).

3. Operator introduces left rotation against the restricted barrier (Fig. 13.46).

4. Patient instruction is to turn the head to the right against the operator's resisting right hand with a light isometric contraction.

5. After a 3- to 5-second contraction and subsequent relaxation, the operator increases left rotation to the next resistent barrier.

6. Patient repeats right rotational effort against resistance three to five times.

7. Retest.

Note: Eye movement activating force is looking to the right.

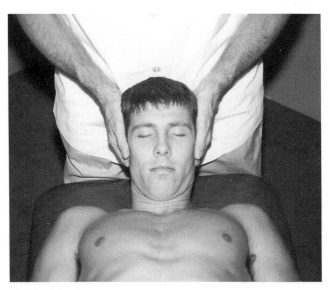

Figure 13.45.

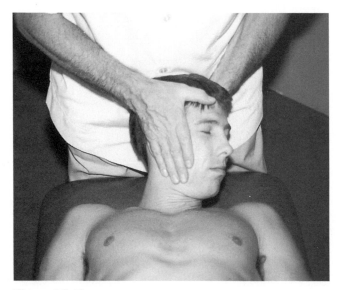

Figure 13.46.

Cervical Spine Muscle Energy Technique

Occipitoatlantal (C0–1)

Diagnosis
Position: Flexed, sidebent right, rotated left
($FS_R R_L$)
Motion restriction: Backward-bending, left sidebending, right rotation

1. Patient supine on table with operator sitting or standing at head.

2. Operator's left hand controls the patient's occiput with the web of the thumb and index finger along the soft tissues at the cervicocranial junction (Fig. 13.47).

3. Operator's right hand holds the patient's chin with the index finger in front and the middle finger below the tip of the ramus and with the right forearm in contact with the right side of the patient's head (Fig. 13.48).

4. The backward-bending barrier is engaged by the operator's two hands rotating the head posteriorly around a transverse axis through the external auditory meati (Fig. 13.49).

5. Left sidebending is introduced through the operator's right forearm by slight left to right translation (Fig. 13.50). Note: Rotation is not actively introduced.

6. The patient is instructed to look down at the feet or pull the chin toward the chest against resistance offered by the operator's right hand for a 3- to 5-second light isometric muscle contraction.

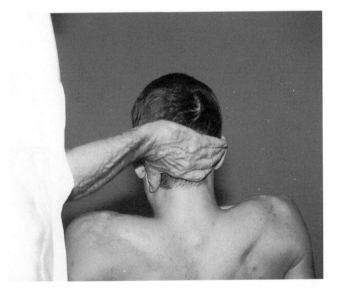

Figure 13.47.

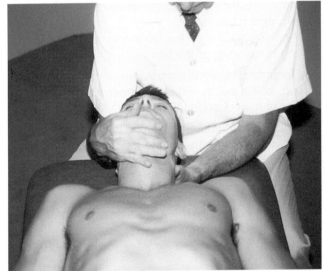

Figure 13.49.

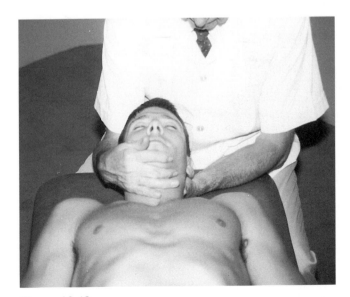

Figure 13.48.

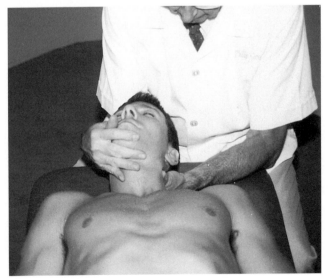

Figure 13.50.

7. After relaxation, the new backward-bending, left sidebending, and right rotational barrier are engaged.

8. Operator's muscle contraction is repeated three to five times with the operator relocalizing against the resisted barrier after each effort.

9. Retest.

Note: The eye movement of looking toward the feet is usually sufficient force for correction of this dysfunction.

Cervical Spine Muscle Energy Technique

Occipitoatlantal (C0–1)

Diagnosis
Position: Extended, sidebent right, rotated left ($ES_R\ R_L$)
Motion restriction: Forward-bending, left sidebending, right rotation

1. Patient is supine on the table with the operator sitting or standing at the head.

2. Operator's left hand controls the occiput with the web of the thumb and index finger along the soft tissue of the suboccipital area (Fig. 13.47).

3. The operator's right hand cups the chin with the index finger in front and the middle finger below the tip of the ramus. The operator's right forearm is placed along the right side of the patient's head (Fig. 13.51).

4. Forward-bending is introduced by rotating the head forward by the operator's two hands around a transverse axis through the external auditory meati (Fig. 13.52).

5. Sidebending and right rotation are introduced by the operator's right forearm and with slight left to right translation of the patient's head to engage the restrictive barrier (Fig. 13.53). Note: Right rotation is not actively introduced.

6. Patient instruction is to push the head directly posteriorly toward the table into the hand offering resistance for 3–5 seconds of a mild isometric muscle contraction.

7. After relaxation, the operator engages the forward-bending, left sidebending, and right rotational barriers.

8. Patient repeats the isometric contractions three to five times.

9. Retest.

Note: An eye motion activating force is to look up toward the operator or toward the eyebrows.

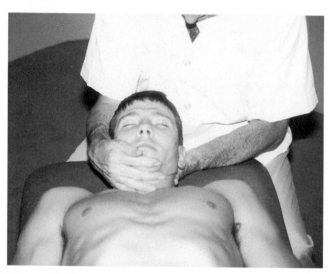

Figure 13.52.

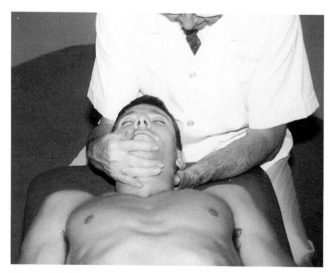

Figure 13.51.

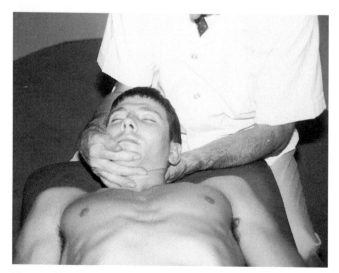

Figure 13.53.

Cervical Spine Muscle Energy Technique

Occipitoatlantal (C0–1)

1. Patient supine on table with operator sitting at head.

2. Operator's left thumb and index finger grasp the posterior arch of the atlas and the occiput lies in the palm of the operator's left hand (Fig. 13.54).

3. Operator's right hand spans the frontal region of the patient's head.

4. For a dysfunction that resists forward-bending, left sidebending, and right rotation (ES_RR_L), the operator rolls the head into forward-bending and with the right hand introduces left sidebending and right rotation against the resistance of the atlas held by the operator's left hand (Fig. 13.55).

5. A 3- to 5-second slight mild isometric contraction of the patient's head into backward-bending or right sidebending is resisted by the operator's two hands.

6. After relaxation, the new barriers are engaged and the patient repeats the isometric contraction three to five times.

7. Retest.

8. For a dysfunction showing restriction of backward-bending, right sidebending, and left rotation, the operator introduces backward-bending through rotation, sidebending to the right, and rotation to the left with the right hand (Fig. 13.56).

9. The patient provides a mild isometric contraction in the direction of forward-bending or left sidebending against resistance offered by the operator's right hand and against the atlas stabilized by the operator's left hand.

10. After relaxation, the new backward-bending (extension), right sidebending, and left rotation barrier is engaged and the patient repeats the isometric contraction three to five times.

11. Retest.

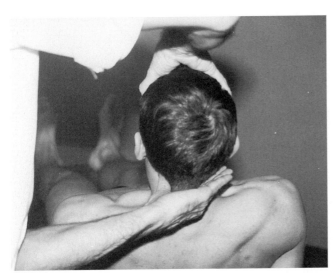

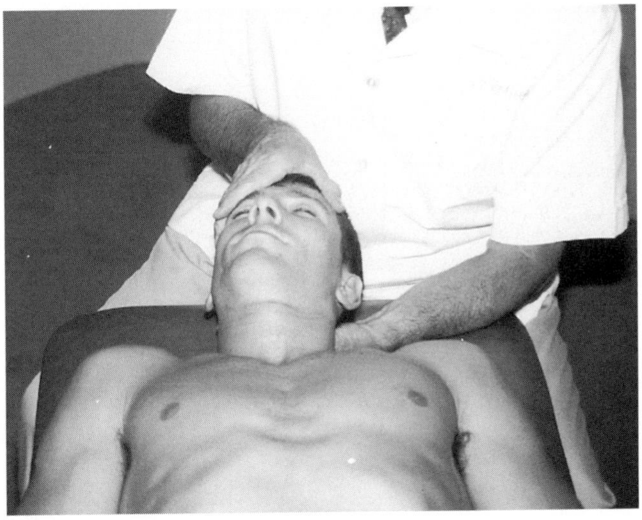

Figure 13.54.

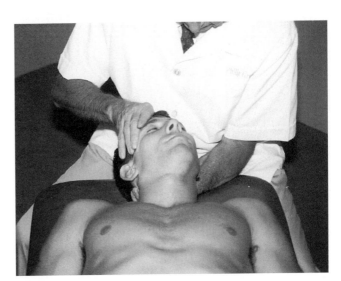

Figure 13.55.

Figure 13.56.

Cervical Spine Mobilization with Impulse Technique

Typical Cervical Vertebra C5–6 Example

Diagnosis
Position: Flexed, rotated left, sidebent left (FRS_left)
Motion restriction: Extension, right rotation, right sidebending

1. Patient supine on table with operator sitting or standing at head.

2. Operator's left hand controls left side of the patient's head and proximal neck.

3. Operator's right second metacarpophalangeal joint contacts the articular pillar of C5 (the superior vertebra of the dysfunctional vertebral motion segment) (Fig. 13.57).

4. Backward-bending and right sidebending is introduced to the restricted barrier (Fig. 13.58).

    Note: Even though the head is sidebent right and rotated left through the upper cervical complex, C5 is rotating right in response to the right sidebending of C5 on C6.

5. A high velocity, low amplitude thrust is applied in a caudad direction toward the spinous process of T1 (Fig. 13.59).

6. Retest.

    Note: Regardless of which cervical segment is dysfunctional, the thrust is always in the direction of the spinous process of T1.

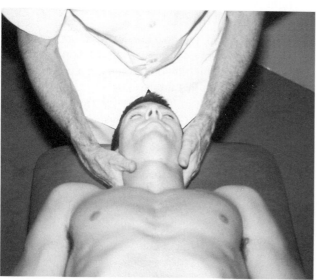

Figure 13.57.

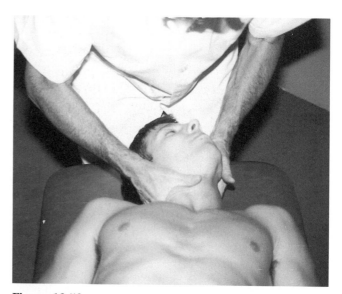

Figure 13.59.

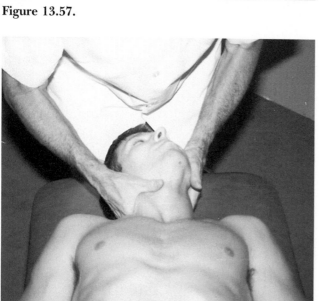

Figure 13.58.

Cervical Spinal Mobilization with Impulse Technique

C2–3 Example

Diagnosis
Position: Extended, rotated left, sidebent left (ERS$_{left}$)
Motion restriction: Forward-bending, right rotation, right sidebending
Opening facet thrust variation 1

1. Patient supine with operator standing at head of table.

2. Operator's right second metacarpophalangeal joint contacts the right zygapophysial joint of C2–3. The operator's left hand controls the patients head and neck (Fig. 13.60).

3. The head is flexed and sidebent right localized at C2–3 (Fig. 13.61).

4. A high velocity, low amplitude thrust is applied horizontally in the plane of the involved C2–3 joint, resulting in a "gapping" opening of the left zygapophysial joint (Fig. 13.62).

5. Retest.

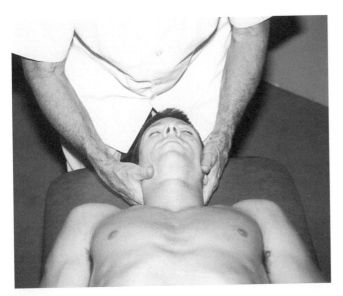

Figure 13.60.

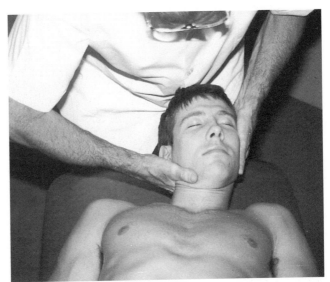

Figure 13.62.

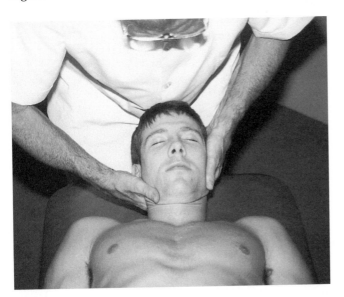

Figure 13.61.

Cervical Spine Mobilization with Impulse Technique

Typical Cervical Segments C2–3 Example

Diagnosis
Position: Extended, rotated left, sidebent left (ERS$_{left}$)
Motion restriction: Forward-bending, right rotation, right sidebending
Opening facet thrust variation 2

1. Patient supine with operator sitting or standing at head of table.

2. Operator controls the head through both hands with the left second metacarpophalangeal joint overlying the left pillar of C2 (Fig. 13.63). The second and third fingers of the operator's right hand contact the right zygapophysial joint of C2–3 to serve as a blocking pivot (Fig. 13.64).

3. Using both hands, the operator forward bends the head down to the flexion barrier of C2–3 (Fig. 13.65).

4. Operator right rotates and right sidebends the patient's head over the fulcrum established by the right second and third fingers to the barrier (Fig. 13.66).

   Note: Be sure to maintain the right sidebending component as the left hand introduces right rotation (Fig. 13.67).

5. A high velocity, low amplitude rotary thrust is applied through the operator's left hand by elevating the left elbow toward the ceiling (Fig. 13.68).

6. Retest.

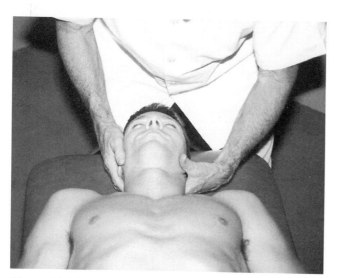

Figure 13.63.

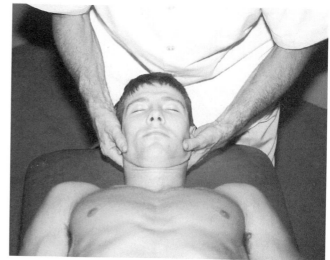

Figure 13.65.

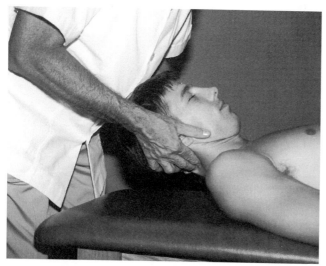

Figure 13.64.

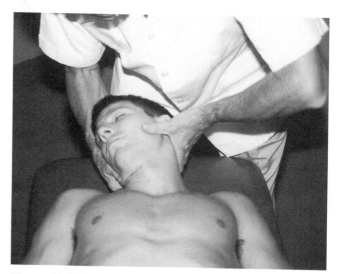

Figure 13.66.

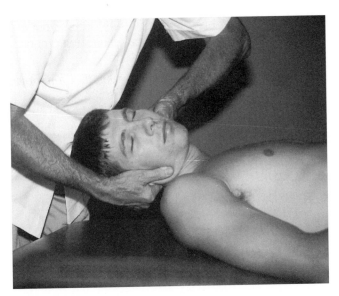

Figure 13.67.

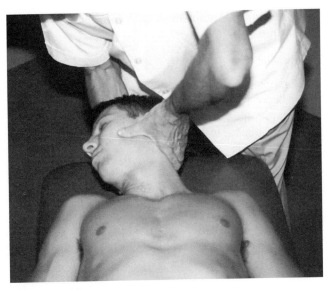

Figure 13.68.

Cervical Spine Mobilization with Impulse Technique

Atlantoaxial (C1–2)

Diagnosis
Position: Atlas rotated right
Motion restriction: Atlas resists left rotation on axis

1. Patient supine with operator sitting or standing at head of table.

2. Operator's right second metacarpophalangeal joint contacts the right posterior arch of the atlas. The operator's left hand controls the left side of the head and neck.

3. Head is flexed approximately 30–45° to take out the flexion mobility of the typical cervical segments below (Fig. 13.69).

4. Operator's two hands rotate the atlas to the right to its restrictional barrier and fine-tune the forward-bending and backward-bending and right and left sidebending components to maximum ease (Fig. 13.70).

5. A rotary thrust is applied through both hands in a left rotational direction (Fig. 13.71).

6. Retest.

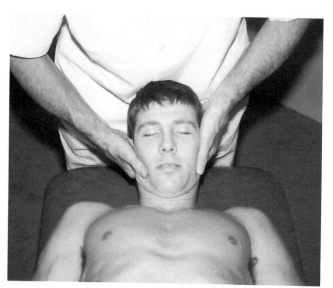

Figure 13.69.

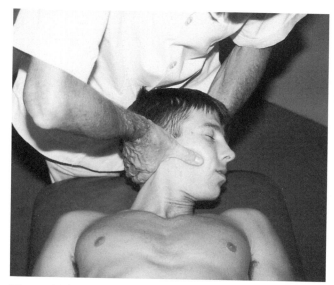

Figure 13.71.

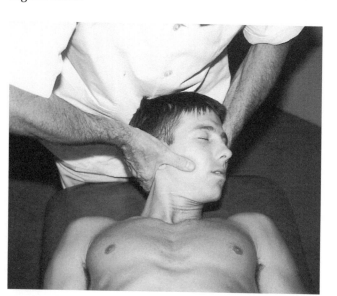

Figure 13.70.

Cervical Spine Mobilization with Impulse Technique

Occipitoatlantal (C0–1)

Diagnosis
Position: Flexed, sidebent right, rotated left
(FS$_R$ R$_L$)
Motion restriction: Backward-bending, left sidebending, right rotation

1. Patient supine with operator sitting at head of table.

2. Operator's left hand cradles the occiput between the web of the thumb and index finger with bony contact at suboccipital region. Do not compress the posterior occipitoatlantal membrane (Fig. 13.72).

3. Operator's right hand cradles the patient's chin with the right forearm along the right side of the patient's mandible and temporal regions (Fig. 13.73). Extension is introduced through both hands by posterior rotation around a transverse axis through the external auditory meati. Left sidebending and right rotation are introduced through the operator's right forearm and with slight left to right translation (Fig. 13.74). Note: Rotation is not actively introduced but follows sidebending.

4. When all three barriers are engaged, a high velocity, low amplitude thrust is applied through both operator's hands in a cephalic long axis extension direction (Fig. 13.75).

Note: The left forearm is caudad to the left hand contact on the occiput for better control of the long axis extension thrust.

5. Retest.

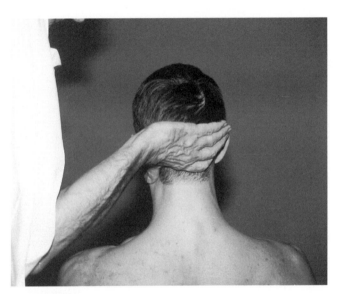

Figure 13.72.

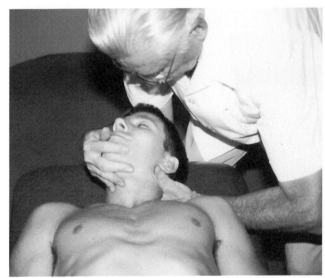

Figure 13.74.

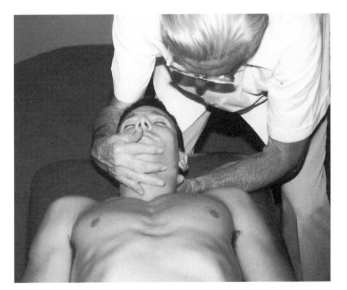

Figure 13.73.

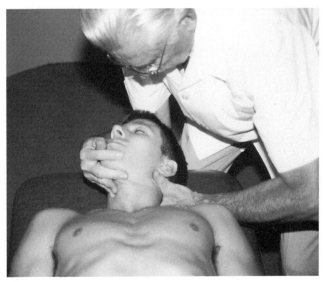

Figure 13.75.

Cervical Spine Mobilization with Impulse Technique

Occipitoatlantal (C0–1)

Diagnosis
Position: Extended, right sidebent, left rotated
Motion restriction: Forward-bending, left sidebending, right rotation

1. Patient supine with operator sitting or standing at head of table.

2. Operator's left hand cradles occiput with web of thumb and index finger on bone to monitor suboccipital tissue tension. Do not compress the posterior occipitoatlantal membrane (Fig. 13.72).

3. Operator's right hand cradles patient's chin with right forearm along right side of patient's face and head (Fig. 13.76).

4. Operator introduces forward-bending by rotating the head anteriorly around a transverse axis through the external auditory meati.

5. Left sidebending and right rotation are introduced through the operator's right forearm and slight left to right translation (Fig. 13.77). Note: Right rotation is not actively introduced.

6. When the flexion, left sidebending, and right rotational barriers are engaged, a high velocity, low amplitude thrust is applied in a cephalic long axis extension, direction simultaneously by both hands (Fig. 13.78).

Note: The operator's left forearm to elbow are below the occipital contact giving better control of the long axis extension thrust.

7. Retest.

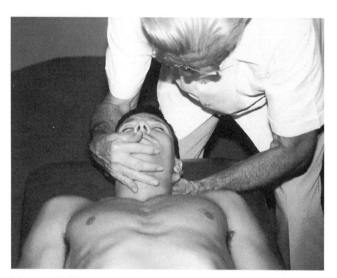

Figure 13.76.

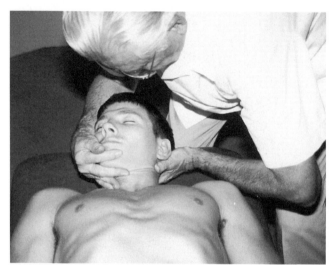

Figure 13.78.

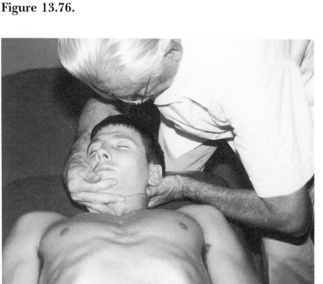

Figure 13.77.

Cervical Spine Combined Soft Muscle Inhibition and Craniosacral Condylar Decompression

Craniooccipital Junction

1. Patient supine with operator sitting at head of table.

2. Operator cradles head in both hands with finger-pads along the insertion of extensor cervical muscles in the occiput.

3. Flexion of the operator's distal interphalangeal joints place inhibitory pressure against muscle insertion in the occiput (Fig. 13.79).

4. When softening of muscle hypertonicity occurs, the operator places the two middle fingers on each side of the external occipital protuberance (inion) with the heels of the hands together.

5. With the operator's forearms on the table, the middle fingers are moved anteriorly along bone as far forward as possible with contact on the condylar portion of the occipital bone (Fig. 13.80).

6. With flexion of the distal interphalangeal joints of the middle finger putting compressive force on the occipital condylar portion, the elbows are brought together, resulting in a posterolateral distraction of each condylar portion of bone (Fig. 13.81).

7. Operator enhances the amount of compressive force on the condylar portion of the occiput that has less resilience until softening occurs.

8. The goal of treatment is relaxation of suboccipital muscles and symmetrical resiliency of bone in the occipital condylar parts.

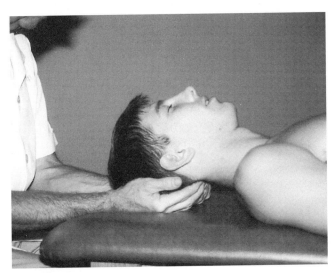

Figure 13.79.

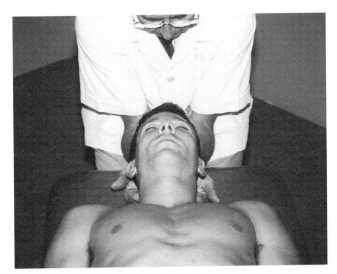

Figure 13.81.

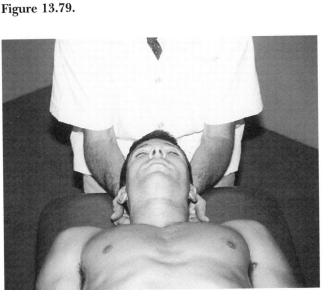

Figure 13.80.

CONCLUSION

There are a number of structural diagnostic and manual medicine therapeutic interventions for the cervical spine. Only five somatic dysfunctions occur in the cervical spine, namely, flexion or extension restriction with coupled sidebending and rotation to the same side in the typical cervical segments, rotational restriction of the atlas on the axis, and either flexion or extension with sidebending and rotational restriction to opposite sides at the occipitoatlantal articulation. There are many combinations of these dysfunctions. Remember that the upper cervical complex functions as an integrative unit and dysfunction of the occipitoatlantal, atlantoaxial, and C2 on C3 are very common. The muscle energy and mobilization with impulse techniques described in this chapter have been most effective and safe in the hands of the author. Mastery of the diagnostic and manual medicine treatment procedures for the cervical spine is useful in managing the myriad of head, neck, and upper extremity problems presenting to the manual medicine practitioner. A thorough understanding of the functional anatomy and biomechanics of the cervical spine is essential for effective and safe manual medicine technique.

14

Twelve vertebrae comprise the thoracic spine and are noted for their posterior kyphosis. The thoracic spine is intimately related to the rib cage and essentially works as a single unit. Alteration in thoracic spine function influences the rib cage, and alteration in rib cage function alters the thoracic spine. Hence, from the respiratory-circulatory model of manual medicine, the thoracic spine assumes major importance in providing optimal functional capacity to the thoracic cage for respiration and circulation. The thoracic spine takes on additional importance from the neurological perspective because of the relationship with the sympathetic division of the autonomic nervous system. All 12 segments of the thoracic spinal cord give origin to preganglionic sympathetic nerve fibers, which exit through the intervertebral canals of the thoracic vertebra and either synapse in or traverse through the lateral chain sympathetic ganglion lying on the anterior aspect of the costovertebral articulations. Recall that the preganglionic sympathetic nerve innervation to the soma and viscera above the diaphragm takes origin from the first four to five segments of the thoracic cord. All of the viscera and soma below the diaphragm receive their preganglionic sympathetic nerve fibers from the spinal cord below T5. Many of the tissue texture abnormalities used in the diagnosis of somatic dysfunction appear to be manifestations of altered secretomotor, pilomotor, and vasomotor functions of the skin viscera. Because the sympathetic nervous system is segmentally organized, skin viscera and internal viscera share many sympathetic nervous system reflexes. It has been clinically noted that internal viscera sharing preganglionic innervation origin in the spinal cord with somatic segments demonstrating tissue texture abnormality may be involved in dysfunctional or diseased states.

FUNCTIONAL ANATOMY

The typical thoracic vertebra has a body roughly equal in its transverse and anteroposterior diameters. The vertebral bodies have demifacets, located posterolaterally at the upper and lower margins of the body, which articulate with the head of the rib. These demifacets are true arthrodial joints with a capsule and articular cartilage. The posterior arch of the thoracic vertebra has zygapophysial joints on the superior and inferior articular pillars. The superior zygapophysial joints face backward, laterally, and slightly superiorly, and the inferior zygapophysial joints face just the reverse. Theoretically, this facet facing would provide a great deal of rotation to the thoracic vertebra, but rotation is restricted by the attachment of the ribs. The transverse processes are unique, with the anterior surface having a small articular facet for articulation with the posterior-facing facet of the tubercle of the adjacent rib. The relationship of the costovertebral and costotransverse articulations greatly influences the type and amount of rib motion. The posterior aspects of the transverse processes are valuable anatomical landmarks for structural diagnosis of thoracic spine dysfunction. The spinous processes project backward and inferiorly and, in the midportion, are severely shingled one upon the other (see rule of 3s, Chapter 5).

Atypical Thoracic Vertebrae

The atypical thoracic vertebrae are those that are transitional between the cervical and thoracic spines and the thoracic and lumbar spines. T1 has the broadest transverse processes in the thoracic spine. The lateral portion of the vertebral body has a unifacet for articulation with the head of the first rib. Although the inferior zygapophysial joint facing is typically thoracic, the superior zygapophysial joint facing is transitional from the cervical spine and may have typical cervical characteristics. T1 is also the junction of the change in anteroposterior curve between the cervical and thoracic spine. Dysfunction of T1 profoundly affects the functional capacity of the thoracic inlet and related structures.

T12 is the location of transition to the lumbar spine. The superior zygapophysial joint facing is usually typically thoracic, whereas the inferior zygapophysial joint facing tends toward lumbar characteristics. There is a unifacet on the lateral side of the body for articulation with the 12th rib. The transverse processes are quite short and rudimentary and are difficult to palpate with certainty. T12 is the location for the change in the anteroposterior curve between the thoracic kyphosis and the lumbar lordosis, a location of change in mobility of two areas of the spine, and a point of frequent dysfunction.

Thoracic Kyphosis

Thoracic kyphosis is normally a smooth posterior convexity without severe areas of increased convexity or "flattening." The observation of "flat spots" within the thoracic kyphosis should alert the diagnostician to evaluate this area carefully for nonneutral type II vertebral somatic dysfunction. The thoracic kyphosis changes at its upper and lower extremities (at the transitional zones) to flow into the cervical and lumbar lordoses. Because of this, frequently the upper segments of the thoracic spine are viewed from the perspective of the cervical spine, whereas the lower thoracic segments are viewed as an extension of the lumbar spine. Many techniques for cervical dysfunction are highly appropriate and effective in the upper thoracic spine, and many lumbar techniques are effective in the lower thoracic spine.

THORACIC SPINE MOTION

The attachment of the ribs through the costovertebral and costotransverse articulations reduce the amount of mobility within the thoracic spine. Thoracic segments have forward-bending and backward-bending movement, as well as coupled movements of sidebending and rotation to the same side and to opposite sides. The coupling of sidebending and rotation in the thoracic spine is complex. Vertebral coupling depends on many factors, including whether the segments involved are above or below the apex of the thoracic kyphosis and whether sidebending or rotation is introduced first. As a general rule, if sidebending is introduced with the thoracic spine in a neutral kyphosis, rotation occurs to the opposite side after neutral (type I) vertebral motion. If rotation is introduced first in the presence of a normal thoracic kyphosis, sidebending and rotation occur to the same side after the rule of nonneutral (type II) vertebral mechanics. T1 through T3 most commonly follows nonneutral vertebral mechanics as a carryover from the lower cervical spine.

Despite the complexity of thoracic spine motion, clinical evaluation identifies that the thoracic spine can become dysfunctional with nonneutral single segment (type II) dysfunctions and neutral (type I) group dysfunction. The screening and scanning examination can lead the examiner to pursue specific segmental diagnosis in the thoracic spine. Identification of the dysfunctional segment begins by palpating soft tissue changes of hypertonicity in the fourth layer of the erector spinae muscle mass by palpating in the medial groove between the spinous process and the longissimus. Palpable muscle hypertonicity of the deepest muscle layers, including the multifidi and levator costales, is pathognomonic of vertebral motion segment dysfunction at that level (Fig. 14.1).

MOTION TESTING

Vertebral motion testing and the diagnosis of restriction of vertebral motion are described in Chapter 6. The most useful test is to monitor change in the relationship of pairs of transverse processes through an arc of forward-bending to backward-bending. For the upper thoracic spine from T1 to T5, the introduction of active forward-bending and backward-bending of the head on the neck is performed while the operator monitors the behavior of the paired transverse processes. With nonneutral (type II) extended, rotated, sidebent (ERS) restriction, the transverse process on one side will become more prominent during forward-bending and the transverse processes become symmetric during backward-bending. In nonneutral (type II) flexed, rotated, sidebent (FRS) restriction, one transverse process becomes more prominent during backward-bending and the transverse processes become symmetric during forward-bending. In the presence of a neutral group (type I) dysfunction, three or more vertebrae, the transverse processes are prominent on one side. During the forward-bending to backward-bending arc, the posterior transverse processes may change a little, but they never become symmetric.

In the middle and lower thoracic spine, the evaluation is performed both in the sitting position with the patient assuming the three positions of forward-

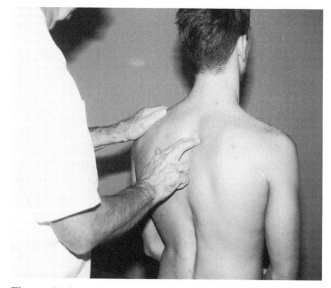

Figure 14.1.
Palpation of hypertonic fourth-layer muscle.

bending, neutral, and backward-bending or in the three static positions of being fully forward bent, prone in neutral on the table, and in backward-bending in the prone prop position.

Structural diagnosis in the presence of a primary structural scoliosis of the thoracic spine becomes quite difficult. The segments involved in a primary scoliosis behave as a neutral group (type I) dysfunction. Patients with a primary structural scoliosis of the thoracic spine have few symptoms of back pain until a relatively minor traumatic episode occurs. Pain and restriction of motion become quite evident. A non-neutral (type II) dysfunction within the primary scoliotic curve is frequently found in this situation. The diagnosis of these nonneutral (type II) dysfunctions is quite difficult, but if the examiner is diligent in searching from one segment to the other, one frequently observes a nonneutral single segment vertebral somatic dysfunction within the curve. The usual observation is a single vertebral motion segment with rotation into the concavity. Single segment fourth layer muscle hypertonicity is a valuable finding in making a diagnosis as to the presence and location of a nonneutral dysfunction within the primary curve.

Thoracic Spine

Upper Thoracic Spine (T1-5)

Diagnosis

1. Patient is sitting on table with operator standing behind.

2. Operator's thumbs palpate the posterior aspect of the transverse processes of the segment under diagnosis (Fig. 14.2).

3. The operator follows the pair of transverse processes during the backward-bending arc as the patient is asked to look up toward the ceiling (Fig. 14.3).

4. The operator follows the pair of transverse processes through a forward-bending arc while asking the patient to look down at the floor (Fig. 14.4).

Note: It is easier to follow a pair of transverse processes during backward-bending than during forward-bending.

5. Based on the behavior of the transverse processes during the forward-bending, neutral, and backward-bending arc, an appropriate single segment vertebral motion somatic dysfunction is made.

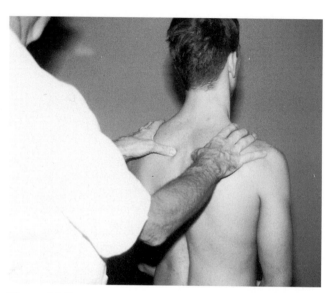

Figure 14.2.

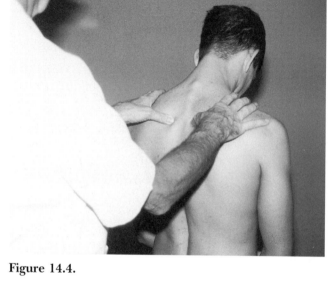

Figure 14.4.

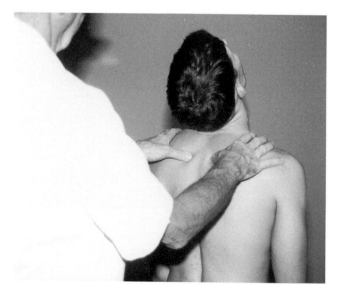

Figure 14.3.

Thoracic Spine Diagnosis

Middle to Lower Thoracic Spine

Dynamic Process

1. The patient is sitting on table with operator standing behind.

2. The operator palpates the posterior aspect of a pair of transverse processes at the segment under diagnosis (Fig. 14.5).

3. Patient is asked to look up at the ceiling and arch the back by pushing the abdomen anteriorly as the operator follows a pair of transverse processes into backward-bending (Fig. 14.6).

4. Patient is asked to slump the back and forward bend the trunk as the operator follows a pair of transverse processes into flexion (Fig. 14.7).

5. Operator evaluates the behavior of the transverse processes through the forward-bending and backward-bending arc, making a diagnosis of a single segment vertebral somatic dysfunction of the ERS or FRS type.

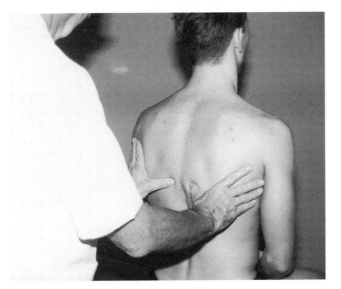

Figure 14.5.

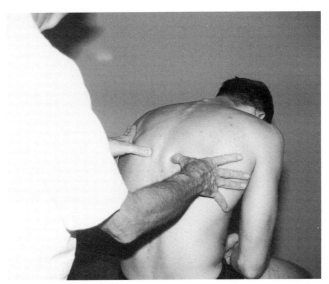

Figure 14.7.

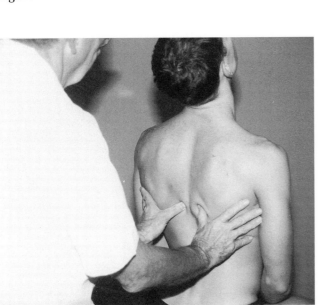

Figure 14.6.

Thoracic Spine Diagnosis

Middle to Lower Thoracic Spine Static Three Positions

1. Patient prone on the table with the operator standing at the side with thumbs palpating a pair of transverse processes (Fig. 14.8).

2. Operator monitors the posterior aspect of the paired transverse processes in the backward bent (prone prop) position (Fig. 14.9).

3. Operator evaluates the pair of transverse processes in the static forward bent position (Fig. 14.7).

4. Evaluation of a single segment nonneutral vertebral dysfunction is identified by comparing the behavior of the paired transverse processes through the three static positions of neutral, backward bent, and forward bent.

MANUAL MEDICINE TECHNIQUE FOR THORACIC SPINE DYSFUNCTION

In the treatment sequence of a patient presenting with multiple areas of somatic dysfunction, the thoracic spine is treated before the treatment of dysfunction of the ribs. This fundamental rule is broken only if resolution of restriction from rib cage dysfunction assists in the treatment process of the thoracic spine dysfunction. Most muscle energy procedures for thoracic spine somatic dysfunctions are performed with the patient sitting, but all can be modified for a patient in the horizontal position supine, lateral recumbent, or prone. As in the cervical spine, muscle energy techniques are usually performed as the initial intervention. If the muscle energy procedure is ineffective and the structural diagnostic process has identified the presence of a chronic deep motion restrictor in the articular and periarticular structures, a mobilization with impulse technique becomes indicated.

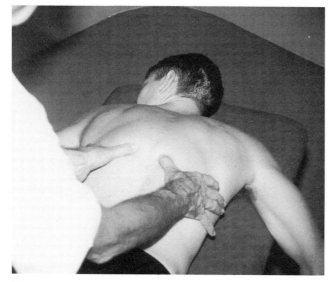

Figure 14.8.

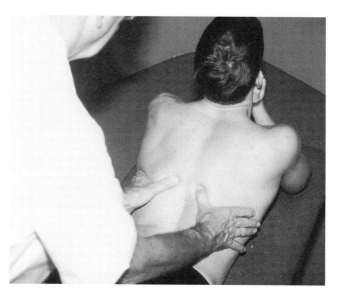

Figure 14.9.

Thoracic Spine

Muscle Energy Technique
T1-5
Sitting (Example: T4-5)
Diagnosis
Position: Extended, rotated left, sidebent left
(ERS$_L$)
Motion restriction: Forward-bending, right rotation, right sidebending

1. Patient sitting on the table with the operator behind.

2. Operator's left hand monitors the T4-5 segment with the left index finger in the interspinous space and the left middle finger overlying the posterior left transverse process of T4 (Fig. 14.10).

3. Operator's right hand is on the top of the patient's head, and the operator's trunk is against the posterior aspect of the patient's body.

4. Operator introduces forward-bending to the T4-5 segment by anterior to posterior translation of the patient's body localized at the T4-5 level (Fig. 14.11).

5. Operator engages the right sidebending and right rotational barrier at the T4-5 level by introducing right to left translation through the trunk with localization at the T4-5 level (Fig. 14.12).

6. Operator resists either a backward-bending, left sidebending, or left rotational effort of the patient's head and neck by giving resistance with the right

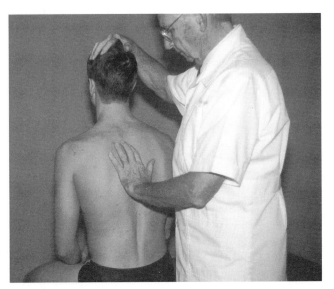

Figure 14.10.

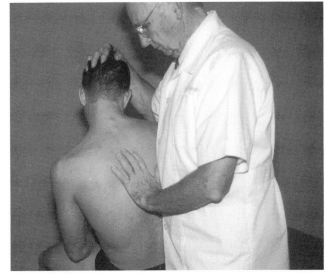

Figure 14.12.

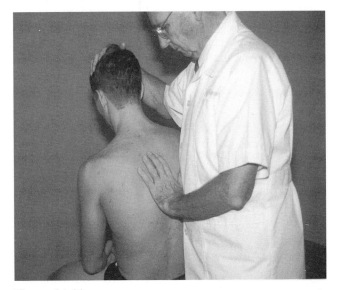

Figure 14.11.

hand (Fig. 14.13). A 3- to 5-second isometric muscle contraction is resisted by the operator's right hand.

7. After relaxation, the operator engages the new forward-bending, right sidebending, and right rota-

tional barrier and the patient performs three to five repetitions of the isometric muscle contraction (Fig. 14.14).

8. Retest.

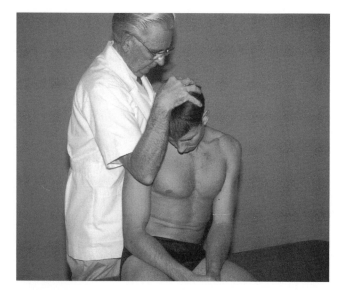

Figure 14.13.

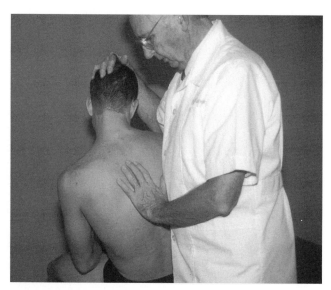

Figure 14.14.

Thoracic Spine

Muscle Energy Technique
T1-5
Sitting (Example: T2-3)
Diagnosis
    Position: Flexed, sidebent left, rotated left
    (FRS$_L$)
    Motion restriction: Backward-bending, right
    sidebending, and right rotation

1. Patient is sitting with the operator behind.

2. Operator's right index finger palpates the interspace between T2 and T3 and the right middle finger palpates over the right transverse process of T2 (Fig. 14.15).

3. Operator's left hand and forearm control the patient's head and neck with the operator's trunk against the posterior aspect of the left trunk of the patient (Fig. 14.16). Operator's left hand introduces a small amount of right rotation to gap the right zygapophysial joint at T2-3.

4. Operator translates the trunk forward with localization of the thumb over the middle to lower scapular region. The patient is asked to tuck the chin in and carry the head into posterior translation localizing extension at the T2-3 segment (Fig. 14.17). Translation right to left engages right sidebending, right rotation barrier.

5. The patient is instructed to perform a mild isometric contraction of forward-bending, left sidebending, or left rotation of the head and neck against the resisting left hand and forearm of the operator for a 3- to 5-second contraction.

6. After relaxation, a new backward-bending, right sidebending, and right rotational barrier is engaged, and the patient is instructed to repeat the isometric contraction three to five times (Fig. 14.18).

7. Retest.

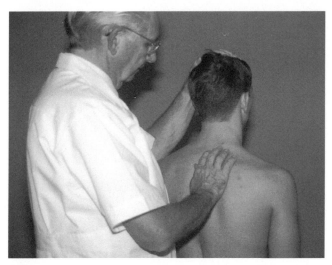

Figure 14.15.

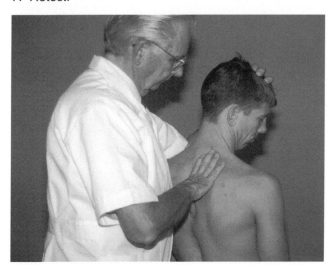

Figure 14.17.

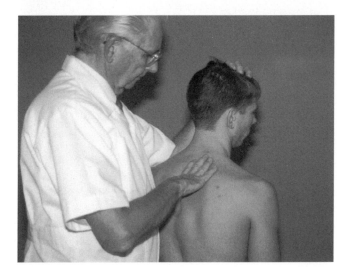

Figure 14.16.

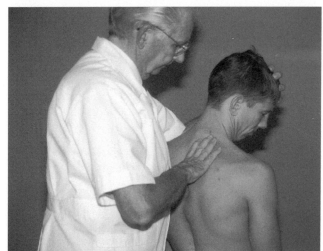

Figure 14.18.

Thoracic Spine

Muscle Energy Technique
T1-5
Sitting
Diagnosis
Dysfunction: Neutral, sidebent right, rotated left
(NS_RR_L) or (EN_L).
Motion restriction: Sidebending left, rotation right.

1. Patient sits erect with operator standing behind.
2. Operator's left thumb is localized to the apex of the left convexity (Fig. 14.19).
3. Operator's right hand controls the patient's head and stabilizes the cervical spine (Fig. 14.20).

4. Left sidebending and right rotation are introduced by translation by the localizing thumb from left to right (Fig. 14.21).
5. Patient is instructed to sidebend the head to the right against the resistance offered by the operator's right hand and forearm (Fig. 14.22).
6. After relaxation, left sidebending and right rotational barriers are again engaged, and the patient repeats the isometric muscle contraction of right sidebending.
7. Three to five repetitions are made of a 3- to 5-second isometric contraction.
8. Retest.

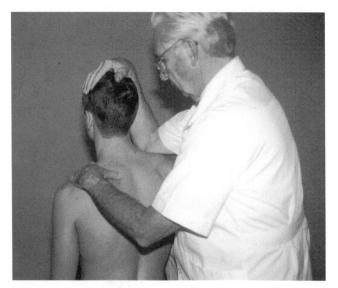

Figure 14.19.

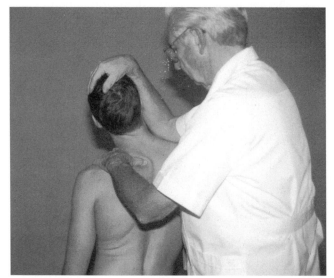

Figure 14.21.

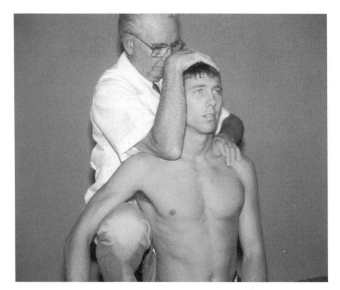

Figure 14.20.

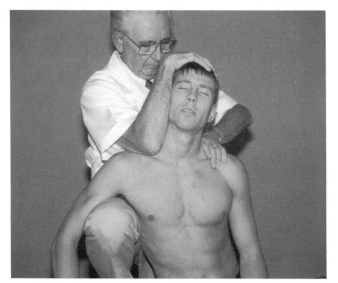

Figure 14.22.

Thoracic Spine

Muscle Energy Technique
T5-12
Sitting (Example: T8-9)
Diagnosis
    Position: Extended (backward bent), right
    rotated, right sidebent (ERS$_R$)
    Motion restriction: Flexion (forward-bending),
    left sidebending, left rotation

1. Patient sitting with operator behind.

2. Patient's left hand holds the right shoulder. Operator's left arm controls the patient's trunk with the left hand grasping the right shoulder and the left shoulder resting in the operator's left axilla (Fig. 14.23).

3. Operator's right index finger monitors the interspinous space at T8-9 and right middle finger monitors the right transverse process of T8 (Fig. 14.24).

4. The forward-bending (flexion) barrier is engaged by an anterior to posterior translation of the trunk at the T8-9 level (Fig. 14.25).

5. The left sidebending and left rotational barrier are engaged by translation of the patient's trunk from left to right at the T8-9 level (Fig. 14.26).

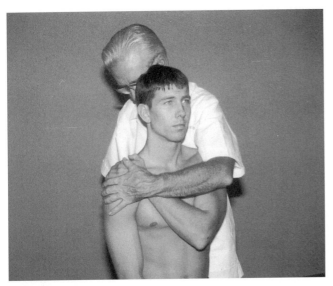

Figure 14.23.

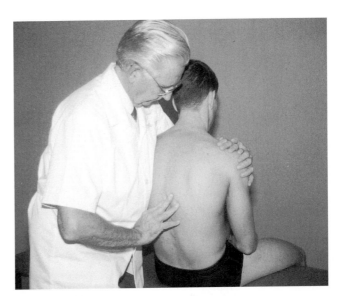

Figure 14.25.

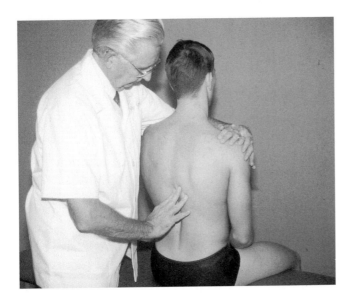

Figure 14.24.

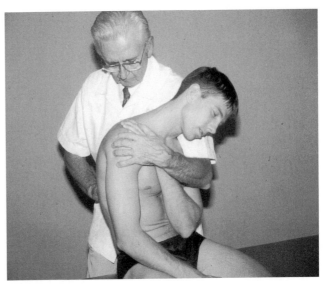

Figure 14.26.

6. Patient is instructed to perform a right sidebending isometric contraction against resistance offered by the operator's left hand and arm for 3–5 seconds (Fig. 14.27).

7. After relaxation, all three barriers are reengaged and the patient performs three to five repetitions of a 3- to 5-second isometric contraction.

8. Retest.

    Note: This technique can be adapted into the upper lumbar spine.

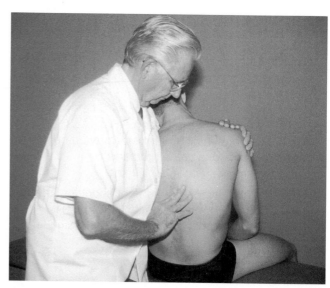

Figure 14.27.

Thoracic Spine

Muscle Energy Technique
T5-12 (Example: T8-9)
Diagnosis

Position: Flexed (forward bent), rotated right, sidebent right (FRS$_R$)

Motion restriction: Extension (backward-bending), sidebending left, rotation left

1. Patient sitting with operator behind.

2. Operator's left hand controls the patient's trunk through a contact on the left shoulder. Operator's right index finger monitors the interspinous space of T8-9 and the middle finger monitors the right transverse process of T8 (Fig. 14.28).

3. With the spine in the erect neutral position, rotation left of T8 is introduced by right to left translation of T8-9 with the patient dropping the right shoulder and shifting the weight to the left buttock (Fig. 14.29).

4. Patient is instructed to perform a left sidebending isometric contraction against resistance offered by the operator's left hand. This is repeated two to three times to enhance left rotation of T8.

5. Left sidebending and extension barriers are engaged by the operator depressing the patient's left shoulder and the patient shifting the body weight to the right buttock after the operator's instruction of projecting the abdomen over the right knee (Fig. 14.30).

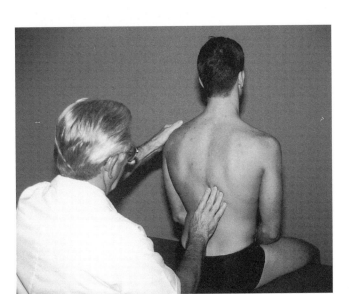

Figure 14.28.

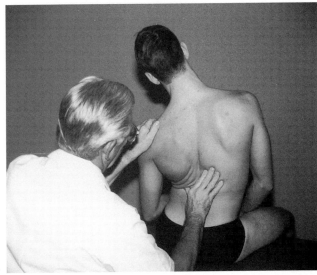

Figure 14.30.

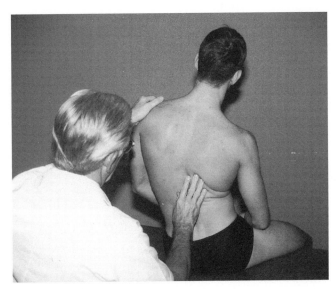

Figure 14.29.

6. The patient is instructed to lift the left shoulder toward the ceiling (right sidebending effort) or pull the left shoulder forward (right rotational effort) for 3–5 seconds and three to five repetitions.

7. After each effort, extension, left sidebending, and left rotational barriers are reengaged by projecting the abdomen over the right knee and translating the trunk from left to right at T8-9.

8. Patient's trunk is now returned to midline with operator's right hand blocking the T9 segment (Fig. 14.31).

9. Operator resists trunk forward-bending by the patient's shoulders with the resisting left arm (Fig. 14.32).

10. Retest.

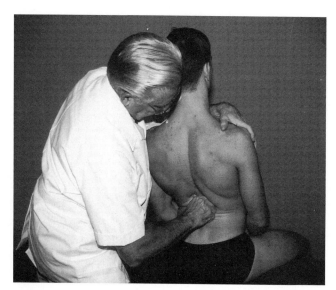

Figure 14.31.

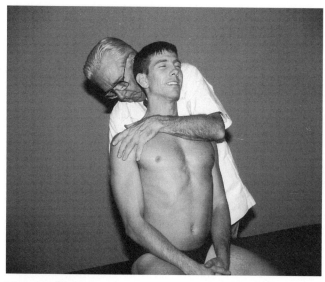

Figure 14.32.

Thoracic Spine

Muscle Energy Technique
T5-12
Group Dysfunction
Diagnosis
  Position: Neutral, sidebent left, rotated right
  ($NS_L R_R$) or (EN_R).
  Motion restriction: Sidebending right, rotation left.

1. Patient sitting with operator behind.

2. Operator's right thumb is localized at the apex of the right convexity with a vector of force anteromedially (Fig. 14.33).

3. Patient's left hand grasps the right shoulder and the operator places the left arm through the patient's left axilla and grasps the right shoulder (Fig. 14.34).

4. With the spine in neutral, sidebending right and rotation left barriers are engaged by a right to left translatory movement at the apex of the convexity (Fig. 14.35).

5. Operator's left arm resists a 3- to 5-second isometric contraction of left sidebending by the patient (Fig. 14.36).

6. After each isometric effort, a new right sidebending and left rotational barrier is engaged and the patient repeats the left sidebending isometric contraction with three to five repetitions.

7. Retest.

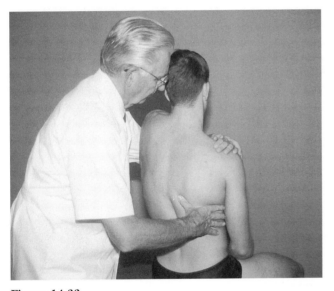

Figure 14.33.

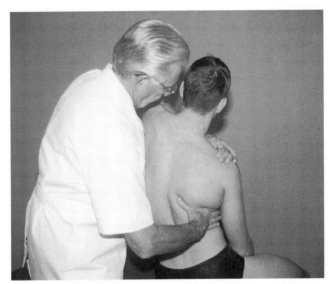

Figure 14.35.

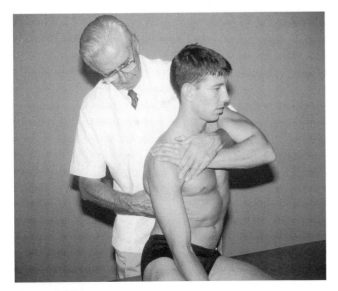

Figure 14.34.

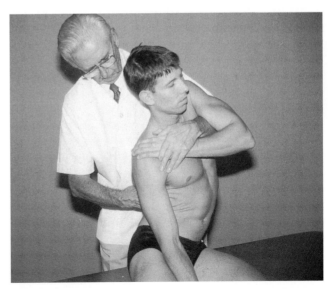

Figure 14.36.

Thoracic Spine

Mobilization with Impulse Technique
T1-5
Sitting (Example: T3-4)
Diagnosis
> Position: Extended (backward bent), left rotated, left sidebent (ERS$_L$)
> Motion restriction: Flexion (forward-bending), right rotation, right sidebending

1. Patient sitting with operator standing behind.

2. Operator's left hand and forearm control the patient's head and left side of neck. Operator's right hand is over the right shawl area with the thumb contacting the right side of the spinous process of T3 (the superior segment of the dysfunctional vertebral motion unit) (Fig. 14.37).

3. Operator's left hand introduces flexion, right side-bending, and right rotation of the patient's head and neck through translation from before backward and from right to left localizing at the T3-4 level (Fig. 14.38).

4. When all barriers are engaged, a high velocity, low amplitude thrust is introduced through the operator's right thumb against the spinous process in a right to left translatory movement (Fig. 14.39).

5. Retest.

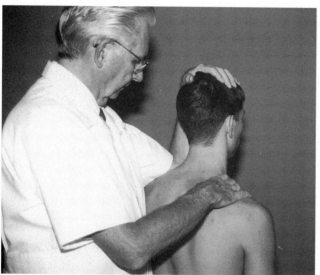

Figure 14.37.

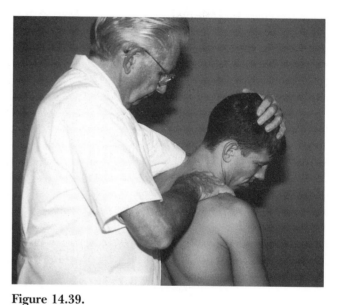

Figure 14.39.

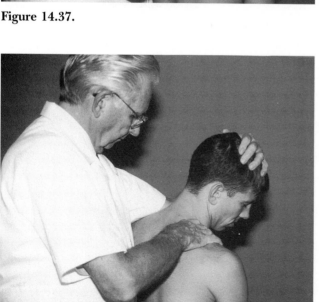

Figure 14.38.

Thoracic Spine

Mobilization with Impulse Technique
T1-5
Sitting
Diagnosis (Example: T3-4)

   Position: Flexed (forward bent), sidebent left, rotated left (FRS_L)

   Motion restriction: Extension (backward-bending), right sidebending, right rotation.

1. Patient sitting with operator standing behind. Patient's left arm may be draped over the operator's left thigh with the left foot on the table.

2. Patient's head and left side of the neck are controlled by the operator's left hand and forearm. Operator's right hand overlies the patient's right shawl area with the thumb in contact with the right side of the spinous process of T3 (the superior segment of the dysfunctional vertebral motor unit) (Fig. 14.40).

3. Operator's left forearm and hand introduce extension (backward-bending), right sidebending, right rotation of the patient's head and neck to T3-4 by translation from behind forward and from right to left (Fig. 14.41).

4. With the extension, right sidebending, and right rotational barriers engaged, a high velocity, low amplitude thrust is introduced from right to left through the thumb contact with the spinous process of T3 (Fig. 14.42).

5. Retest.

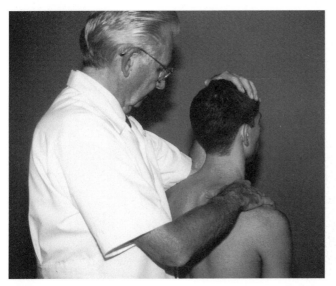

Figure 14.40.

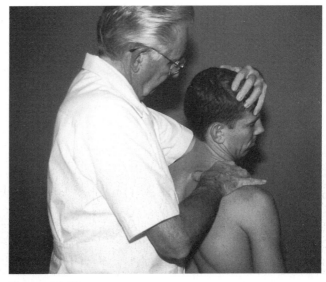

Figure 14.42.

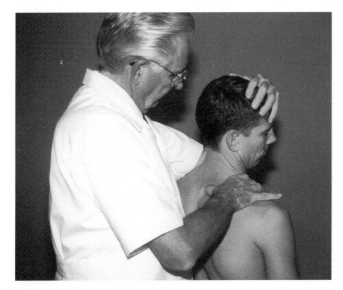

Figure 14.41.

Thoracic Spine

Mobilization with Impulse Technique
T1-5
Sitting (Example: T1-4)
Diagnosis: Group Dysfunction (Type I)
    Position: Neutral, sidebent right, rotated left
    (NS_RR_L) or (EN_L).
    Motion restriction: Sidebending left, rotation
    right.

1. Patient sitting with operator behind. Patient's right arm is draped over the operator's right leg with the right foot on the table.

2. Operator's right hand and forearm control the patient's head and right side of the neck. Operator's left hand is placed over the patient's left shawl area with the left thumb at the intertransverse space between T2 and T3 (Fig. 14.43).

3. Operator's right hand and forearm introduce left sidebending and right rotation with localization at the apex of the left convexity through the left thumb with an anteromedial vector of force (Fig. 14.44).

4. Left sidebending and right rotational barrier is engaged by a left to right translatory movement of the operator's left hand and forearm (Fig. 14.45).

5. A high velocity, low amplitude thrust is introduced through the operator's left hand and thumb in an anteromedial direction from left to right (Fig. 14.46).

6. Retest.

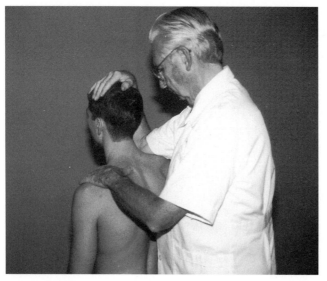

Figure 14.43.

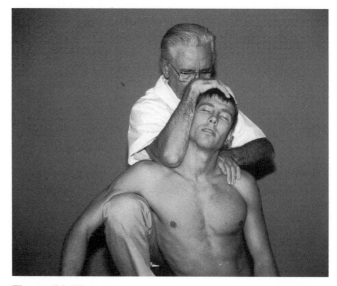

Figure 14.45.

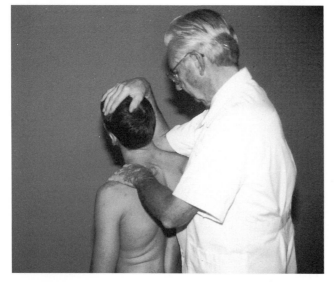

Figure 14.44.

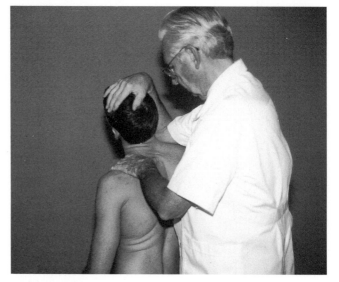

Figure 14.46.

Thoracic Spine

Mobilization with Impulse Technique
T1-5
Prone (Example: T3-4)
Diagnosis
Position: Flexed (forward bent) rotated left, sidebent left (FRS$_L$)
Motion restriction: Extension (backward-bending), right rotation, right sidebending

1. Patient prone with operator standing at head (Fig. 14.47).

2. Operator's hands move patient's chin to the right (introducing right sidebending) and rotate the face to the right (Fig. 14.48).

3. Operator's right pisiform is placed on the right transverse process of T4 (inferior segment of the dysfunctional vertebral motor unit) (Fig. 14.49).

4. A high velocity, low amplitude thrust is applied through the pisiform of the right hand with the operator's left hand stabilizing the head and neck in right sidebending and right rotation. The thrust direction is ventral, rotating T4 to the left with extension, resulting in closure of the right zygapophysial joint at T3-4.

5. Retest.

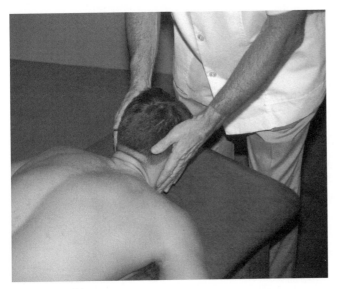

Figure 14.47.

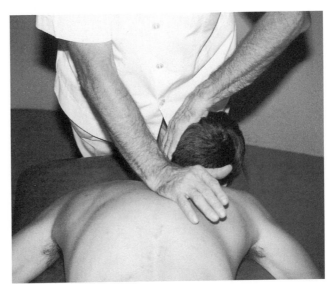

Figure 14.49.

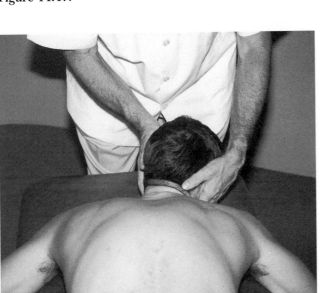

Figure 14.48.

Thoracic Spine

Mobilization with Impulse Technique
T1-5
Prone (Example: Group Dysfunction T1-4)
Diagnosis

Position: Neutral, sidebent right, rotated left
(NS_RR_L) or (EN_L).
Motion restriction: Sidebending left, rotation
right.

1. Patient prone with operator standing with hand controlling patient's head (Fig. 14.50).

2. With chin staying at the midline, operator's left hand introduces left sidebending and right rotation to the apex of the group dysfunction (Fig. 14.51).

3. With the thumb at the intertransverse space of T2-3, a high velocity, low amplitude thrust is performed with an anteromedial thrust of the thumb with the left hand holding the patient's head and neck stable or an exaggeration of the left sidebending and right rotation of the head and neck through the operator's left hand against a stable fulcrum of the right thumb.

4. An alternative contact is with the operator's right pisiform bone at the intertransverse space of T2-3 on the left with similar thrusting force anteromedially with the right hand or exaggeration of the left sidebending right rotation of the head and neck against the fulcrum of the right pisiform (Fig. 14.52).

5. Retest.

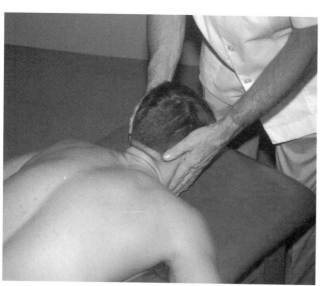

Figure 14.50.

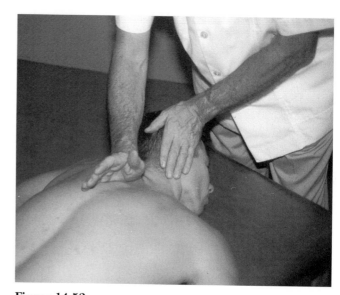

Figure 14.52.

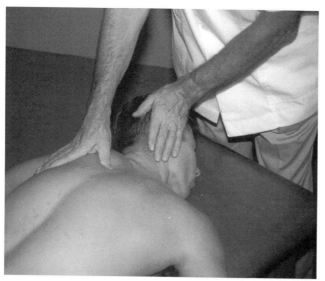

Figure 14.51.

Thoracic Spine

Mobilization with Impulse Technique
T5-10
Prone (Example: T6-7)
Diagnosis
    Position: Flexed (forward bent), rotated right, sidebent right (FRS$_R$)
    Motion restriction: Extension (backward bending), left rotation, left sidebending

1. Patient prone with operator standing on patient's left side.

2. Operator's left pisiform contacts the superior aspect of the left transverse process of T6 in a caudad direction (Fig. 14.53).

3. Operator's right pisiform contacts the right transverse process of T6 with anterior compression introducing left rotation of T6 (Fig. 14.54).

4. The restrictive barrier is engaged by a caudad movement with the operator's left pisiform and an anterior movement of the operator's right pisiform.

5. A high velocity, low amplitude thrust is made through both hands in a ventral direction introducing extension, left sidebending and left rotation of T6 (Fig. 14.55).

6. Retest.

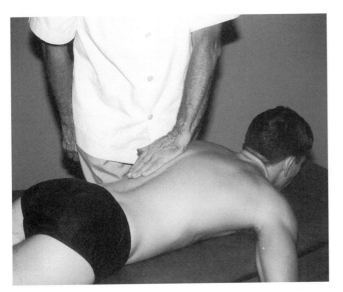

Figure 14.53.

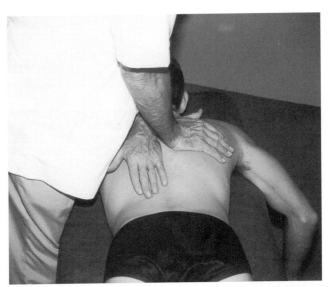

Figure 14.55.

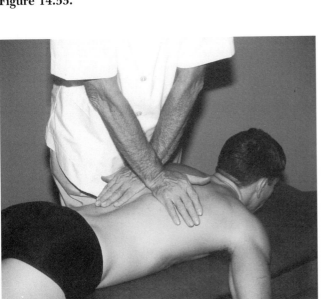

Figure 14.54.

Thoracic Spine

Mobilization with Impulse Technique
T3-12
Supine
Principles of the Technique

Principle 1. Establish lever arm

1. Patient supine with operator standing at side.

2. Patient crosses arms over chest and holds the opposite shoulder. The arm opposite the operator is the superior (Fig. 14.56).

3. Alternative arm position two has the patient clasp the two hands together behind the cervical spine (not the head). This arm position is particular useful in the lower thoracic region (Fig. 14.57).

4. Alternative arm position three is unilateral using the arm opposite the operator grasping the patient's opposite shoulder (Fig. 14.58).

5. Alternative arm position four has patient grasp the right shoulder with the left hand and the left elbow with the right hand (Fig. 14.59).

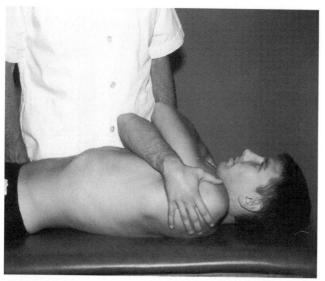

Figure 14.56.

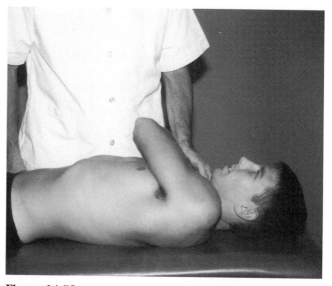

Figure 14.58.

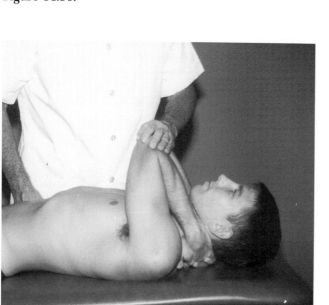

Figure 14.57.

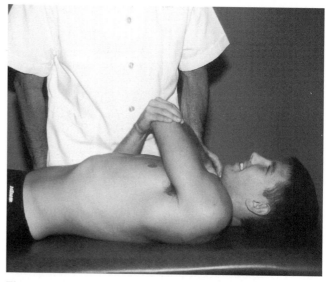

Figure 14.59.

Principle 2. Establish fulcrum

1. The hand is placed to control the inferior segment of the dysfunctional vertebral motion segment with the spinous processes placed in the palm of the hand and with the thumb along the side of the spinous processes (Fig. 14.60).

2. Alternative hand position two is the use of the flexed second, third, fourth, and fifth fingers on one side of the spinous process and the thenar and hypothenar eminence on the other side of the spinous process (Fig. 14.61). This hand position may be uncomfortable both to the patient and operator.

3. A third alternative hand position uses flexion of the proximal and distal interphalangeal joints of the index finger against one transverse process of the inferior segment and the metacarpophalangeal joint of the thumb on the opposite transverse process (Fig. 14.62). This hand position is preferred because it provides a contact of the thenar eminence against the rib shaft of a dysfunctional rib associated with nonneutral (ERS) dysfunctions of the thoracic spine.

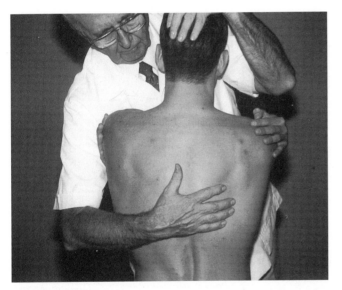

Figure 14.60.

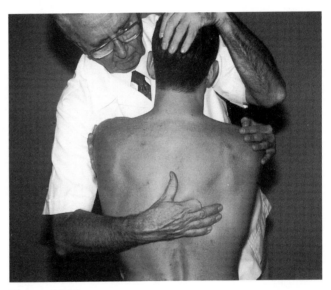

Figure 14.62.

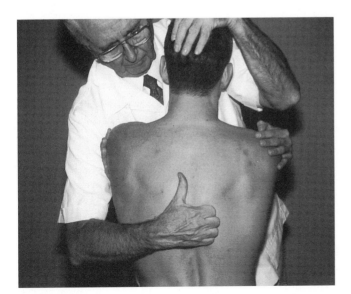

Figure 14.61.

Principle 3. Localization of the lever arm to the fulcrum

1. The operator rolls the patient toward him or her to place the fulcrum on the inferior vertebra of the dysfunctional vertebral motor motion segment.

2. The patient is returned to the neutral position and a body contact is made with the crossed arm lever arm. This preferably is the epigastrium. Care should be taken not to put compressive force against the operator's rib cage or, in a female operator, against breast tissue. A folded towel or small pillow can be used to cushion the patient's elbows against the operator's trunk (Fig. 14.63).

Principle 4. Localization of thrust

1. The fulcrum holds the inferior segment so that the superior segment can be moved in the appropriate direction to engage the barrier.

2. The thrusting force is directed at the superior aspect of the fulcrum.

Thoracic Spine

Mobilization with Impulse Technique
T3-12
Supine
Diagnosis
    Position: Bilaterally extended (both facets in the closed position)
    Motion restriction: Sagittal plane flexion

1. Patient supine with operator standing at side.

2. The lever arm is established by crossing both arms over the chest (or one of the alternative lever arm positions).

3. Operator places the fulcrum hand under the patient's torso localized to the inferior segment of the dysfunctional vertebral unit.

4. Patient returned to neutral midline position with localization of lever arm to fulcrum. Operator's cephalic hand controls patient's head and neck to introduce flexion (Fig. 14.64).

5. Operator flexes thoracic spine down to the superior vertebra of the dysfunctional vertebral motion unit (Fig. 14.65).

6. A high velocity, low amplitude thrust is performed by dropping the operator's body weight through the lever arm to the fulcrum with slight exaggeration of the patient's flexed position.

7. Retest.

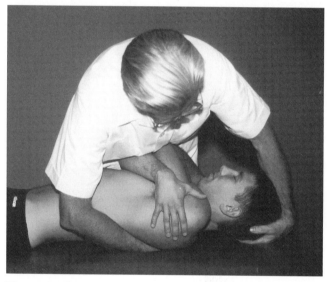

Figure 14.64.

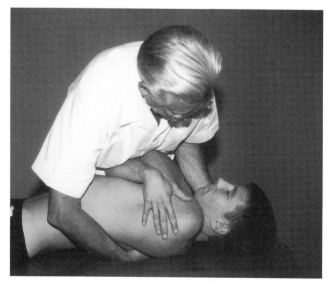

Figure 14.63.

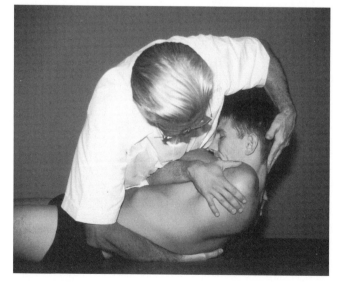

Figure 14.65.

Thoracic Spine

Mobilization with Impulse Technique
T3-12
Supine
Diagnosis
    Position: Bilaterally flexed (both facets in the open position)
    Motion restriction: Sagittal plane extension

1. Patient supine with operator standing at side.

2. Lever arm is established by crossing the arms across the patient's chest holding each shoulder.

3. Operator's hand is placed as the fulcrum on the lower segment of the dysfunctional vertebral motion unit.

4. Patient returned to midline with operator controlling the patient's upper trunk, neck, and head.

5. Patient flexes upper trunk just past the fulcrum (Fig. 14.66).

6. Operator drops patient's head, neck, and upper trunk into extension just over the fulcrum.

7. A high velocity, low amplitude thrust through the operator's trunk against the lever arm takes the superior segment into extension over the fulcrum (Fig. 14.67).

8. Retest.

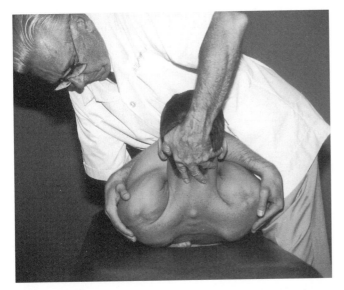

Figure 14.66.

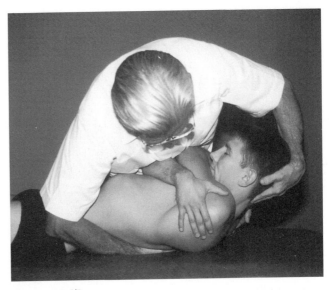

Figure 14.67.

Thoracic Spine

Mobilization with Impulse Technique
T3-12
Supine
Diagnosis (Example: T4-5)
Position: Extended (backward bent), rotated left, sidebent left (ERS$_L$)
Motion restriction: Flexion (forward-bending), right rotation, and right sidebending

1. Patient supine with operator standing on patient's right side.

2. Patient established lever arm by crossing hands over chest.

3. Operator's right hand establishes a fulcrum on both transverse processes of T5.

4. Patient returned to neutral position and lever arm is localized to the fulcrum.

5. Operator's left hand introduces flexion, right side-bending, and right rotation of the neck and upper thoracic spine down to T4 (Fig. 14.68).

6. A high velocity, low amplitude thrust is made by the operator's body weight on the lever arm to the fulcrum, resulting in flexion, right sidebending, and right rotation of T4 and opening of the left zygapophysial joint (Fig. 14.69).

7. Retest.

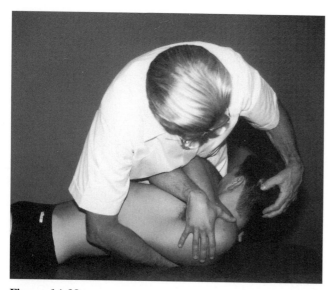

Figure 14.68.

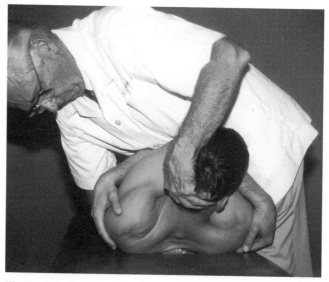

Figure 14.69.

Thoracic Spine

Mobilization with Impulse Technique
T3-12
Supine
Diagnosis (Example: Group dysfunction T3-6)
    Position: Neutral, sidebent right, rotated left
    (NS_RR_L) or (EN_L).
    Motion restriction: Sidebending left, rotation
    right.

1. Patient supine on table with operator standing on right side.

2. Patient establishes the lever arm by crossing the arms over the chest.

3. Operator's right hand establishes the fulcrum with the metacarpophalangeal joint localized to the left intertransverse space of T4-5 using the hand position shown in Figure 14.60.

4. Operator localizes lever arm to fulcrum and with the left hand flexes and extends the head and upper trunk to ensure neutral mechanics at the dysfunctional segments (Fig. 14.70).

5. Operator's left hand introduces left sidebending and right rotation down to the dysfunctional segments (Fig. 14.71).

6. Operator's torso provides a thrusting force through the lever arm to the fulcrum, resulting in left sidebending and right rotation of the dysfunctional segments.

7. Retest.

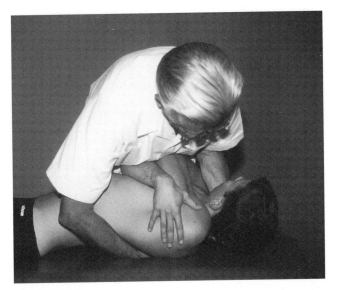

Figure 14.70.

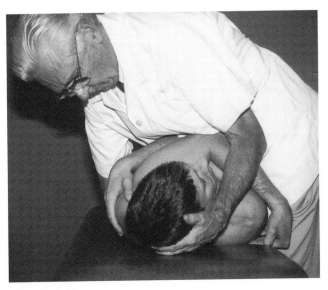

Figure 14.71.

Thoracic Spine

Mobilization with Impulse Technique
T5-12
Sitting

Principle 1. Establish a lever arm

1. Patient sitting on a step ladder treatment stool clasps both hands together against the cervical spine (not occiput) (Fig. 14.72).

2. Operator threads both hands under the patient's axilla and grasps each forearm, providing control of the patient's trunk (Fig. 14.73).

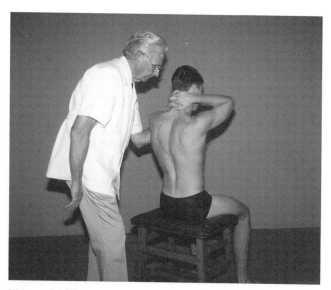

Figure 14.72.

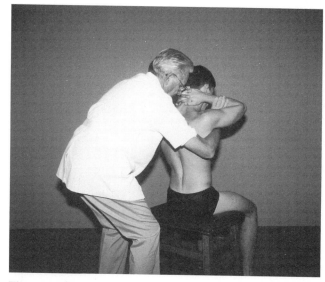

Figure 14.73.

Principle 2. Establish a fulcrum

1. Operator places the knee on the inferior vertebra of the dysfunctional vertebral motion unit, either against the spinous process or a transverse process (Fig. 14.74).

2. Operator places foot on appropriate step of the step ladder treatment stool to localize the knee at the dysfunctional vertebral motion unit.

3. Alternatively, a rolled towel can be used as the fulcrum with the edge against the inferior segment of the dysfunctional vertebral motion unit (Fig. 14.75).

4. The operator's trunk is placed against the towel fulcrum to control the inferior vertebra (Fig. 14.76).

Principle 3. Thrust through the lever arm to the fulcrum

1. Operator's two arms pull the patient's trunk toward the fulcrum or lift the trunk over the fulcrum, depending on whether a flexion or an extension thrust is necessary.

2. The thrusting procedure occurs with operator's both arms controlling the patient's trunk through the operator's hand contact on the forearms.

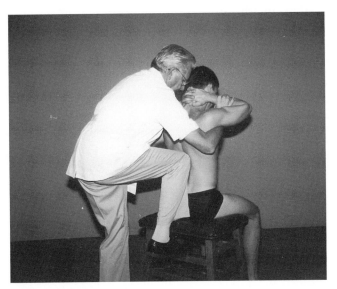

Figure 14.74.

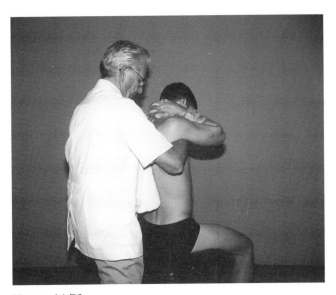

Figure 14.76.

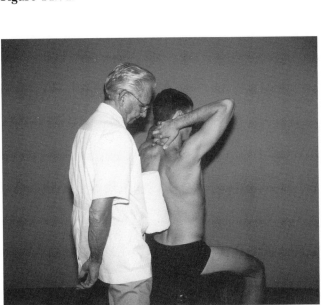

Figure 14.75.

Thoracic Spine

Mobilization with Impulse Technique
T5-12
Sitting
Diagnosis
    Position: Bilateral extended
    Motion restriction: Bilateral flexion

1. Operator seated on stool with hands grasped behind neck.

2. Operator places the knee or towel fulcrum on the spinous process of the inferior vertebra of the dysfunctional vertebral motion unit.

3. Operator threads both hands through the axilla and grasps each forearm of the patient.

4. Flexion is introduced until localized at the dysfunctional segment (Fig. 14.77).

5. A high velocity, low amplitude thrust is made by the operator pulling directly posteriorly toward the fulcrum, enhancing flexion from above against the fixed lower vertebra.

6. Retest.

Thoracic Spine

Mobilization with Impulse Technique
T5-12
Sitting
Diagnosis
    Position: Bilateral flexed
    Motion restriction: Bilateral extension

1. Patient sitting with hands clasped behind neck.

2. Operator stands behind patient with knee or rolled towel as fulcrum on spinous process of inferior vertebra of dysfunctional vertebral motion unit.

3. Operator threads both hands under patient's axilla grasping patient's forearms.

4. Localization to the dysfunctional segment is made by extending the patient's trunk over the fulcrum (Fig. 14.78).

5. A high velocity, low amplitude thrust is applied by a lifting motion by the operator extending the patient's upper trunk over the fulcrum.

6. Retest.

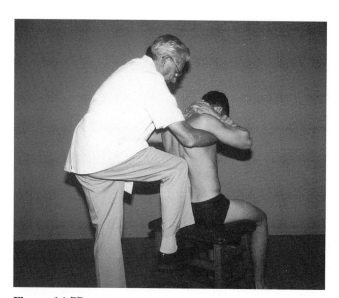

Figure 14.77.

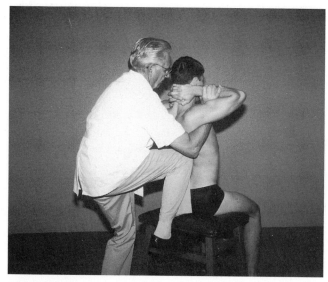

Figure 14.78.

Thoracic Spine

Mobilization with Impulse Technique
T5-12
Sitting
Diagnosis (Example: T8-9)
   Position: Extended (backward bent), left side-bent, left rotated (ERS$_L$)
   Motion restriction: Flexion (forward-bending), right sidebending, right rotation

1. Patient sitting with hands clasped behind neck.

2. Operator stands behind patient and establishes the fulcrum against the right transverse process of T9 (the inferior vertebra).

3. Operator threads arms through patient's axillae and grasps each forearm.

4. Operator localizes patient's upper trunk to the barrier of flexion, right sidebending, and right rotation (Fig. 14.79).

5. A flexion type high velocity, low amplitude thrust is made by the operator pulling the patient's upper trunk toward the fulcrum.

6. Retest.

Thoracic Spine

Mobilization with Impulse Technique
T5-12
Sitting
Diagnosis (Example: T8-9)
   Position: Flexed (forward bent), rotated left, sidebent left (FRS$_L$)
   Motion restriction: Extension (backward-bending), right rotation, right sidebending

1. Patient sitting with hands clasped behind neck.

2. Operator establishes fulcrum against the right transverse process of T9 (the inferior segment).

3. Operator threads arms through patient's axillae and grasps patient's forearms.

4. Operator engages extension, right sidebending, and right rotational barrier at the dysfunctional segment (Fig. 14.80).

5. A high velocity, low amplitude thrust is made, with the operator lifting and posteriorly translating the patient's trunk over the fulcrum.

6. Retest.

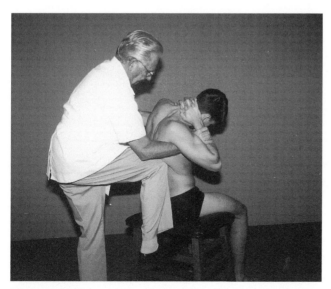

Figure 14.79.

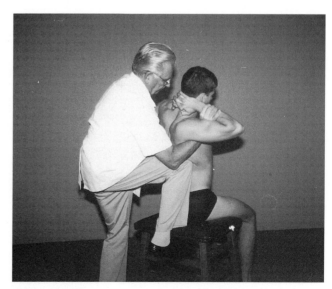

Figure 14.80.

Thoracic Spine

Mobilization with Impulse Technique
T5-12
Sitting
Diagnosis (Example: Group dysfunction T7-10)
    Position: Neutral, sidebent left, rotated right
    (NS_LR_R) or (EN_R).
    Motion restriction: Right sidebending, left
    rotation.

1. Patient sitting with hands clasped behind neck.

2. Operator establishes the fulcrum at the intertransverse space on the right of T8-9.

3. Operator threads arms through patient's axillae and grasps patient's forearms.

4. Operator flexes and extends to neutral, then introduces right sidebending and left rotation to localize at the apex of the dysfunctional segments (Fig. 14.81).

5. A high velocity, low amplitude thrust by the operator through the patient's upper trunk through the fulcrum enhances right sidebending and left rotation of the dysfunctional vertebra.

6. Retest.

CONCLUSION

In the treatment sequence, the thoracic spine should be evaluated and treated before evaluation and treatment of rib function. Occasionally, it is found useful to treat a major rib dysfunction first to better evaluate and treat dysfunction of the thoracic spine.

In the seated middle to lower thoracic mobilization with impulse technique, this author prefers to use the knee or rolled towel as a fulcrum on the inferior vertebra of the dysfunctional vertebral motion unit. Other practitioners and authors will occasionally apply the fulcrum against the posterior transverse process of the superior vertebra of the dysfunctional vertebral motion unit and thrust forward with the knee, or the trunk through the rolled up towel, to derotate the dysfunctional vertebra. In either instance it is imperative that there be good localization of the thrusting force to the fulcrum.

It should be noted that the prone mobilization with impulse technique for T5-12 is only used for FRS dysfunctions. This technique is contraindicated in an ERS dysfunction. Although it is possible to adapt the supine mobilization with impulse techniques for T5-12 for FRS dysfunctions, it is difficult to perform. It is recommended for FRS dysfunctions in this region that the prone technique be used. In the prone and sitting mobilization with impulse techniques, it is important the localization to the transverse processes be precise and not against the adjacent rib shaft because repetitive thrusting on a rib shaft can cause hypermobility of the costovertebral and costotransverse articulations resulting in chronic structural rib dysfunction.

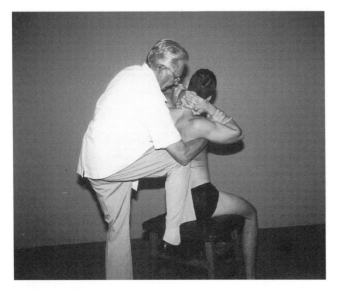

Figure 14.81.

The thoracic cage consists of the 12 thoracic vertebra, the paired 12 ribs, the sternum, and the related ligaments and muscles. The ribs maintain the contour of the thoracic cage, much like a cylinder, and house the thoracic viscera, primarily the heart and great vessels, the lungs, trachea, and esophagus. The thoracoabdominal diaphragm (Fig. 15.1) functions as the piston within the cylinder of the thoracic cage, changing the relative negative interthoracic pressure for respiration. In addition to being the main muscle of respiration, the diaphragm is the major "pump" of the low pressure venous and lymphatic systems.

FUNCTIONAL ANATOMY

Thoracic Inlet

At the cephalic end of the thoracic cage is the thoracic inlet (Fig. 15.2) that is bounded by the body of T1, the medial margins of the right and left first rib, the posterior aspect of the manubrium of the sternum, and the medial end of the right and left clavicle. Through the thoracic inlet pass the esophagus, trachea, and major vessels of the neck and upper extremity.

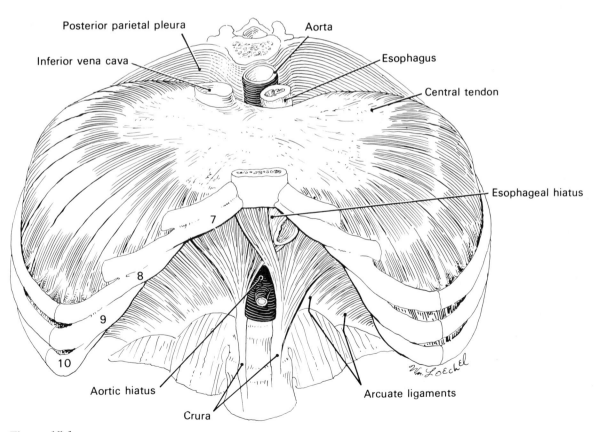

Figure 15.1.
Diaphragm.

Lymphatic Drainage

The thoracic inlet is of importance in lymphatic drainage as the lymphatic system for the whole body drains into the venous system immediately posterior to the medial end of the clavicle and first rib (Fig. 15.3). Altered rib cage function influences respiratory activity, circulatory activity (arterial, venous, and lymphatic), and neural activity (particularly of the intercostal nerves and the brachial plexus superior to rib one).

Sympathetic Trunk

The thoracic lateral chain ganglia of the sympathetic division of the autonomic nervous system lies anterior to the capsule of the costovertebral articulations and is tightly bound down to the posterior thoracic wall by heavy dense fascia.

Rib cage dysfunction is frequently a major component of dysfunction in the musculoskeletal system and is frequently painless. These dysfunctions are frequently described as respiratory restrictions and contribute to the persistence and recurrence of dysfunction within the thoracic spine and can contribute as long restrictors to dysfunction of the musculoskeletal system elsewhere.

INTERCOSTAL NEURALGIA

Other rib dysfunctions are found in association of pain in the intercostal space, commonly described as intercostal neuralgia. These rib dysfunctions are de-scribed as structural rib dysfunctions. They contribute to restriction of respiratory activity of the rib cage as well, but they primarily are found as the dysfunctions associated with chest wall pain. Intercostal neuralgic symptoms in the absence of structural rib dysfunctions should alert the physician to search for organic causes of intercostal neuralgia, for example, herpes zoster, cord tumor, and primary or secondary inflammatory or neoplastic disease of the thoracic viscera.

RIB ANATOMY

Ribs are described as typical or atypical. The atypical ribs are those with the numbers one and two, namely rib 1, 2, 11, and 12. The first rib is broad, flat, and articulates with T1 by a unifacet. It is the lateral boundary of the thoracic inlet and has multiple types of dysfunction. The second rib articulates by two demifacets with T1 and T2. Anteriorly it articulates by a strong cartilaginous attachment with the manubriogladiolar junction of the sternum at the angle of Louis. Alteration in function of the second rib profoundly influences the function of the sternum and frequently contributes to pain syndromes in the upper extremity (Fig. 15.4). Ribs 11 and 12 articulate by unifacets with the 11th and 12th vertebra. They do not have typical costotransverse articulations. They are both associated with the muscles of the posterior abdominal wall. The quadratus lumborum muscle attaches to the inferior margin of rib 12. The

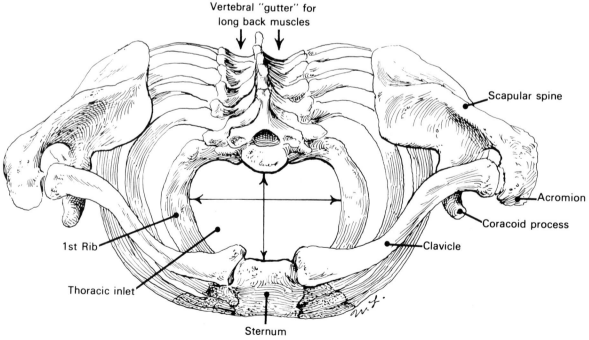

Figure 15.2.
Thoracic inlet.

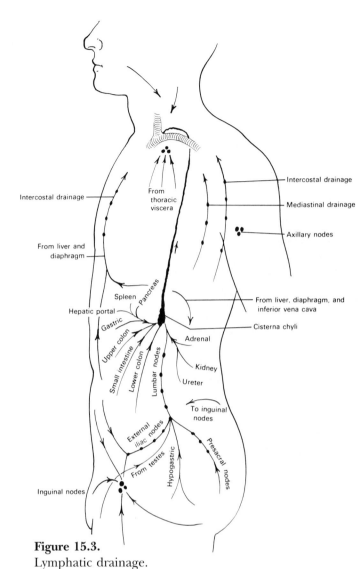

Figure 15.3.
Lymphatic drainage.

12th rib is frequently asymmetrical in length. Neither rib attaches to the costal arch.

The typical ribs, 3–10, have three articulations. The posterior articulations are the costovertebral, with the rib head attaching to demifacets of the thoracic vertebra above and below, and through a strong ligamentous attachment, to the annulus of the intervertebral disk. The second posterior articulation is the costotransverse. This synovial joint incorporates the anterior surface of the transverse process and the articular surface of the posterior aspect of the rib. As an example, the costovertebral articulation of rib 4 attaches to the inferior demifacet of T3 and the superior demifacet of T4, whereas the costotransverse articulation is at the T4 level. The anterior articulation is the costochondral. Each rib attaches either to the sternum directly or through the costal arch. Normal rib motion requires mobility of the thoracic vertebra and mobility at the costovertebral, costotransverse, and costochondral articulations. The rib angle of the

typical ribs is the most posterior aspect of the rib shaft and is the attachment of the iliocostalis muscles.

DIAPHRAGM

The diaphragm (Fig. 15.1) is the primary muscle of respiration. When it contracts, it descends and increases the negative intrathoracic pressure, enhancing inspiration. As it relaxes, the passive recoil of the thoracic cage results in exhalation. Other inspiratory muscles include the external intercostals, the sternocostalis, and the accessory muscles of inspiration. These include the sternocleidomastoid, scalenes, pectoralis major and minor, and, occasionally, the serratus anterior and latissimus dorsi, serratus posterior superior, and the superior fibers of the iliocostalis. The primary exhalation muscles are the internal intercostals and the accessory exhalation muscles that are the abdominals, lower fibers of the iliocostalis, serratus posterior inferior, and quadratus lumborum. The external and internal intercostal muscles are frequently viewed as respiratory muscles, but in large measure their function is to maintain the integrity of the contour of the thoracic cylinder and prevent invagination during increasing negative intrathoracic pressure.

RIB MOTIONS

The primary rib motion is that of inhalation and exhalation. Inhalation and exhalation are further described as pump handle and bucket handle (Fig. 15.5). During inhalation, the anterior extremity of a rib moves superiorly in a pump-handle fashion and the lateral aspect of the rib goes superiorly in a bucket-handle fashion. During exhalation both the pump-handle and bucket-handle components move in a caudad direction. All ribs have both pump-handle and bucket-handle movement. The more cephalic ribs have more pump-handle motion and the more caudal ribs have more bucket-handle motion. The major determinant of this bucket-handle, pump-handle movement is the axis of motion between the costovertebral and the costotransverse articulation. In the upper ribs, this axis is more transverse, providing more pump-handle activity, whereas in the lower ribs, this axis is more anteroposterior, providing for more bucket-handle motion. In a true bucket-handle motion, the anterior and posterior ends of the ribs should be fixed. This is not true in the normal chest wall as the anterior extremity of the rib moves laterally and somewhat superiorly during inhalation and medially and inferiorly during exhalation. Nonetheless, the descriptors of pump-handle and bucket-handle movement are good for describing the characteristics of chest wall motion.

A third rib motion occurs at the 11th and 12th ribs. As they have no articular attachments anteriorly

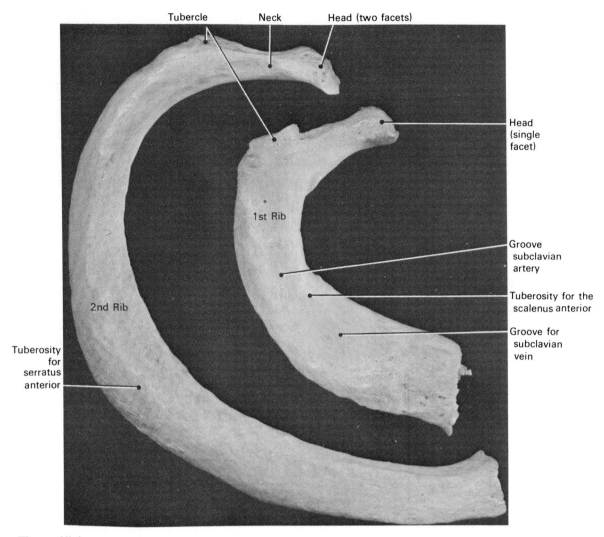

Figure 15.4.
Ribs 1 and 2.

and no costotransverse articulations, their motion is primarily posterior and lateral during inhalation and anterior and medial during exhalation. This motion has been described as caliper motion, simulating the action of a set of ice tongs.

A fourth rib motion is that which accompanies rotation of the thoracic spine. Torsional movement results when a pair of typical ribs are attached to two thoracic vertebra involved in a rotational movement. For example, when T5 rotates to the right in relation to T6, the posterior aspect of the right sixth rib turns externally and the posterior aspect of the left sixth rib turns internally. The rib appears to twist on this long axis. This torsional movement continues around the rib cage to the sternal attachment with the anterior extremity of the right sixth rib being more flat with its inferior border sharp and the anterior extremity of the left sixth rib having its superior margin accentuated. As the thoracic spine returns to neutral,

the rib torsional movement should return to bilateral symmetry.

When the rib cage is subjected to traumatic insult, abnormal rib motions can occur. After a single traumatic episode or multiple microtrauma, one or more ribs may become subluxed anteriorly or posteriorly. These subluxations are abnormal hypermobile ribs with the rib being carried either more anteriorly or posteriorly along the axis of motion between the costovertebral and the costotransverse articulations. A third subluxation is the possibility of rib 1 being carried cephalward at its unifacet on the lateral side of T1, resulting in the rib shaft sitting on top of the transverse process.

Rib shafts also have a great deal of pliability and are built to sustain anteroposterior and lateral compression loads as they maintain the integrity of the chest wall cylinder. Occasionally, after trauma from an anteroposterior or a lateral direction, one or

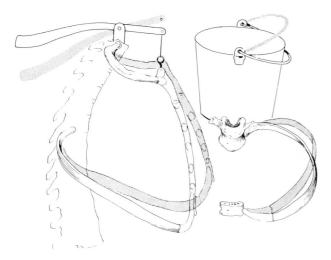

Figure 15.5.
Pump-handle and bucket-handle motion.

more ribs lose this plasticity and become restricted in a deformed state.

STRUCTURAL DIAGNOSIS OF THE RIB CAGE

Structural diagnosis of the rib cage assesses for the diagnostic triad of asymmetry, altered range of motion, and tissue texture abnormality. The examiner assesses the symmetry or asymmetry of the chest wall by palpation anteriorly, posteriorly, and laterally. Concurrently, the examiner can assess for tissue texture abnormality, particularly hypertonicity of the iliocostalis attachment at the rib angle and the intercostal muscles. Motion characteristics are identified by symmetrically palpating ribs, both in groups and singly, and following respiratory activity of inhalation and exhalation.

Rib Cage

Diagnosis
Sitting
Posterior palpation

1. Patient sitting with operator standing behind.

2. Operator palpates the posterior convexity of the thorax in the upper region (Fig. 15.6), midregion (Fig. 15.7), and lower region (Fig. 15.8).

3. Assessment is made of the participation of each rib angle in the posterior convexity. Is one more prominent or less prominent than another?

4. Assessment is made of the hypertonicity and tenderness of the iliocostalis muscle at the rib angle.

5. Assessment is made of the posterior contour of the rib shaft. There is a normal posterior convexity with the lower border of the rib being somewhat more easily palpable than the superior.

6. Assessment is made of the width of the intercostal space and the intercostal muscle hypertonicity and tenderness. Each interspace should be symmetrical with its fellow on the opposite side and with one above and below.

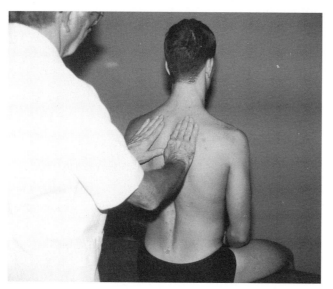

Figure 15.6.

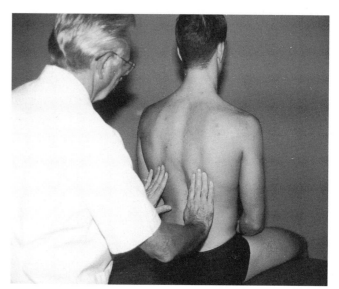

Figure 15.8.

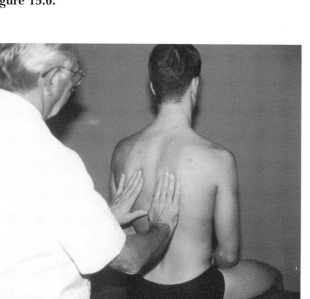

Figure 15.7.

Rib Cage

Diagnosis
Sitting
Anterior palpation

1. Patient sitting on table with operator standing in front.

2. Operator palpates the anterior contour of the chest wall and its anterior convexity beginning at the upper region (Fig. 15.9) with the longest finger palpating the costal cartilage of rib one under the medial extremity of the clavicle. The middle ribs (Fig. 15.10) and lower ribs (Fig. 15.11) are palpated.

3. Assessment is made for the participation of the anterior aspect of each rib in the normal convexity.

4. Assessment is made of the intercostal spaces and the tissue tension and tenderness of intercostal muscles.

5. Assessment is made of the costochondral junction (Fig. 15.12) assessing for prominence, depression, tissue reaction, and tenderness.

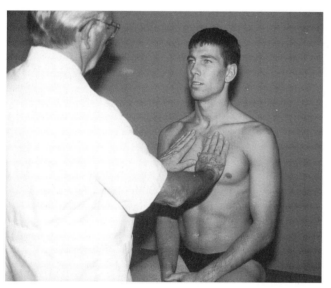

Figure 15.9.

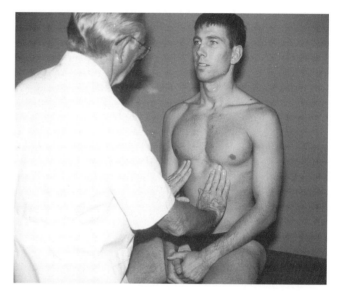

Figure 15.11.

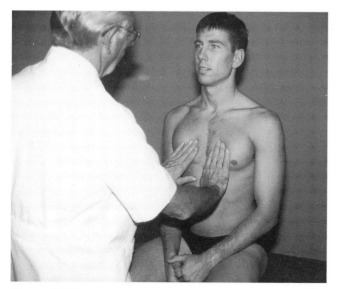

Figure 15.10.

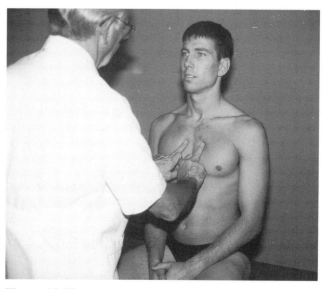

Figure 15.12.

Rib Cage

Diagnosis
Sitting
First rib for superior subluxation

1. Patient sitting on table with operator standing behind.

2. Operator grasps anterior aspect of the superior trapezius on each side and pulls posteriorly (Fig. 15.13).

3. With posterior retraction of the upper trapezius, the long fingers are directed caudally onto the posterior shaft of the first rib.

4. Unleveling of one rib in comparison with the other by 5 mm is a positive finding (Fig. 15.14).

5. The dysfunctional rib is markedly tender on its superior aspect.

6. The dysfunctional rib has significant exhalation restriction.

7. There is usually hypertonicity of the ipsilateral scalene muscles.

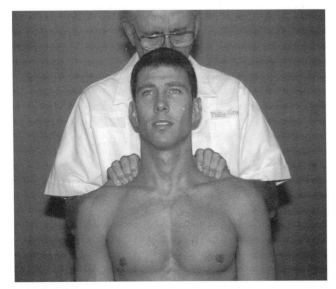

Figure 15.13.

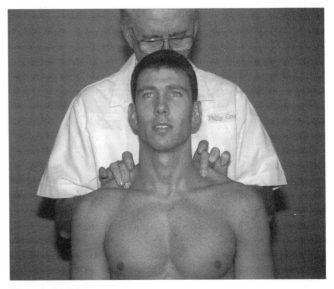

Figure 15.14.

Rib Cage

Diagnosis
Supine
Respiratory motion restriction

1. Patient supine with operator standing at side of table with dominant eye over the midline.

2. Operator symmetrically places hands over lateral aspect of lower rib cage with fingers in interspaces (Fig. 15.15).

3. Operator follows inhalation and exhalation effort looking for symmetry of full inhalation and exhalation excursion.

4. Palpation is performed on the anterior extremity of the lower ribs (Fig. 15.16), assessing pump-handle motion.

5. Similar assessment of bucket-handle movement (Fig. 15.17) and pump-handle movement (Fig. 15.18) is made of the middle ribs.

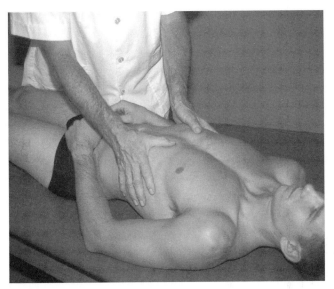

Figure 15.15.

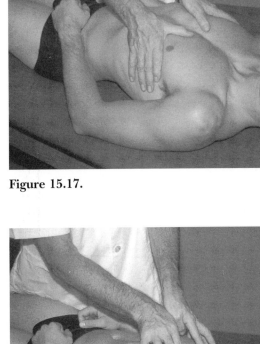

Figure 15.17.

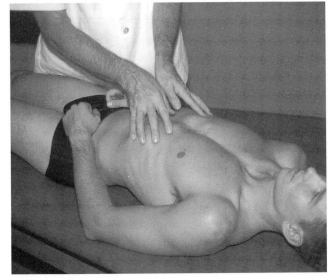

Figure 15.16.

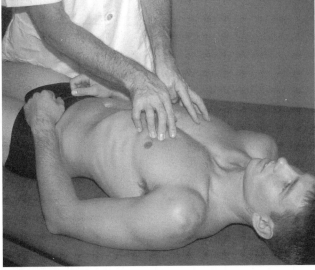

Figure 15.18.

6. Similar assessment of the bucket-handle movement (Fig. 15.19) and pump-handle movement (Fig. 15.20) of the upper ribs is made. Note that the long finger is in contact with the anterior extremity of the first rib.

Rib Cage

Diagnosis
Supine
Identification of "key rib"

1. Patient supine with operator standing at side with dominant eye over the midline.

2. Operator symmetrically places a finger on the superior aspect of a pair of ribs and follows inhalation and exhalation effort (Fig. 15.21).

3. A rib that stops first during inhalation effort has inhalation restriction.

4. A rib that stops first during exhalation effort has exhalation restriction.

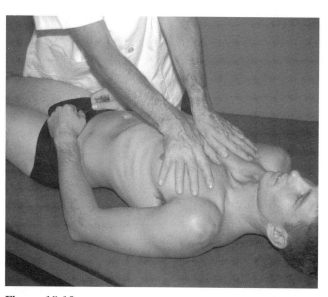

Figure 15.19.

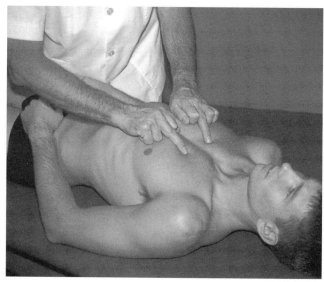

Figure 15.21.

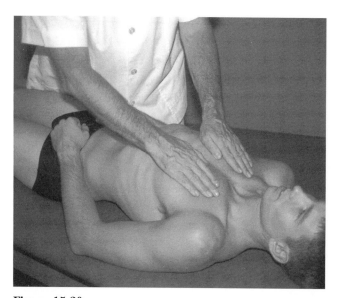

Figure 15.20.

Rib Cage

Diagnosis
Prone
Respiratory movement of the 11th and 12th ribs

1. Patient prone on table with operator standing at side and dominant eye over the midline.

2. Operator identifies the tip of the 11th rib usually found in the midaxillary line just superior to the iliac crest.

3. Operator follows the contour of the 11th rib medially and places the thumbs and thenar eminences over the posterior shaft of the 11th and 12th ribs (Fig. 15.22).

4. Operator follows inhalation exhalation effort of the patient.

5. The 11th and 12th ribs, which do not move posteriorly during inhalation, have inhalation restriction.

6. The 11th and 12th ribs, which do not move anteriorly during exhalation, have exhalation restriction.

7. The 12th rib is notoriously asymmetric but always follows the 11th rib.

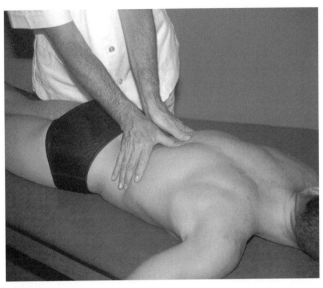

Figure 15.22.

RIB CAGE SOMATIC DYSFUNCTION

Rib dysfunctions are classified as structural and respiratory. The structural rib dysfunctions include anterior and posterior subluxation and, in the instance of the first rib, a superior subluxation. Another structural rib dysfunction is rib torsion, usually accompanying a nonneutral dysfunction of the thoracic spine, particularly of the extended, rotated, and sidebent (ERS) variety. Rib torsional dysfunctions will frequently resolve when the nonneutral thoracic spine dysfunction has been successfully treated. In other instances, the rib torsional dysfunction persists and will need to be treated appropriately to prevent recurrence of the thoracic spine dysfunction. Another structural rib dysfunction is rib compression. These are either in an anteroposterior or lateral direction and follow trauma. Fortunately, they are quite rare. They are frequently associated with motor vehicle accidents and sports injuries. Their presentation is similar to that of a rib fracture, but fracture is not demonstrated by appropriate imaging techniques. A structural dysfunction frequently observed at rib 2 is described as being "laterally flexed." In this dysfunction, the rib behaves as though the anterior and posterior ends of the second rib were fixed in a true bucket-handle fashion, and the traumatic episode results in the rib being laterally flexed. This usually occurs in a superior direction. Some authors describe this as a major bucket-handle exhalation restriction, but they do not respond to the usual respiratory rib techniques. They usually result from acute sidebending injuries to the cervical thoracic junction. Shortening and hypertonicity of the posterior scalene muscles is an important associated finding.

The diagnostic criteria for structural rib dysfunctions are as follows.

1. Anterior Subluxation
   a. Rib angle less prominent in posterior rib cage contour.
   b. Rib angle tender with tension of iliocostalis muscle.
   c. Prominence of anterior extremity of the rib in the anterior rib cage contour.
   d. Marked motion restriction of inhalation and exhalation.
   e. Frequently present with complaint of "intercostal neuralgia" in adjacent interspace.
2. Posterior Subluxation
   a. Rib angle more prominent in posterior rib cage contour.
   b. Rib angle tender with tension of iliocostalis muscle.
   c. Anterior extremity of the rib less prominent in anterior rib cage contour.
   d. Marked restriction of rib in inhalation and exhalation movement.
   e. Frequent complaint of intercostal neuralgia in adjacent interspace.
3. Superior First Rib Subluxation
   a. Palpation of superior aspect of first rib anterior to the upper trapezius muscle shows dysfunctional rib to be 5–6 mm cephalic in relation to contralateral side.
   b. Marked tenderness of superior aspect of first rib.
   c. Restriction of respiratory motion primarily exhalation.
   d. Hypertonicity of scalene muscles on ipsilateral side.
4. External Rib Torsion
   a. Superior border of dysfunctional rib more prominent.
   b. Inferior border of dysfunctional rib less prominent.
   c. Tension and tenderness at iliocostalis muscle attachment at rib angle.
   d. Widened intercostal space above and narrowed intercostal space below dysfunctional rib with tension of the intercostal muscles on the inferior interspace.
   e. Respiratory motion restriction primarily of exhalation.
   f. These dysfunctions are frequently the key rib in exhalation group rib restrictions.

Note: External torsional dysfunctions are commonly associated with ERS dysfunction to the ipsilateral side. Internal torsional dysfunction has the reverse findings and is usually found on the contralateral side. Rib torsion dysfunctions are seldom found associated with flexed, rotated, and sidebent (FRS) dysfunctions.

5. Anteroposterior Rib Compression
   a. Less prominence of the rib shaft in the anterior and posterior convexities of the thoracic cage.
   b. Prominence of the rib shaft in the midaxillary line.
   c. Tenderness and tension of the intercostal space above and below dysfunctional rib.
   d. Frequent complaint of chest wall pain of the intercostal neuralgia type.
   e. Motion restriction of respiratory activity.
6. Lateral Rib Compression
   a. Prominence of the rib shaft in the anterior and posterior convexities of the rib cage.
   b. Dysfunctional rib shaft less prominent in the midaxillary line.
   c. Tenderness and tension of the intercostal space above and below dysfunctional rib.

d. Complaint of chest wall pain consistent with intercostal neuralgia.
e. Respiratory motion restriction.

Note: Both anteroposterior and lateral rib compressions simulate rib fracture.

7. Lateral Flexed Rib
   a. Prominence of the rib shaft in the midaxillary line.
   b. Marked respiratory rib restriction usually exhalation.
   c. Asymmetry of interspace above and below dysfunctional rib with the superior usually narrow and the inferior wider.
   d. Marked tenderness of the interspace usually the one above.
   e. Most commonly seen in rib 2 being dysfunctional in a superior position (laterally flexed superiorly).
   f. Marked tenderness of the superior intercostal space of rib 2 at its lateral aspect just beneath the lateral extremity of the clavicle.
   g. Frequently associated with brachialgia-type symptoms in the upper extremity.

RESPIRATORY RIB DYSFUNCTIONS

A single rib, or a group of ribs, can demonstrate restriction of either inhalation or exhalation movement. When a group of ribs have restriction of inhalation or exhalation function, we look for the *key rib*. The key rib is the major restrictor of the group's ability to move into either inhalation or exhalation. The key rib is found at the upper or lower end of the group. In exhalation group rib dysfunction, the key rib is at the bottom of the dysfunctional group. In inhalation group rib dysfunction, the key rib is at the upper end of the group. The key rib is frequently one of the structural rib dysfunctions. If a structural rib dysfunction is identified, it should be appropriately treated before dealing with the respiratory rib dysfunctions. In treating group respiratory rib restrictions of the inhalation and exhalation type, the key rib is usually addressed in the treatment procedure. Caution must be advised for the beginning student when assessing respiratory restrictions. The diagnostic criteria is based on the rib group that stops first during inhalation or exhalation. It is not the rib group that has the alteration in the excursion of range. For example, a group of ribs that has exhalation restriction stops first during the exhalation phase of respiration. Because the ribs are already held in a position of inhalation, they have a reduced range of inhalation. These rib dysfunctions are frequently misdiagnosed as inhalation restrictions because the range is reduced. However, they are really exhalation restrictions because they have reduced range of exhalation when compared with the opposite side. The converse is true of inhalation restrictions. Because they are already held in a position of exhalation, they have a reduced range of exhalation, but their major restriction is in the direction of inhalation.

Diagnostic criteria for respiratory rib dysfunctions are as follows.
1. Exhalation Restriction
   a. A rib or group of ribs that ceases movement first during exhalation effort.
   b. The key rib is at the bottom of the group.
   c. Assessment is made as to which of the pump-handle and bucket-handle components is the most restricted.
2. Inhalation Restriction
   a. A rib or group of ribs that ceases moving first during inhalation effort.
   b. The key rib is at the top of the group.
   c. Assessment is made as to whether the pump-handle or bucket-handle component is most restricted.

In group rib respiratory restrictions, there may be more than one key rib. Each rib must be assessed for its compliance in the overall inhalation and exhalation effort of that group of ribs.

TREATMENT OF RIB CAGE DYSFUNCTION

There are general principles of treatment sequence that should be followed for the successful treatment of rib cage dysfunction. As a general rule, treatment of the thoracic spine should precede treatment of the ribs, either individually or in groups. Torsional rib dysfunction frequently responds simultaneously with the treatment of the associated nonneutral thoracic dysfunction. The unique anatomy at the thoracic inlet, particularly at T1, requires that T1 should be adequately evaluated and treated before addressing dysfunction of ribs 1 and 2. The unifacet for the first rib on the lateral side of T1 allows a great deal of variable motion of the first rib.

The second principle of treating rib dysfunctions is to address the structural rib dysfunctions before treatment of respiratory rib restriction. The key rib of a group respiratory rib dysfunction is usually a structural rib at the top or bottom of the group. Appropriate treatment to the structural rib dysfunction frequently restores normal movement to the group of ribs and their respiratory capacity. After treatment of structural rib dysfunction, the respiratory rib dysfunctions are addressed with the goal of restoration of maximal, symmetrical, inhalation, and exhalation movement.

Technique of rib cage dysfunction is usually direct action with combined activating forces of muscle energy, respiratory effort, and operator guiding.

Rib Cage

Structural Rib Dysfunction
Diagnosis
Superior subluxation first rib (left side example)

1. Patient sitting with operator standing behind.

2. Patient's right arm is draped over the operator's right thigh with foot on the table.

3. Operator's right hand and forearm control the patient's head and neck with the fingers of the left hand overlying the upper trapezius muscle that is pulled posteriorly (Fig. 15.23).

4. Operator's left thumb contacts the posterior shaft of rib 1 through the trapezius muscle (Fig. 15.24).

5. Operator's right hand introduces left sidebending and rotation of the patient's neck to unload the left scalene muscles, and with the tips of the forefin-

gers continuing to maintain the trapezius posteriorly, a caudal force is placed on the shaft of the first rib (Fig. 15.25).

6. Simultaneously, the operator's left thumb maintains an anterior force on the posterior aspect of the shaft of the first rib to slide it forward in relation to the left transverse process of T1 (Fig. 15.26).

7. Patient performs a right sidebending effort of the head and neck against operator's resistance through the right hand, activating the right scalene muscles and resulting in inhibition of the left scalenes.

8. Two to three efforts may be necessary before release is felt of the superior subluxation restoring symmetry with the opposite side.

9. Retest.

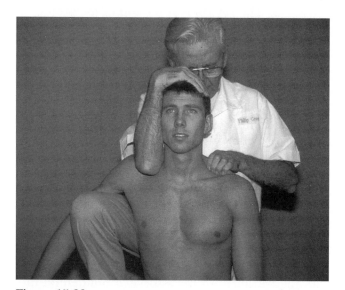

Figure 15.23.

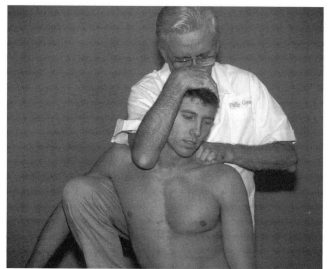

Figure 15.25.

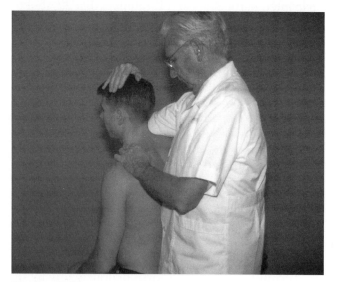

Figure 15.24.

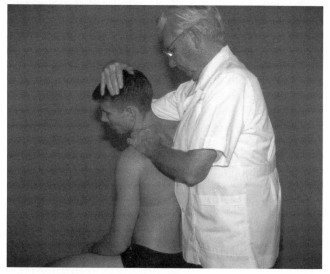

Figure 15.26.

Rib Cage

Structural Rib Dysfunction
Diagnosis
Anterior subluxation (Example: right fifth rib)

1. Patient sitting on table with right hand holding left shoulder.

2. Operator stands behind the patient with the right thumb on the shaft of the fifth rib medial to the rib angle (Fig. 15.27) and with the left hand controlling the patient's right elbow (Fig. 15.28).

3. Operator applies and maintains a posterolateral "pull" force on the rib shaft (Fig. 15.29).

4. Patient is instructed to "pull" the right elbow laterally or caudally (Fig. 15.30). Three to five repetitions are made of a 3- to 5-second muscle contraction of the patient with operator monitoring rib motion.

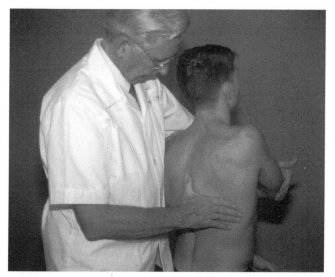

Figure 15.27.

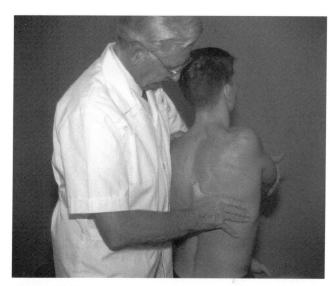

Figure 15.29.

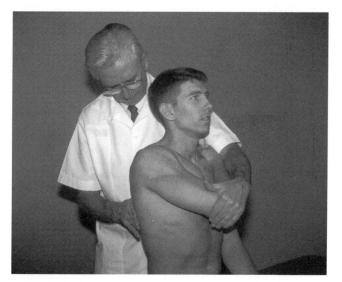

Figure 15.28.

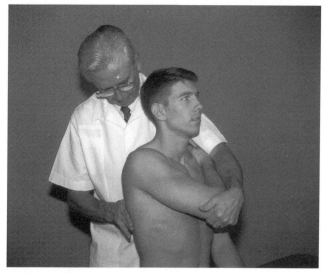

Figure 15.30.

5. Patient's left fist can be applied to the anterior extremity of the dysfunctional rib so that when the caudad pulling motion is performed, there is anterior to posterior force directed on the dysfunctional rib (Fig. 15.31).

6. Retest.

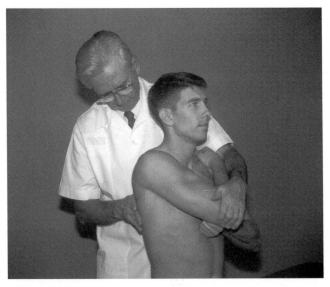

Figure 15.31.

Rib Cage

Structural Rib Dysfunction
Diagnosis
Posterior subluxation (Example: right fifth rib)

1. Patient sitting on table with right hand grasping left shoulder.

2. Operator stands behind patient with thumb placed on shaft of right fifth rib lateral to the angle (Fig. 15.32) and with left hand holding the patient's right elbow (Fig. 15.33).

3. Operator maintains an anteromedial "push" force on the rib shaft and resists the patient's instructed "push" of the elbow to the left (Fig. 15.34) or a "push" of the right elbow toward the ceiling (Fig. 15.35).

4. Three to five repetitions of a 3- to 5-second muscle effort are usually necessary to restore symmetry.

5. Retest.

Note: Rib subluxations are frequently hypermobile, and after treatment stabilization of the rib cage by strapping or a rib belt is frequently useful.

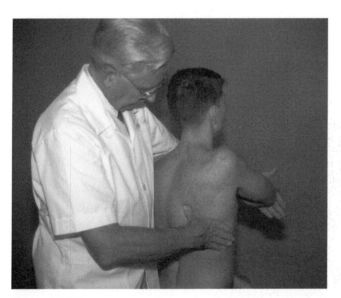

Figure 15.32.

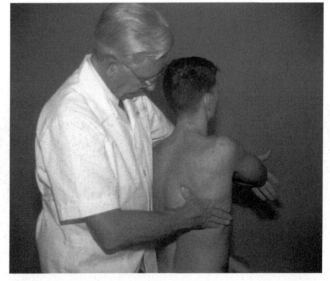

Figure 15.34.

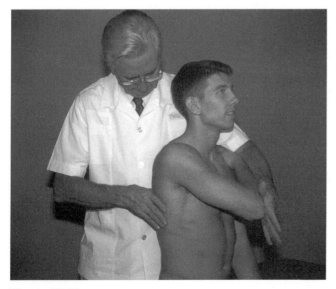

Figure 15.33.

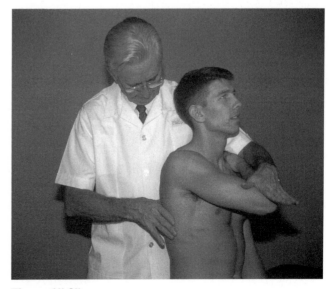

Figure 15.35.

Rib Cage

Structural Rib Dysfunction
Diagnosis
Rib torsion (Example: right fifth rib)

1. Patient sitting on table with right hand holding left shoulder.

2. Operator stands behind with thumb contacting the rib angle of the right fifth rib in a vertical fashion (Fig. 15.36).

3. With external torsional restriction, the thumb applies an anterior force on the superior border of the dysfunctional rib.

4. For internal torsional restriction, the operator's thumb applies an anterior force on the inferior margin of the dysfunctional rib.

5. Patient is instructed to alternately pull the elbow to the lap (Fig. 15.37) and push toward the ceiling (Fig. 15.38) with the operator maintaining the appropriate compressive force on the superior or inferior aspect of the rib shaft.

6. Pulling toward the lap introduces external torsional movement and pushing toward the ceiling introduces internal torsional movement. Operator resists the rib motion during the appropriate muscle effort and takes up the slack to the new barrier during each relaxation.

7. Three to five repetitions of 3- to 5-second contractions are made.

8. Retest.

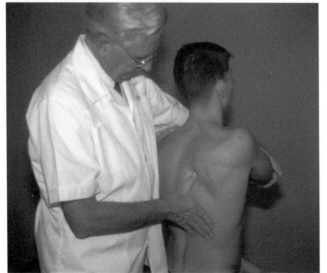

Figure 15.36.

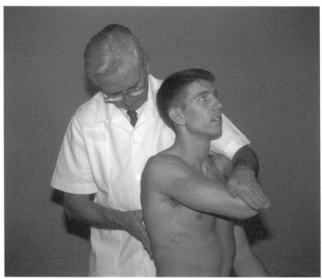

Figure 15.38.

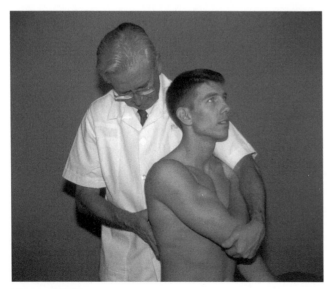

Figure 15.37.

Rib Cage

Structural Rib Dysfunction
Diagnosis
External torsion (Example: right fifth rib)

1. Patient sitting on table with right hand grasping left shoulder.

2. Operator stands behind with the left arm controlling the patient's trunk with the left axilla over the patient's left shoulder and the left hand grasping the right shoulder. Operator's right hand identifies dysfunctional rib angle and shaft (Fig. 15.39).

3. Operator introduces small amount of flexion, left sidebending, and left rotation of the trunk and follows the right fifth rib anteriorly (Fig. 15.40).

4. Operator's thumb and thenar eminence are over the anterior shaft of the right fifth rib, exerting an internal rotary force over the prominent inferior margin of the shaft (Fig. 15.41).

5. Operator increases the forward-bending, left sidebending, and left rotation of the trunk (Fig. 15.42).

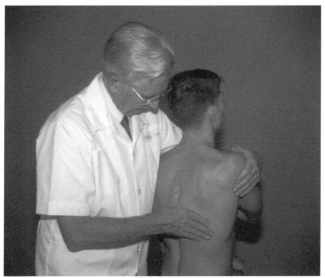

Figure 15.39.

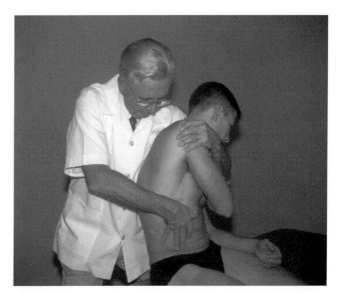

Figure 15.41.

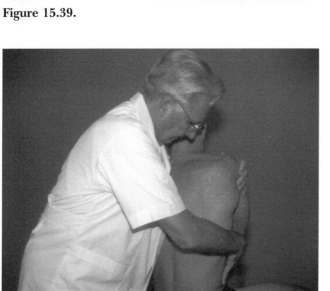

Figure 15.40.

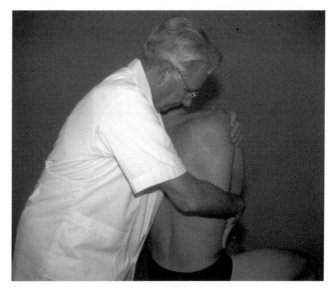

Figure 15.42.

6. Operator resists a right rotation, right sidebending, and extension effort of the patient while maintaining a compressive force on the inferior margin of the anterior shaft of the fifth rib (Fig. 15.43).

7. Three to five repetitions of a 3- to 5-second effort are made with the operator engaging a new barrier after each effort.

8. Retest.

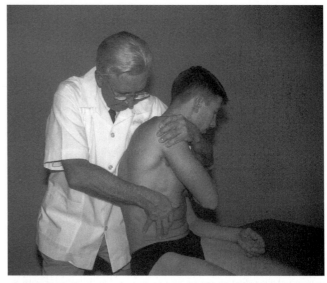

Figure 15.43.

Rib Cage

Structural Rib Dysfunction
Diagnosis
Anterior posterior compression (Example: right sixth rib)

1. Patient sits on end of table with operator standing on the side opposite to the dysfunction and patient's arm is draped over the operator's shoulder (Fig. 15.44).
2. Operator's middle finger of both hands contacts the prominent rib shaft in the midaxillary line (Fig. 15.45).
3. Operator sidebends patient to the right while applying a medial compressive force on the shaft of the dysfunctional rib (Fig. 15.46).
4. Patient is instructed to deeply inhale, hold the breath, and perform a left sidebending effort of the trunk against operator resistance while the operator maintains a medial compressive force on the dysfunctional rib (Fig. 15.47).
5. Three to five repetitions are made.
6. Retest.

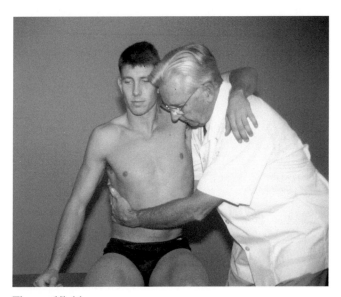

Figure 15.44.

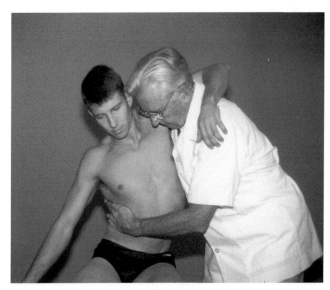

Figure 15.46.

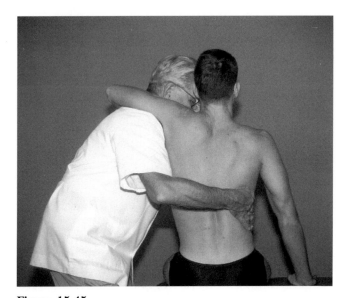

Figure 15.45.

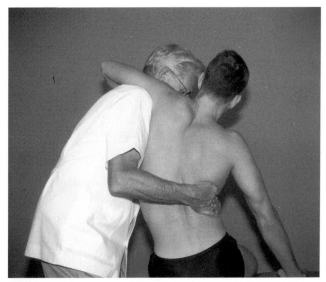

Figure 15.47.

Rib Cage

Structural Rib Dysfunction
Diagnosis
Lateral compression (Example: left fifth rib)

1. Patient sitting on end of table with operator standing on the side of dysfunction with patient's left arm draped over the operator's right shoulder (Fig. 15.48).

2. Operator places the thenar eminence over the prominent posterior and anterior shaft of the dysfunctional fifth rib (Fig. 15.49).

3. Operator sidebends the patient to the right while maintaining an anteroposterior compression on the dysfunctional rib (Fig. 15.50).

4. Patient takes a deep breath in, holds the breath, and performs a left sidebending effort against the resistance of the operator's shoulder (Fig. 15.51).

5. Three to five repetitions of a 3- to 5-second effort are performed with the operator engaging a new barrier after each effort.

6. Retest.

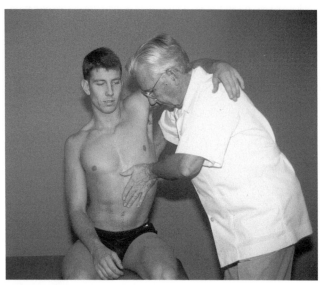

Figure 15.48.

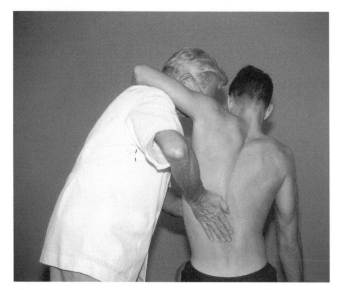

Figure 15.50.

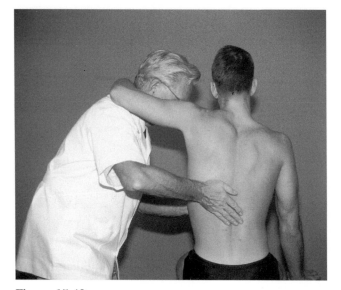

Figure 15.49.

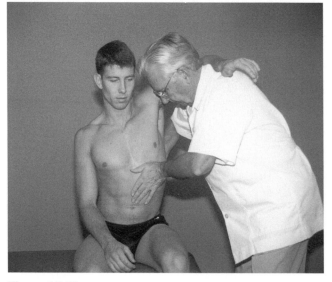

Figure 15.51.

Rib Cage

Structural Rib Dysfunction
Diagnosis
Laterally flexed superior (Example: left second rib)

1. Patient supine on table with operator standing on side of dysfunction facing cephalward with the right hand against the midaxillary line of the patient's thorax (Fig. 15.52).

2. Operator slides right hand cephalically along the lateral rib shaft with the left hand holding the right arm inferiorly (Fig. 15.53).

3. Operator's left hand introduces left sidebending of the head and neck with the patient instructed to fully exhale and reach toward the left knee to increase left sidebending (Fig. 15.54).

4. After several respiratory efforts with increased left sidebending, operator's right hand grasps the superior aspect of the shaft of the second rib and the left hand is switched to the opposite side of the patient's head (Fig. 15.55).

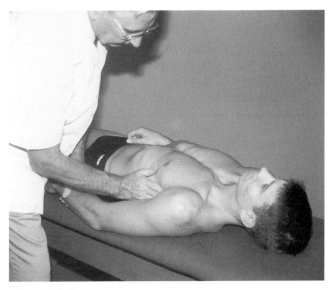

Figure 15.52.

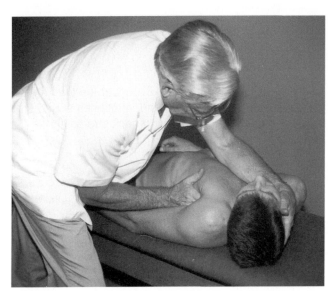

Figure 15.54.

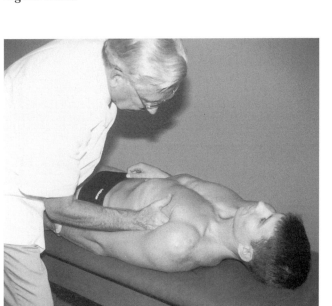

Figure 15.53.

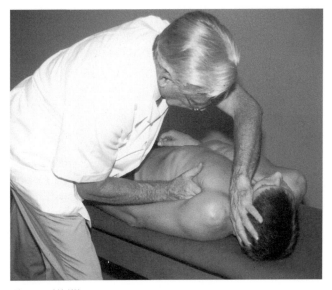

Figure 15.55.

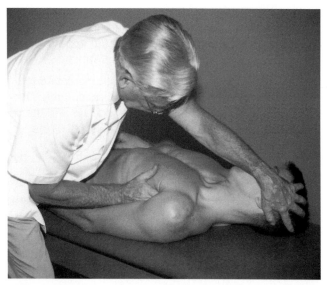

Figure 15.56.

5. While holding the superior aspect of the dysfunctional rib, operator's left hand introduces acute right sidebending of the head and neck stretching the left scalene muscles (Fig. 15.56).

6. Retest.

Note: This dysfunction is exquisitely tender to the patient and the treatment procedure is significantly painful. The patient should be appropriately informed.

RESPIRATORY RIB RESTRICTIONS

After the treatment of structural rib dysfunctions, respiratory rib restrictions are addressed. The practitioner needs to be able to deal with both inhalation and exhalation rib restriction.

PRINCIPLES OF TREATMENT FOR INHALATION RESTRICTION

1. Operator pulls rib angle laterally and caudad to disengage rib head at the costovertebral articulation.
2. Patient inhalation effort.
3. Contraction of muscle groups: ribs 1 and 2, scalenes; ribs 3–5, pectoralis minor; and ribs 3–9, serratus anterior.

PRINCIPLES OF TREATMENT OF EXHALATION RESTRICTION

1. Patient position in combined sidebending and flexion to the side of dysfunction.
2. Patient exhalation effort.
3. Operator contacts superior shaft and costochondral junction of the dysfunctional rib and holds in an exhalation position.
4. Patient returned to neutral trunk position while holding rib in exhalation position.

Rib Cage

Respiratory Restriction
Ribs 1 and 2
Diagnosis
Inhalation restriction (right side example)

1. Patient supine with operator standing on left side of table.

2. The fingers of operator's left hand contact the medial aspect of the first and second rib as close to the transverse process as possible (Fig. 15.57).

3. Patient's trunk is returned to the table with the operator's elbow on the table with a lateral and inferior pull on the first and second rib.

4. Operator's right hand introduces left sidebending and rotation of the head and neck putting the right scalenes on tension (Fig. 15.58).

5. Patient is instructed to deeply inhale and lift the head off the table for pump-handle restriction or sidebend the head to the right for bucket-handle restriction against the resistance of the operator's right hand (Fig. 15.59).

6. Three to five repetitions are made of a 3- to 5-second effort.

7. This can be done in the presence of pathology of the right shoulder. If the right shoulder is normal, an alternate hand position has the patient's forearm resting against the head (Fig. 15.60), reducing the caudad traction on the first and second rib by the fascia of the right upper extremity.

8. Retest.

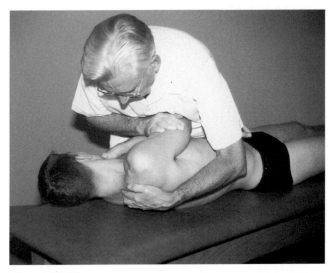

Figure 15.57.

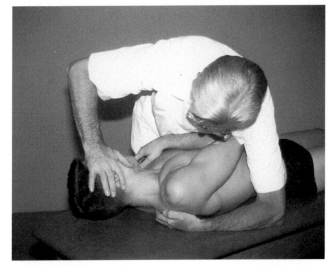

Figure 15.59.

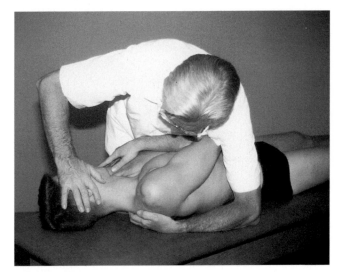

Figure 15.58.

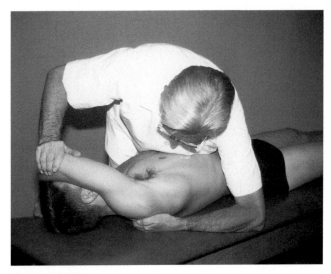

Figure 15.60.

Rib Cage

Respiratory Restriction
Ribs 3–5
Diagnosis
Inhalation restriction (right side example)

1. Patient supine on table with operator standing on left side and with the left hand grasps the shafts of ribs 3, 4, and 5 medial to the angle (Fig. 15.61).

2. Operator returns the patient to neutral on the table and with the left forearm on the table applies a lateral and caudad distraction on the dysfunctional ribs.

3. Patient's right arm is elevated and abducted, putting the pectoralis minor muscle on stretch.

4. Patient is instructed to take a deep breath and hold.

5. Patient performs a muscle effort of adduction against the operator's resistance for bucket-handle restriction (Fig. 15.62) or a flexion effort against operator resistance for a pump-handle restriction (Fig. 15.63).

6. A 3- to 5-second contraction for three to five repetitions is made.

7. In the presence of right shoulder pathology, the alternative procedure finds the operator's thumb medial to the right coracoid process to resist an anterior motion of the right shoulder girdle (Fig. 15.64).

8. Retest.

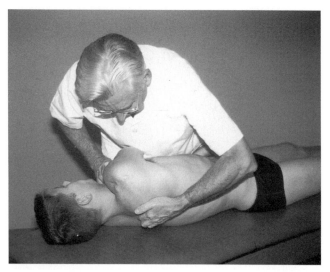

Figure 15.61.

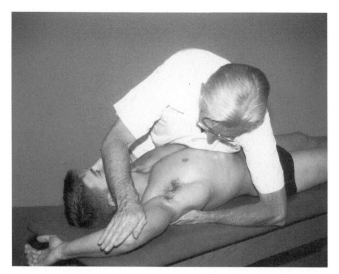

Figure 15.63.

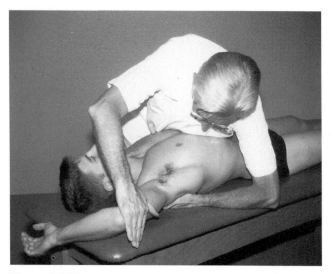

Figure 15.62.

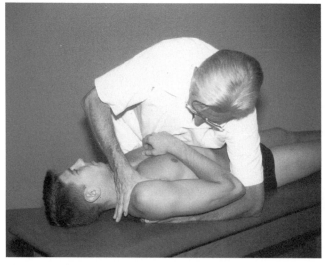

Figure 15.64.

Rib Cage

Respiratory Restriction
Ribs 6–9
Diagnosis
Inhalation restriction (right side example)

1. Patient supine on table with operator standing on left side.

2. The fingers of the operator's left hand contact the sixth, seventh, eighth, and ninth ribs medial to the angle (Fig. 15.65).

3. Operator returns patient to neutral position and with the left elbow on the table puts a lateral and caudad distractive force on the four ribs.

4. Operator's right hand controls the patient's right upper extremity.

5. Patient is instructed to take a deep breath and for a pump-handle restriction flex the upper extremity against operator resistance (Fig. 15.66) or in a lateral direction for bucket-handle restriction (Fig. 15.67).

6. Three to five repetitions of a 3- to 5-second effort are performed.

7. In the presence of shoulder dysfunction, operator resists a protraction action of the right scapula at the inferior scapular angle (Fig. 15.68).

8. Retest.

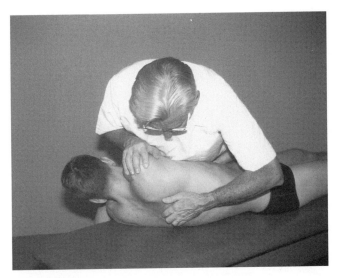

Figure 15.65.

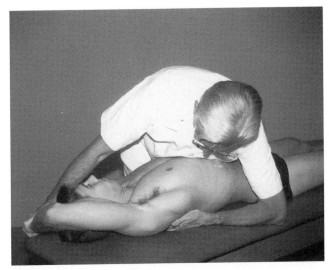

Figure 15.67.

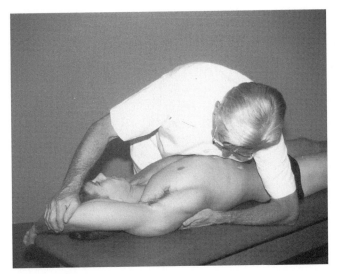

Figure 15.66.

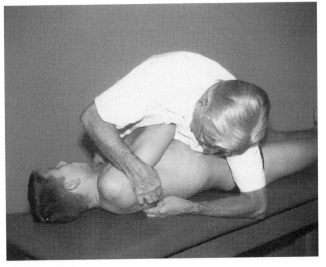

Figure 15.68.

Rib Cage

Respiratory Restriction
Lower Ribs
Diagnosis
Exhalation restriction (left side example)

1. Patient supine on table with operator standing at the left side of the head of the table.

2. Operator's left thumb and thenar eminence contacts the superior aspect of the dysfunctional key rib, including the costochondral junction (Fig. 15.69).

3. Operator's right hand supports head, neck, and upper thorax to control patient body position (Fig. 15.70).

4. Operator introduces left sidebending and flexion of the trunk down to the key rib (Fig. 15.71).

5. Patient is instructed to breath in and exhale completely.

6. Operator follows exhalation movement of the rib and holds it in that position.

7. Patient's inhalation respiratory effort is resisted by the operator and during exhalation a new barrier is engaged by trunk flexion and sidebending (Fig. 15.72).

8. After three to five repetitions with maximum exhalation being obtained, patient's head, neck, and upper trunk are returned to neutral while the operator holds the key rib in an exhalation position.

9. Operator releases the left thumb from the key rib slowly.

10. Retest.

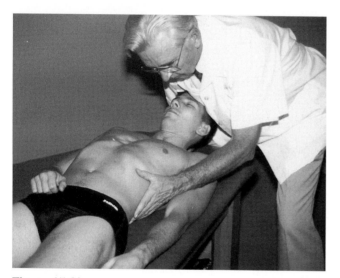

Figure 15.69.

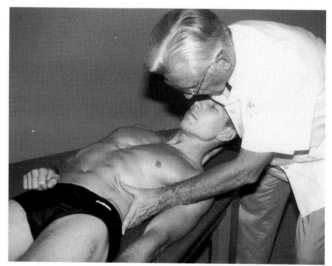

Figure 15.71.

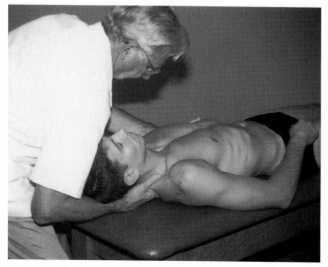

Figure 15.70.

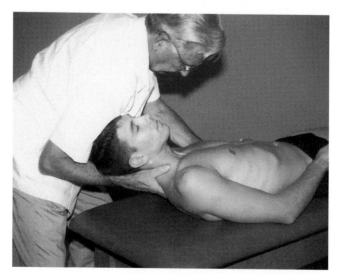

Figure 15.72.

Rib Cage

Respiratory Restriction
Upper Ribs
Diagnosis
Exhalation restriction (left side example)

1. Patient supine on table with operator standing at left side of head of table.

2. Operator's left thumb and thenar eminence contacts the superior aspect of the shaft of the dysfunctional rib spanning the costochondral junction (Fig. 15.73). Note that the more cephalic the rib, the more medial is the costochondral junction.

3. Operator's right hand controls patient's head, neck, and upper thorax and introduces flexion and sidebending to the side of dysfunction (Fig. 15.74).

4. Operator introduces more flexion for pump-handle component and sidebending for the bucket-handle component (Fig. 15.75).

5. Patient is instructed to breath in and exhale completely while operator follows the rib into exhalation with increasing flexion and sidebending (Fig. 15.76).

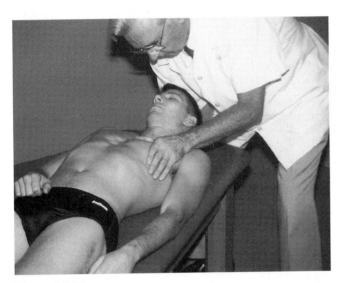

Figure 15.73.

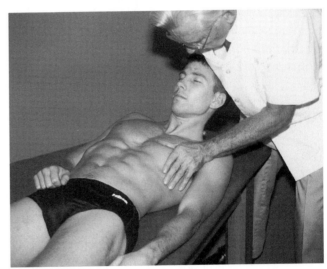

Figure 15.75.

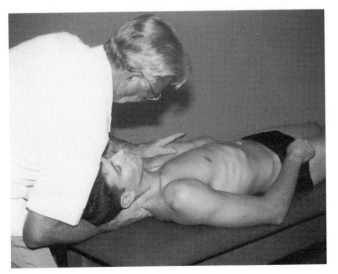

Figure 15.74.

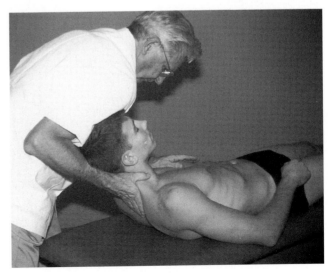

Figure 15.76.

6. Three to five repetitions are performed, and when maximum exhalation movement has been achieved, patient's head and neck are returned to neutral while operator holds dysfunctional rib in exhalation position (Fig. 15.77).

7. Operator releases compressive left thumb very slowly.

8. Retest.

Rib Cage

Respiratory Restriction
Upper Ribs
Diagnosis
Exhalation restriction (left side example)

1. Patient supine with operator standing at head of table.

2. Operator's left hand controls the patient's head and neck while the right thumb and thenar eminence contacts the shaft and costochondral articulation of the dysfunction rib (Fig. 15.78).

3. Operator introduces flexion and sidebending toward the side of dysfunction.

4. Patient is instructed to fully exhale after a short inhalation and the operator follows the dysfunctional rib into an exhalation position and holds it there (Fig. 15.79).

5. After several respiratory efforts with increasing flexion and sidebending, operator returns the head to neutral and slowly releases the compressive force on the dysfunctional rib.

6. Retest.

Note: This alternative position avoids compressive force on breast tissue, particularly in females. It is also particularly valuable for the pump-handle component of upper rib restrictions.

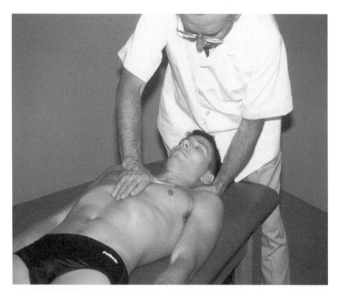

Figure 15.78.

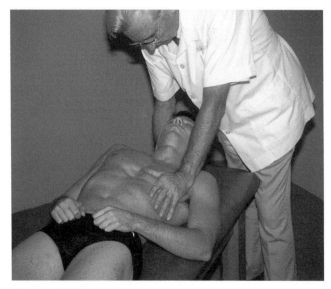

Figure 15.77.

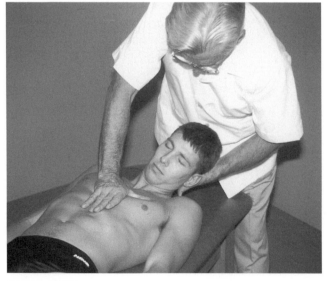

Figure 15.79.

Rib Cage

Respiratory Restriction
First Rib
Diagnosis
Exhalation restriction: pump-handle component
(left side example)

1. Patient supine on table with operator sitting at head.

2. Operator's right hand controls the patient's head while the left thumb contacts the superior aspect of the anterior extremity of the first rib either lateral to or between the heads of the sternocleidomastoid muscle (Fig. 15.80).

3. Operator introduces flexion with some left sidebending (Fig. 15.81).

4. Patient is instructed to perform forced exhalation while operator increases flexion and left sidebending and follows the left first rib into exhalation (Fig. 15.82).

5. Operator resists inhalation movement of the first rib and during exhalation follows the first rib into the exhalation position.

6. Three to five efforts are performed, and when maximum exhalation has been achieved, operator returns the head to neutral and slowly releases the contact on the first rib.

7. Retest.

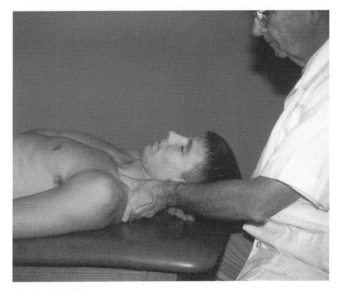

Figure 15.80.

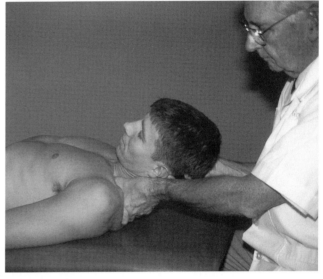

Figure 15.82.

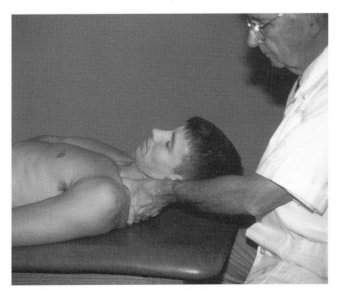

Figure 15.81.

Rib Cage

Respiratory Restriction
First Rib
Diagnosis
Exhalation restriction: bucket-handle component
(left side example)

1. Patient supine with operator sitting at head of table.

2. Operator's right hand grasps patient's head and neck while left thumb contacts the superior aspect of the lateral shaft of the first rib just anterior to the trapezius and posterior to the clavicle (Fig. 15.83).

3. Patient is instructed to take a short inhalation followed by forced exhalation while operator side-bends the head to the left with a small amount of flexion and follows the lateral shaft of the rib into exhalation (Fig. 15.84).

4. Operator continues holding the first rib in exhalation and patient repeats the minimal inhalation and maximal exhalation effort with increasing left side-bending of the head and neck by the operator's right hand (Fig. 15.85).

5. When maximal exhalation effort has been achieved, operator holds first rib in exhalation position and returns head to neutral.

6. Operator's left thumb is released slowly.

7. Retest.

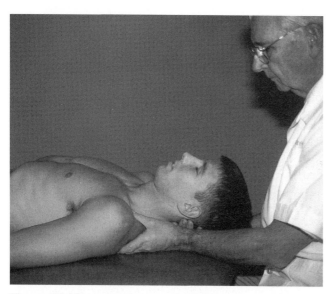

Figure 15.83.

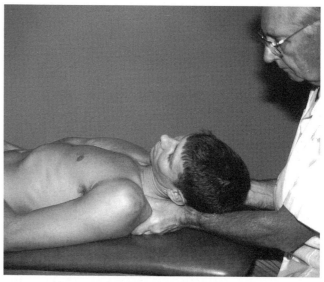

Figure 15.85.

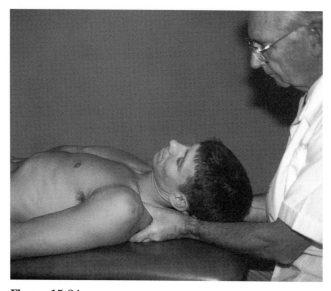

Figure 15.84.

Rib Cage

Respiratory Restriction
Ribs 11 and 12
Diagnosis
Exhalation restriction (right side example)

1. Patient prone on table with operator standing on left side of patient.

2. Operator's heel of left hand contacts the medial side of the shafts of the 11th and 12th ribs (Fig. 15.86).

3. Patient's right arm is placed on the table and reaches toward the feet with trunk sidebending toward the right.

4. Operator's right hand grasps the patient's right anterior superior iliac spine (Fig. 15.87).

5. Patient is instructed to inhale slightly and exhale maximally.

6. Patient's left hand carries the 11th and 12th ribs in a lateral and caudad direction.

7. At the end of full exhalation, patient pulls the right anterior superior iliac spine down toward the table for 3–5 seconds (Fig. 15.88).

8. After each effort, operator engages a new barrier. Three to five repetitions are made.

9. Retest.

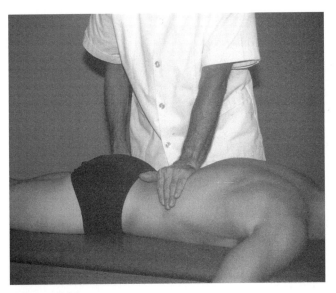

Figure 15.86.

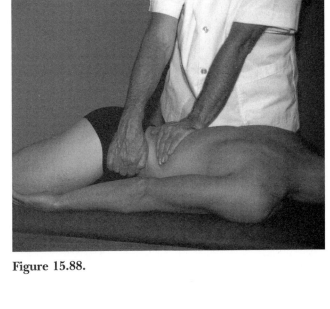

Figure 15.88.

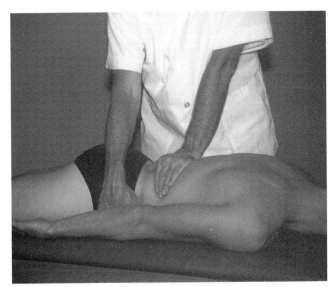

Figure 15.87.

Rib Cage

Respiratory Restriction
Ribs 11 and 12
Diagnosis
Inhalation restriction (right side example)

1. Patient prone on table with operator standing on the left side.

2. Operator's heel of left hand contacts the medial aspect of the patient's 11th and 12th ribs (Fig. 15.89).

3. Operator's right hand exerts a lateral and cephalic force with the patient's right hand over the head and with the feet to the left introducing left side-bending (Fig. 15.90).

4. Operator's right hand grasps the right anterior superior iliac spine.

5. Patient is instructed to take a maximal inhalation effort and hold.

6. Operator lifts patient's right pelvis off table and resists the patient's effort to pull the right anterior superior iliac spine down to the table (Fig. 15.91).

7. Three to five repetitions are made with a new barrier being engaged after each effort.

8. Retest.

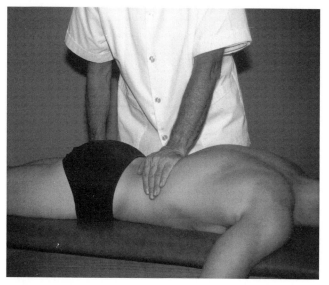

Figure 15.89.

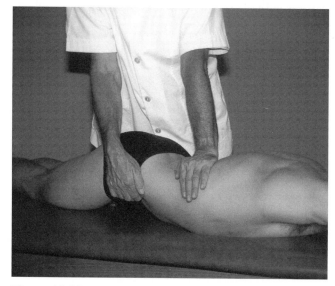

Figure 15.91.

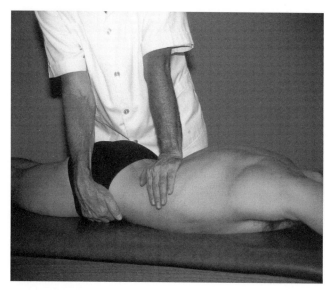

Figure 15.90.

MOBILIZATION WITH IMPULSE (HIGH VELOCITY THRUST) DIRECT ACTION TECHNIQUE FOR RIB DYSFUNCTION

The major restrictors of rib cage dysfunction are primarily myofascial. Occasionally, a rib becomes dysfunctional with palpable characteristics of deep articular and periarticular tissue reaction. Mobilization with impulse technique would then be of assistance in the management of the rib cage. Mobilization with impulse technique can be used to treat single rib and group rib dysfunctions of both the structural and respiratory type. Mobilization with impulse techniques are contraindicated in the presence of rib subluxations. The treatment sequence is the same as previously described.

The structural rib dysfunction most frequently treated with mobilization with impulse technique is external rib torsional dysfunction associated with a nonneutral ERS dysfunction of the thoracic spine.

Rib Cage

Respiratory Restriction
Mobilization with Impulse Technique
Supine
Diagnosis
External torsion dysfunction (Example: left fifth rib)

1. The patient and operator positions are the same as for the thoracic spine, mobilization with impulse technique for an ERS left dysfunction at T4-5 (see Figures 14.68 and 14.69).

2. Operator establishes lever arm.

3. Operator's right hand establishes a fulcrum to stabilize both transverse processes of T5 and with the thenar eminence on the inferior aspect of the left fifth rib.

4. After return of the patient to neutral position and the establishment of the lever arm to the fulcrum, operator's left hand introduces flexion, right side-bending, and right rotation of the neck and upper thoracic spine down to the left fifth rib.

5. The force through the lever arm to the fulcrum is somewhat more to the left side than midline as for the thoracic dysfunction, and a high velocity, low amplitude thrust is made by the body weight of the operator on the lever arm to the fulcrum resulting in flexion, right sidebending, and right rotation of T4 on T5, the opening of the left zygapophysial joint, and the mobilization of the left fifth rib. The thenar eminence of the operator's right hand maintains a cephalic pressure on the inferior aspect of the fifth rib at the time of the thrust.

6. Commonly, two cavitation pop sounds occur in rapid sequence when the thrust is applied.

7. Retest.

Rib Cage

Respiratory Restriction
Mobilization with Impulse Technique
Rib 1
Diagnosis
Inhalation or exhalation restriction (left first rib example)

1. Patient supine on table. Operator stands on right side and slides arm under patient with fingers of the right hand grasping the superior aspect of the left first rib (Fig. 15.92).

2. With exhalation restriction, operator depresses anterior aspect of the rib shaft. With inhalation restriction, operator's depress posterior aspect of first rib.

3. Operator's left hand sidebends patient's head and neck to the left and rotates to the right, with localization to T1 (Fig. 15.93).

4. A mobilization with impulse thrust is performed by the operator with either an acute exaggeration of the head and neck position into left sidebending or stabilizing the head and neck with the left hand and performing an acute caudad thrust through the right hand in the axis of the right forearm.

5. Retest.

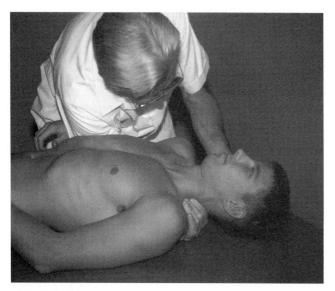

Figure 15.92.

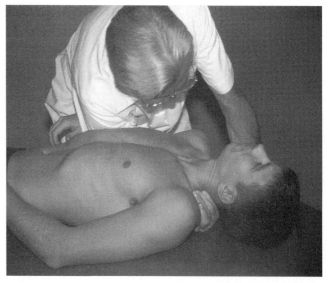

Figure 15.93.

Rib Cage

Respiratory Restriction
Mobilization with Impulse Technique
Rib 1
Diagnosis
Exhalation restriction (left first rib example)

1. Patient sitting on the table with operator standing behind.

2. Operator's right foot is placed on the table and the patient's right extremity is draped over the operator's right thigh.

3. Operator's right hand contacts the right side of the head and neck of the patient while the left hand contacts the left first rib over its anterior and posterior extremity (Fig. 15.94).

4. Operator's left forearm is angled from above downward against the hand contact on the first rib (Fig. 15.95).

5. Operator introduces left sidebending and right rotation of the patient's head and neck localized at T1 (Fig. 15.96).

6. A mobilization with impulse thrust is performed through the operator's left forearm in a caudad and medial direction (Fig. 15.97).

7. Retest.

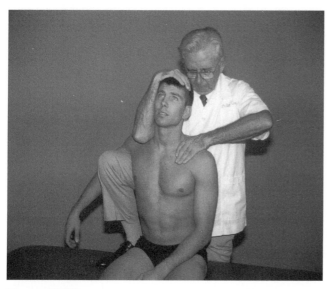

Figure 15.94.

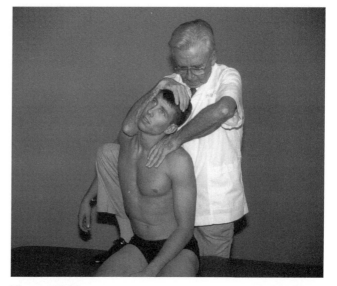

Figure 15.96.

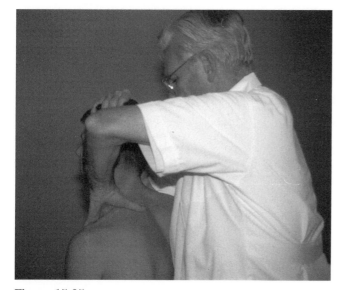

Figure 15.95.

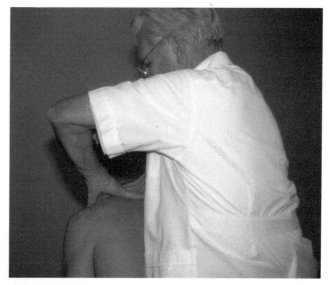

Figure 15.97.

Rib Cage

Respiratory Restriction
Mobilization with Impulse Technique
Rib 2
Diagnosis
Exhalation restriction (left second rib example)

1. Patient sitting on table with operator standing behind with right foot on the table and patient's right arm draped over the operator's right thigh.

2. Operator's right hand controls the right side of the patient's head and neck and the left hand is over the patient's left shoulder (Fig. 15.98).

3. Operator's left thumb is on the posterior shaft of rib 2 (Fig. 15.99).

4. Operator introduces left sidebending and right rotation of the head and neck, and with translation of the trunk from left to right localizes to T1–2 and the left second rib (Fig. 15.100).

5. When the barrier is engaged, a mobilization with impulse technique is performed through the left forearm with an anterior and medial thrust against the resistance of the stabilizing right arm (Fig. 15.101).

6. Retest.

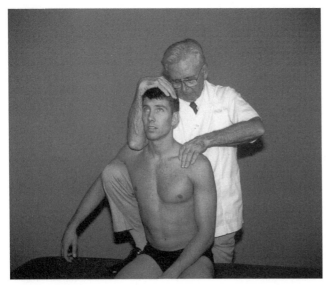

Figure 15.98.

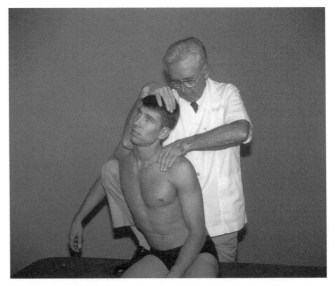

Figure 15.100.

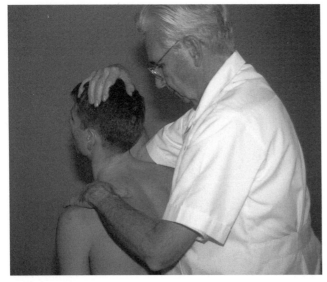

Figure 15.99.

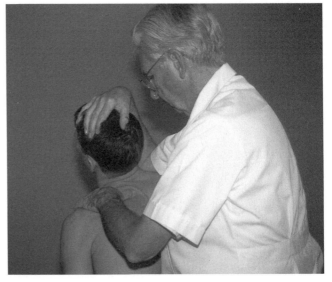

Figure 15.101.

Rib Cage

Respiratory Restriction
Mobilization with Impulse Technique
Typical Ribs (3–10)
Diagnosis
Inhalation or exhalation restriction (Example: left ribs)

1. Operator's thumb and thenar eminence function as the fulcrum. The thumb contacts either the superior or inferior aspect of the dysfunctional rib (Fig. 15.102).

2. For exhalation restriction, the thumb is placed below the rib shaft and exerts a superior force (Fig. 15.103).

3. For inhalation restriction, the thumb and thenar contact is on the superior aspect of the rib shaft with the rib being carried caudad (Fig. 15.104).

4. Patient's left hand grasps the right shoulder, establishing the lever arm (Fig. 15.105).

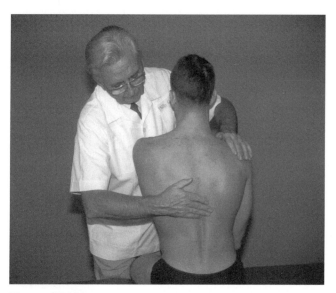

Figure 15.102.

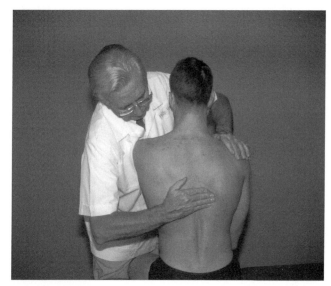

Figure 15.104.

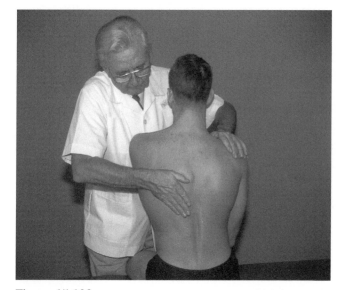

Figure 15.103.

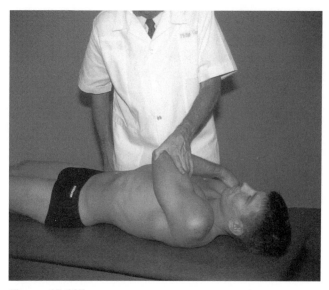

Figure 15.105.

5. Operator places the fulcrum on the dysfunctional rib as appropriate for the respiratory restriction (Fig. 15.106).

6. Patient's trunk is returned to midline, and operator's body (either chest wall or abdomen) localizes to fulcrum through the lever arm (Fig. 15.107).

7. A mobilization with impulse thrust is made by the operator's body dropped through the lever arm to the fulcrum with the right thumb and thenar eminence exerting a cephalic directed force for exhalation restriction and a caudad direction force for inhalation restriction.

8. A respiratory assist of inhalation or exhalation can be made, but usually exhalation for relaxation of the patient is more helpful.

9. Retest.

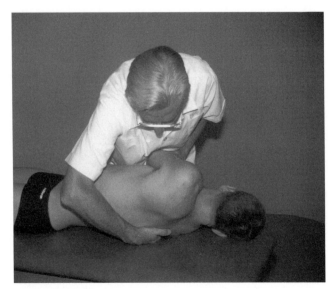

Figure 15.106.

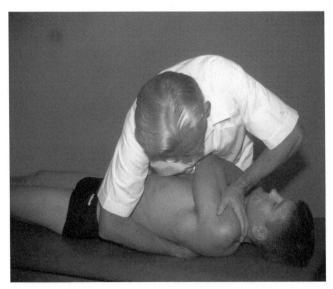

Figure 15.107.

Rib Cage

Respiratory Restriction
Mobilization with Impulse Technique
Lower Typical Ribs and Ribs 11 and 12
Diagnosis
Inhalation or exhalation restriction (left side example)

1. Patient in lateral recumbent position with the dysfunctional side up.

2. Operator stands in front of patient with the pisiform of the right hand in contact with the posterior aspect of the dysfunctional rib (Fig. 15.108).

3. Operator's left hand contacts the anterior aspect of the patient's left shoulder.

4. For exhalation restriction, the pisiform contact is on the inferior aspect of the rib shaft and operator's right forearm directs the rib in an anterior and superior direction (Fig. 15.109).

5. For inhalation restriction, the pisiform contact is on the superior aspect of the rib shaft and operator's right arm carries it caudally (Fig. 15.110).

6. A mobilization with impulse thrust is performed by a body drop of the operator, directing force through the right forearm in the appropriate direction for inhalation or exhalation restriction.

7. Retest.

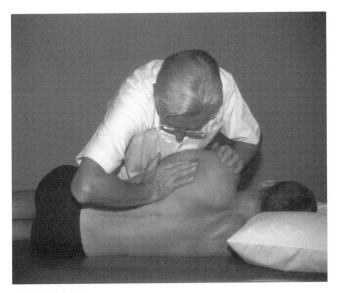

Figure 15.108.

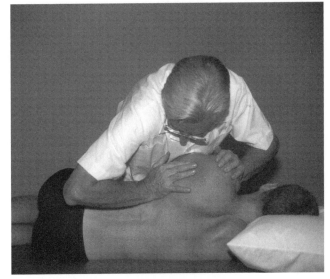

Figure 15.110.

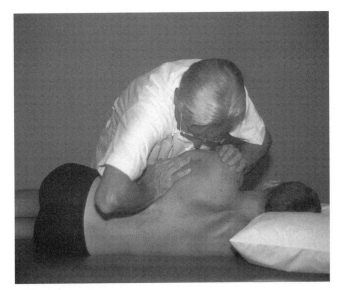

Figure 15.109.

Rib Cage

Respiratory Restriction
Mobilization with Impulse Technique
Diagnosis
Ribs 11 and 12 (right side example)

1. Patient prone on table with operator standing on left side with left hand medial to the shafts of ribs 11 and 12 and the right hand grasping the patient's right anterior superior iliac spine.

2. For exhalation restriction, the patient is sidebent to the right with the right arm reaching toward the right knee (Fig. 15.111).

3. For inhalation restriction, the patient is left sidebent with the right hand over the head (Fig. 15.112).

4. The barrier is engaged by lifting the anterior superior iliac spine from the table.

5. A mobilization with impulse thrust is performed through the operator's left hand in a lateral and inferior direction for exhalation restriction and in a lateral and superior direction for inhalation restriction.

6. Retest.

CONCLUSION

Dysfunction of the rib cage is highly significant in many problems of the musculoskeletal system. The structural rib dysfunctions can be major pain generators. Respiratory rib restriction compromises the patient's capacity for respiration and efficient circulation of the low pressure venous and lymphatic systems. There are extensive muscle attachments to the rib cage that can serve as restrictors of the cervical spine, the upper extremities, the lumbar spine, and even into the pelvis and lower extremity. Restoration of symmetrical thoracic cage function for respiration and circulation is as important as restoring symmetrical mobility of the lumbar spine, pelvis, and lower extremities in the walking cycle.

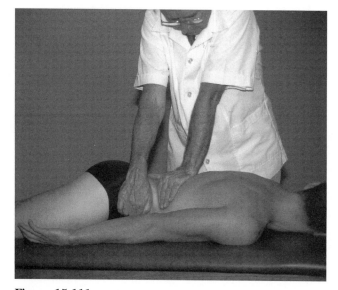

Figure 15.111

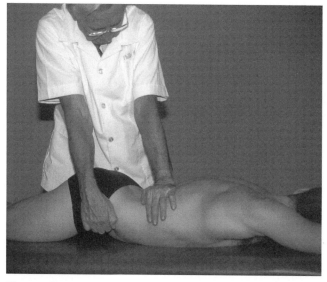

Figure 15.112.

16

LUMBAR SPINE

The lumbar spine and pelvic girdle (see Chapter 17) contain many of the structures incriminated in the complaint of "low back pain." The classic report of Mixter and Barr in 1934 brought the lumbar intervertebral disk to the attention of physicians in many disciplines. The differential diagnosis of low back pain continues to be a dilemma for the examining physician, and 60–80% of cases are still classified as idiopathic. After the exclusion of organic and pathological conditions by orthodox orthopedic and neurological testing, the examiner is left with the difficulty of determining any other treatable source for the back pain. It is in these patients that the ability to identify and treat functional abnormalities of the musculoskeletal system has been found clinically effective. It is strongly recommended that the structural diagnostic procedures identified here and in Chapter 17 should be used concurrently with orthopedic and neurological testing of the lower trunk and lower extremities. Including functional diagnosis in these patients greatly reduces the number that need to be classified as idiopathic. More clinical research is needed into the origin of pain in dysfunctions of the lumbar spine and pelvis and the efficacy and mechanisms of manual medicine therapeutic applications.

FUNCTIONAL ANATOMY

The five lumbar vertebrae are the most massive in the vertebral column. The vertebral bodies are kidney shaped and are solidly constructed to participate in weight bearing of the superincumbent vertebral column. The posterior arches are strongly developed with large spinous processes projecting directly posterior from the vertebral bodies. The transverse processes are quite large, and those at L3 are usually the broadest. The lumbar lordosis has an anterior convexity with L3 usually the most anterior segment. L4 and L5 have limited motion because of the strong attachments of the iliolumbar ligaments to the osseous pelvis; therefore, L3 becomes the first lumbar segment that is freely movable.

The articular pillar has a superior zygapophysial

joint that faces posteriorly and medially and an inferior zygapophysial joint that faces laterally and anteriorly. The superior facet is somewhat concave and the inferior facet somewhat convex. The facing of the lumbar zygapophysial joint is variable and asymmetry is quite common. Because of the shape of the zygapophysial joints, only a small amount of axial rotation movement is present. When the plane of the zygapophysial joints is more sagittal, there appears to be increased stability of the lumbar spine. The more coronal facing the lumbar zygapophysial joints are, the more mobility and potential hypermobility appears to be present. In the presence of asymmetry, with one zygapophysial joint being sagittal and the other being coronal, there appears to be an increase in the risk of disk degeneration and herniation, with a tendency toward herniation to the side of the coronal facing facet. Asymmetrical zygapophysial joints also appear to influence the motion characteristics of the segment and are frequently found in patients with recurrent and refractory dysfunctional problems in the lumbar spine. Between the superior and inferior zygapophysial joints lies the structure called the pars interarticularis. Disruption through the pars without separation is called spondylolysis. With separation at this level, the body, pedicle, and superior articular pillar slide anteriorly, whereas the spinous process, laminae, and inferior articular pillar are held posteriorly, resulting in spondylolisthesis.

The lower lumbar region is frequently the site of developmental variations. In addition to asymmetrical development of the zygapophysial joints, other variations in the posterior arch occur, resulting in unilateral and bilateral changes in size and shape of the transverse process and culminating in a transitional lumbosacral vertebra that may have lumbar or sacral characteristics (previously referred to as lumbarization and sacralization). Failure of closure of the posterior arch is not infrequently seen, and occasionally the spinous process of L5 is missing. Absence of these structures must result in alteration of the usual ligamentous and muscular attachments in the region.

LUMBAR MOTION

The motions available in the lumbar spine are primarily flexion and extension. There is a small amount of right and left sidebending and a minimal amount of rotation. The coupled movements of sidebending and rotation available in the lumbar spine are both neutral (type I) and nonneutral (type II). In the absence of dysfunction, when in neutral and backward-bending position, sidebending and rotation are coupled to opposite sides. In the forward-bending position, sidebending and rotation couple to the same side. The intimate attachments of the iliolumbar ligaments from L4 and L5 to the osseous pelvis result in these two segments having less mobility than the upper three lumbar vertebrae.

MOTION AT LUMBOSACRAL JUNCTION

During neutral vertebral mechanics and in the absence of dysfunction, L5 and the sacrum move in opposite directions. With sidebending right and rotation left of the sacrum between the innominates, L5 adapts by sidebending left and rotating right. As the sacrum moves into anterior nutation (flexion of the sacrum between the innominates), L5 moves into backward-bending (extension) in relation to the sacrum. With the sacrum moving into posterior nutation (extension of the sacrum between the innominates), L5 moves into forward-bending (flexion) in relation to the sacrum. In the absence of dysfunction, all lumbar segments should follow the segment below during the forward-bending and backward-bending arc. The paired transverse processes of each segment should remain in the same plane as the segment below. Loss of the normal neutral relationship of L5 to the sacrum is of great clinical significance and is termed "nonadaptive lumbar response" to sacral function. Restoration of this normal relationship at L5 to S1 is one of the major reasons for diagnosing and treating lumbar spine dysfunctions before addressing the two sacroiliac joints. Many of the techniques to be described in Chapter 17 require the normal neutral relationship of L5 to the sacrum.

STRUCTURAL DIAGNOSIS OF LUMBAR SPINE DYSFUNCTION

The lumbar spine can become dysfunctional with nonneutral (type II) dysfunctions of either the extended, rotated, and sidebent (ERS) or flexed, rotated, and sidebent (FRS) type. The lumbar spine can have neutral (group) dysfunctions, particularly in the upper lumbar segments carrying over into the lower segments of the thoracic spine. When one finds flattening of the lumbar lordosis, the probability of FRS dysfunction with extension restriction is high. If the lumbar lordosis is increased, the probability of ERS dysfunction with flexion restriction is high. The diagnosis of lumbar segmental dysfunction combines tissue texture changes of the deeper layers of paravertebral muscle, particularly hypertonicity of the multifidi, rotatores, and intertransversariae, and alteration in motion characteristics. Evaluation of lumbar segmental motion can be done in a variety of ways. For the reasons described in Chapter 6, the recommended process is to evaluate the location of the posterior aspect of the transverse processes in three positions. This process requires the assessment of the superior segment in relation to the inferior. In the lumbar spine, this requires that L5 be assessed in relation to the sacrum. Therefore, assessment of the lumbar spine begins by identifying the sacral base, the posterior aspect of the transverse processes of S1. Because of the anatomy of the lumbosacral junction, it is not possible to palpate the transverse processes of L5. Instead, the examiner identifies the symmetrical portions of the posterior arch of L5, as far laterally as possible, to assess rotation of L5 in relation to S1.

The diagnostic procedure requires the assessment of the paired transverse processes in neutral, forward bent, and backward bent positions. A sequence that is the easiest for the beginning student is to first assess in the prone (neutral) position on the table (Fig. 16.1). Beginning at the sacral base, each lumbar vertebra is assessed for its relationship to the one below up to the thoracolumbar junction. Assessment is now made in the backward bent (extended) prone prop position on the table (sphinx position) (Fig. 16.2). Despite the mass size of the lumbar musculature, the transverse processes are quite easily palpated in this position. Assessment is

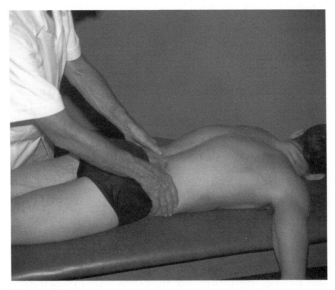

Figure 16.1.
Transverse process palpation neutral position.

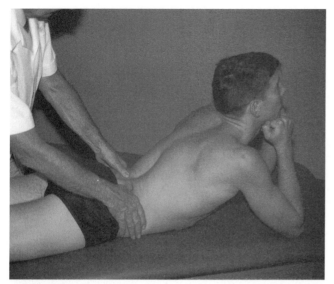

Figure 16.2.
Transverse process palpation backward bent (extended) position (prone prop).

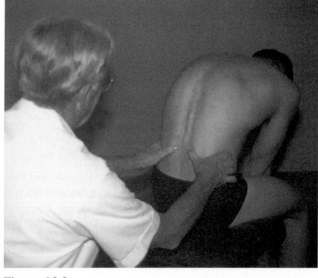

Figure 16.3.
Transverse process palpation forward bent position.

then made in the fully forward bent position with the patient seated with the feet on the floor or a stool. Assessment is made from below upward in similar fashion. It is more difficult to palpate transverse processes in this position because of the tension through the lumbar muscles and the lumbodorsal fascia (Fig. 16.3). If one transverse process is more posterior in the fully forward bent position and becomes symmetric in the prone prop (sphinx position), a nonneutral (type II) ERS dysfunction is present at this level. If one transverse process is more prominent in the prone prop (sphinx position) and becomes symmetric in the forward bent position, a nonneutral (type II) FRS restriction is present. If three or more transverse processes remain prominent throughout all three positions, a neutral (type I) dysfunction is present. It is difficult to evaluate the functional capacity of the upper lumbar segments until those identified as dysfunctional in the lower region are successfully treated. Nonneutral dysfunctions are common at L4 and L5, as well as at the thoracolumbar junction. Nonneutral dysfunctions at L4 and L5 are frequently seen in association with dysfunction of the sacroiliac joints.

In the presence of unleveling of the sacrum, in the absence of dysfunction of the lumbar spine, there will be sidebending and rotation to opposite sides of the lumbar vertebra to compensate and maintain the trunk erect. This adaptive response is only found in neutral. The longer this is present, the more likely it is to develop a neutral (group) dysfunction.

MANUAL MEDICINE PROCEDURES FOR DYSFUNCTIONS OF LUMBAR SPINE

The treating clinician needs to have manual medicine techniques to treat group (type I) dysfunctions and the nonneutral (type II) ERS and FRS dysfunctions. In the treatment sequence, it is recommended that nonneutral dysfunctions be treated first and group dysfunctions last. Usually, one begins by treating the lower segments first and then sequentially from below upward. Exceptions to this below upward rule are those cases in which the major restrictor is higher in the lumbar spine or those cases in which the lowest segment is so acute it is difficult to directly address. One should be able to treat a patient in the erect sitting posture or recumbent on the table.

Lumbar Spine

Muscle Energy Technique
Sitting
Nonneutral Dysfunction (Example: L4 ERS$_L$)
    Position: Backward bent (extended), left side-
    bent, left rotated (ERS$_L$)
    Motion restriction: Forward bending (flexion),
    right sidebending, right rotation

1. Patient sitting on stool with left hand holding the
   right shoulder and right arm dropped at the side.

2. Operator stands at left side of patient straddling the
   patient's left knee with the left hand grasping patient's right shoulder and controlling the left shoulder with the left axilla (Fig. 16.4). Operator's middle
   finger monitors the L4-5 interspinous space and the
   right index finger monitors the left transverse process of L4.

3. The forward-bending (flexion) barrier is engaged by
   an anterior to posterior translatory movement at
   L4-5 (Fig. 16.5).

4. Right sidebending and right rotation are introduced
   at L4-5 by the operator's left arm, asking the patient to reach to the floor with the right hand
   (Fig. 16.6).

5. Patient is instructed to sidebend to the left against
   equal resistance for 3–5 seconds. After relaxation,

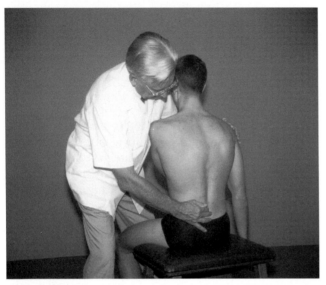

Figure 16.4.

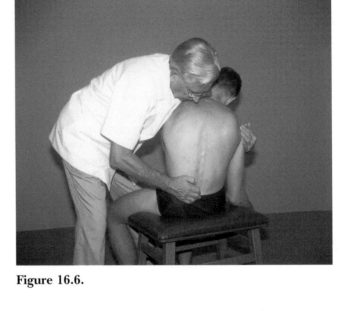

Figure 16.6.

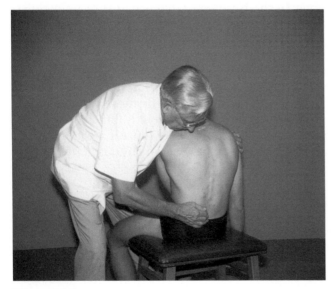

Figure 16.5.

the new forward-bending, right sidebending, and right rotational barrier are engaged and three to five repetitions are made of the left sidebending effort.

6. When all right rotation and right sidebending restriction is removed, operator forward bends the patient while maintaining right rotation (Fig. 16.7).

7. Operator's left hand resists a patient trunk extension effort, fully forward-bending the segment and opening both zygapophysial joints at L4-5 (Fig. 16.8).

8. Retest.

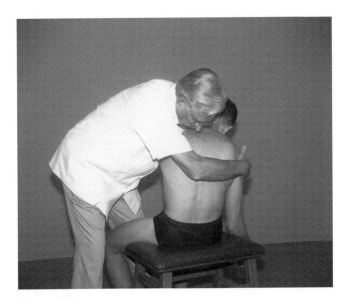

Figure 16.7.

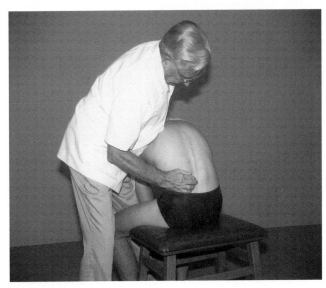

Figure 16.8.

Lumbar Spine

Muscle Energy Technique
Sitting
Nonneutral Dysfunction (Example: L3 FRS$_L$)
  Position: Forward bent (flexed), rotated left, sidebent left (FRS$_L$)
  Motion restriction: Backward bending (extension), right sidebending, right rotation

1. Patient sitting on stool with operator sitting behind controlling patient's trunk with the right hand and monitoring the interspinous space of L3-4 with the left index finger and the left transverse process of L3 with the left middle finger.

2. Operator introduces sidebending left and rotation right in neutral mechanics by the patient dropping the left shoulder and shifting the weight to the right buttock.

3. Three to four repetitions of a right sidebending effort by the patient pushing the right shoulder into the operator's right hand introduces right rotation at L3 on L4 (Fig. 16.9).

4. Operator introduces extension and right sidebending while right rotated by pressing inferiorly on the right shoulder while the patient shifts the weight to the left buttock and projects the abdomen over the left knee (Fig. 16.10).

5. Operator resists a series of three to five isometric contractions of 3–5 seconds with the patient either pulling the right shoulder forward against resistance or lifting the right shoulder toward the ceiling against resistance (Fig. 16.11). After each repetition, a new barrier is engaged.

6. When all right sidebending and right rotation restriction is removed, operator maintains extension and straightens patient's shoulders while blocking the L4 segment bilaterally with the left hand (Fig. 16.12). Operator right hand resists flexion effort by the patient's trunk to fully extend L3 on L4 closing both zygapophysial joints.

7. Retest.

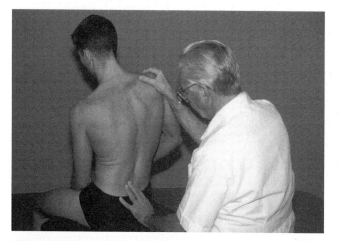

Figure 16.9.

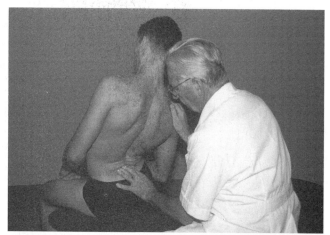

Figure 16.11.

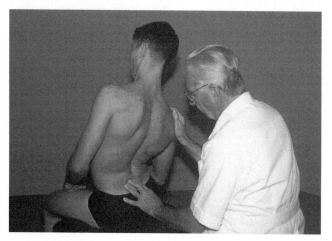

Figure 16.10.

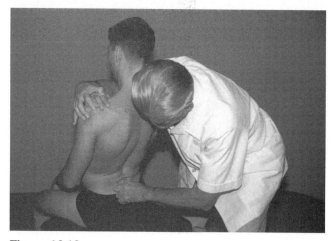

Figure 16.12.

Lumbar Spine

Muscle Energy Technique
Sitting
Neutral (Group) Dysfunction
Variation 1

    Position: Neutral, sidebent right, rotated left (NS_RR_L) or (EN_L).

    Motion restriction: Sidebending left, rotation right.

1. Patient sitting on table with right hand grasping the left shoulder. Operator standing behind with right arm under patient's right axilla and grasping patient's left shoulder to control upper trunk (Fig. 16.13).

2. Operator's left thumb is placed at the apex of the left lumbar convexity for localization (Fig. 16.14).

3. Operator introduces left sidebending and right rotation localized to the thumb contact at the apex of the left lumbar convexity (Fig. 16.15).

4. Operator resists a series of 3- to 5-second right sidebending efforts against operator's resistance through the right arm (Fig. 16.16). The localizing thumb maintains a force anteromedially against the left lumbar curve.

5. Retest.

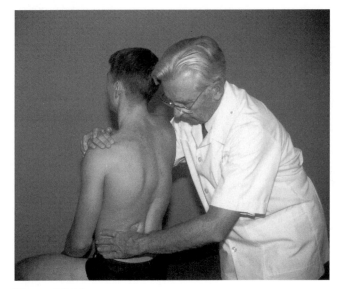

Figure 16.13.

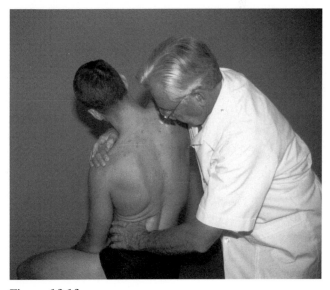

Figure 16.15.

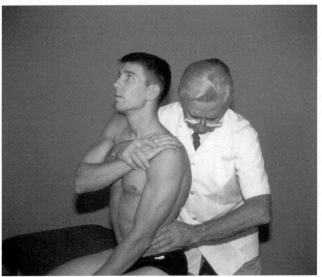

Figure 16.14.

Figure 16.16.

Lumbar Spine

Muscle Energy Technique
Sitting
Neutral (Group) Dysfunction
Variation 2

   Position: Neutral, sidebent right, rotated left (NS_RR_L) or (EN_L).
   Motion restriction: Sidebending left, rotation right.

1. Patient sitting on table with left hand holding the right shoulder. Operator standing behind with the left hand grasping patient's right shoulder and with left axilla over patient's left shoulder. Operator's right thumb is at the apex of the left lumbar convexity pressing anteromedially (Fig. 16.17).

2. Operator introduces left sidebending and right rotation through the left arm contact with translation from left to right at the apex of the curve monitored by the right thumb (Fig. 16.18).

3. Operator resists patient's right sidebending effort of 3–5 seconds repeated three to five times (Fig. 16.19).

4. After each effort, the operator engages the new left sidebending right rotational barrier with left to right translation localized at the apex.

5. Retest.

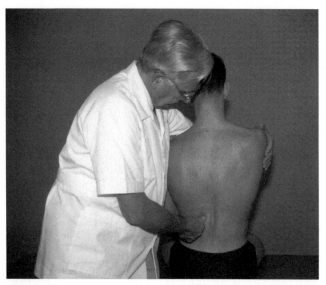

Figure 16.17.

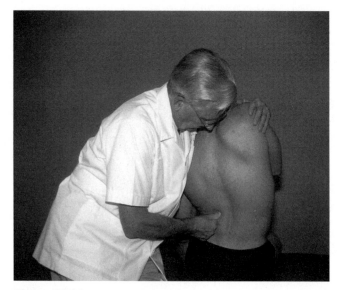

Figure 16.19.

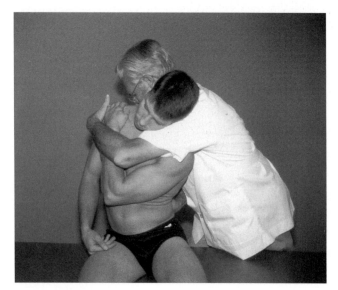

Figure 16.18.

Lumbar Spine

Muscle Energy Technique
Sitting
Bilateral Extension Restriction (Example: L1-2)
Position: Bilaterally flexed
Motion restriction: Bilateral extension

1. Patient sitting on table with hands holding opposite shoulder. Operator standing behind with left hand holding both elbows to control patient's trunk (Fig. 16.20).

2. Operator's hand blocks the L2 segment in the midline (Fig. 16.21).

3. Operator engages extension barrier by backward-bending the trunk while translating from posterior to anterior through the right hand (Fig. 16.22). Note the blocking of the right elbow against the operator's trunk.

4. Operator's left arm resists a forward-bending effort by the patient with a 3- to 5-second contraction repeated three to five times (Fig. 16.23).

5. The extension barrier is engaged after each patient effort.

6. Retest.

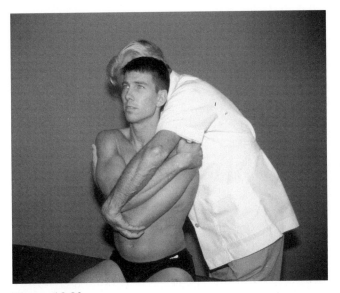

Figure 16.20.

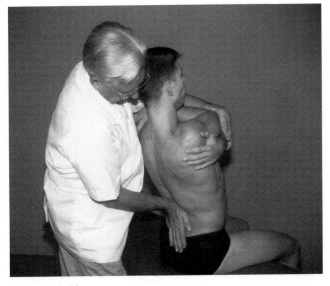

Figure 16.22.

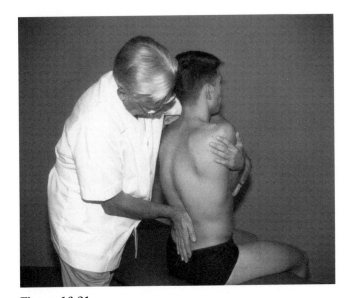

Figure 16.21.

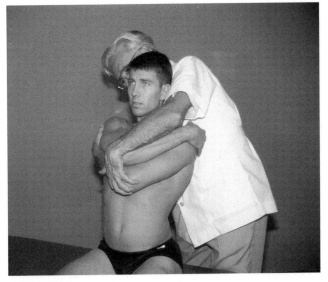

Figure 16.23.

Lumbar Spine

Muscle Energy Technique
Lateral Recumbent (Sims Position) (Example: L4 ERS$_R$)

> Position: Backward bent (extended), rotated right, sidebend right (ERS$_R$)
> Motion restriction: Forward-bending (flexion), rotation left, sidebending left

1. Patient prone on table with operator standing at left side. Operator flexes patient's knees, rolls lower extremity onto left hip into the Sims position (Fig. 16.24).

2. Operator's left middle finger palpates the L4-5 interspace with the index finger over the right trans- verse process of L4. Operator's right hand intro- duces left rotation of the trunk down to L4. Patient assists by reaching toward the floor (Fig. 16.25).

3. Operator switches hands with right hand monitoring the L4-5 level as the left arm and left thigh flex the patient's knees up to L5 engaging the flexion bar- rier (Fig. 16.26).

4. While continuing to monitor the L4-5 level, operator drops both feet to the floor, introducing left side- bending to the barrier (Fig. 16.27). Note that the pa- tient's knees are resting on the operator's left thigh.

5. Operator resists a muscle effort by the patient to lift the feet to the ceiling, attempting to introduce a

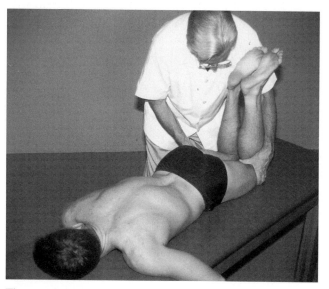

Figure 16.24.

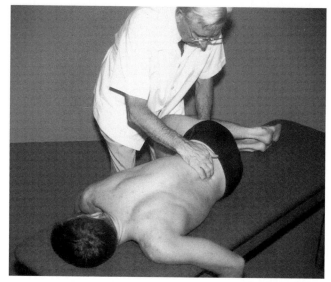

Figure 16.26.

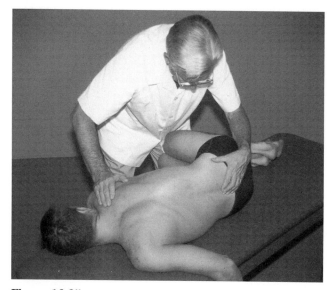

Figure 16.25.

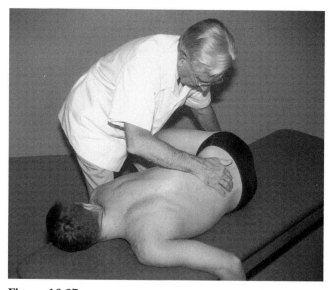

Figure 16.27.

right sidebending effort against resistance (Fig. 16.28). Operator's right hand monitors over the L4-5 level, ensuring localization of muscle contraction at that level.

6. Three to five repetitions of a 3- to 5-second muscle contraction are performed by the patient with the operator engaging a new flexion, left rotation, and left sidebending barrier after each effort.

7. Retest.

Note: Caution must be used to protect the lateral aspect of the patient's left thigh against the edge of the table. If the operator is unable to stabilize the patient's legs against the left thigh, a rolled towel or small pillow can be placed between the patient's thighs and the edge of the table. Another option is for the operator to sit on the end of the table with the left hand monitoring the L4-5 level and controlling the lower extremities with the right hand and with the patient's left knee over the operator's left thigh.

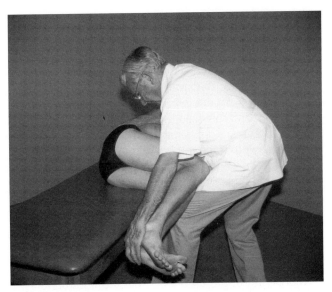

Figure 16.28.

Lumbar Spine

Muscle Energy Technique
Lateral Recumbent
Nonneutral Dysfunction (Example: L4 ERS$_L$)
>   Position: Backward bent (extended), rotated left, sidebent left (ERS$_L$)
>   Motion restriction: Forward-bending (flexion), rotation right, sidebending right

1. Patient lying in the left lateral recumbent position with the feet and knees together and shoulders and hips perpendicular to the table. Operator stands in front of patient and with right hand flexes patient's trunk down to L4 from above maintaining the shoulders perpendicular to the table for right sidebending (Fig. 16.29).

2. Operator flexes the lower extremities up to L5 while monitoring at the L4-5 level with the right hand (Fig. 16.30).

3. Operator introduces right rotation through the right forearm, rotating the patient's right shoulder posteriorly while monitoring at the L4-5 level with the right hand (Fig. 16.31).

4. Operator introduces right sidebending by lifting both feet toward the ceiling and engaging the combined right rotation, right sidebending barrier.

5. Operator resists patient effort of pulling the feet back toward the table (a left sidebending effort) while monitoring for contraction of the erector spinae muscles at the L4-5 level.

6. Three to five repetitions of a 3- to 5-second effort are performed by the patient. During each relaxation phase, the operator reengages the forward-bending, right rotation, right sidebending barrier.

7. Retest.

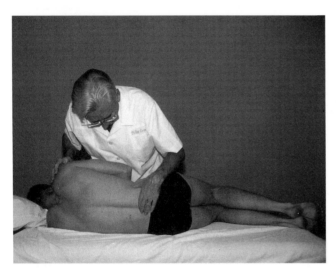

Figure 16.29.

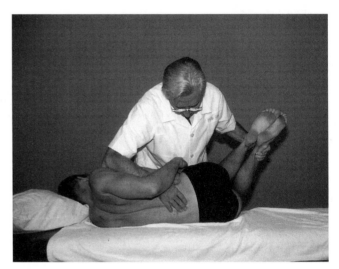

Figure 16.31.

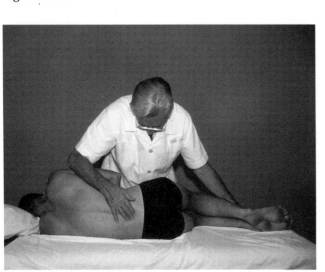

Figure 16.30.

Lumbar Spine

Muscle Energy Technique
Lateral Recumbent (Example: L4 FRS$_L$)

    Position: Forward bent (flexed), rotated left, sidebent left (FRS$_L$)

    Motion restriction: Backward bending (extension), right rotation, right sidebending

1. Patient in the left lateral recumbent position with the knees and feet together and with shoulders and pelvis perpendicular to the table (begins right sidebending by position).

2. Operator stands in front of the patient and with two hands contacts the L4-5 level (Fig. 16.32).

3. Operator engages first backward-bending (extension) barrier by translating the L4-5 level from posterior to anterior (Fig. 16.33). Note: Patient is lying on a sheet or towel so that sliding on the table is facilitated.

4. Operator fine-tunes backward-bending (extension) barrier from above by translating the left shoulder posteriorly, maintaining both shoulders perpendicular to the table, and monitoring with the left hand for motion down to L4 (Fig. 16.34).

5. Operator fine-tunes backward-bending (extension) barrier from below by extending the lower extremities and monitoring with the right hand for movement up to L5 (Fig. 16.35).

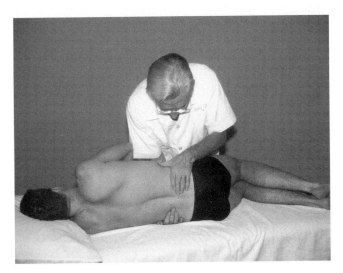

Figure 16.32.

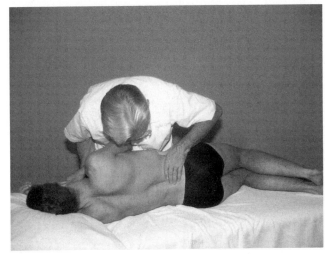

Figure 16.34.

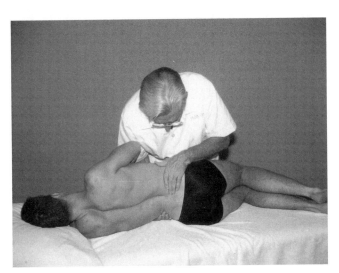

Figure 16.33.

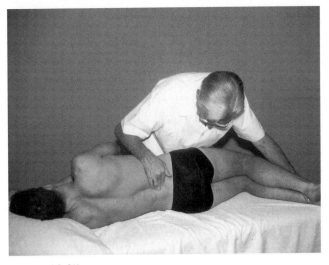

Figure 16.35.

6. Operator engages right rotation barrier by rotating the right shoulder posteriorly with the right hand monitoring rotation to L4 with the left hand (Fig. 16.36). Patient grasps the edge of the table to maintain the right rotation and to introduce more extension.

7. Operator's left hand lifts the right leg to engage the right sidebending barrier while monitoring with the right hand at the L4-5 level (Fig. 16.37).

8. Patient pulls right knee down toward the left knee for three to five repetitions of a 3- to 5-second muscle contraction against resistance provided by the operator's left hand. After each effort, increased engagement of the right sidebending barrier is performed by the operator by lifting the knee toward the ceiling and the backward-bending barrier by translating L4-5 anteriorly by the right hand.

9. Operator returns patient's right knee to the table and places right forearm against the patient's right shoulder, maintaining right rotation. Right hand monitors at the L4-5 level. Operator's left hand on patient's right buttock engages right sidebending barrier by cephalic translation (Fig. 16.38). Operator resists with the right forearm a left rotation effort of the patient's trunk by pushing the right shoulder into the operator's right forearm or a left sidebending effort by pushing the right buttock caudad. Again, three to five repetitions are performed.

10. Retest.

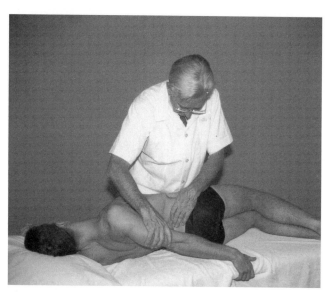

Figure 16.36.

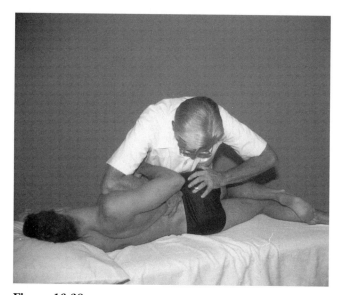

Figure 16.38.

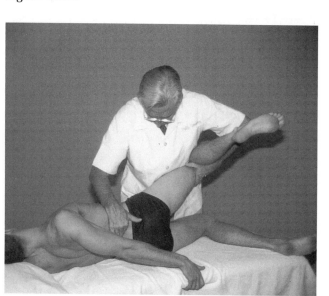

Figure 16.37.

Lumbar Spine

Lateral Recumbent Position
Neutral (Group) Dysfunction (Example: L1-4 convex left)

Position: Neutral, sidebent right, rotated left (NS_RR_L) or (EN_L).
Motion restriction: Left sidebending, right rotation.

1. Patient in right lateral recumbent position with shoulders and pelvis perpendicular to the table and with knees and feet together. Operator stands in front.

2. Operator flexes and extends the lower extremities to ensure the point of maximum ease of the forward-bending and backward-bending movement of the L1-4 lumbar neutral curve. Operator monitors with the left hand (Fig. 16.39).

3. Operator lifts both feet toward the ceiling, introducing a left sidebending, right rotational movement to the lumbar spine (Fig. 16.40).

4. Operator's right hand resists patient's effort of pulling the feet back to the table for 3–5 seconds and three to five repetitions (a right sidebending effort).

5. Operator's left hand monitors the muscle contraction and postcontraction stretch of the right paravertebral muscles (the concavity).

6. Retest.

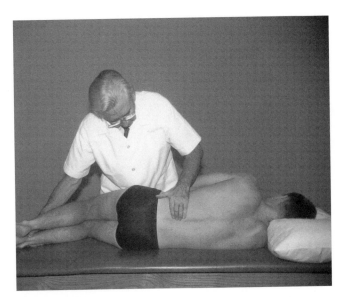

Figure 16.39.

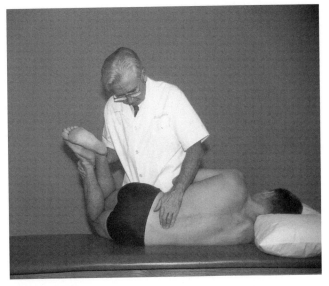

Figure 16.40.

Lumbar Spine

Mobilization with Impulse Technique
Lateral Recumbent Position
Neutral (Group) Dysfunction (Example: L1-4 convex left)

Position: Neutral, sidebent right, rotated left (NS_RR_L) or (EN_L).
Motion restriction: Sidebending left, rotation right.

1. Patient in the left lateral recumbent position (most posterior transverse processes toward the table) with operator standing in front.
2. Patient's lower extremities are flexed and extended to the point of maximum ease of the forward-bending and backward-bending range of the lumbar lordosis.
3. Operator monitors dysfunctional lumbar segments with the left hand and grasps the patient's left elbow (Fig. 16.41).
4. Operator pulls patient's left elbow forward and caudad (Fig. 16.42), introducing left sidebending and right rotation from above (Fig. 16.43).
5. Operator's right forearm in contact with the patient's right axilla and pectoral region maintains right rotation from above while operator's left forearm pulls patient's pelvis into left rotation (Fig. 16.44). The transverse processes of the apex of

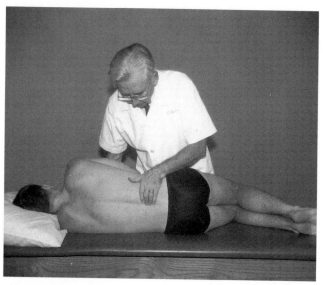

Figure 16.41.

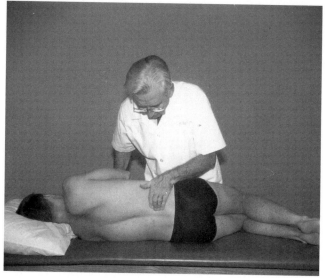

Figure 16.43.

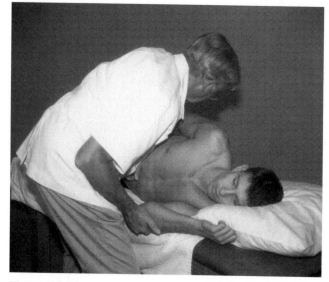

Figure 16.42.

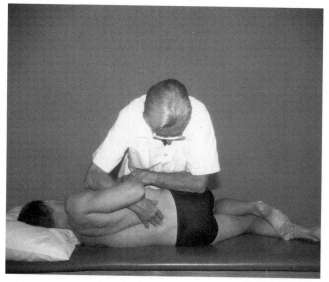

Figure 16.44.

the dysfunctional group are perpendicular to the table.

6. A mobilization with impulse thrust is made through the left forearm by the operator's body drop, rotating the pelvis anteriorly into left rotation.

7. An alternate arm position finds the operator's right forearm stabilizing the patient's right shoulder and pectoral region and both hands monitoring at the dysfunctional lumbar segments. Again, an anterior rotary thrust is applied through the left forearm by an operator body drop (Fig. 16.45).

8. An alternate arm position has operator's right hand stabilizing the anterior aspect of the pectoral region and the left forearm incorporated as part of the operator's body provides the anterior rotational thrust. Note operator's left hand monitoring dysfunctional segments (Fig. 16.46).

9. Retest.

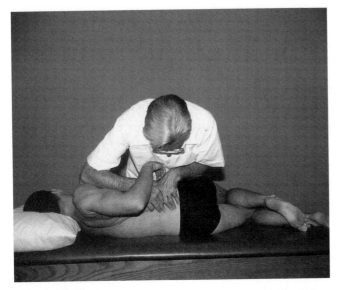

Figure 16.45.

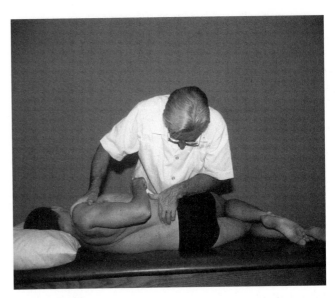

Figure 16.46.

Lumbar Spine

Mobilization with Impulse Technique
Lateral Recumbent Position
Nonneutral Dysfunction (Example: L4 ERS$_L$)
> Position: Backward bent (extended), rotated left, sidebent left (ERS$_L$)
> Motion restriction: Forward-bending (flexion), right rotation, right sidebending

1. Patient in the left lateral recumbent position (most posterior transverse process toward the table) with knees and feet together and shoulders and pelvis perpendicular to the table (initiating beginning right sidebending). Operator stands in front monitoring L4-5 level with the left hand (Fig. 16.47).

2. While maintaining the patient's shoulders perpendicular to the table, operator introduces forward-bending down to L4 from above by curling the patient's trunk forward (Fig. 16.48).

3. Operator now monitors the L4-5 segment with the right hand and flexes the lower extremities up to L5 (Fig. 16.49).

4. Operator's left hand places the patient's right foot in the left popliteal space. Operator's right forearm introduces right rotation down to L4 (Fig. 16.50).

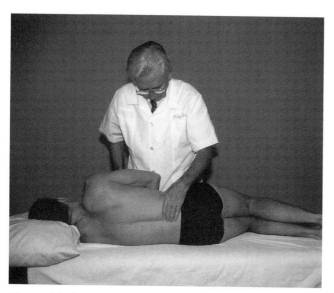

Figure 16.47.

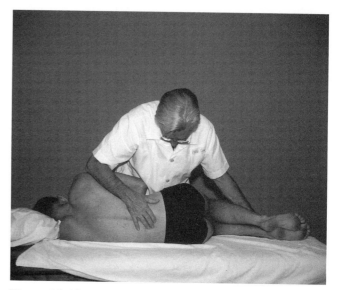

Figure 16.49.

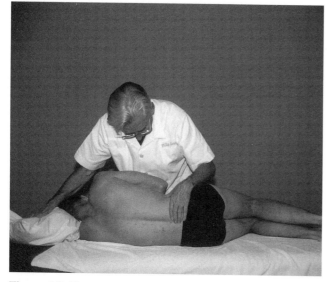

Figure 16.48.

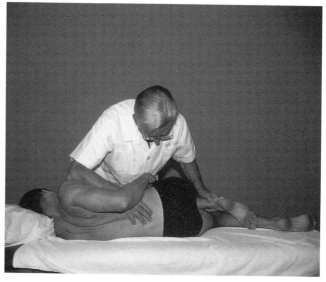

Figure 16.50.

5. Operator's left forearm in contact with the patient's right buttock rotates the pelvis anteriorly and superiorly (Fig. 16.51).

6. Operator fine-tunes forward-bending, right rotation, and right sidebending to the elastic barrier and provides an anterior and cephalward thrust through the left forearm by a body drop. The localization attempts to maintain the transverse processes of L4 perpendicular to the table.

7. Retest.

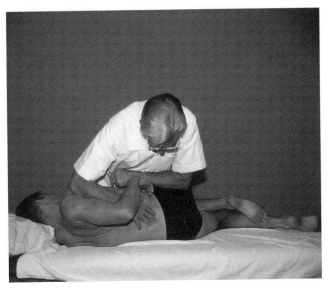

Figure 16.51.

Lumbar Spine

Mobilization with Impulse Technique
Lateral Recumbent Position
Nonneutral Dysfunction (Example: L4 FRS$_L$)
Position: Forward bent (flexed), rotated left, sidebent left (FRS$_L$)
Motion restriction: Backward-bending (extension), right rotation, right sidebending

1. Patient lies in the left lateral recumbent position (most posterior transverse process toward the table) with the knees and feet together, shoulders and pelvis perpendicular to the table.

2. Operator stands in front and grasps the L4-5 segment level between the two hands (Fig. 16.52).

3. Operator's hands localizes to the first backward-bending barrier by translating the patient's trunk from posterior to anterior (Fig. 16.53).

4. Operator fine-tunes extension barrier from above by translating patient posteriorly through the operator's right forearm (Fig. 16.54) while monitoring with the left hand over the L4-5 segment (Fig. 16.55).

5. Operator fine-tunes extension barrier from below by extending the lower extremities with the left arm for

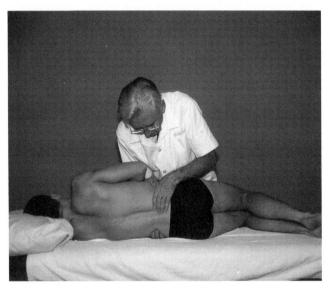

Figure 16.52.

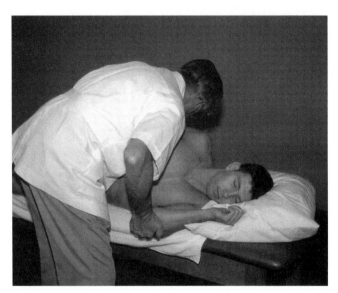

Figure 16.54.

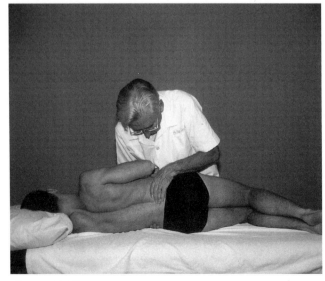

Figure 16.53.

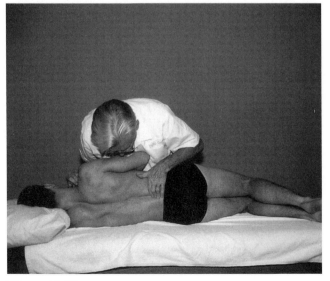

Figure 16.55.

movement up to L5 being monitored by the right hand (Fig. 16.56).

6. Operator's left hand places patient's right foot in the left popliteal space while the right forearm in contact with the patient's right pectoral region introduces right rotation from above monitoring with the right fingers over the L4-5 level (Fig. 16.57).

7. Operator's left forearm contacts patient's right buttock and introduces anterior and cephalad rotation

of the pelvis engaging the barrier at the L4-5 level (Fig. 16.58).

8. Operator introduces mobilizing thrust through the left forearm by a body drop in an anterior and cephalward direction.

9. Retest.

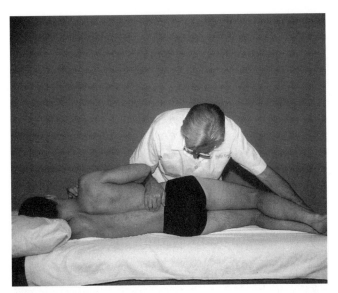

Figure 16.56.

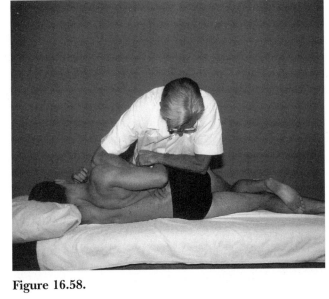

Figure 16.58.

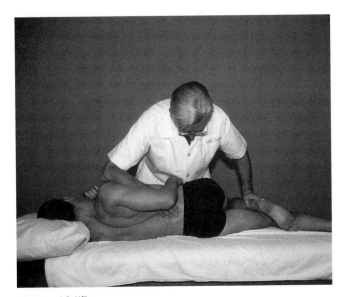

Figure 16.57.

Lumbar Spine

Mobilization with Impulse Technique
Sitting
Sagittal Plane Restriction (Example: L1 bilaterally
flexed)

Position: Bilaterally forward bent (flexed)
Motion restriction: Bilateral backward-bending
(extension)

1. Patient sitting on table with arms crossed holding
the opposite shoulder. Operator stands behind
grasping patient's elbows for trunk control (Fig.
16.59).

2. Heel of operator's right hand is placed in the midline over the spinous process of L2 with localization
to the inferior segment (Fig. 16.60).

3. Operator applies a backward-bending (extension)
thrust by lifting the patient's trunk through the elbows over the fulcrum applied by the right hand on
L2 (Fig. 16.61).

4. An alternate thrust is a body drop of the operator's
body through a lever arm of the right forearm in an
anterior direction against the right hand contact on
L2 (Fig. 16.62).

5. When using either of the thrust options, the operator tries to thrust with one hand only while the other
maintains stabilization. However, both options require two-handed coordination.

6. Retest.

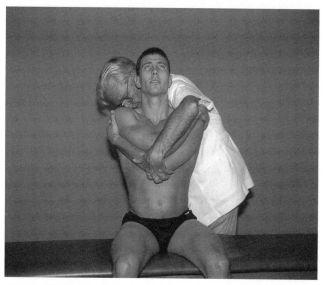

Figure 16.59.

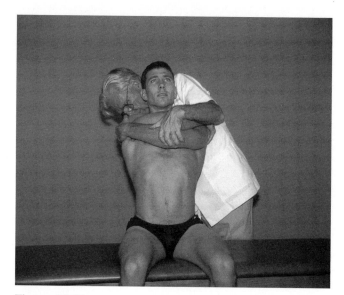

Figure 16.61.

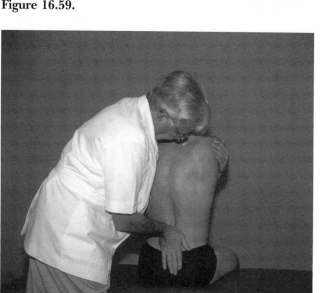

Figure 16.60.

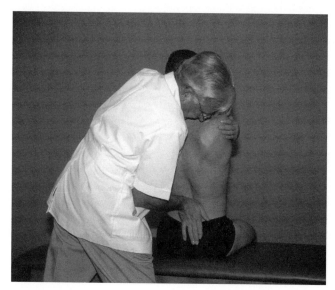

Figure 16.62.

Lumbar Spine

Mobilization with Impulse Technique
Sitting
Nonneutral Dysfunction (Example: L3 ERS$_L$)
    Position: Backward bent (extended), rotated left, sidebent left (ERS$_L$)
    Motion restriction: Forward-bending (flexion), right rotation, right sidebending

1. Patient sitting astride the table with arms crossed holding each shoulder.

2. Operator stands at right side of patient with right hand grasping patient's left shoulder and right axilla over patient's right shoulder. Reinforced thumb is in contact with the right side of the spinous process of L3 (Fig. 16.63).

3. Operator engages the forward-bending, right side-bending, and right rotational barrier through movement of the patient's trunk by the right arm and with right to left pressure of the right thumb on the spinous process of L3 (Fig. 16.64).

4. The mobilizing thrust is applied by exaggerating the patient's body position by dropping the operator's weight toward the floor while simultaneously thrusting from right to left with the left thumb on the spinous process of L3.

5. An alternative localizing hand position is the use of the left pisiform through the operator's hypothenar eminence on the right side of the spinous process of L3 (Fig. 16.65). Note the blocking of the operator's left forearm against the left hip.

6. Retest.

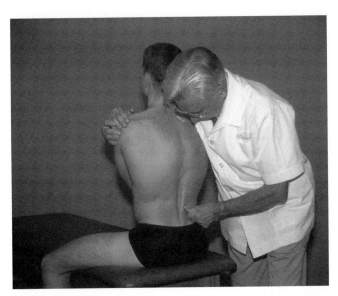

Figure 16.63.

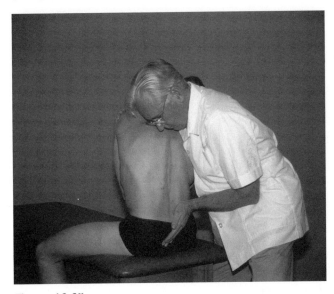

Figure 16.65.

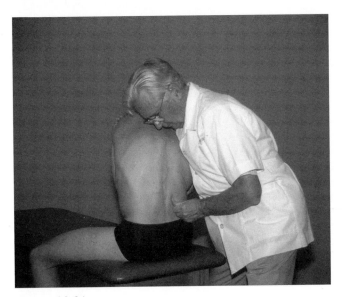

Figure 16.64.

Lumbar Spine

Mobilization with Impulse Technique
Sitting
Nonneutral Dysfunction (Example: L3 FRS$_L$)
    Position: Forward bent (flexed), rotated left, sidebent left
    Motion restriction: Backward-bending (extension), right rotation, right sidebending

1. Patient sitting astride the table with the right hand holding the left shoulder.

2. Operator stands at the right side with the right hand holding patient's left shoulder and the right axilla on top of the patient's right shoulder. Operator's reinforced left thumb is on the right side of the spinous process of L3 (Fig. 16.66).

3. Operator introduces backward-bending, right side-bending, and right rotation through the right arm contact with the patient's trunk while pressing from right to left on the spinous process of L3 (Fig. 16.67).

4. The mobilizing thrust is introduced by inferior body drop of the operator on the patient's right shoulder and a right to left force through the left thumb.

5. An alternative hand contact is the operator's pisiform through the left hypothenar eminence on the right side of the spinous process of L3 (Fig. 16.68). Note operator's left elbow is in contact with the left hip providing a lever arm to the contact on L3.

6. Retest.

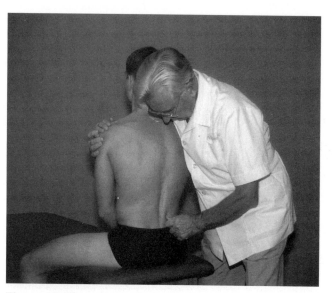

Figure 16.66.

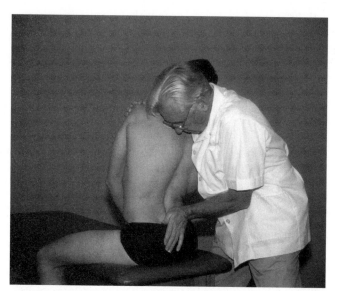

Figure 16.68.

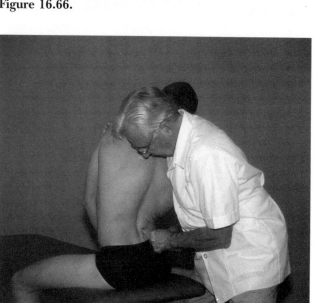

Figure 16.67.

Lumbar Spine

Mobilization with Impulse Technique
Sitting
Neutral (Group) Dysfunction (Example: L1-4 convex left)

Position: Neutral, sidebent right, rotated left (NS_RR_L) or (EN_L).

Motion restriction: Sidebending left, rotation right.

1. Patient sitting astride the table with the left hand on the right shoulder.

2. Operator stands at the left side of the patient with the left hand holding the right shoulder and the left axilla on top of the patient's left shoulder with the reinforced thumb in the intertransverse space between L2 and L3 (Fig. 16.69).

3. Operator engages the left sidebending and right rotation barrier through the control of the patient's trunk with the left arm while maintaining an anteromedial localizing fulcrum with the right thumb (Fig. 16.70).

4. The mobilizing thrust is a body drop of the operator toward the floor, enhancing the left sidebending and right rotation with localization at the apex of the curve.

5. An alternate hand position is the use of the right pisiform and right hypothenar eminence at the apex of the lumbar curve (Fig. 16.71).

6. Retest.

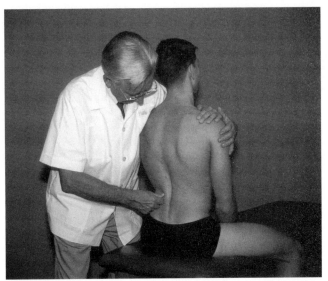

Figure 16.69.

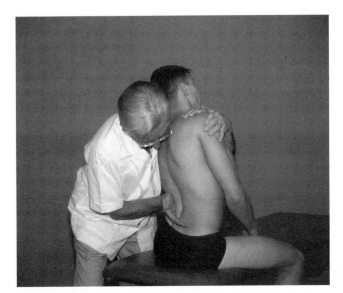

Figure 16.71.

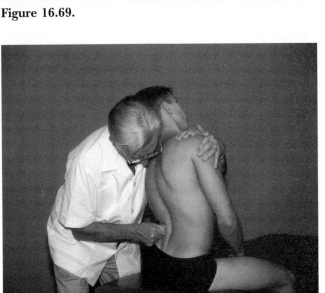

Figure 16.70.

Lumbar Spine

Mobilization without Impulse (Articulatory) Technique
Activating Force Variations

1. All previous mobilization with impulse techniques can be modified using a mobilization without impulse activating force.

2. Patient and operator positions remain the same.

3. Follow the principles found in Chapter 7.

4. Use repetitive oscillatory operator efforts in the direction of the restrictive barrier gradually increasing the range of movement.

5. This technique is frequently applied before the use of final mobilizing with impulse thrust.

6. Retest.

Lumbar Spine

Muscle Energy Activating Force

1. Any of the mobilizing with impulse techniques can be modified to use a muscle intrinsic activating force.

2. Patient's activating force is in the direction opposite to the operator localized position.

3. Three to five repetitions of a 3- to 5-second muscle contraction are used with the operator reengaging the new barrier after each patient effort.

4. Frequently two or three muscle energy efforts are used before the mobilization with impulse thrust activating force.

5. Retest.

17

PELVIC GIRDLE DYSFUNCTION

The sacroiliac joints remain controversial in the production of musculoskeletal pain syndromes. Motion at the sacroiliac joints has been reported in the medical literature since the mid-19th century. However, for many years authorities viewed that no movement occurred at the sacroiliac joints and therefore were not clinically significant. Recent contributions from both the basic and clinical sciences caused a change in perception of the role of the sacroiliac joint in clinical pain syndromes. Movement within the sacroiliac joint is now generally recognized, although it is only a small amount. Controversy continues as to the type of motion available and the axes of motion. Sacroiliac arthrography has demonstrated that some sacroiliac joints are painful on injection and pain relief occurs after installation of local anesthetic. Normal sacroiliac joints do not appear to respond with pain on injection. Controversy continues as to the ability of a clinician to identify a significant sacroiliac dysfunction. More basic and clinical research is clearly needed.

It is beyond the scope of this volume to review all of the work on sacroiliac motion. The diagnostic and therapeutic system for pelvic girdle dysfunction to be described would allow the clinician to diagnosis and treat all of the physical findings available in pelvic girdle dysfunctions. The system builds on the current knowledge of pelvic girdle movement and adds a theoretical construct and terminology to describe the various physical findings encountered during examination of the pelvic girdle.

MODELS OF PELVIC GIRDLE DYSFUNCTION

Structural diagnosis and management of the pelvic girdle are important to the postural structural model. The pelvis links the highly mobile extremities with the trunk in the highly complex mechanism of ambulation. Manual medicine management of the pelvic girdle restores functional symmetry to the three bones and joints of the pelvic girdle during the walking cycle. The superior surface of the body of the sacrum supports the vertebral column. Alteration in the sacrum has a significant effect on the vertebral function above.

The pelvic girdle is important in the respiratory circulatory model because of relationship to the pelvic diaphragm. Dysfunction of the osseous pelvis alters the functional capacity of the muscles of the pelvic diaphragm in a similar fashion to thoracic spine and rib dysfunction on the thoracoabdominal diaphragm.

The sacral component of the pelvis is of importance within the craniosacral system. The sacrum has inherent mobility between the two innominates as part of craniosacral rhythm. Alterated mechanical function of the pelvic girdle can negatively influence the craniosacral mechanism, and, vice versa, alterated craniosacral mechanics can influence the biomechanical function of the osseous pelvis. The osseous pelvis has a significant contribution to the functional capacity of the musculoskeletal system and warrants appropriate investigation and management in all patients.

FUNCTIONAL ANATOMY

The pelvic girdle consists of three bones and three joints (Fig. 17.1). The sacrum is formed by the fused elements of the sacral vertebrae and articulates superiorly with the last lumbar vertebra and caudally with the coccyx. The sacrum should be viewed as a component part of the vertebral axis. In many instances, the sacrum functions as an atypical lumbar vertebra between the two innominate bones, with the sacroiliac joints as atypical zygapophysial joints. The right and left innominate bones consist of the fused elements of the ilium, ischium, and pubis. The two innominates are joined anteriorly by the symphysis pubis joint. Each innominate bone articulates cephalically with the sacrum at the ipsilateral sacroiliac joint and caudally with the femur at the hip joint. Functionally, the innominate bone should be viewed as a lower extremity bone and the two sacroiliac joints as the junction of the vertebral axis and the lower extremity.

The joints of the pelvic girdle consist of the symphysis pubis and the two sacroiliac joints. The symphysis pubis is an amphiarthrosis with strong superior and inferior ligaments and a thinner posterior liga-

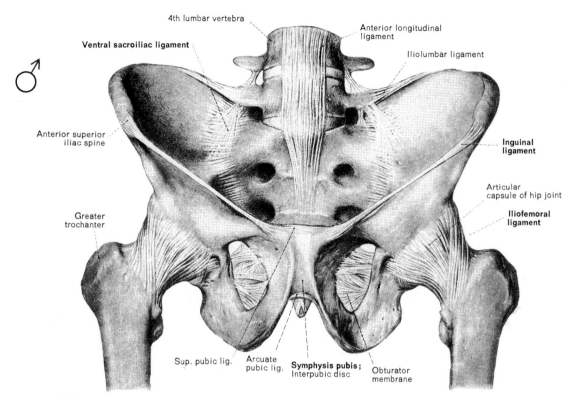

Figure 17.1.
Pelvic girdle.

ment. The opposing surfaces can range from symmetrically flat to quite asymmetrical and interlocking. The minimal amount of motion available at this joint is strongly influenced by the shape of the joint, the ligamentous integrity of the joint (particularly under the influence of hormonal changes), and the action of the abdominal muscles from above and the adductor muscles of the lower extremity below.

The sacroiliac joints are true arthrodial joints with a joint space, articular capsule, and articular cartilage. They are unique in that the cartilage on the sacral side is hyaline cartilage and on the ilial side is fibrocartilage. The articular cartilage on the sacral side is much thicker than that on the ilial side. They are L-shaped in contour, with a shorter upper arm and a longer lower arm. The joint contour usually has a depression on the sacral side at approximately S2 and a corresponding prominence on the ilial side. The shape of the sacroiliac joint varies markedly from individual to individual and from side to side in the same individual. During the aging process, there is an increase in the grooves on the opposing surfaces of the sacrum and ilium that appears to reduce available motion. It is of interest to note that the age with highest incidence of disabling back pain (25–45 years) is the same age where the greatest amount of motion is available in the sacroiliac joints. Asymmet-

ric dysfunction of this movement may well contribute to disabling back pain. The sacroiliac joint usually has change in anteroposterior bevelling at approximately the junction of the upper and lower arm. The plane of the upper portion is convergent from behind forward, whereas the lower portion is divergent from behind forward, resulting in an interlocking mechanism centering at approximately S2. Occasionally, the opposing joint surfaces are quite flat and do not have the interlocking joint bevel change at S2 or the ilial prominence within the sacral depression. This type of sacroiliac joint is much less stable, and the possibility of superior and inferior translatory movement, or shearing, exists. Occasionally, the sacral concavity is replaced by a convexity with the ilial side being more concave. This joint structure provides for increased mobility, primarily in rotation medially and laterally, around a vertical axis.

Much of the integrity of the sacroiliac joint depends on ligamentous structures. The iliolumbar ligaments attach to the transverse processes of L4 and L5 and to the anterior surface of the iliac crest. The lower fibers extend inferiorly and blend with the anterior sacroiliac ligaments. The anterior sacroiliac ligaments are two relatively flat and thin bands. They can be viewed as providing a sling from the two innominate bones for the anterior surface of the sacrum (Fig. 17.2). The posterior sacroiliac ligaments have three layers. The deepest layer consists of short interosseous ligaments running from the sacrum to the ilium. The intermediate layer runs from the posterior arches of the sacrum to the medial side of the ilium, occupying most of the space overlying the posterior aspect of the sacroiliac joint. The long posterior sacroiliac ligaments blend together and course vertically from the sacral crest to the ilium. Inferiorly, these posterior sacroiliac ligaments blend with the accessory sacroiliac ligaments, the sacrotuberous and the sacrospinous. The sacrotuberous ligament runs from the inferior lateral angle of the sacrum to the ischial tuberosity and has a crescent-shaped medial border. The sacrospinous ligament lies under the sacrotuberous and runs from the inferior lateral angle of the sacrum to the ischial spine. These two accessory ligaments contribute to the formation of the greater and lesser sciatic notches, which are divided by the sacrospinous ligament.

Muscular attachment to the pelvic girdle is extensive, but muscles that directly influence sacroiliac motion are difficult to identify. Movement of the sacroiliac mechanism appears to be mainly passive in response to muscle action in the surrounding areas.

The abdominal muscles, including the two obliques, the intermedius, and the rectus abdominus, insert on the superior aspect of the pelvic girdle and are joined posteriorly by the quadratus lumborum, the lumbodorsal fascia, and the erector spinae mass. Six groups of hip and thigh muscles attach to the pelvic girdle and lower extremities. These hip muscles strongly influence the movement of the two innominates within the pelvic girdle. Anterior to the sacroiliac joints are two highly significant muscles, the psoas and piriformis. The psoas crosses over the anterior aspect of the sacroiliac joints in its travel from the lumbar region to insert into the lesser trochanter of the femur. The right and left piriformis muscles originate from the anterior surface of the sacrum, travel through the sciatic notch, and insert into the greater trochanter of the femur.

Muscle imbalance in any of these groups affects pelvic girdle function. Imbalance in piriformis length and strength strongly influences movement of the sacrum between the innominates. Imbalance of the pelvic diaphragm is significant in patients with rectal, gynecological, and urological problems. The reader is encouraged to review the anatomy of all these muscles in a standard anatomical text.

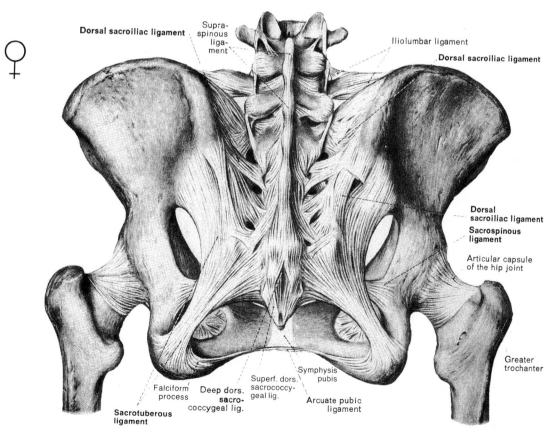

Figure 17.2.
Sacroiliac joint.

MOTION IN THE PELVIC GIRDLE

The pelvic girdle functions as an integrated unit with all three bones moving at all three joints, influenced by the lower extremities below and the vertebral column and trunk above. This integration results in torsional movement, both left and right, around a vertical (*y*) axis. In torsional movement to the left, the symphysis turns left of the midline, the right innominate is carried forward, the left innominate is carried backward, and the sacrum faces somewhat to the left (counterclockwise pelvic rotation). Torsion to the right (clockwise rotation) is just the reverse. A simple screening test for this global torsional movement involves the patient in the supine position with the operator placing the palm of the hands over each anterior superior iliac spine. Alternate rocking of the osseous pelvis by pushing posteriorly on each anterior superior iliac spine results in a sensation of symmetry or asymmetry. If movement seems to be more restricted when pushing posteriorly on the right anterior superior iliac spine than with the left, one can presume that the pelvic girdle is torsioned to the left and that there is some restrictor in the mechanism that needs to have further evaluation.

The amount of movement present at the symphysis pubis and at both sacroiliac joints is certainly not great, and more biomechanical research is needed to identify the specific motions available and to determine their axes. The descriptions that follow are based on current biomechanical information and clinical observations. Many of the clinical observations cannot be adequately explained by current biomechanical information. A theoretical construct is offered to explain some of the clinical observations and to establish a vocabulary to describe both available normal motions and dysfunctions.

MOVEMENT AT SYMPHYSIS PUBIS

Movement at the symphysis pubis is quite small. It occurs in one-legged standing and during the walking cycle. The normal integrity of the joint is maintained by strong ligaments, primarily superiorly and inferiorly. The ligaments become more lax as a result of hormonal change in females, particularly during pregnancy and delivery, and separation occurs to widen the internal pelvic diameter during delivery. There is a normal superior shearing movement if one-legged standing is maintained for several minutes. After standing on the opposite leg, or with prolonged standing on both legs, the shearing movement returns to normal. During normal walking, the symphysis pubis serves as the anterior axis for innominate rotation. Symphysis pubis dysfunction alters anterior and posterior innominate rotation during walking.

SACROILIAC MOTION

Sacroiliac motion is movement of the sacrum between the two innominate bones and requires the participation of both sacroiliac joints. Nutation and counternutation (anterior nutation-posterior nutation) is the sacral motion about which the most is known from biomechanical and radiographical research. Nutation is a nodding movement of the sacrum between the innominates with the sacral base moving anteriorly and inferiorly and the sacral apex moving posteriorly and superiorly. Counternutation occurs when the sacral base moves posteriorly and superiorly and the sacral apex moves anteriorly and inferiorly. This is the sacroiliac movement that occurs in two-legged stance with trunk forward-bending and backward-bending. Many other structures participate in trunk forward-bending and backward-bending, but the sacroiliac motion is described as nutation and counternutation. For the purposes of structural diagnosis, nutation is described as anterior or forward and counternutation is described as backward or posterior. The axis around which this anterior-posterior nutation occurs has been described differently by various investigators but appears to be related to the upper and lower limbs of the sacroiliac joint and their junction somewhere around S2. A superior to inferior translatory movement accompanies the anterior and posterior nutation. During anterior nutation (nutation), there is an inferior translatory movement of the sacrum. During posterior nutation (counternutation), there is a superior translatory movement. Bilateral symmetry of anterior-posterior nutation depends on the symmetry of the two sacroiliac joints. With asymmetry of a patient's two sacroiliac joints being so common, asymmetry of this anterior-posterior nutation is also quite common. Anterior nutation is called sacral flexion in the biomechanical model and sacral extension in the craniosacral model. Posterior nutation is called sacral extension in the biomechanical model and sacral flexion in the craniosacral model.

Movement of the sacrum between the two innominates during walking is more complex and less well understood. If one palpates the right side of the sacral base with the right thumb, the right inferior lateral angle with the right index finger, and the left sacral base and left inferior lateral angle with the left thumb and index finger and follows movement of the sacrum during walking, the sacrum appears to have an oscillatory movement, first left and then right. The right base appears to move anteriorly, whereas the left inferior lateral angle moves posteriorly, and then the reverse occurs, with the left sacral base moving anteriorly and the right inferior lateral angle moving posteriorly. This sacral motion has been described as torsion to describe the coupling of sidebending and rotation to opposite sides.

In one cadaveric study, the coupling of sacral sidebending and rotation appeared to depend on whether sidebending or rotation was introduced first. Clinical observation of the walking cycle demonstrates that sacral sidebending and rotation couple to opposite sides. In left torsional movement, the anterior surface of the sacrum rotates to face left (left rotation), whereas the superior surface of S1 (sacral base plane) declines to the right (right sidebending). Right torsion is the exact opposite. For descriptive purposes, this complex, polyaxial, torsional movement is considered to occur around an oblique axis. By convention, the left oblique axis runs from the upper extremity of the left sacroiliac joint to the lower end of the right sacroiliac joint, and the right oblique axis runs from the upper end of the right sacroiliac joint to the lower extremity of the left sacroiliac joint. Although the exact biomechanics of the torsional movements of the sacrum are unknown, the hypothetical left and right oblique axes are useful for descriptive purposes.

In the normal walking cycle, the sacrum appears to move with left torsion on the left oblique axis, return to neutral, rotate in right torsion on the right oblique axis, and then return to neutral. With left torsion on the left oblique axis, the sacrum rotates left and sidebends right, with the right sacral base moving into anterior nutation. In right torsional movement on the right oblique axis, the sacrum rotates right and sidebends left, with the left sacral base moving into anterior nutational movement. Because the nutational component of this normal walking movement is anterior in direction, left torsion on the left oblique axis (L on L) and right torsion on the right oblique axis (R on R) are described as anterior torsional movements. The nutational movement in normal walking is anterior on one side, return to neutral, and anterior to the opposite side, and return to neutral. Posterior nutational movement does not appear past neutral in the normal walking cycle.

Because much of the activity of the musculoskeletal system involves the walking cycle, maintenance of normal L-on-L and R-on-R sacral movement is an important therapeutic objective. Because walking occurs with the vertebral column in the neutral (neither flexed nor extended) position, the anterior torsional sacral movements are called neutral mechanics. During walking, the thoracolumbar spine sidebends left and rotates right and then sidebends right and rotates left with each step. This neutral movement of the vertebral column requires normal segmental mobility and starts with the response of L5 at the lumbosacral junction. As the sacrum sidebends

right and rotates left, L5 sidebends left and rotates right. Each vertebra above L5 should appropriately respond as part of the adaptive neutral curve. A vertebra, particularly in the lower lumbar spine, with nonneutral dysfunction results in a "nonadaptive" vertebral response to the sacrum. Treatment of lumbar spine dysfunction should always precede treatment of sacroiliac dysfunction because many sacroiliac treatments require the use of the lumbar spine as a lever.

A third sacral movement occurs when the trunk is forward bent and sidebent or rotated to one side. This maneuver results in the nonneutral behavior of the lumbar spine with sidebending and rotation being coupled to the same side. The sacrum between the innominates participates in this maneuver by backward or posterior torsional movement. Posterior torsional movement occurs on either the left or right oblique axes, and the coupling of sidebending and rotation occurs to opposite sides. In posterior torsional movement, one side of the sacral base moves beyond neutral into posterior nutation. In posterior or backward torsion to the right on the left oblique axis, the sacrum rotates right, sidebends left, and the right base moves into posterior nutation. In backward or posterior torsion to the left on the right oblique axis, the sacrum rotates left, sidebends right, and the left base goes into posterior nutation. These posterior torsional movements can be described as nonneutral sacroiliac mechanics and are not part of the normal walking cycle.

The sacroiliac joint is at risk for injury like the lumbar spine when the trunk is forward bent and sidebending and rotation are introduced. In this posture the lumbar spine is at risk for annular tear of the disc, strain of deep lumbar muscles, and sprain of the zygapophysial joints. The posterior torsional movement of the sacrum appears to sprain the posterior sacroiliac ligaments. Nonneutral dysfunction of the lower lumbar spine and backward torsional dysfunction of the sacroiliac joint occurs in the well-known syndrome of "the well man bent over and the cripple stood up."

ILIOSACRAL MOVEMENT

The sacroiliac mechanism can be viewed from the perspective of each innominate articulating with the sacrum. The motion can be described as one innominate moving on one side of the sacrum (iliosacral movement). Each innominate in the walking cycle rotates anteriorly and posteriorly around the anterior axis at the symphysis pubis and anteriorly and posteriorly with each side of the sacrum in a posterior axis. In anterior innominate rotation, the innominate rotates forward in relation to the sacrum with the anterior superior iliac spine being carried anterior and inferior, the posterior superior iliac spine being carried anterior and superior, and the ischial tuberosity being carried posterior and superior. In posterior innominate rotation, the anterior superior iliac spine is carried superior and posterior, the posterior superior iliac spine is carried posterior and inferior, and the ischial tuberosity is carried anterior and superior. Anterior and posterior innominate rotation occurs in the presence of normal sacroiliac joint contour. If the opposing surfaces of the sacrum and ilium at the sacroiliac joint are altered, atypical movements appear clinically. A superior-inferior translatory shearing movement occurs when the opposing joint surfaces are flatter and more parallel. If the sacral side is convex and the ilial concave, internal and external rotation around a vertical axis appears possible. These movements are termed in-flare and out-flare, describing the medial and lateral rotation observed clinically.

Somatic dysfunction can occur with any of these motions within the pelvic girdle. Each of these motions is quite small, but when lost, each has a significant clinical effect. In dysfunctions within the pelvic girdle, it is not uncommon to find restriction of several movements within the mechanism.

STRUCTURAL DIAGNOSIS OF PELVIC GIRDLE SOMATIC DYSFUNCTION

In the structural diagnosis of the pelvic girdle, the examiner looks for the diagnostic triad of asymmetry, range of motion alteration, and tissue texture abnormality. Evaluation is made of asymmetry of paired anatomical landmarks within the pelvic girdle and lower extremity, altered range of motion (by the standing and seated flexion tests, the stork test, and various springing movement tests of the sacroiliac joints), and tissue texture abnormality in the deep fascia and ligaments over the sacroiliac joints, within the sacrotuberous ligament and the gluteal and perineal muscles. Combinations of findings within the asymmetry, range of motion, tissue texture abnormality (ART) diagnostic triad leads to the diagnosis of pelvic girdle dysfunction. The diagnostic process identifies dysfunction at the symphysis pubis (dysfunction between the two pubic bones), the sacroiliac joints (sacrum between the two innominates), and the iliosacral joints (each innominate as it articulates with its respective side of the sacrum). The diagnostic sequence is standing, sitting with feet on floor or supported, supine, prone, and supine.

Pelvic Girdle

Diagnosis: Standing

1. Patient stands with weight equally distributed on both feet acetabular distance apart.

2. Operator stands or sits behind patient.

3. Operator palpates superior aspect of each iliac crest, evaluating relative height (Fig. 17.3).

4. Operator palpates superior aspect of greater trochanter of each femur, evaluating relative height (Fig. 17.4).

5. One crest and greater trochanter higher than the other is presumptive evidence of anatomical shortening of lower extremity.

6. Level crest height but unlevel trochanters or unlevel crests and equal trochanters are presumptive evidence of bony asymmetry of the pelvic girdle.

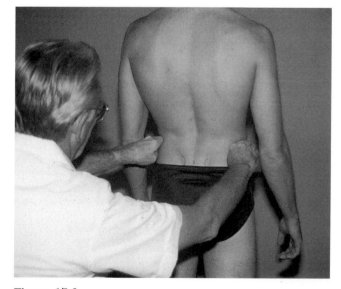

Figure 17.3.

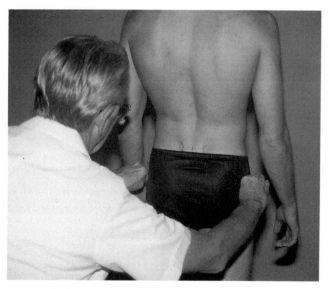

Figure 17.4.

Pelvic Girdle

Diagnosis: Standing Flexion Test

1. Patient stands with weight equally distributed on both feet acetabular distance apart.

2. Operator stands or sits behind patient.

3. Operator palpates inferior slope of each posterior superior iliac spine (Fig. 17.5).

4. Patient bends forward in a smooth fashion as far as possible without bending knees (Fig. 17.6).

5. Examiner follows the excursion of each posterior superior iliac spine. The test is positive on the side that the posterior superior iliac spine appears to move more cephalward and/or ventral.

6. The test is sensitive but not specific for restricted motion of the sacroiliac joint on the positive side. False positives are found with asymmetric tightness of the contralateral hamstring and of the ipsilateral quadratus lumborum.

7. Operator observes the response of the vertebral column for dysrhythmia and presence of altered lateral curvatures.

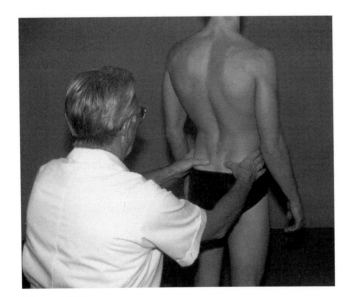

Figure 17.5.

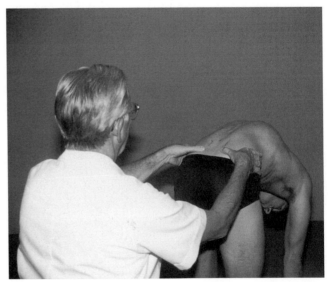

Figure 17.6.

Pelvic Girdle

Diagnosis: One-Legged Stork Test (Gillet)

1. Operator stands or sits behind the standing patient.

2. Operator's right thumb on posterior aspect of the right posterior superior iliac spine with left thumb over the sacral crest at the same level (Fig. 17.7).

3. Patient raises right knee toward the ceiling.

4. Normal response is the thumb on the posterior superior iliac spine moving caudad in relation to the thumb on the sacrum (Fig. 17.8).

5. A positive response finds the thumb on the posterior superior iliac spine moving cephalically (Fig. 17.9).

6. Comparison is made with the opposite side by reversing the procedure.

7. Lower pole movement is tested by placing the left thumb on the sacral hiatus and the right thumb at the same level on the posterior inferior aspect of the iliac bone (Fig. 17.10).

8. Patient lifts right knee toward ceiling.

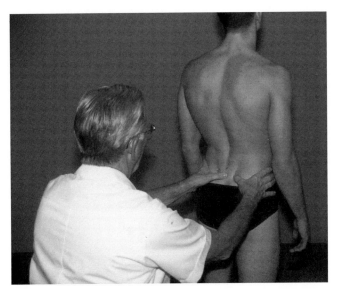

Figure 17.7.

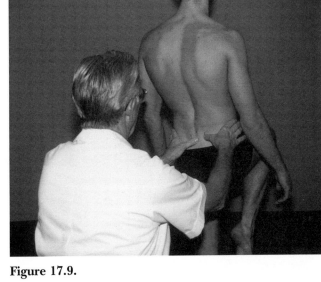

Figure 17.9.

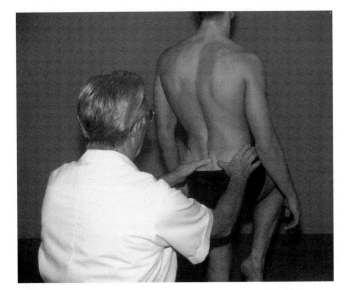

Figure 17.8.

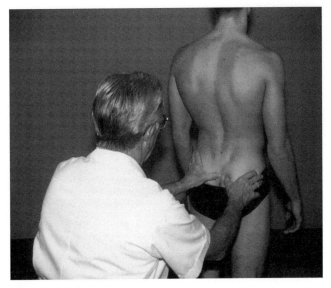

Figure 17.10.

9. The normal response is the right thumb moving laterally, caudally, and ventrally (Fig. 17.11).

10. Positive response means the right thumb moving cephalward in relation to the left thumb on the sacrum (Fig. 17.12).

11. If the patient is unable to do the one-legged standing required for this test, suspect sensory motor balance dysfunction and assess accordingly (see Chapter 20).

12. Standing flexion test is used to identify the side of dysfunction for symphysis pubis and iliosacral motion.

Note: The one-legged stork test is more specific for sacroiliac joint restriction than the standing flexion test. It is helpful in differentiating a bilateral positive standing flexion test from a negative standing flexion test.

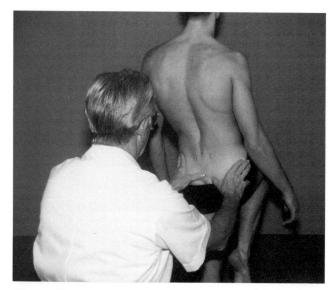

Figure 17.11.

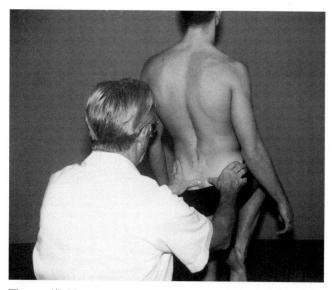

Figure 17.12.

Pelvic Girdle

Diagnosis: Standing
　　　Trunk Sidebending

1. Operator stands or sits behind patient standing with feet acetabular distance apart.

2. Operator palpates each posterior superior iliac spine with the thumbs (Fig. 17.13).

3. Patient sidebends trunk to the left (Fig. 17.14) while operator observes a behavior of the induced lumbar curve and the pelvic motion.

4. Patient sidebending of trunk to the right is performed (Fig. 17.15).

5. Operator observes symmetry of induced sidebending curve. A normal response is a smooth C curve with fullness of the side of the convexity. A positive finding is a straightening of the lumbar curve and/or fullness of the side of concavity.

6. Operator observes behavior of the pelvis during trunk sidebending. The normal response is pelvic rotation opposite to the induced lumbar rotation above. A positive response is any other pelvic motion.

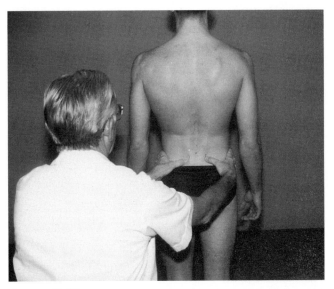

Figure 17.13.

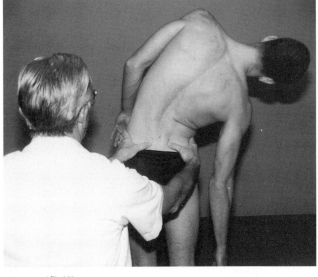

Figure 17.15.

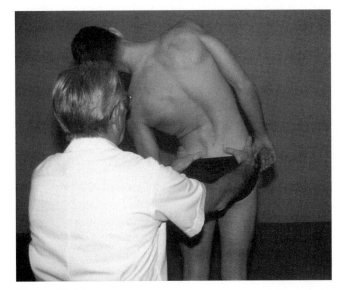

Figure 17.14.

Pelvic Girdle

Diagnosis: Sitting

Sitting Flexion Test

1. Patient sits on examining stool with feet on the floor or on the table with feet supported.

2. Operator sits or kneels behind the patient with the thumbs on the inferior aspect of the posterior superior iliac spines and the index fingers on the iliac crests (Fig. 17.16).

3. Unleveling of the crest in the seated position is strong evidence of osseous asymmetry in the bony pelvis.

4. Patient is asked to smoothly forward bend as far as possible with the arms between the knees (Fig. 17.17).

5. A positive finding finds the posterior superior iliac spine on one side moving more cephalward and/or more ventral. A false-positive response is found in the presence of ipsilateral quadratus lumborum tightness.

6. Operator observes the behavior of the lumbar and lower thoracic spine for dysrhythmia and abnormal lateral curves. Comparison is made with that observed while standing.

7. With the patient in the fully forward-bent position, operator palpates the posterior aspect of the inferior lateral angle of the sacrum to find whether they are symmetrically in the coronal plane or whether one is more posterior than the other (Fig. 17.18). This finding will be used in sacroiliac diagnosis.

Note: If altered vertebral mechanics is more severe during the standing flexion test than seated, major restriction in the lower extremities is suggested. If vertebral dysrhythmia is worse during the seated flexion test, major restriction above the pelvic girdle is suggested.

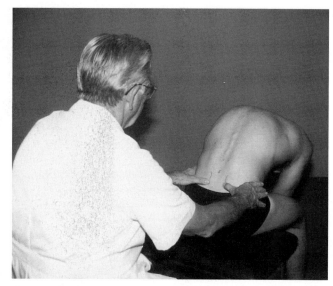

Figure 17.17.

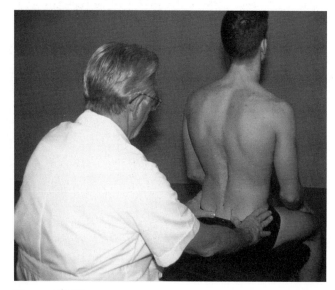

Figure 17.16.

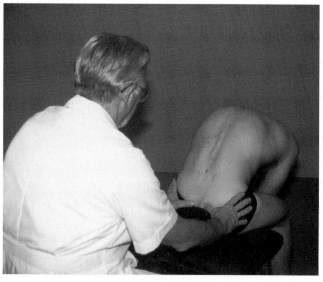

Figure 17.18.

Pelvic Girdle

Diagnosis: Supine
Pubic Symphysis Height

1. Patient supine on table.

2. Operator stands at side of table with dominant eye over the midline.

3. Operator places palm of hand on abdomen and moves caudally until the heel of the hand strikes the superior aspect of the symphysis pubis (Fig. 17.19).

4. Operator places the pads of the index fingers on the superior aspect of the symphysis pubis (Fig. 17.20).

5. Operator moves index finger pads laterally approximately 2 cm, palpating the superior aspect of the pubic tubercles (Fig. 17.21).

6. One pubic tubercle more superior or inferior than the other and tension and tenderness of the medial attachment of the inguinal ligament are positive findings.

Note: If a positive finding for dysfunction of the pubic symphysis is made, it should be appropriately treated before proceeding with the diagnostic process.

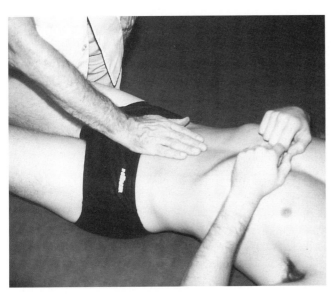

Figure 17.19.

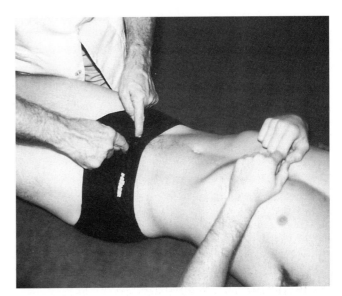

Figure 17.21.

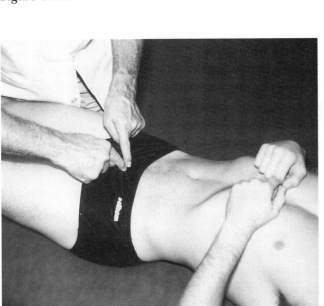

Figure 17.20.

Pelvic Girdle

Diagnosis: Supine and Prone
Iliac Crest Height

1. Patient supine on table with operator standing at side with dominant eye over the midline.

2. Operator palpates the superior aspect of each iliac crest in relation to the horizontal plane by symmetric placements of the index fingers (Fig. 17.22).

3. Patient prone on table with operator standing at side with dominant eye over the midline.

4. Operator palpates the superior aspect of each iliac crest in relation to the horizontal plane with the index fingers (Fig. 17.23).

5. If one crest is higher than the other, operator is highly suspicious of the presence of an innominate shear dysfunction. If subsequently verified, it should be treated before proceeding with the remaining examination of the pelvic girdle.

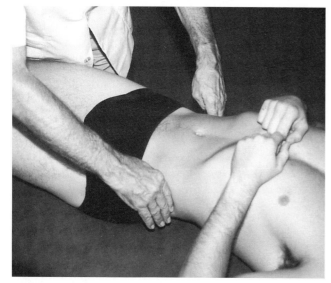

Figure 17.22.

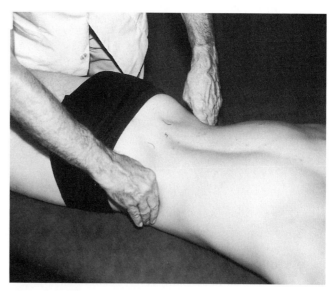

Figure 17.23.

Pelvic Girdle

Diagnosis: Prone
   Leg Length at Medial Malleolus

1. Patient prone on table with dorsum of the foot free and distal tibia and fibula at edge of table.

2. Operator stands at end of table and palpates the most inferior aspect of each medial malleolus, determining whether one is longer or shorter (Fig. 17.24).

3. A confirmatory test is to dorsiflex the feet and sight down perpendicularly on the pads of each heel to determine which is longer or shorter.

4. Inequality may be a function of asymmetric leg length.

5. In the presence of symmetrical leg length, inequality in the medial malleolus is usually a function of the adaption of the lumbar spine to sacral base unleveling in sacroiliac dysfunction.

Pelvic Girdle

Diagnosis: Prone
   Ischial Tuberosity Level

1. Patient prone on table with operator standing at side with dominant eye over the midline.

2. Operator places the side of the thumbs in gluteal fold and presses ventrally into the posterior aspect of the hamstring fascia (Fig. 17.25).

3. Operator's thumbs move superiorly until the pad strikes the inferior aspect of the ischial tuberosity (Fig. 17.26).

4. Evaluation is made of the level of the ischial tuberosities against the horizontal plane.

5. Unleveling of the ischial tuberosity by the width of the thumb (6 mm) is considered positive.

Note: Care must be exercised to palpate the most inferior aspect of the ischial tuberosity because the structure is quite round.

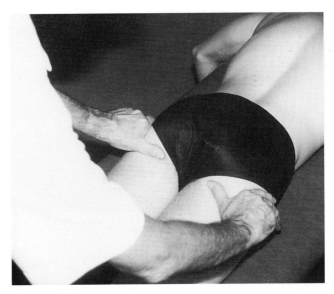

Figure 17.25.

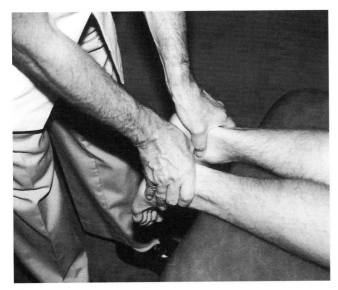

Figure 17.24.

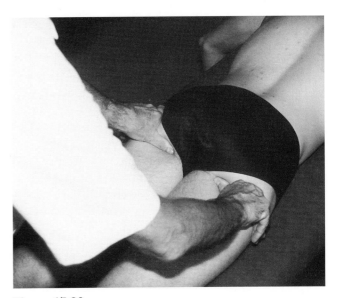

Figure 17.26.

Pelvic Girdle

Diagnosis: Prone
Sacrotuberous Ligament Tension

1. Patient prone with operator standing at side with dominant eye over the midline.

2. Operator's thumbs are placed on the inferior aspect of the ischial tuberosities (Fig. 17.26).

3. Operator's thumbs stay on bone and move medially, curl cephalward, and hook out posterolaterally on each side under each sacrotuberous ligament (Fig. 17.27).

4. Operator assesses the symmetry of tone of the sacrotuberous ligament. Laxity or increased tension with associated tenderness is interpreted as a positive finding.

5. Unleveling of the ischial tuberosity and asymmetric tension of the sacrotuberous ligaments are positive findings for innominate shear dysfunction.

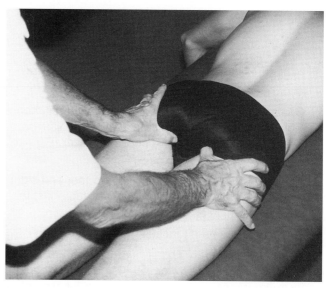

Figure 17.27.

Pelvic Girdle

Diagnosis: Prone
Inferior Lateral Angle

1. Patient prone on table with operator standing at side with dominant eye over the midline.

2. Operator palpates the sacral hiatus at the caudal end of the sacral crest (Fig. 17.28).

3. At 1.5–2.0 cm lateral to the sacral hiatus, the posterior aspect of the inferior lateral angle is identified (Fig. 17.29).

4. Operator places the pad of each thumb over the posterior aspect of the inferior lateral angle, evaluating the level against the coronal plane. A small depression of bone makes this landmark easily palpable (Fig. 17.30).

5. Without lifting thumbs off of bony contact, operator's thumbs are turned under the inferior aspect of the inferior lateral angle for evaluation of the level against the horizontal plane (Fig. 17.31).

6. In the presence of a symmetrically shaped sacrum, a posterior inferior lateral angle is always inferior and an inferior lateral angle is always posterior. The finding is occasionally more posterior than inferior or more inferior than posterior.

7. While palpating the inferior aspect of the inferior lateral angle, tension and tenderness of the superior attachment of the sacrotuberous ligament is assessed. Sacrotuberous ligament is palpably tense and usually tender in the presence of many sacroiliac dysfunctions.

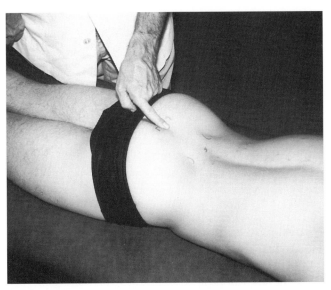

Figure 17.28.

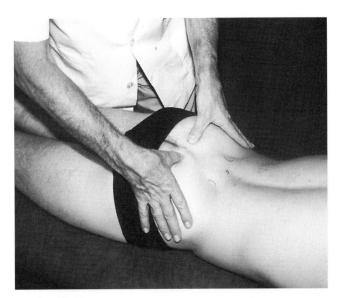

Figure 17.30.

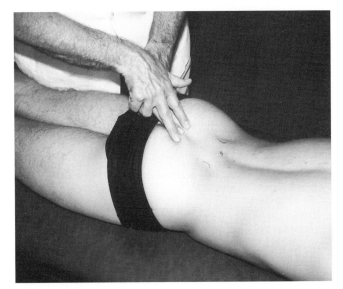

Figure 17.29.

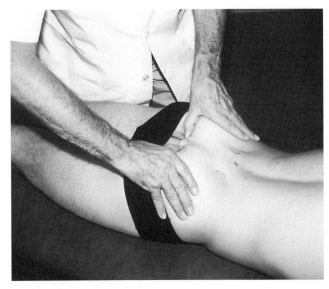

Figure 17.31.

Pelvic Girdle

Diagnosis: Prone
    Posterior Superior Iliac Spine, Sacral Base
    and L5

1. Patient prone on the table with operator standing at side with dominant eye over the midline.

2. Operator places thumb pads on the inferior slope of the posterior superior iliac spine to assess level against the horizontal plane (Fig. 17.32).

3. Operator places thumb pads on the most posterior aspect of the posterior superior iliac spine and curls thumbs medially and caudally approximately 30° until the tip of the thumb strikes the sacral base. Assessment is made for level against the coronal plane (Fig. 17.33).

4. Operator's thumbs begin at the same most posterior aspect of the posterior superior iliac spine and curl medially and cephalward approximately 30° to strike the posterior arch of L5 (Fig. 17.34). Assessment is made for level against the coronal plane.

5. The level of the sacral base is frequently referred to as "depth of the sacral sulcus." If one sacral base is more anterior than the other, the sacral sulcus is said to be "deep" on that side. The term "depth of the sacral sulcus" should be reserved to a finding of depth difference from the posterior superior iliac spine to a sacral base that is level in the coronal plane.

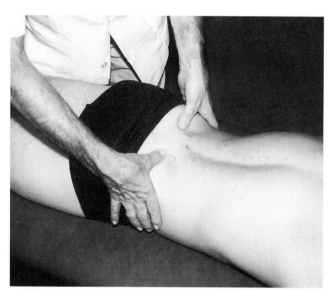

Figure 17.32.

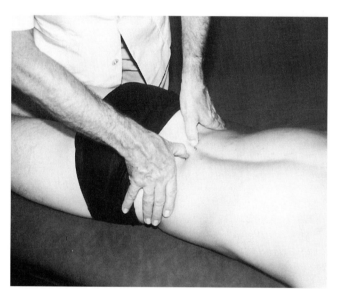

Figure 17.34.

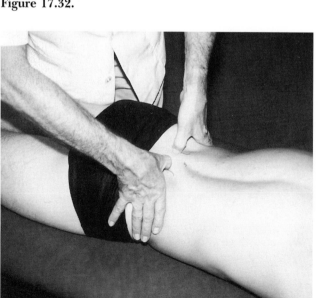

Figure 17.33.

Pelvic Girdle

Diagnosis: Prone
  Four-Point Sacral Motion

1. Patient prone on table with operator standing at side with dominant eye over the midline.

2. Operator's thumbs are on the posterior aspect of each inferior lateral angle and the index fingers are over each side of the sacral base (Fig. 17.35). Assessment is made of the level of the inferior lateral angle and the sacral base against the coronal plane.

3. Operator monitors the movement of the four-point contact on the sacrum while the patient deeply inhales and exhales several times. Normal function finds the sacral base to move dorsally and the sacral inferior lateral angle ventrally during deep inhalation; the reverse is found during exhalation.

4. Patient is asked to assume trunk extension through the prone prop position with the chin in the hands (Fig. 17.36). Assessment is made as to the level of the inferior lateral angles and sacral base against the coronal plane in comparison with the prone neutral position.

5. The level of the inferior lateral angle during trunk forward-bending has previously been assessed (see Figure 17.18).

6. The behavior of the inferior lateral angle and sacral base during the three positions of neutral, backward bent (prone prop position), and forward bent (during seated flexion) is the most reliable sign of sacroiliac dysfunction.

Pelvic Girdle

Diagnosis: Prone
  Spring Test

1. Patient prone on table with operator standing at side with dominant eye over the midline.

2. Operator places the palm of the hand over the midline of the lumbar region with the heel of the hand over the lumbosacral junction and the middle finger over the lumbar spinous processes.

3. Operator evaluates the lumbar lordosis for normal, increased, or flattened.

4. Operator provides a short quick push with the heel of the hand toward the table, evaluating for yielding of the lumbar spine.

5. Yielding of the lumbar lordosis with no resistance felt is recorded as negative.

6. A lumbar spine resisting this maneuver is recorded as positive.

7. The status of the lumbar lordosis and the presence of a positive or negative spring test are useful findings in the diagnosis of sacroiliac dysfunction.

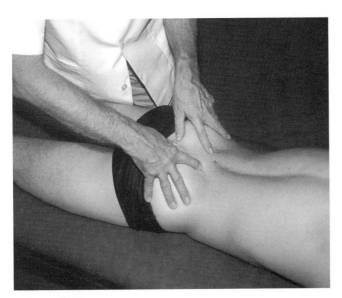

Figure 17.35.

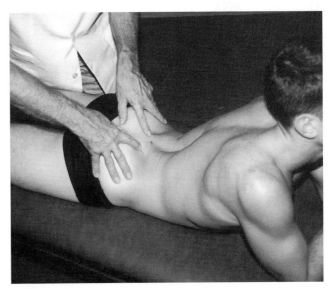

Figure 17.36.

Pelvic Girdle

Diagnosis: Prone
Sacroiliac Rocking Test

1. Patient prone on table with operator standing at side.

2. Operator places right thumb over the left inferior lateral angle and the left thumb over the left sacral base (Fig. 17.37).

3. Alternate ventral pressure of each thumb tests the capacity of the left sacroiliac joint to nutate anteriorly and posteriorly.

4. Operator's thumbs are placed over the right inferior lateral angle and sacral base (Fig. 17.38), and the right sacroiliac joint is similarly tested for nutation anteriorly and posteriorly across the transverse axis.

5. Operator's right thumb is over the posterior aspect of the left inferior lateral angle, and the left thumb is over the right sacral base (Fig. 17.39).

6. Alternate ventral pressure by the thumbs tests the capacity of the sacrum's torsional movement around the left oblique axis.

7. Operator's right thumb is over the right inferior lateral angle and the left thumb of the left sacral base (Fig. 17.40). A similar ventral pressure motion tests the capacity of the sacrum to move around the right oblique axis.

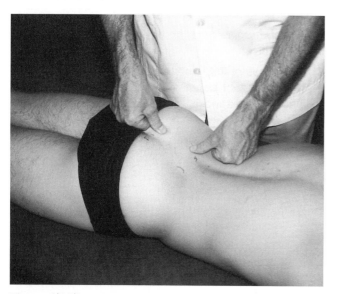

Figure 17.37.

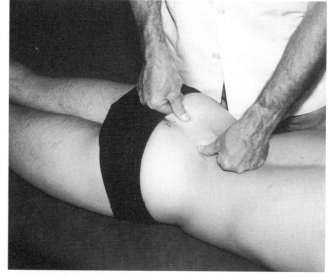

Figure 17.39.

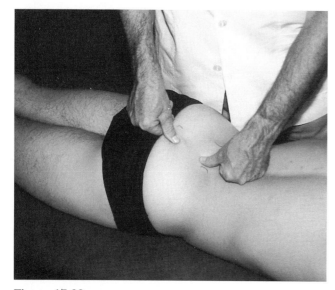

Figure 17.38.

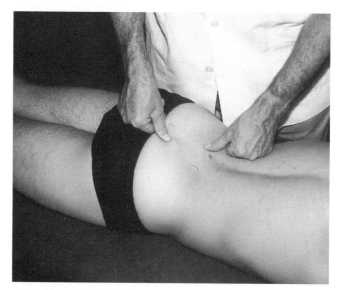

Figure 17.40.

Pelvic Girdle

Diagnosis: Prone
Sacroiliac Motion Spring Test

1. Patient prone on table with operator standing at side.

2. Operator's thenar eminence is over the left inferior lateral angle and the index and middle fingers of the left hand are over the left sacral base (Fig. 17.41).

3. Ventral pressure through the right hand while monitoring movement at the left fingers tests for posterior nutation capacity of the left sacroiliac joint.

4. The right sacroiliac joint can be similarly tested by placing the thenar eminence over the right inferior lateral angle and the left fingers over the right sacral base.

5. Operator's right thenar eminence is over the left inferior lateral angle and the monitoring left fingers are over the right sacral base (Fig. 17.42).

6. Ventral springing through the right thenar eminence with monitoring of motion of the right sacral base identifies coupled sidebending and rotational torsional movement around the left oblique axis.

7. Operator's right thenar eminence is over the right inferior lateral angle and the left fingers monitor the left sacral base (Fig. 17.43). Ventral pressure through the right hand monitored at the left base identifies torsional movement around the right oblique axis.

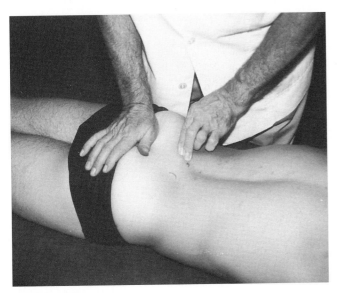

Figure 17.41.

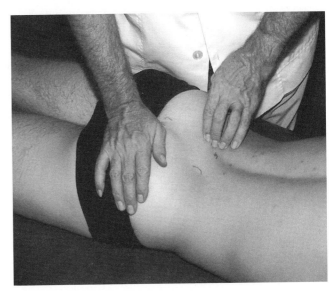

Figure 17.43.

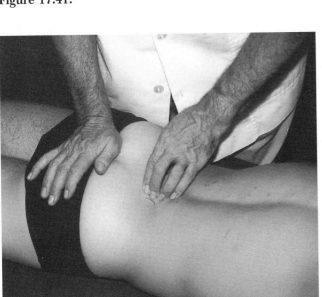

Figure 17.42.

Pelvic Girdle

Diagnosis: Prone
Sacroiliac Motion Test by Gapping

1. Patient prone on table with operator standing at side.

2. Operator's fingers of the left hand overlie the posterior aspect of the left sacroiliac joint while the right hand controls the left lower extremity with contact at the ankle (Fig. 17.44).

3. With knee below 90° of flexion, operator introduces internal rotation of the lower extremity through the femur, hip joint, and innominate while monitoring movement of the left sacroiliac joint.

4. The normal motion is gapping of the joint posteriorly.

5. Internal rotation of the leg with the knee below 90° primarily tests the lower pole of the left sacroiliac joint.

6. Operator repeats the maneuver with the knee flexed above 90° (Fig. 17.45), which primarily tests movement of the upper pole.

Pelvic Girdle

Diagnosis: Supine
Leg Length

1. Patient supine with operator standing at end of table.

2. Operator grasps patient's feet and ankles with the thumbs under the inferior aspect of each medial malleolus (Fig. 17.46).

3. Operator sights down perpendicular to each thumb to identify which leg appears longer or shorter.

4. In the absence of anatomical difference in leg length, inequality of leg length in the supine position is a function of innominate rotation due to iliosacral dysfunction.

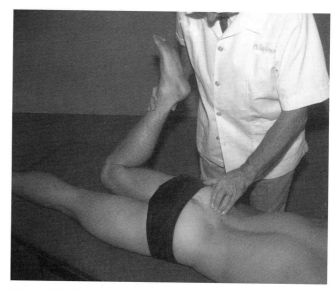

Figure 17.45.

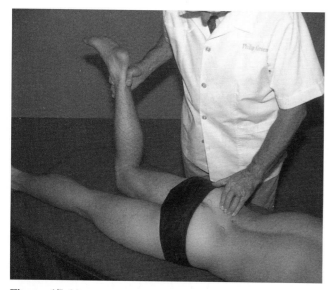

Figure 17.44.

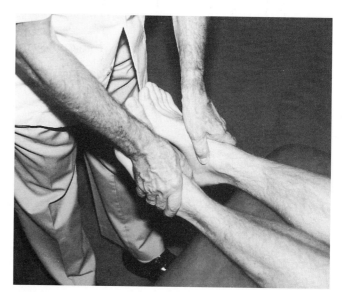

Figure 17.46.

Pelvic Girdle

Diagnosis: Supine
    Anterior Superior Iliac Spine

1. Patient supine with operator standing at side with dominant eye over the midline.

2. Operator places the palms of the hands over each anterior superior iliac spine for precise localization (Fig. 17.47).

3. Operator places both thumbs on the inferior aspect of the anterior superior iliac spine, testing against the horizontal plane for innominate rotation (Fig. 17.48).

4. Operator places each thumb on the anterior aspect of the anterior superior iliac spine, testing against the coronal plane to determine whether one innominate is more anterior or posterior than the other (Fig. 17.49).

5. Operator's thumbs are placed on the medial side of the anterior superior iliac spine, testing their relationship to the midsagittal plane to see whether one is more medial or lateral than the other (Fig. 17.50).

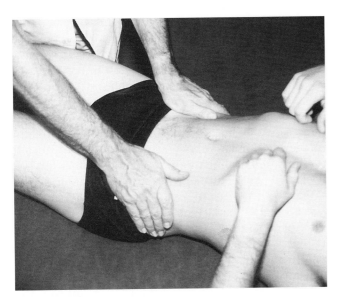

Figure 17.47.

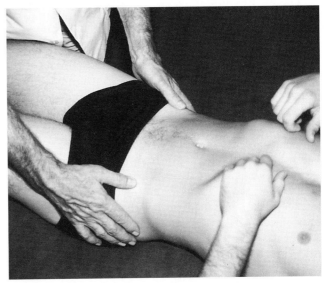

Figure 17.49.

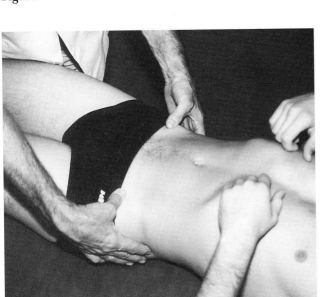

Figure 17.48.

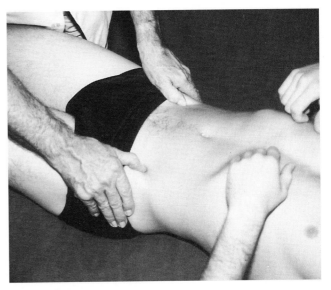

Figure 17.50.

PELVIC GIRDLE DYSFUNCTIONS

There are 14 different dysfunctions possible within the pelvic girdle (Table 17.1). It is seldom that one finds a single dysfunction within the pelvis. Combinations of dysfunctions of the pubis, sacroiliac, and iliosacral mechanisms are quite common.

Diagnosis of these dysfunctions is made from a combination of physical findings of asymmetry of osseous parts, asymmetric range of motion of the right and left side of the pelvis, and tissue texture abnormalities primarily of ligamentous tension and tenderness.

Pubic Symphysis Dysfunction

Dysfunction of the symphysis pubis is very common and frequently overlooked. Muscle imbalance between the abdominals above and the adductors below are major contributors to the presence and persistence of this dysfunction. They frequently result from the chronic posture of standing with more load on one leg (one-legged standing). Pubic dysfunction restricts symmetrical motion of the innominate bones during the walking cycle. The diagnostic criteria for pubic dysfunction is found in Table 17.2.

Sacroiliac Dysfunctions

Sacroiliac dysfunctions are frequently associated with muscle imbalance of the piriformis and psoas muscles (Table 17.3). The sacrum becomes dysfunctional between the two iliac bones through alteration of motion across the transverse axis, the unilateral and bilateral nutational restrictions, or around the oblique axis, the anterior and posterior torsions. Occasionally, more than one sacroiliac dysfunction is identified. A diagnostic finding helpful in differentiating the torsions from the nutated sacrums is the

Table 17.1
Pelvic Girdle Dysfunctions

Pubis
1. Superior
2. Inferior

Sacroiliac
1. Bilaterally nutated anteriorly
2. Bilaterally nutated posteriorly
3. Unilaterally nutated anteriorly (sacrum flexed)
4. Unilaterally nutated posteriorly (sacrum extended)
5. Torsioned anteriorly (left on left or right on right)
6. Torsioned posteriorly (left on right or right on left)

Iliosacral
1. Rotated anteriorly
2. Rotated posteriorly
3. Superior (cephalic) shear
4. Inferior (caudad) shear
5. Rotated medially (inflare)
6. Rotated laterally (outflare)

Table 17.2
Pubic Symphysis Dysfunction

Diagnosis		Standing Flexion Test Positve	Pubic Tubercle Height	Tension and Tenderness of Inguinal Ligament
Superior	Right	Right	Right superior	Right
	Left	Left	Left superior	Left
Inferior	Right	Right	Right inferior	Right
	Left	Left	Left inferior	Left

sacral base and inferior lateral angle will always be posterior on the same side in the torsions, either anterior or posterior. If an inferior lateral angle is posterior but the base is anterior of the same side, one has either an anteriorly nutated (flexed) on that side or a posteriorly nutated (extended) sacrum on the opposite. A bilaterally nutated anterior or posterior sacrum is quite rare. The motion of the inferior lateral angle is a valuable diagnostic test in determining sacroiliac dysfunction. In an anterior torsion, the usual finding is of an inferior lateral angle posterior on one side (along with the base posterior on the same side) in the neutral position. If the asymmetry of the inferior lateral angle becomes greater during the forward-bending movement and becomes level in backward-bending, one is ensured of an anterior torsional restriction to the side of the posterior inferior lateral angle. Similarly, in the backward torsions, an inferior lateral angle will be posterior in neutral (along with the sacral base) and becomes more asymmetric during backward-bending of the trunk but becomes symmetric when fully forward bent. This is the most valuable physical finding in identifying the torsions. In the unilateral anteriorly nutated or posteriorly nutated sacrum, one inferior lateral angle will be more posterior in neutral, but its base will be anterior on the same side. In a unilateral anteriorly nutated (flexed) sacrum, the inferior lateral angle appears to be somewhat more posterior during forward-bending but does not become symmetric in backward-bending. In the unilateral posteriorly nutated (extended) sacrum, the inferior lateral angle appears to be more posterior in neutral and becomes more prominent during the trunk extended motion than during the trunk flexed. However, it never becomes symmetric either.

Iliosacral Dysfunctions

The examiner cannot make an accurate diagnosis of iliosacral dysfunction until the sacroiliac dysfunctions are treated because iliosacral dysfunction is the result of a unilateral problem with one side of the sacrum that must be midline to assess relation of the ilium to the sacrum (Table 17.4). The physical findings of

Table 17.3
Sacroiliac Dysfunctions

Diagnosis	Seated Flexion Test Positive	Base of Sacrum	Inferior Lateral Angle Position	Inferior Lateral Angle Motion	Lumbar Scoliosis	Lumbar Lordosis*	Medial Malleolus Prone
Unilateral nutated anteriorly (flexed)							
Right	Right	Anterior right	Inferior right		Convex right	Normal to increased	Long right
Left	Left	Anterior left	Inferior left		Convex left	Normal to increased	Long left
Unilateral nutated posteriorly (extended)							
Right	Right	Posterior right	Superior right		Convex left	Reduced	Short right
Left	Left	Posterior left	Superior left		Convex right	Reduced	Short left
Anterior torsion							
Left on left	Right	Anterior right	Posterior left	Left, increased on forward-bending	Convex right	Increased	Short left
Right on right	Left	Anterior left	Posterior right	Right, increased on forward-bending	Convex left	Increased	Short right
Backward torsion							
Right on left	Right	Posterior right	Posterior right	Right, increased on backward-bending	Convex left	Reduced	Short right
Left on right	Left	Posterior left	Posterior left	Left, increased on backward-bending	Convex right	Reduced	Short left
Bilateral nutated anterior (flexed)	Bilateral	Anterior	Posterior			Increased	Even
Bilateral nutated posterior (extended)	Bilateral	Posterior	Anterior			Reduced	Even

*Reduced is also a positive spring test.

greatest importance are the relationship of each anterior superior iliac spine and the length of the medial malleolus in the supine position. The finding of a right anterior superior iliac spine being more caudad than the left could occur with either a right anteriorly rotated innominate or a left posteriorly rotated innominate. The differentiation is based on the motion tests, primarily the standing flexion test. Iliosacral dysfunctions of the rotational type are very common and appear to be the result of muscle imbalance during the walking cycle. The shear dysfunctions occur only in those individuals with sacroiliac joints that have less change in bevel and convex concave relationship at the junction of the upper and lower poles of the joint. The shear dysfunctions are usually traumatically induced and are major contributors to lower back and lower extremity pain syndromes. The medially and laterally rotated iliosacral dysfunctions are quite rare, and the diagnosis can only be made after the anterior or posterior rotational component of the iliosacral mechanism is restored to symmetry. The medially and laterally rotated innominates are frequently misdiagnosed because there is a small amount of medial and lateral rotational component to every anterior and posterior rotation of the innominate. As an innominate rotates anteriorly during the walking cycle and with an anteriorly rotated dysfunction, it also rotates somewhat laterally (outflare). The reverse is true with the posteriorly rotated innominate as it medially rotates both during the walking cycle and when dysfunctional. This medial to lateral rotational component of an anterior or posterior innominate is what is frequently diagnosed as an inflare or outflare dysfunction.

MANAGEMENT OF PELVIC GIRDLE DYSFUNCTION

The goal of manual medicine treatment to pelvic girdle dysfunction is to restore the mechanics of the normal walking cycle. In the overall treatment of the patient, one should treat the lumbar spine before the treatment of the pelvis because many sacroiliac techniques require the use of the lumbar spine as a lever arm. The pelvis is the bony attachment of many muscles of the trunk above and the extremities below. Treatment of the pelvic girdle should always be accompanied by the diagnosis and treatment of muscle imbalance above and below the pelvis to prevent recurrence of dysfunction and to enhance the therapeutic outcome.

Table 17.4
Iliosacral Dysfunctions

Diagnosis	Standing Flexion Test Positive	Anterior Superior Iliac Spine Supine	Medial Malleolus Supine	Posterior Superior Iliac Spine Prone	Sacral Sulcus Prone	Ischial Tuberosity Prone	Sacrotuberous Ligament Prone
Anterior rotated							
Right	Right	Inferior right	Long right	Superior right	Shallow right		
Left	Left	Inferior left	Long left	Superior left	Shallow left		
Rotated posterior							
Right	Right	Superior right	Short right	Inferior right	Deep right		
Left	Left	Superior left	Short left	Inferior left	Deep left		
Rotated lateral (outflare)							
Right	Right	Lateral right		Medial right	Narrow right		
Left	Left	Lateral left		Medial left	Narrow left		
Rotated medial (inflare)							
Right	Right	Medial right		Lateral right	Wide right		
Left	Left	Medial left		Lateral left	Wide left		
Superior shear (upslip)							
Right	Right	Superior right	Short right	Superior right		Superior right	Lax right
Left	Left	Superior left	Short left	Superior left		Superior left	Lax left
Inferior shear (downslip)							
Right	Right	Inferior right	Long right	Inferior right		Inferior right	Tight right
Left	Left	Inferior left	Long left	Inferior left		Inferior left	Tight left

Treatment Sequence

The recommended treatment sequence is pubic symphysis, innominate shear dysfunction, sacroiliac dysfunction, and iliosacral dysfunction. In the diagnostic sequence, one assesses for pubic dysfunctions early that, if found, should be treated before proceeding with the diagnostic sequence. Recall that the major criteria for sacroiliac dysfunction is identified with the patient in the prone position. If there is residual dysfunction of the symphysis pubis in front, the patient is not symmetrical in the prone position on the tripod of the two anterior superior iliac spines and the symphysis pubis.

After the diagnosis and treatment of the pubic dysfunction, the next major assessment is for the presence of innominate shear dysfunction. The major index of suspicion occurs with unleveling of the iliac crests in the unloaded position. When an innominate shear dysfunction is present, it appears to restrict all other motions within that sacroiliac joint. Therefore, it deserves attention early in the diagnostic and treatment process. A second reason for treating the innominate shear early is the need to have two symmetrical innominates available to assess the sacrum's position in between. Sacroiliac dysfunction is then addressed to restore its symmetry to the coronal plane when the patient is supine on the examining table to allow assessment of each innominate in relation to the fixed sacrum on the table.

Pelvic Girdle

Symphysis Pubis

Muscle Energy Technique
Supine
Diagnosis
Position: Symphysis either superior or inferior ("shotgun technique")

1. Patient supine with hips and knees flexed and feet together.

2. Operator stands at side of table holding patient's knees together.

3. Operator resists two to three patient efforts of knee abduction for 3–5 seconds (Fig. 17.51).

4. Operator places forearm between patient's knees (Fig. 17.52).

5. A series of adduction efforts of both knees attempts to distract the symphysis pubis.

6. Retest.

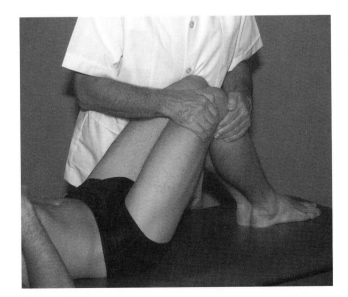

Figure 17.51.

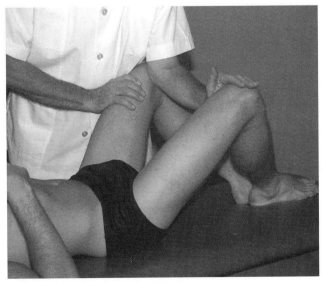

Figure 17.52.

Pelvic Girdle

Symphysis Pubis

Muscle Energy Technique
Supine
Diagnosis
      Position: Left superior symphysis

1. Patient supine on table with operator standing on left side (Fig. 17.53).

2. Operator slides patient's pelvis to the left side of the table, maintaining the left innominate on the edge. Patient's left arm holds right shoulder for trunk stability (Fig. 17.54).

3. Operator's legs support the patient's freely hanging left leg.

4. Operator's left hand stabilizes patient's right side of pelvis, and right hand is placed above the patella over patient's distal left femur.

5. Patient performs a series of three to five repetitions of 3- to 5-second muscle contractions of hip flexion against operator's right hand (Fig. 17.55).

6. After each patient effort, operator engages new barrier by additional left leg extension.

7. Retest.

Note: With patient's leg in an abducted and extended position, hip flexion activates left adductor muscle group, pulling left symphysis inferiorly by concentric isotonic muscle contraction.

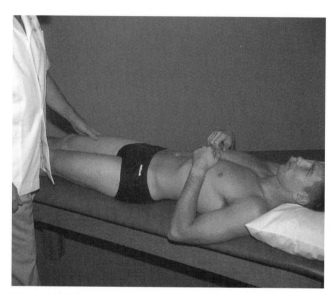

Figure 17.53.

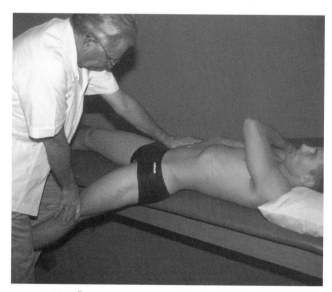

Figure 17.55.

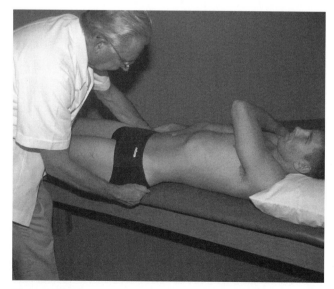

Figure 17.54.

Pelvic Girdle

Symphysis Pubis

Muscle Energy Technique
Supine
Diagnosis
  Position: Right symphysis inferior

1. Patient supine on table with right knee and hip flexed, adducted, and slightly internally rotated.

2. Operator stands on left side and rolls patient's pelvis to the left to place operator's left hand to control patient's right innominate (Fig. 17.56).

3. Operator places patient's right posterior superior iliac spine between the operator's left middle and ring fingers with heel of hand in contact with the ischial tuberosity (Fig. 17.57).

4. Operator returns patient's pelvis to the table with the right innominate in contact with the left hand, and a superior and medial compressive force of the heel of the left hand is applied against the ischial tuberosity (Fig. 17.58).

5. Operator resists three to five efforts of a 3- to 5-second muscle contraction of the patient to straighten the right leg in the caudad direction.

6. After each effort, the operator engages new barriers by more hip flexion and compression against the right ischial tuberosity.

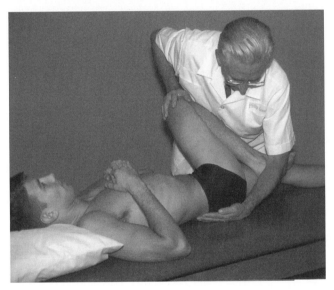

Figure 17.56.

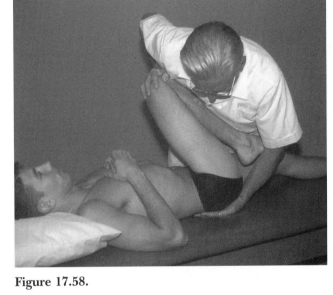

Figure 17.58.

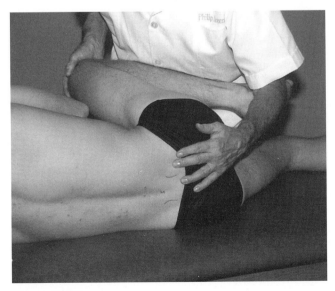

Figure 17.57.

7. Alternative operator position with the patient's right knee in the operator's right axilla with right hand holding edge of table (Fig. 17.59).

8. Retest.

   Note: Flexion, internal rotation, and adduction of the right hip close packs the right sacroiliac joint so that hip extension effort transmits operator force against the ischial tuberosity in a cephalward and medial direction toward the symphysis pubis.

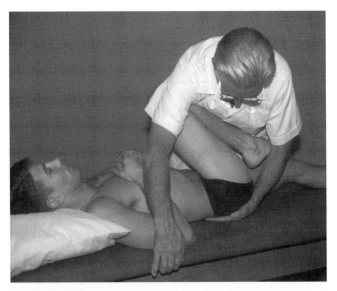

Figure 17.59.

Pelvic Girdle

Iliosacral

Muscle Energy Technique
Supine
Diagnosis
Position: Left superior innominate shear dysfunction

1. Patient supine with feet off end of table.

2. Operator stands at end of table with left thigh against patient's right foot and both hands grasping patient's left leg just proximal to the ankle (Fig. 17.60).

3. Operator abducts the extended left leg 10–15° to loose pack the left sacroiliac joint (Fig. 17.61).

4. Operator internally rotates the extended abducted left leg to close pack the left hip joint (Fig. 17.62).

5. Operator puts long axis extension on the left leg while the patient performs a series of inhalation and exhalation efforts (Fig. 17.63).

6. Three to four respiratory cycles are performed, and during the last exhalation effort the patient is instructed to cough while simultaneously the operator tugs left leg in a caudad direction.

7. Retest.

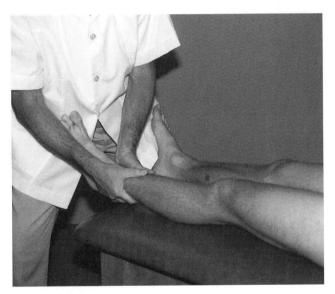

Figure 17.60.

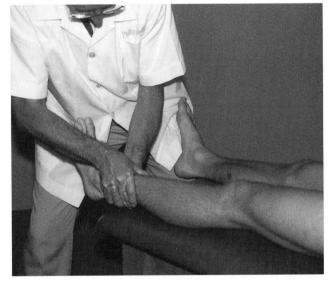

Figure 17.62.

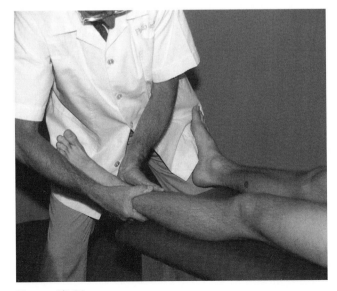

Figure 17.61.

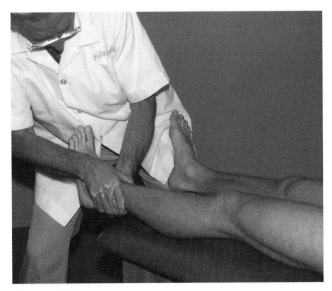

Figure 17.63.

Pelvic Girdle

Iliosacral

Muscle Energy Technique
Lateral Recumbent
Diagnosis: Right inferior innominate shear

1. Patient lies in the left lateral recumbent position.

2. Operator stands in front (or back) of patient with right arm and shoulder supporting the weight of the right lower extremity (an assistant may help by holding the weight of the right leg).

3. Operator's left hand grasps the posterior aspect of the right innominate from the ischial tuberosity to the posterior superior iliac spine (Fig. 17.64).

4. Operator's right hand grasps the right innominate from the ischial tuberosity to the inferior pubic ramus (Fig. 17.65).

5. Operator's two hands distract the right innominate laterally (toward the ceiling) and exerts a cephalic directional force on the right innominate.

6. Patient performs a series of deep inhalation and exhalation efforts while operator maintains distraction of the right innominate in a cephalic direction.

7. Retest.

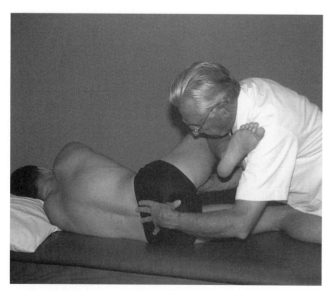

Figure 17.64.

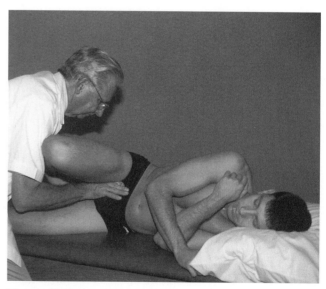

Figure 17.65.

Pelvic Girdle

Iliosacral

Muscle Energy Technique
Prone
Diagnosis
> Position: Right inferior innominate shear

1. Patient prone on table with operator standing on the right side.

2. Operator places patient's right foot between the knees and extended right arm and hand controls right knee to loose pack the right sacroiliac joint (Fig. 17.66).

3. Operator's left hand contacts the right ischial tuberosity and maintains a force in a cephalic direction.

4. Patient performs a series of deep inhalation and exhalation efforts.

5. Patient attempts to straighten right arm against a hand contact on the table leg, resulting in a caudad force through the trunk.

6. A combination of the operator force on ischial tuberosity, patient's right arm muscle effort against trunk, and respiratory effort provides superior shearing movement of the right innominate against the sacrum.

7. Retest.

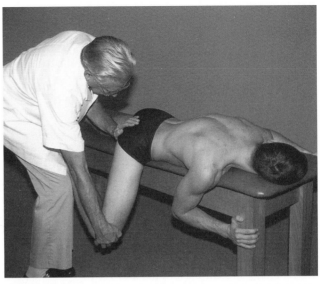

Figure 17.66.

Pelvic Girdle

Sacroiliac

Muscle Energy Technique
Prone
Diagnosis
Position: Left unilateral anterior nutated sacrum (left sacrum flexed)
Motion restriction: Left unilateral posterior nutation

1. Patient prone with operator standing on left side.

2. Operator's left hand monitors left sacral base while right arm introduces abduction of patient's left leg to approximately 15° (Fig. 17.67).

3. Operator internally rotates left leg, gapping the posterior aspect of the left sacroiliac joint. Patient holds leg in that position (Fig. 17.68).

4. With right arm straight, operator places heel of hand on left inferior lateral angle and springs sacrum from above and below and from side to side until point of maximum motion is identified at the left sacral base (Fig. 17.69).

5. Patient takes a maximum inhalation and holds breath as operator maintains a ventral and cephalic compressive force on the left inferior lateral angle.

6. As patient exhales, operator maintains pressure.

7. A series of forced inhalation efforts are made by the patient while operator maintains force on inferior lateral angle.

8. Retest.

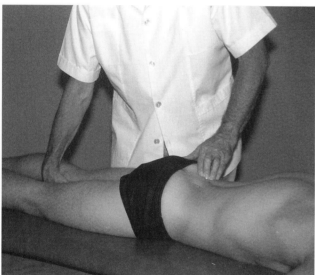

Figure 17.67.

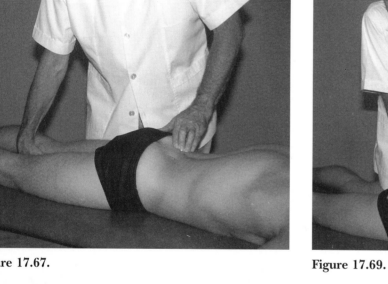

Figure 17.69.

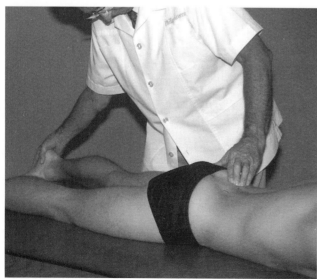

Figure 17.68.

Pelvic Girdle

Sacroiliac

Muscle Energy Technique
Prone
Diagnosis
  Position: Right posterior nutated sacrum
  (right extended sacrum)
  Motion restriction: Anterior nutation of right
  sacrum

1. Patient prone on table with operator standing on right side.

2. Operator's right hand monitors the right sacroiliac joint as the left hand abducts right leg to approximately 15°, loose packing right sacroiliac joint (Fig. 17.70).

3. Operator externally rotates right abducted leg, gapping the anterior aspect of the right sacroiliac joint. Patient instructed to hold right leg in that position (Fig. 17.71).

4. Patient's trunk extended by prone prop position while operator's right pisiform in contact with the right sacral base maintains a ventral and caudad directional force (Fig. 17.72).

5. Operator's left hand on the right anterior superior iliac spine provides a counterforce against the compression through the right hand (Fig. 17.73).

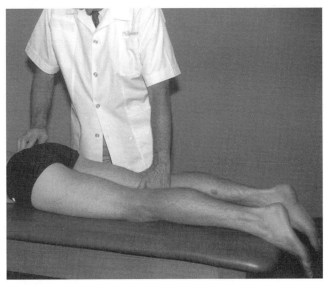

Figure 17.70.

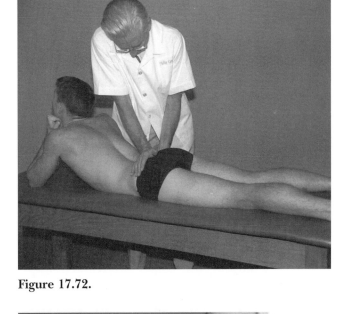

Figure 17.72.

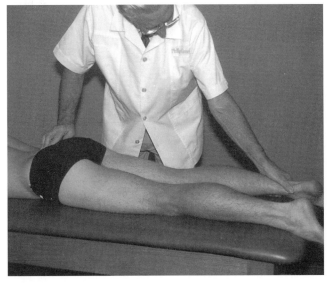

Figure 17.71.

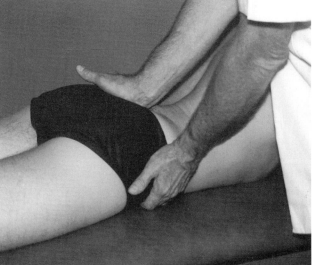

Figure 17.73.

6. Patient performs a series of forced exhalation efforts while operator maintains ventral and caudad compressive force against the right sacral base.

7. At the end of each exhalation effort, patient is instructed to pull the right anterior superior iliac spine toward the table as a muscle activating force.

8. After three to five repetitions, the operator maintains the sacral compression against the counterforce on the anterior superior iliac spine and the patient is instructed to return to the neutral position (Fig. 17.74).

9. Retest.

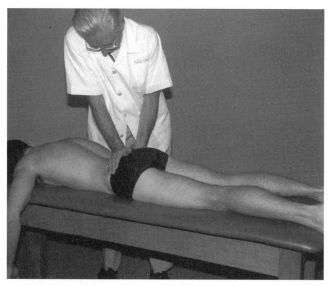

Figure 17.74.

Pelvic Girdle

Sacroiliac

Muscle Energy Technique
Sims Position
Diagnosis: Left arm left sacral torsion
    Position: Sacrum left rotated, right sidebent, and anteriorly nutated at right base
    Motion restriction: Right rotation, left sidebending, and posterior nutation of right base

1. Patient prone on table.

2. Operator stands on right side and flexes patient's knees to 90° (Fig. 17.75).

3. Operator rolls patient onto left hip, introducing Sims position (Fig. 17.76).

4. Operator controls patient's knees on left thigh, monitors lumbosacral junction with left hand, and introduces trunk rotation to the left through the right hand until L5 begins to rotate left (Fig. 17.77).

5. Operator's right hand now monitors the lumbosacral junction and right sacral base while left hand introduces left sidebending (Fig. 17.78).

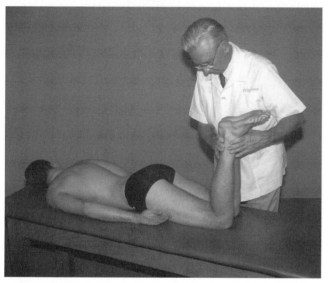

Figure 17.75.

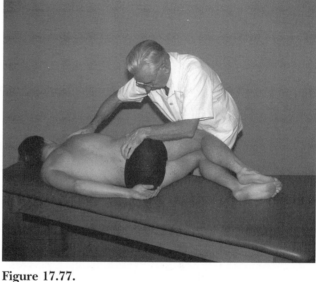

Figure 17.77.

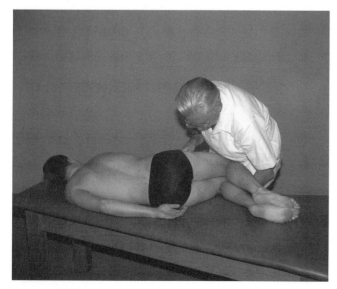

Figure 17.76.

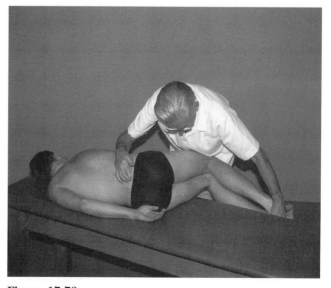

Figure 17.78.

6. Operator flexes lower extremities until right sacral base begins to move posteriorly and then resists an effort by the patient of lifting both feet toward the ceiling against resistance offered by the left hand (Fig. 17.79).

7. Patient performs three to five muscle contractions of lifting feet to ceiling for 3–5 seconds against resistance offered by the operator with engagement of the flexion and sidebending barrier between each effort.

8. Retest.

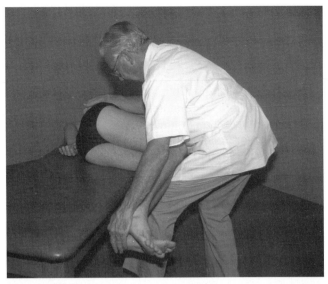

Figure 17.79.

Pelvic Girdle

Sacroiliac

Muscle Energy Technique
Lateral Recumbent
Diagnosis: Left on left sacral torsion
> Position: Left rotated, right sidebent, and anteriorly nutated right sacral base
> Motion restriction: Right rotation, left sidebending, and posterior nutation to right sacral base

1. Patient in right lateral recumbent position with operator standing in front monitoring the lumbosacral junction (Fig. 17.80).
2. Operator introduces neutral sidebending right, rotation left, through the lumbar spine until L5 first begins to rotate left (Fig. 17.81).
3. Operator flexes thighs and pelvis until first posterior movement of the right sacral base.
4. Operator introduces left sidebending by lifting the feet toward the ceiling (Fig. 17.82).
5. Patient performs three to five muscle contractions for 3–5 seconds by pulling the feet down toward the table.
6. Operator engages new barrier by increasing hip flexion and sidebending by lifting knees to the ceiling between each muscle effort.
7. Retest.

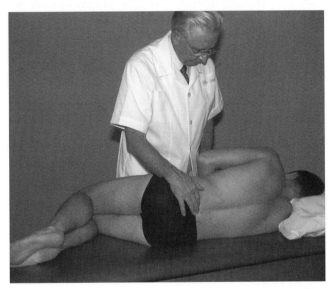

Figure 17.80.

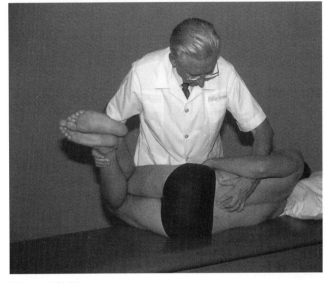

Figure 17.82.

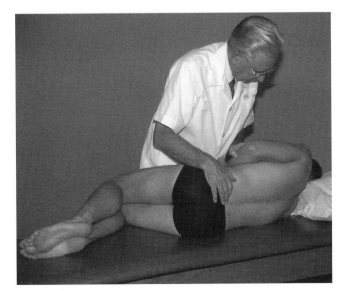

Figure 17.81.

Pelvic Girdle

Sacroiliac

Muscle Energy Technique
Lateral Recumbent
Diagnosis: Right on left sacral torsion
Position: Right rotated, left sidebent, and posteriorly nutated right sacral base
Motion restriction: Left rotation, right sidebending, and anterior nutation of right sacral base

1. Patient in left lateral recumbent position with operator standing in front monitoring the lumbosacral junction with the left hand (Fig. 17.83).

2. Operator pulls patient's left arm anterior and caudad, introducing neutral left sidebending and right rotation of the lumbar spine until L5 first rotates to the right (Fig. 17.84).

3. Operator introduces extension of both legs through the left hand while the right hand monitors the right sacral base until the base first moves anteriorly (Fig. 17.85).

4. Operator drops right leg in front of left knee and places left hand against the patient's distal right femur (Fig. 17.86).

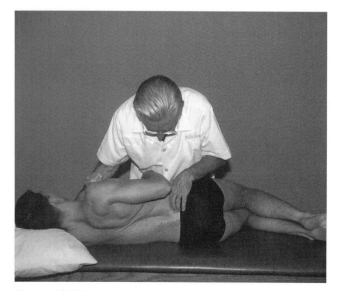

Figure 17.83.

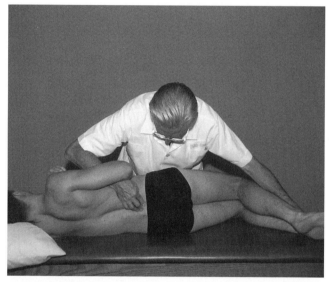

Figure 17.85.

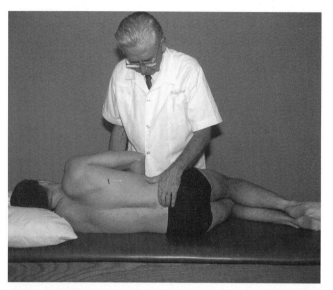

Figure 17.84.

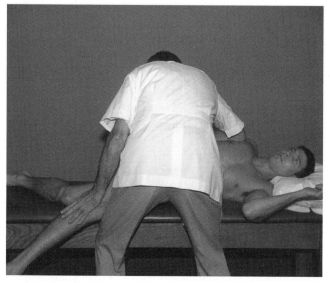

Figure 17.86.

5. Operator's right forearm maintains L5 rotation to the right while left hand resists patient's effort of lifting the right knee toward the ceiling (Fig. 17.87).

6. Three to five muscle contractions for 3–5 seconds are performed by the patient with the operator engaging the new barriers between each effort by further extending the bottom leg and dropping the right leg more toward the floor.

7. Retest.

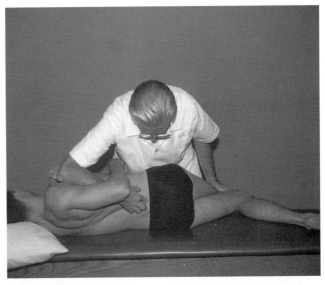

Figure 17.87.

Pelvic Girdle

Sacroiliac

Muscle Energy Technique
Sitting
Diagnosis: Bilateral sacrum flexed
  Position: Bilateral anterior nutated
  Motion restriction: Bilateral posterior nutation

1. Patient sits on stool with feet apart and legs internally rotated (Fig. 17.88).

2. Patient flexes trunk forward.

3. Operator places heel of right hand over apex of the sacrum and left hand over the patient's thoracic spine (Fig. 17.89).

4. Operator maintains ventral pressure on the sacral apex and resists patient's instruction to lift shoulders toward the ceiling.

5. Three to five efforts of 3–5 seconds by the patient restores posterior nutational movement of the sacral base.

6. Retest.

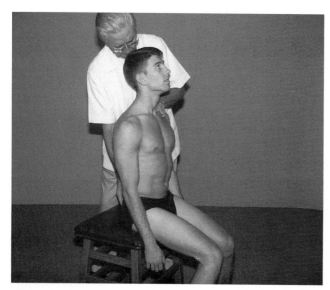

Figure 17.88.

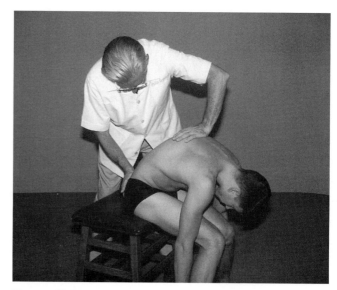

Figure 17.89.

Pelvic Girdle

Sacroiliac

Muscle Energy Technique
Sitting
Diagnosis: Sacrum bilateral extended
    Position: Bilaterally posterior nutated
    Motion restriction: Bilateral anterior nutation

1. Patient sitting on stool with feet together and knees apart, externally rotating legs. Arms are crossed.

2. Operator stands at side with right hand on sacral base and left hand controlling patient's trunk (Fig. 17.90).

3. Patient is instructed to arch the back by pushing abdomen toward the knees while operator maintains a ventral compressive force with the right hand on the sacral base (Fig. 17.91).

4. Operator's left hand resists three to five repetitions of 3- to 5-second muscle contraction of trunk flexion.

5. An exhalation effort assists in moving the sacral base anteriorly.

6. An inhalation effort assists in moving the sacral base posteriorly.

7. Retest.

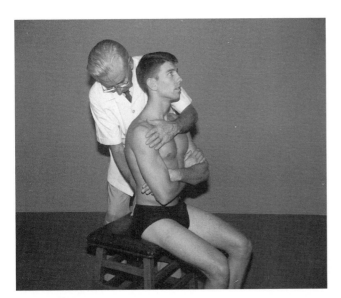

Figure 17.90.

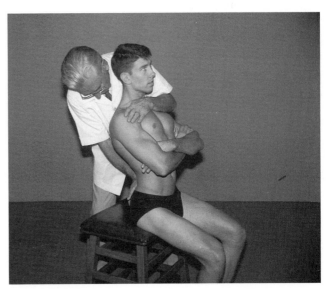

Figure 17.91.

Pelvic Girdle

Iliosacral

Muscle Energy Technique
Supine
Diagnosis: Left posterior innominate
Position: Innominate rotated posteriorly
Motion restriction: Anterior rotation of innominate

1. Patient supine on table with operator standing on left side.

2. Operator slides patient's pelvis until sacrum is at the edge of the table (Fig. 17.92).

3. Operator controls left lower extremity between the knees.

4. Operator stabilizes right side of pelvis at right anterior superior iliac spine (Fig. 17.93).

5. Operator's right hand contacts distal femur above the patella.

6. Operator resists patient's hip flexion effort for 3–5 seconds.

7. Operator engages new barrier by dropping the patient's left leg toward the floor and repeats resistance to hip flexion effort three to five times.

8. Retest.

Note: This procedure is similar to that for a superior pubic symphysis dysfunction with the difference being that the sacrum and not the posterior aspect of the innominate is the fixed point on the edge of the table.

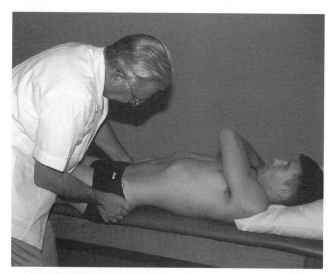

Figure 17.92.

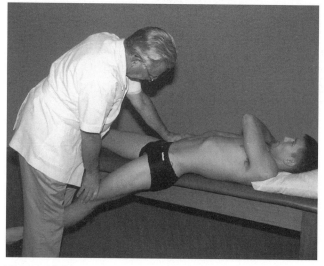

Figure 17.93.

Pelvic Girdle

Iliosacral

Muscle Energy Technique
Prone
Diagnosis: Left posterior innominate
    Position: Left innominate rotated posteriorly
    Motion restriction: Anterior rotation of left innominate

1. Patient prone on table with operator standing on right side.

2. Operator controls patient's left leg by grasping flexed knee in the left hand. Left leg abducted to loose pack left sacroiliac joint.

3. Operator's right hand is on left iliac crest 5–6 cm anterior to the posterior superior iliac spine (Fig. 17.94).

4. Operator extends patient's leg to barrier while exerting pressure with right hand in the direction of the iliac crest (Fig. 17.95).

5. Patient's muscle effort is a series of three to five contractions for 3–5 seconds of hip flexion (pull leg to table) against operator resistance.

6. After each muscle effort operator engages new extension barrier.

7. Retest.

Note: This dysfunction frequently accompanies a left sacrum flexed (anteriorly nutated). A combination technique can be performed as the last step of the muscle energy procedure for the left sacrum flexed. While holding the sacrum in the posteriorly nutated position with the right hand, the operator's left extends the left hip, rotating the left innominate anteriorly, and resists the muscle effort of pulling the knee to the table (Fig. 17.96).

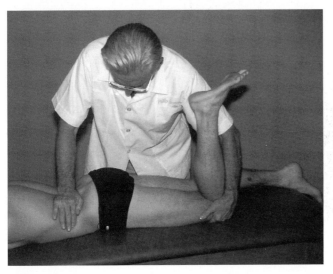

Figure 17.94.

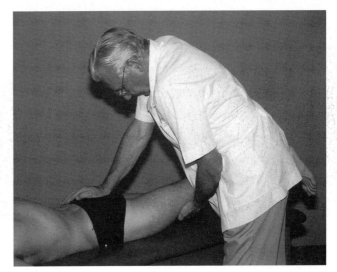

Figure 17.96.

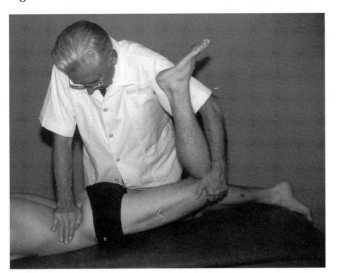

Figure 17.95.

Pelvic Girdle

Iliosacral

Muscle Energy Technique
Lateral Recumbent
Diagnosis: Left posterior innominate
  Position: Left innominate rotated posteriorly
  Motion restriction: Left innominate anterior rotation

1. Patient lies in the right lateral recumbent position with operator standing behind.

2. Operator's right hand placed on iliac crest 5–6 cm anterior to the posterior superior iliac spine (Fig. 17.97).

3. Operator grasps patient's flexed left knee in the left hand and by supporting the left lower extremity loose packs the left sacroiliac joint (Fig. 17.98).

4. Operator extends patient's leg to barrier while exerting anterior pressure along the iliac crest with right hand (Fig. 17.99).

5. Patient provides muscle contraction to pull leg anteriorly against operator resistance for 3–5 seconds and three to five repetitions.

6. Operator engages new extension barrier after each muscle effort.

7. Retest.

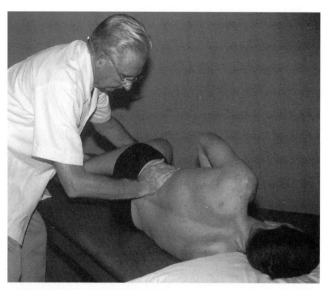

Figure 17.97.

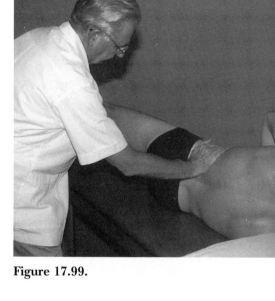

Figure 17.99.

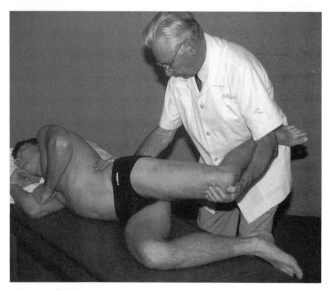

Figure 17.98.

Pelvic Girdle

Iliosacral

Muscle Energy Technique
Prone
Diagnosis: Right anterior innominate
    Position: Right innominate anteriorly rotated
    Motion restriction: Posterior rotation of right innominate

1. Patient in prone position with operator standing at right side.

2. Operator grasps pelvis and slides patient's lower trunk to the right edge of the table (Fig. 17.100).

3. Operator controls patient's right leg by placing the foot between operator's knees and grasping the right knee with the right hand.

4. Operator's left hand stabilizes the sacrum in the midline with the left index finger monitoring the right sacroiliac joint (Fig. 17.101).

5. Operator controls patient's right leg with abduction, external rotation, and flexion to engage barrier to posterior rotational movement (Fig. 17.102).

6. Patient performs muscle effort for 3–5 seconds with three to five repetitions of extending the right leg by pushing the right foot against operator's thigh.

7. Operator engages new barrier of posterior rotation between each patient contraction.

8. Retest.

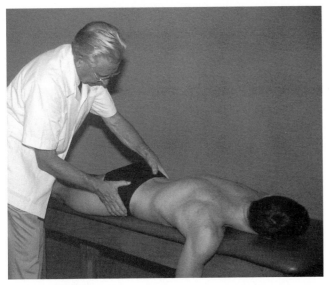

Figure 17.100.

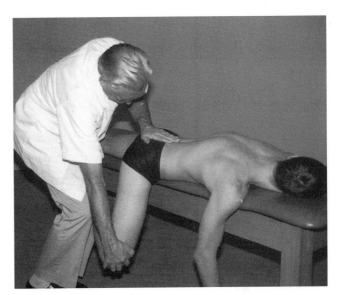

Figure 17.102.

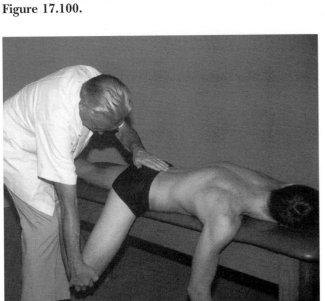

Figure 17.101.

Pelvic Girdle

Iliosacral

Muscle Energy Technique
Supine
Diagnosis: Right anterior innominate
    Position: Right innominate anteriorly rotated
    Motion restriction: Posterior rotation of right
    innominate

1. Patient in the supine position with the right hip and knee flexed.

2. Operator stands on patient's left side with the heel of the left hand contacting the right ischial tuberosity and with the fingers of the left hand monitoring motion of the sacroiliac joint (Fig. 17.103).

3. Operator flexes, externally rotates, and abducts patient's right leg.

4. Operator exerts a cephalward and lateral force against the right ischial tuberosity.

5. Patient performs three to five muscle contractions for 3–5 seconds to extend the right leg against resistance offered by the operator's right hand and trunk (Fig. 17.104).

6. Between each patient effort, operator increases posterior rotation of the right innominate while monitoring loose packed position of the right sacroiliac joint with the left hand.

7. Retest.

Note: This procedure is similar to that for an inferior pubic symphysis dysfunction. The difference is loose packing the right sacroiliac joint and the cephalward and lateral force of the left hand on the ischial tuberosity that directs innominate rotation rather than force toward the symphysis pubis.

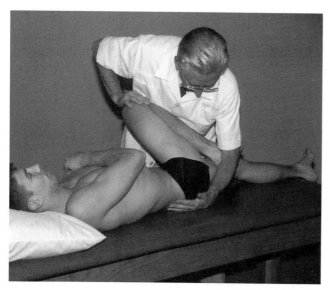

Figure 17.103.

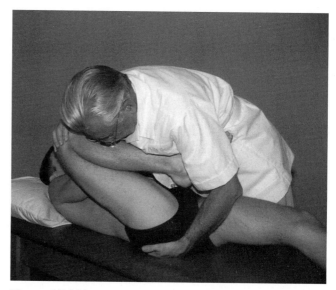

Figure 17.104.

Pelvic Girdle

Iliosacral

Muscle Energy Technique
Lateral Recumbent
Diagnosis: Right anterior innominate
Position: Right innominate anteriorly rotated
Motion restriction: Posterior rotation right innominate

1. Patient in left lateral recumbent position with operator facing patient.

2. Patient's right leg flexed at hip and knee with foot placed against operator's hip.

3. Operator's left hand is placed on the right innominate with the fingers monitoring motion at the right sacroiliac joint and the heel of the hand against the ischial tuberosity (Fig. 17.105).

4. Operator engages barrier by introducing abduction, external rotation, and flexion of the right leg (Fig. 17.106).

5. Patient performs three to five muscle contractions of 3–5 seconds, attempting to straighten the right leg against operator resistance.

6. Operator engages new barrier after each patient relaxation.

7. Retest.

Note: Muscle efforts other than hip extension can be adduction or abduction of the right knee against operator resistance.

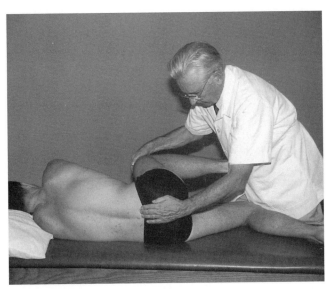

Figure 17.105.

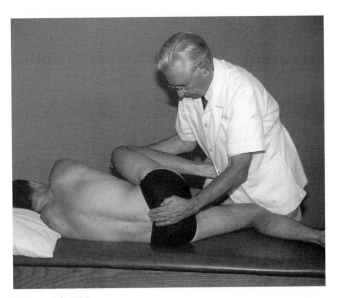

Figure 17.106.

Pelvic Girdle

Iliosacral

Muscle Energy Technique
Supine
Diagnosis: Right innominate internally rotated (inflare)

      Position: Right innominate internally rotated
      Motion restriction: External rotation of right innominate

1. Patient supine on table with operator standing on right side.

2. Operator flexes patient's right hip and knee, placing the right foot on the left knee (Fig. 17.107).

3. Operator's left hand stabilizes left pelvis at the left anterior superior iliac spine.

4. Operator's right hand on medial side of patient's right knee externally rotates hip until barrier is engaged (Fig. 17.108).

5. Patient performs three to five muscle contractions for 3–5 seconds, attempting to internally rotate right leg against resistance by operator.

6. Operator engages new external rotation barrier after each patient contraction.

7. Retest.

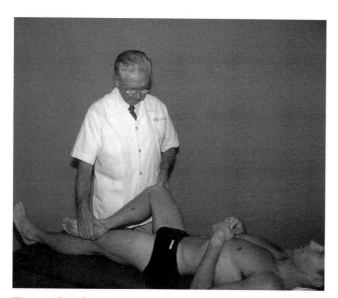

Figure 17.107.

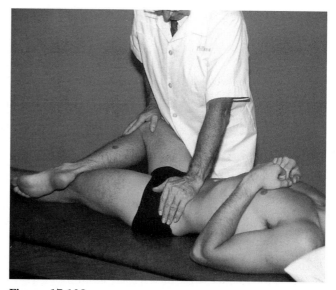

Figure 17.108.

Pelvic Girdle

Iliosacral

Muscle Energy Technique
Supine
Diagnosis: Left innominate externally rotated
(outflare)
    Position: Left innominate externally rotated
    Motion restriction: Internal rotation of left
    innominate

1. Patient supine on table with operator standing on left side.

2. Operator flexes patient's left hip and knee, rolling patient's pelvis to the right. Operator's fingers of the right hand grasp the medial side of the left posterior superior iliac spine (Fig. 17.109).

3. Patient's pelvis returned to neutral with left innominate resting in operator's hand.

4. Operator's left hand adducts the left femur to the internal rotational barrier of the left innominate while maintaining lateral traction on the left posterior superior iliac spine by the right hand.

5. Patient performs three to five muscle efforts for 3–5 seconds, attempting to abduct and externally rotate the left leg against resistance of operator's left hand (Fig. 17.110).

6. Operator engages new internal rotational barrier after each patient relaxation.

7. Retest.

Note: Operator's left hand also maintains pressure through the left thigh toward the table to prevent the pelvis from rotating to the right during muscle contraction.

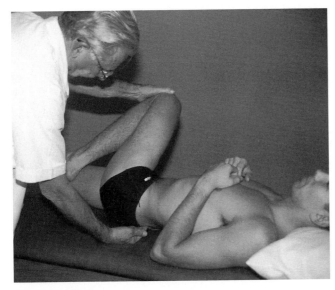

Figure 17.109.

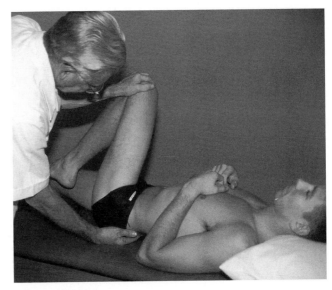

Figure 17.110.

Pelvic Girdle

Symphysis Pubis

Mobilization with Impulse Technique
Supine
Diagnosis: Pubic dysfunction either superior or inferior ("shotgun technique")

1. Patient supine on table with operator standing at side.

2. Operator's knees and hip flexed with feet on the table.

3. Operator's two hands between patient's knees (Fig. 17.111).

4. Patient is instructed to hold knees together.

5. Operator provides mobilization with impulse thrust by separating both knees with both hands against patient resistance (Fig. 17.112).

6. Retest.

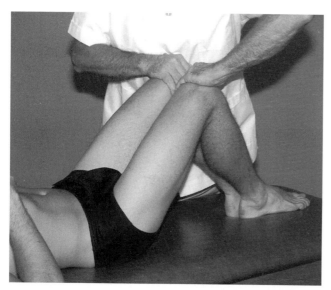

Figure 17.111.

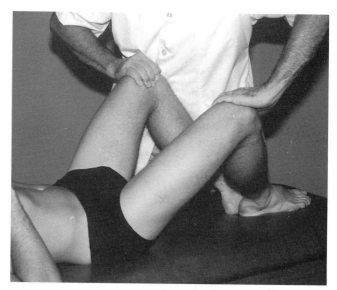

Figure 17.112.

Pelvic Girdle

Sacroiliac

Mobilization with Impulse Technique
Lateral Recumbent
Diagnosis: Left sacrum flexed
    Position: Left sacrum anteriorly nutated
    Motion restriction: Posterior nutation left
    sacral base

1. Patient in left lateral recumbent position with knees and feet together.
2. Operator stands in front and monitors lumbosacral junction with left hand (Fig. 17.113).
3. Operator's right hand pulls patient's left shoulder anterior and caudad, introducing neutral left side-bending right rotation of the lumbar spine until L5 begins to rotate to the right.
4. Operator's left hand contacts the sacrum with the pisiform on the left inferior lateral angle and with left forearm parallel to the table (Fig. 17.114).
5. Operator's right hand and forearm stabilizes trunk and monitors at lumbosacral junction.
6. Operator performs mobilizing thrust through the left arm in a cephalic direction parallel to the table.
7. Alternate right hand position stabilizes right shoulder for the thrust through the left forearm (Fig. 17.115). This position may offer better leverage for the cephalic thrust through the left arm.
8. Retest.

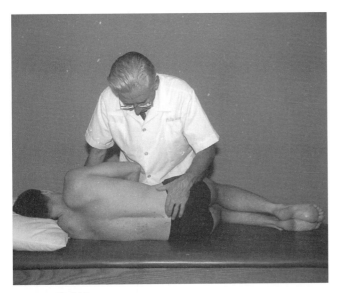

Figure 17.113.

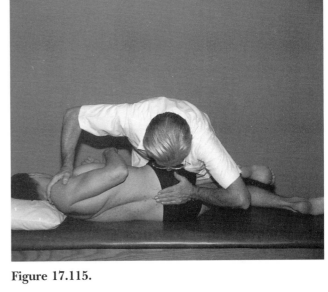

Figure 17.115.

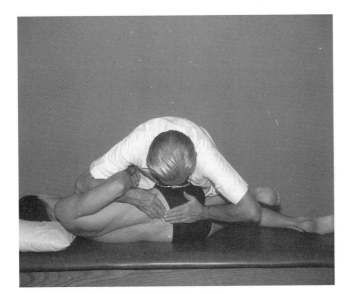

Figure 17.114.

Pelvic Girdle

Sacroiliac

Mobilization with Impulse Technique
Prone
Diagnosis: Left sacrum flexed
Position: Left sacrum anteriorly nutated
Motion restriction: Posterior nutation of left sacral base

1. Patient prone on table with operator standing on left side.

2. Operator's left hand monitors left sacroiliac joint while right hand abducts left leg to loose pack position (approximately 15–20°). Left leg internally rotated and held by patient (Fig. 17.116).

3. Operator's right thenar eminence contacts left inferior lateral angle.

4. Operator engages posterior nutational barrier by springing the sacrum.

5. Patient deeply inhales and operator delivers a mobilization with impulse thrust in an anterior and superior direction through the right hand (Fig. 17.117).

6. Retest.

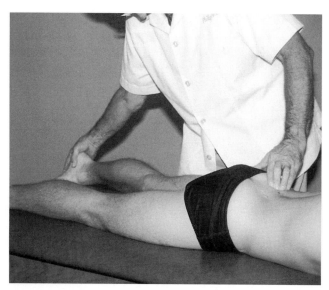

Figure 17.116.

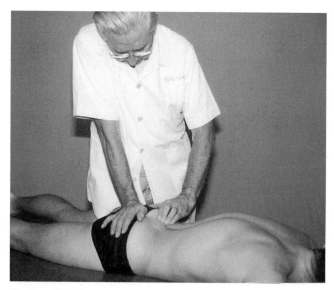

Figure 17.117.

Pelvic Girdle

Sacroiliac

Mobilization with Impulse Technique
Left Lateral Recumbent
Diagnosis: Left on left sacral torsion
    Position: Sacrum left rotated, right sidebent, and anteriorly nutated right base
    Motion restriction: Sacral right rotation, left sidebending, and posterior nutation right base

1. Patient in left lateral recumbent position with knees and feet together and shoulders perpendicular to the table.

2. Operator stands in front and flexes and extends lower extremities, maintaining neutral mechanics in the lumbar spine and engaging the first posterior nutational barrier of the sacrum (Fig. 17.118).

3. Operator's right hand on right shoulder introduces sidebending right and rotation left of the lumbar spine until L5 rotates left.

4. Operator's left hand contacts sacrum with left pisiform against the left inferior lateral angle (Fig. 17.119).

5. The barrier is engaged through the operator's left forearm and hand in contact with the sacrum with the left pisiform in the direction of the right shoulder.

6. A mobilization with impulse thrust is provided in a scooping fashion of the left hand on the left inferior lateral angle in the direction of the resistant right hand on the right shoulder.

7. Retest.

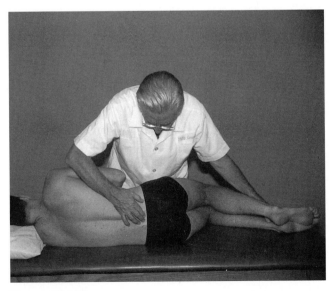

Figure 17.118.

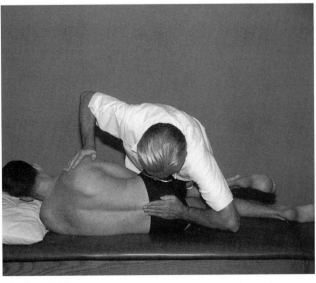

Figure 17.119.

Pelvic Girdle

Sacroiliac

Mobilization with Impulse Technique
Supine
Diagnosis: Right on left sacral torsion
   Position: Sacrum right rotated, left sidebent, and posteriorly nutated right base
   Motion restriction: Left rotation, right sidebending, and anterior nutation of the right sacral base

1. Patient supine with operator standing on left side of table.

2. Operator translates pelvis from right to left, introducing right sidebending of the trunk (Fig. 17.120). Patient clasps hands behind neck.

3. Operator sidebends trunk to the right through the lumbar spine and including the sacrum (Fig. 17.121).

4. Operator threads right forearm through patient's right arm. Operator's back of right hand is against sternum (Fig. 17.122).

5. Operator stabilizes right innominate through left hand contact on right anterior superior iliac spine.

6. Operator engages barrier by left rotation of the trunk without losing right sidebending (Fig. 17.123).

7. Operator performs mobilization with impulse thrust by enhanced trunk rotation to the left against the stabilized right innominate resulting in left rotation, right sidebending, and anterior nutation of the right sacral base.

8. Retest.

Note: This technique is effective for a unilateral right sacrum extended.

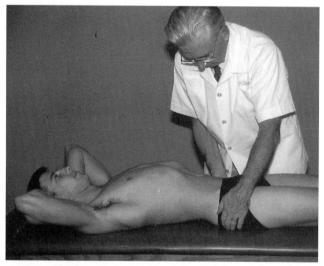

Figure 17.120.

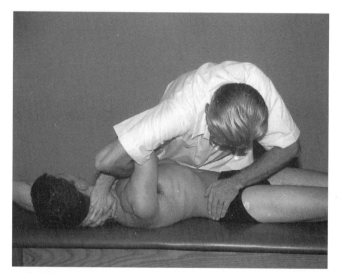

Figure 17.122.

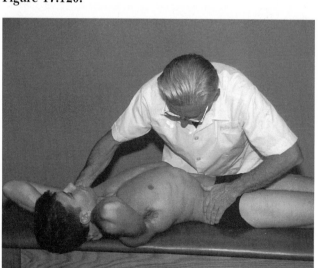

Figure 17.121.

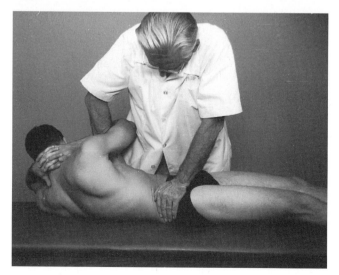

Figure 17.123.

Pelvic Girdle

Sacroiliac

Mobilization with Impulse Technique
Sitting
Diagnosis: Left on left sacral torsion
   Position: Sacrum left rotated, right sidebent, and anteriorly nutated right sacral base
   Muscle restriction: Right rotation, left sidebending, and posterior nutation right sacral base

1. Patient sitting astride table with left hand grasping the right shoulder.

2. Operator stands at right side with right hand grasping patient's left shoulder and right axilla controlling right shoulder.

3. Operator's left pisiform contact is on the left sacral base (Fig. 17.124).

4. Operator's right arm introduces lumbar forward-bending, right sidebending, and right rotation while left hand prevents left rotation of the left sacral base (Fig. 17.125).

5. Operator's right arm maintains trunk right sidebending as nonneutral mechanics are released into neutral lumbar spine (Fig. 17.126).

6. Left rotation is introduced through the trunk while right sidebent and an anterior thrust is delivered by the left forearm through the contact of the left pisiform on the left sacral base (Fig. 17.127).

7. Retest.

Note: Initially, nonneutral lumbar mechanics are used and then released into neutral mechanics so that L5 rotates left and the sacrum rotates to the right, bringing the right sacral base posteriorly.

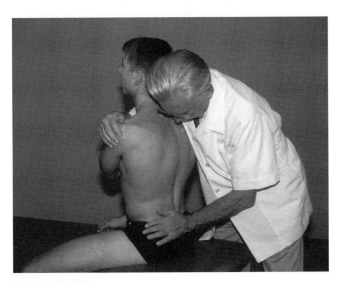

Figure 17.124.

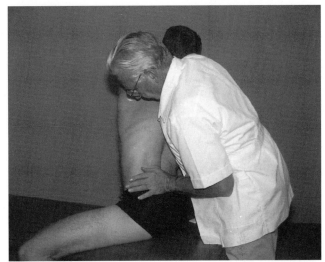

Figure 17.126.

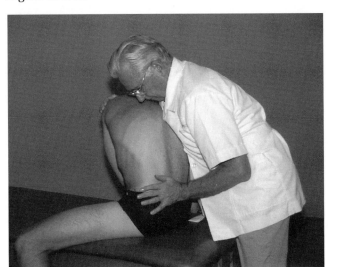

Figure 17.125.

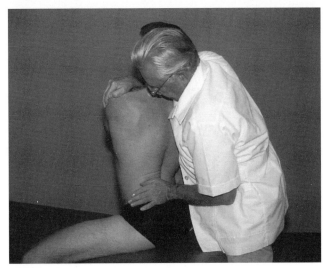

Figure 17.127.

Pelvic Girdle

Sacroiliac

Mobilization with Impulse Technique
Sitting
Diagnosis: Right on left sacral torsion
    Position: Sacrum right rotated, left sidebent, and posteriorly nutated right sacral base
    Motion restriction: Left rotation, right sidebending, and anterior nutation right sacral base

1. Patient sitting astride the table with left hand grasping right shoulder.

2. Operator stands at left side with left hand grasping patient's right shoulder and left axilla controlling patient's left shoulder. Operator's right pisiform contacts right sacral base (Fig. 17.128).

3. Operator introduces left sidebending and right rotation of the trunk down to L5, rotating the sacrum to the left. Operator puts anterior compression on right sacral base (Fig. 17.129).

4. Operator reverses trunk mechanics into right sidebending and left rotation down to and including the sacrum (Fig. 17.130).

5. Operator performs mobilizing with impulse thrust through the right forearm to pisiform contact on right sacral base while exaggerating trunk extension while sidebent right and rotated left.

6. Retest

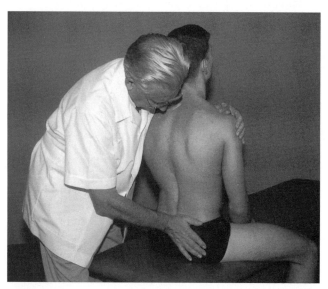

Figure 17.128.

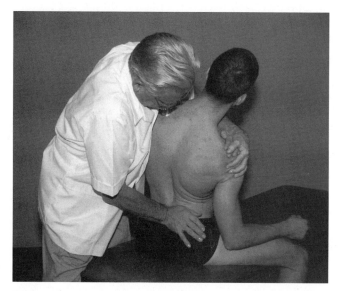

Figure 17.130.

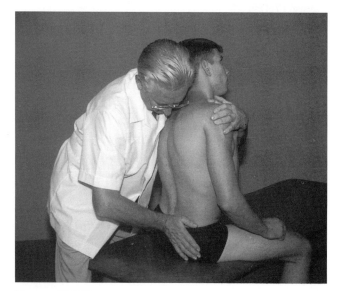

Figure 17.129.

Pelvic Girdle

Iliosacral

Mobilization with Impulse Technique
Supine
Diagnosis: Right superior innominate shear

1. Patient supine with operator standing at end of table.

2. Operator grasps distal tibia and fibula above ankle (Fig. 17.131).

3. Patient flexes knee and hip with slight abduction of the left lower extremity but without rotation (Fig. 17.132).

4. When left leg is controlled with left sacroiliac joint plane loose packed, operator provides mobilization with impulse thrust by long axis extension, carrying knee extension and hip extension to left sacroiliac joint (Fig. 17.133).

5. Retest.

Note: This procedure is not indicated in the presence of knee or hip joint pathology.

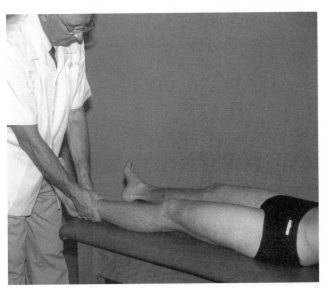

Figure 17.131.

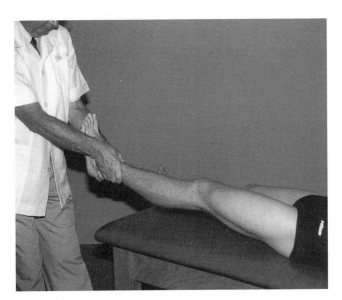

Figure 17.133.

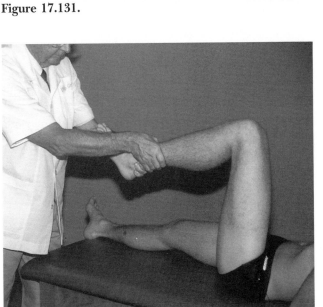

Figure 17.132.

Pelvic Girdle

Iliosacral

Mobilization with Impulse Technique
Lateral Recumbent
Diagnosis: Right inferior innominate shear dysfunction

1. Patient in left lateral recumbent position with operator standing in front monitoring lumbosacral junction (Fig. 17.134).

2. Operator introduces neutral left sidebending right rotation of the lumbar spine down to and including the lumbosacral junction (Fig. 17.135).

3. Operator places patient's right foot in left popliteal space (Fig. 17.136).

4. Operator stabilizes trunk with the right forearm and right hand monitoring at the right sacroiliac joint.

5. Operator's forearm contacts inferior aspect of the patient's right ischial tuberosity (Fig. 17.137).

6. Operator provides mobilization with impulse thrust in a cephalic direction against the right ischial tuberosity with the plane of the right sacroiliac joint parallel to the table, resulting in superior translatory movement of the right innominate.

7. Retest.

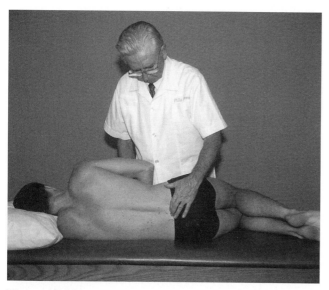

Figure 17.134.

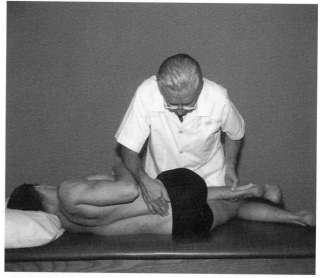

Figure 17.136.

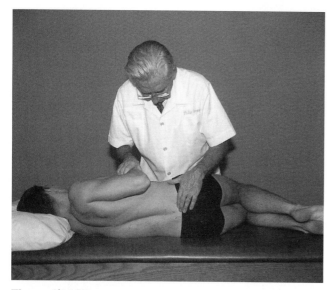

Figure 17.135.

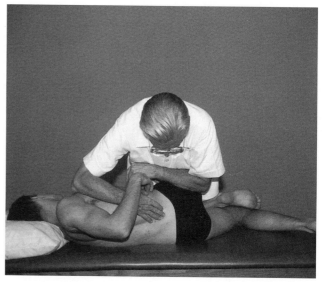

Figure 17.137.

Pelvic Girdle

Iliosacral

Mobilization with Impulse Technique
Lateral Recumbent
Diagnosis: Right anterior innominate
    Position: Right innominate anteriorly rotated
    Motion restriction: Posterior rotation right
    innominate

1–4. These steps are identical to the technique for right inferior innominate shear (Figs. 17.134 to 17.136).

5. Operator's right hand grasps right anterior superior iliac spine while the left hand grasps the right ischial tuberosity.

6. With the plane of the right sacroiliac joint parallel to the table, operator rotates innominate posteriorly to the barrier and provides a mobilization with impulse thrust with both hands in a counterclockwise direction (Fig. 17.138).

7. Alternate hand position finds operator's left forearm on the right ischial tuberosity. Right hand stabilizes the trunk with right sacroiliac joint plane parallel to the table. A mobilization thrust is made by the left forearm in an anterior and superior direction, rotating the left innominate posteriorly (Fig. 17.139).

8. Retest.

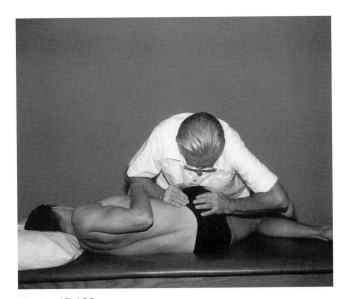

Figure 17.138.

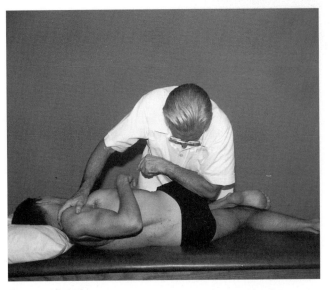

Figure 17.139.

Pelvic Girdle

Iliosacral

Mobilization with Impulse Technique
Lateral Recumbent
Diagnosis: Left posterior innominate
   Position: Left innominate posteriorly rotated
   Motion restriction: Anterior rotation left innominate

1. Patient in right lateral recumbent position with operator standing in front monitoring lumbosacral junction (Fig. 17.140).
2. Operator introduces neutral sidebending right rotation left lumbar curve to include the lumbosacral junction.
3. Operator extends lower extremities until sacral base first starts to move forward (Fig. 17.141).

Patient's left knee is placed in right popliteal space.

4. With the left arm stabilizing the trunk and maintaining the plane of the left sacroiliac joint parallel to the table, operator's right pisiform contacts the left posterior superior iliac spine (Fig. 17.142).
5. A mobilization with impulse technique is provided by operator's body through the right forearm, turning the left innominate anteriorly.
6. Alternate hand contact is the operator's right forearm along the posterior aspect of the patient's left iliac crest (Fig. 17.143).
7. A mobilization with impulse thrust is provided by the operator's body through the left forearm contact, rotating the left innominate anteriorly.
8. Retest.

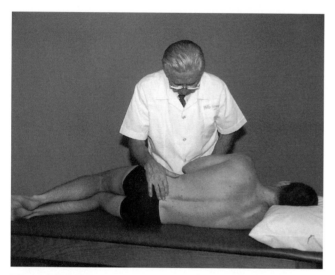

Figure 17.140.

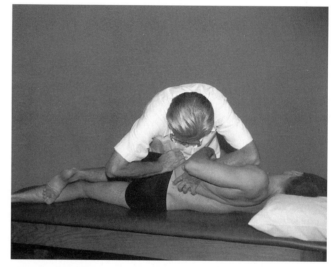

Figure 17.142.

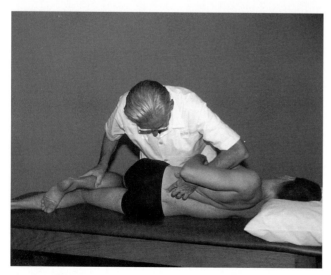

Figure 17.141.

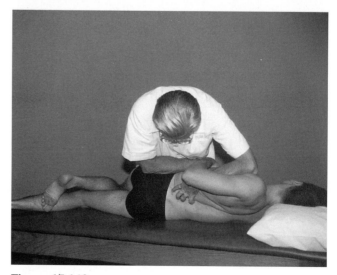

Figure 17.143.

MUSCLE DYSFUNCTIONS OF THE PELVIC GIRDLE

Dysfunctions of the pelvic girdle always involve the many muscles to which it is related. Frequently seen is alteration in the pelvic diaphragm. This is particularly common in dysfunctions of the pubic symphysis and the innominate shear dysfunctions. Widespread symptoms of the lower urinary tract, genitalia, and rectum are frequently present. Restoration of the function of the pelvic diaphragm is described in Chapter 7. Dysfunction of the muscles of the lower extremity and trunk need to be assessed and treated appropriately. These are described in Chapter 20.

CONCLUSION

Dysfunction of the pelvic girdle is complex and not easily understood. It is common to find several dysfunctions within the same pelvic girdle. Each needs to be individually diagnosed and appropriately treated. The diagnostic and therapeutic system described allows the operator to deal with any combination of physical findings that are found within the pelvic girdle. Restoration of pelvic girdle function within the walking cycle is a major therapeutic goal, particularly from the biomechanical postural-structural model.

18

Highly developed hand dexterity is one of the distinguishing characteristics of humans. Upper extremity function places the hand in positions that allow it to perform its unique intricate movements. The upper extremity is attached to the trunk primarily through muscular attachments. The only articulation of the upper extremity with the trunk is the sternoclavicular joint. The arrangement of the muscular attachments allows the extremity a wide range of movement in relation to the trunk. The multiple muscle relationships of the upper extremity account for its strong interrelationship with the cervical spine, thoracic spine, and thoracic cage.

In approaching dysfunctions within the upper extremity, the operator should first examine and treat any dysfunctions within the cervical spine, thoracic spine, and thoracic cage. The cervicothoracic junction is one of the major transitional regions of the body, and the relationship of T1 with the first rib and with the sternoclavicular joint is of major significance in upper extremity problems. T1 dysfunctions influence the first rib and lead to dysfunctions there. Dysfunctions of the first rib influence the manubrium of the sternum and the sternoclavicular joint. Evaluation of symptoms in the upper extremity should proceed from proximal to distal because of the influence of the cervical spine and thoracic inlet on circulatory and neural functions. Whether the practitioner is using a circulatory or a neurological model, evaluation of the cervical and thoracic spine is appropriate before moving distally to the upper extremity.

BRACHIALGIA

A common operator mistake in upper extremity complaints is to evaluate only at the joint where the symptom is present and proximal thereto. From the structural diagnostic perspective, a patient with pain in the upper extremity under the general rubric of "brachialgia" has five potential entrapment sites for elements of the brachial plexus.

1. The cervical roots are at risk at the intervertebral foramen as they exit from the vertebral canal. Productive change of the uncovertebral joint of Luschka and posterolateral protrusion of intervertebral disk material may narrow the intervertebral canal anteriorly, reducing the space available for the roots. Dysfunction or disease of the zygapophysial joints may negatively affect the foraminal size and shape from the posterior direction, reducing space for the nerve roots. In addition to significant osseous change, swelling and congestion from acute or chronic inflammation can also cause entrapment.

2. The roots are transported through the intertransversariae muscles between the transverse processes of the cervical vertebra. Hypertonicity of these short fourth-layer spinal muscles, with accompanying chronic passive congestion, may also be a site of potential entrapment.

3. The roots forming the brachial plexus pass through the scalene muscles. Hypertonicity and passive congestion of these muscles, commonly found in cervical and upper rib cage dysfunction, negatively influence the brachial plexus.

4. As the plexus traverses laterally, it passes through the costoclavicular canal. This triangular-shaped region is bounded by the lateral portion of the second rib and the posterior aspect of the clavicle. Dysfunctions of the second rib, particularly where it is held in an inhalation position in the lateral bucket-handle range, and dysfunction of the sternoclavicular and acromioclavicular articulations can result in potential entrapment at the costoclavicular canal. A large amount of soft tissue occupies space within this region, and if congested, the costoclavicular canal can narrow.

5. More laterally, the neurovascular bundle passes under the insertion of the pectoralis minor tendon to the coronoid process of the scapula. Hypertonicity, shortening, and thickening of the pectoralis muscle and its tendon can compress the nerves as they pass distally.

In addition to the neural structures, the vascular and lymphatic channels are also at risk at the scalenes, first rib, costoclavicular canal, and underlying the pectoralis minor tendon. The examiner must thoroughly evaluate the cervical, upper thoracic, and upper rib cage before proceeding with the evaluation and management of the distal region of the upper extremity.

The screening examination (see Chapter 2) for the upper extremities involves the patient actively abducting the upper extremities with the elbows extended and attempting to bring the backs of the hands together over the head. Inability to symmetrically accomplish this maneuver demands further diagnostic evaluation. The upper extremities should be evaluated by traditional orthopedic and neurological testing. A recent addition to testing of the neural structures is the neural dynamic testing of the nervous system for neural and dural restriction. Neural dynamic examination of the upper extremity (Upper Limb Tension Test) are frequently useful in the assessment of the upper extremities.

There are many systems for the structural diagnosis and manual medicine treatment of the extremities. This author has found many of the procedures found in Mennell's *Joint Pain* to be of considerable therapeutic value. Only a few of these procedures are repeated here, and the reader is encouraged to study Mennell's text.

The shoulder, elbow, and wrist are not single joints; each of the regions contains several articulations. For that reason we approach the upper extremity on a regional basis and evaluate the specific articulations individually.

SHOULDER REGION

The shoulder region consists of the sternoclavicular, acromioclavicular, and glenohumeral articulations.

The scapulocostal junction is not a true articulation. The ability of the concave costal surface of the scapula to smoothly move over the thoracic cage is of major importance in upper extremity function, particularly the shoulder region. The direct restrictors of scapulocostal motion are the muscles and fascia, which hold the scapula to the trunk. These myofascial elements are best approached by soft tissue and myofascial release techniques. Particular attention must be given to the trapezius, sternocleidomastoid, levator scapulae, rhomboids, and latissimus dorsi muscles and their fascias. Evaluation and treatment of these muscles should precede the articulations in the shoulder region.

Sternoclavicular Joint

The medial end of the clavicle articulates with the manubrium of the sternum. Within this joint is found a meniscus. The medial end of the clavicle is intimately related to the anterior aspect of the first rib. The joint is polyaxial in its movement, with the primary motions being abduction, horizontal flexion, and rotation. As the clavicle is abducted, it externally (posteriorly) rotates, and as it returns to neutral, it internally (anteriorly) rotates. Rotation then becomes a coupled movement with abduction.

Upper Extremity

Sternoclavicular Joint

Diagnosis
Test for Restricted Abduction

1. Patient supine on table with arms resting easily at the side.

2. Operator stands at side or head of table with paired fingers over the superior aspect of the medial end of the clavicle (Fig. 18.1).

3. The patient is asked to actively "shrug the shoulders" by bringing the shoulder tip to the ear bilaterally (Fig. 18.2).

4. The operator's palpating fingers follow the movement at the medial end of the clavicle.

5. The normal finding is equal movement of the medial end of both clavicles in a caudad direction.

6. A positive finding is the failure of one clavicle to move caudad when compared with the opposite. It appears to be held in the original starting position.

Note: This test can also be done with patient sitting.

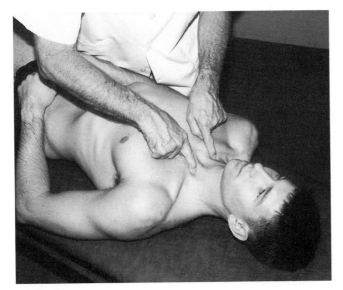

Figure 18.1.

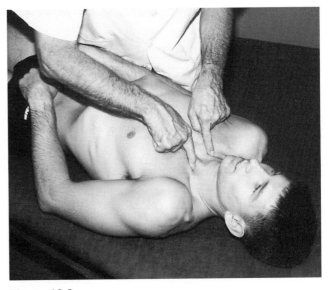

Figure 18.2.

Upper Extremity

Sternoclavicular Joint

Mobilization Without Impulse (Articulatory) Treatment

Diagnosis: Restricted Abduction

1. Patient sits on the examining table or stool.

2. Operator stands behind patient with the thenar eminence of one hand over the superior aspect of the medial end of the dysfunctional clavicle; the other hand grasps the patient's forearm (Fig. 18.3).

3. The operator abducts the extended upper extremity to the resistant barrier (Fig. 18.4) and sweeps it across the patient's torso in the direction of the opposite knee while constant caudad pressure is maintained by the thenar eminence on the medial end of the clavicle (Fig. 18.5).

4. Several repetitions are done, increasing the abduction movement of the patient's extended arm. (A high-velocity thrust by the thenar eminence may be used.)

5. Retest.

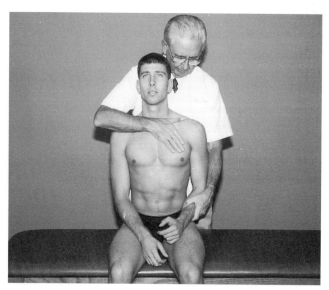

Figure 18.3.

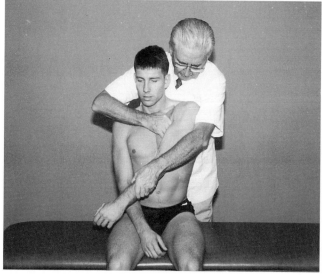

Figure 18.5.

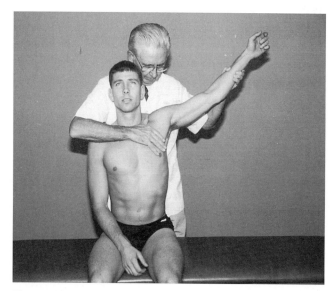

Figure 18.4.

UPPER EXTREMITY

Sternoclavicular Joint

Muscle Energy Technique
Supine
Diagnosis: Restricted Abduction

1. Patient supine on table with the dysfunctional upper extremity at the edge of the table.

2. Operator stands on the side of dysfunction facing cephalward.

3. Operator places one hand over the medial end of the dysfunctional clavicle while the other grasps the patient's forearm just above the wrist (Fig. 18.6).

4. Operator internally rotates the dysfunctional upper extremity into extension off the edge of the table to the resistant barrier while monitoring with the opposite hand at the sternoclavicular region (Fig. 18.7).

5. Patient performs 3- to 5-second muscle contraction for three to five times to extend the arm toward the ceiling against operator resistance.

6. After relaxation, the operator increases the extension of the upper extremity to a new resistant barrier and patient again repeats the effort of lifting the arm toward the ceiling.

7. Retest.

Note: This procedure also increases internal (anterior) rotation at the sternoclavicular joint.

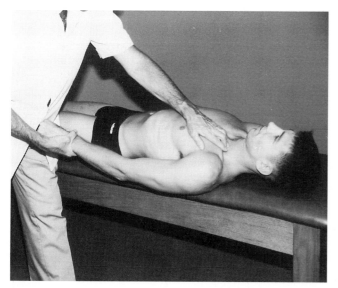

Figure 18.6.

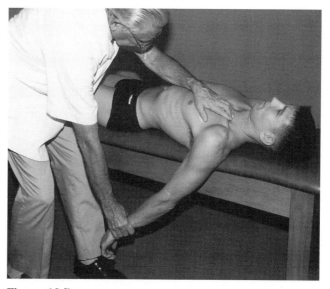

Figure 18.7.

Upper Extremity

Sternoclavicular Joint

Muscle Energy Technique
Sitting
Diagnosis: Restricted Abduction

1. Patient sitting on table or stool.

2. Operator standing behind patient with the thenar eminence of one hand in contact with the superior aspect of the medial end of the dysfunctional clavicle and the other hand controlling the dysfunctional upper extremity at the elbow (Fig. 18.8).

3. With the elbow at 90°, the upper extremity is externally rotated and abducted to approximately 90° with additional abduction until the resistant barrier is engaged (Fig. 18.9).

4. Patient performs muscle contraction to adduct the upper extremity for 3–5 seconds and three to five repetitions against resistance offered at the elbow by the operator.

5. After relaxation, operator engages new barrier.

6. Retest.

Note: This procedure also enhances the external (posterior) rotation at the sternoclavicular joint.

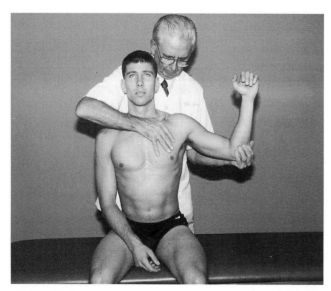

Figure 18.8.

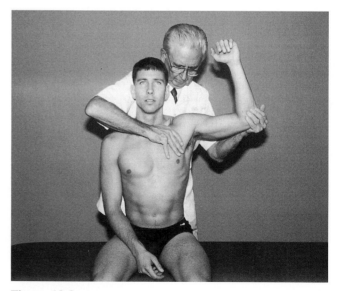

Figure 18.9.

Upper Extremity

Sternoclavicular Joint

Diagnosis

Test for Restricted Horizontal Flexion

1. Patient supine on table.

2. Operator stands at side or head of table with fingers symmetrically placed on the anterior aspect of the medial end of each clavicle (Fig. 18.10).

3. Patient extends the upper extremities in front of the body by reaching toward the ceiling.

4. Operator evaluates movement of the medial end of each clavicle (Fig. 18.11).

5. The normal finding is for each clavicle to move symmetrically in a posterior direction as the lateral end of the clavicle moves anteriorly.

6. A positive finding is for one clavicle not to move in a posterior direction during the reaching effort.

Note: This test can also be done with the patient sitting.

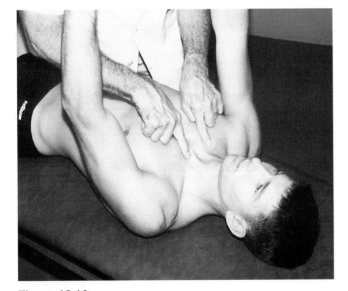

Figure 18.10.

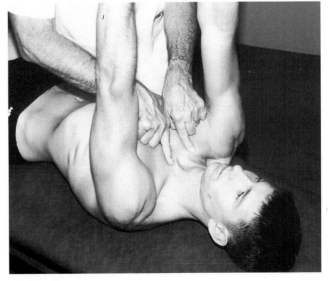

Figure 18.11.

Upper Extremity

Sternoclavicular Joint

Mobilization Without Impulse (Articulatory) Treatment
Sitting
   Diagnosis: Restricted Horizontal Flexion

1. Patient sitting on table.

2. Operator standing behind with one hand on the anterior aspect of the medial end of the dysfunctional clavicle and the lateral hand grasping the forearm (Fig. 18.12).

3. Operator takes the upper extremity into horizontal extension (Fig. 18.13) and sweeps it forward in horizontal flexion (Fig. 18.14) with increasing arcs of movement while the thenar eminence of the opposite hand maintains a posterior compressive force on the medial end of the dysfunctional clavicle. (A high-velocity thrust by the thenar eminence may be substituted.)

4. Retest.

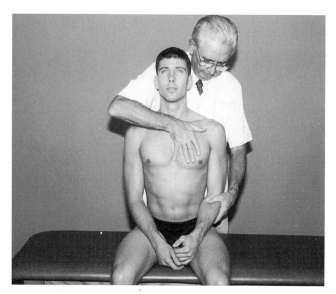

Figure 18.12.

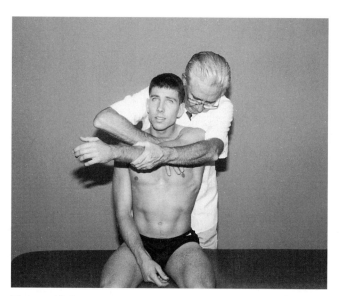

Figure 18.14.

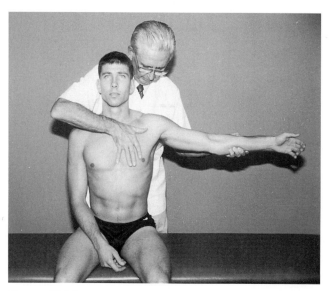

Figure 18.13.

Upper Extremity

Sternoclavicular Joint

Muscle Energy Technique
Supine
Diagnosis: Restricted Horizontal Flexion

1. Patient supine on table.

2. Operator stands on side of table opposite the dysfunctional sternoclavicular joint.

3. Operator places cephalic hand over the medial end of the dysfunctional clavicle and the caudad hand grasps the patient's shoulder girdle over the posterior aspect of the scapula (Fig. 18.15).

4. Patient's hand grasps back of operator's neck with an extended arm.

5. Operator engages the horizontal flexion barrier by standing more erect and lifting the dysfunctional scapula (Fig. 18.16).

6. Patient pulls down on the operator's neck by 3- to 5-second muscle effort with three to five repetitions while operator maintains posterior compression on the anterior aspect of the medial end of the dysfunctional clavicle.

7. Operator engages new barrier after each patient muscle contraction.

8. Retest.

Upper Extremity

Sternoclavicular Joint

Mobilization Without Impulse (Articulatory) Technique
Diagnosis: Restricted Horizontal Flexion

1. Patient is supine, and operator stands on opposite side of dysfunction.

2. Operator places caudad forearm on table between chest and humerus.

3. Patient's opposite hand grasps wrist of dysfunctional extremity. A pull places traction on the clavicle.

4. Operator's cephalic hand applies pressure on medial end of dysfunctional clavicle (Fig. 18.17).

5. Patient pulls on wrist, distracting the clavicle, while operator springs the medial end of the clavicle posteriorly.

6. Retest.

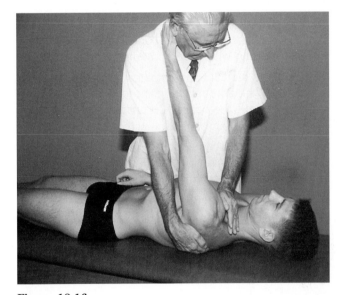

Figure 18.16.

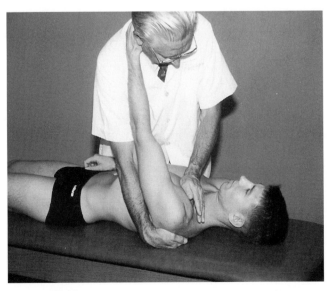

Figure 18.15.

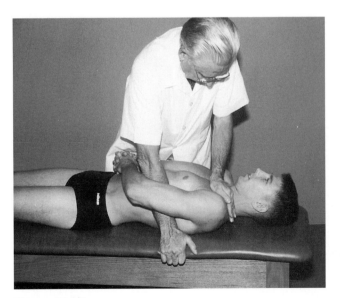

Figure 18.17.

ACROMIOCLAVICULAR JOINT

The acromioclavicular joint contributes a small amount of motion to the shoulder region. The joint depends largely on ligaments for its integrity and frequently separates during trauma. Productive change at this joint is common. Clinical experience has shown that loss of acromioclavicular joint function is highly significant, particularly the loss of abduction. The primary movements of this articulation are abduction and internal and external rotation. The joint is angled laterally at approximately 30° from before backward. This is important to remember during motion testing of the shoulder girdle. Dysfunction of this joint is frequently overlooked.

Upper Extremity

Acromioclavicular Joint

Diagnosis
  Test for Restricted Abduction and Adduction
1. Patient sitting with operator standing behind.

2. Operator's medial hand palpates the superior aspect of the acromioclavicular joint and the lateral hand controls the patient's proximal forearm (Fig. 18.18).

3. Operator introduces adduction and external rotation of the forearm, monitoring a gapping movement at the acromioclavicular joint (Fig. 18.19).

4. Absence of the gapping movement is evidence of restriction of adduction movement.

5. Comparison is made with the opposite side.

6. Operator introduces abduction movement while monitoring at the joint for movement (Fig. 18.20).

7. Comparison is made with the opposite side.

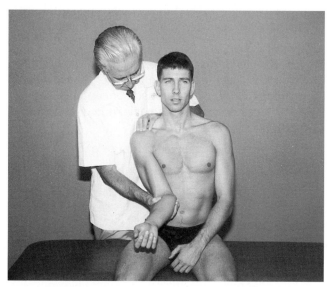

Figure 18.19.

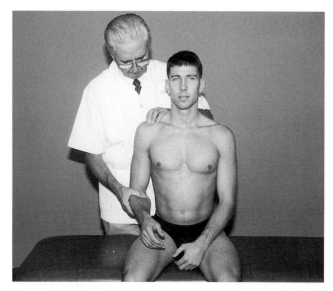

Figure 18.18.

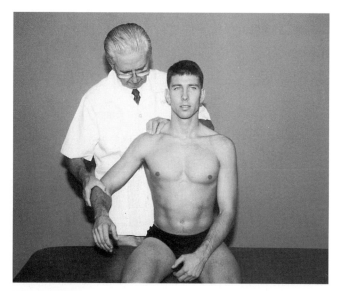

Figure 18.20.

Upper Extremity

Acromioclavicular Joint

Muscle Energy Technique
Sitting
Diagnosis: Restricted Abduction

1. Patient sitting on table or stool with operator standing behind.

2. Operator maintains compressive force on lateral end of the clavicle, medial to the acromioclavicular joint.

3. Operator's lateral hand takes patient's upper extremity to horizontal flexion of 30° and abducts to the barrier (Fig. 18.21).

4. Patient pulls elbow to the side against resistance offered by the operator for 3–5 seconds and three to five repetitions.

5. Operator engages new abduction barrier after each muscle effort.

6. Retest.

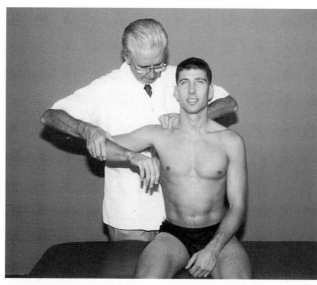

Figure 18.21.

Upper Extremity

Acromioclavicular Joint

Diagnosis: Test for Restricted Internal and External Rotation

1. Patient sitting on table or stool with operator standing behind.

2. Operator's medial hand palpates the superior aspect of the acromioclavicular joint.

3. Operator's lateral hand moves the upper extremity into horizontal flexion to 30° and abduction to the first barrier (Fig. 18.22).

4. Operator introduces internal rotation (Fig. 18.23) and external rotation (Fig. 18.24) while monitoring mobility of the acromioclavicular joint.

5. Comparison is made with the opposite side.

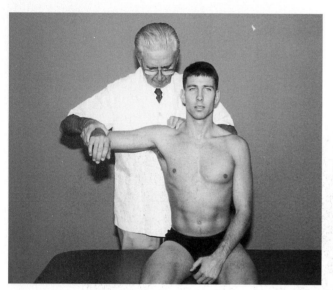

Figure 18.22.

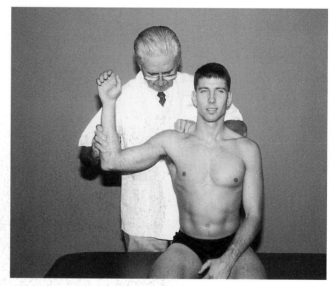

Figure 18.24.

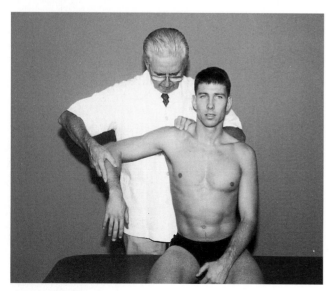

Figure 18.23.

Upper Extremity

Acromioclavicular Joint

Muscle Energy Technique
  Diagnosis: Restricted Internal or External Rotation

1. Patient sitting on table or stool with operator standing behind.

2. Operator's medial hand stabilizes the lateral aspect of the clavicle and monitors the acromioclavicular joint.

3. Operator takes upper extremity to 30° of horizontal flexion and abduction to 90°.

4. External rotational barrier is engaged with the operator's lateral hand grasping the patient's wrist and forearm to forearm (Fig. 18.25).

5. Operator engages internal rotation barrier by threading lateral forearm under patient's elbow and grasping distal forearm (Fig. 18.26).

6. Patient provides muscle contraction for 3–5 seconds and three to five repetitions against resistance of either internal or external rotation.

7. Operator engages new barrier after each muscle contraction.

8. Retest.

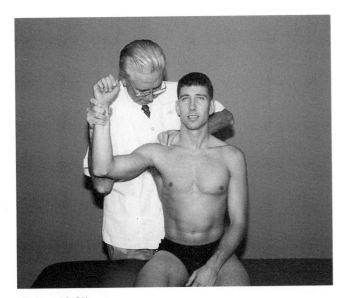

Figure 18.25.

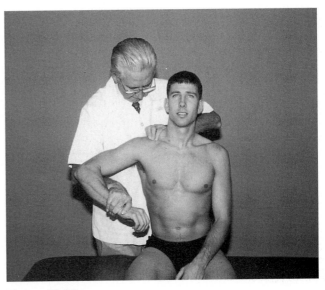

Figure 18.26.

GLENOHUMERAL JOINT

The glenohumeral joint has one of the widest ranges of movement of any joint within the body. The depth of the glenoid is increased by the cartilaginous glenoidal labrum. The articular capsule is normally quite lax and loose, particularly inferiorly, providing for a wide range of movement. Joint integrity is maintained by the intimate attachment of the rotator cuff muscles (supraspinatus, infraspinatus, terres minor, and subscapularis) to the articular capsule.

The extensive movements of this joint are described in relation to the vertical and horizontal planes. In the vertical or neutral plane, the humerus is at the side of the body. Movement then occurs in flexion, extension, internal rotation, and external rotation. In the horizontal plane, with the humerus at 90° to the trunk, it is also possible to have flexion, extension, internal rotation, and external rotation. Adduction moves the humerus toward the body and in front of the chest, and abduction moves the arm away from the body with full-range extending so that the elbow can touch the ear. All of these motions should be tested and compared with the opposite side. The primary movement loss in the glenohumeral joint involves the function of external rotation and abduction. The humeral head must move from cephalad to caudad on the glenoid during abduction. Loss of this ability to track from superior to inferior during abduction results in major restriction at the glenohumeral joint.

Because the vast majority of dysfunctions within the glenohumeral joint are muscular in origin, muscle energy diagnostic and therapeutic techniques are most effective. The principles of diagnosis and treatment are (a) to evaluate range of motion in all of the motion directions described above, (b) to evaluate the strengths of each of the muscle groups, (c) to treat restricted range of movement by isometric technique at the restrictive barrier, and (d) if weakness is identified, to treat by means of a series of concentric isotonic contractions. Each motion should be compared with that available on the opposite side.

Glenohumeral Joint

Muscle Energy Procedure

1. Patient sits on table or stool with operator standing behind.

2. Range of motion is tested in all directions by engaging the restrictive barrier. Comparison is made with the opposite side.

3. If motion is restricted, operator engages resistant barrier. Patient performs three to five repetitions of a 3- to 7-second isometric contraction against operator resistance.

4. Strength testing is done by having the patient contract in the direction of operator resistance. Comparison is made with the opposite side. If one muscle group is found to be weak, a series of three to five

concentric isotonic contractions through total range of movement is performed against progressively increasing resistance by the operator.

5. Operator's medial hand stabilizes the shoulder girdle with the fingers on the coracoid process, the web of the hand over the acromioclavicular joint, and the thumb posterior and inferior over the spine of the scapula.

6. Operator's lateral hand controls patient's elbow and forearm.

7. Operator introduces the following motions and treats accordingly:
   - Neutral flexion (Fig. 18.27);
   - Neutral extension (Fig. 18.28);
   - Neutral external rotation (Fig. 18.29);
   - Neutral internal rotation stage 1 (Fig. 18.30);

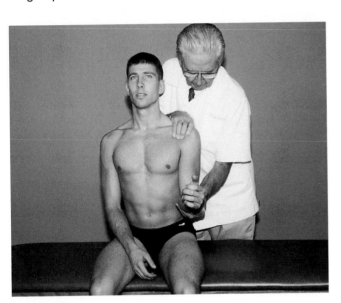

Figure 18.27.

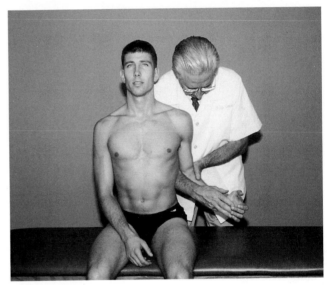

Figure 18.29.

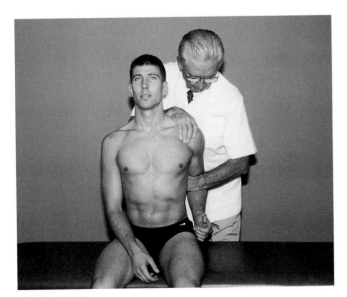

Figure 18.28.

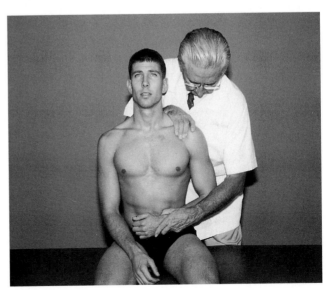

Figure 18.30.

- Neutral Internal rotation stage 2 (Fig. 18.31);
- Adduction (Fig. 18.32);
- Abduction (Fig. 18.33);
- Horizontal flexion (Fig. 18.34);

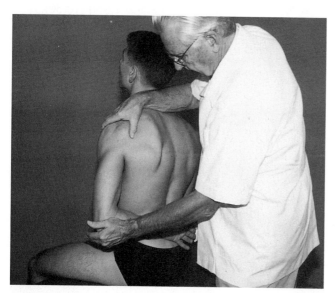

Figure 18.31.

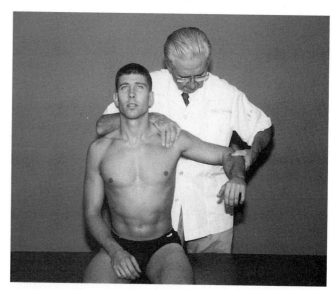

Figure 18.33.

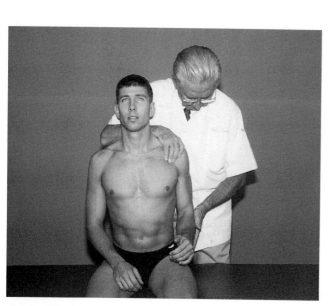

Figure 18.32.

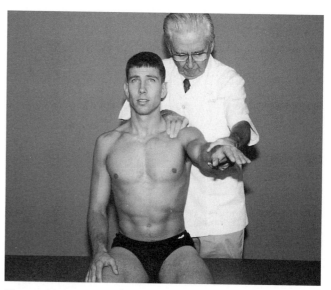

Figure 18.34.

- Horizontal extension (Fig. 18.35);
- Horizontal internal rotation (Fig. 18.36);
- Horizontal external rotation (Fig. 18.37).

8. Retest.

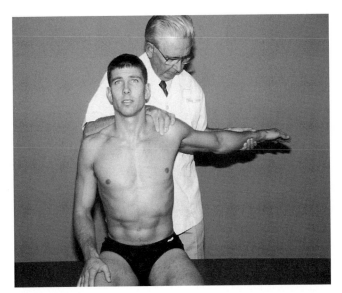

Figure 18.35.

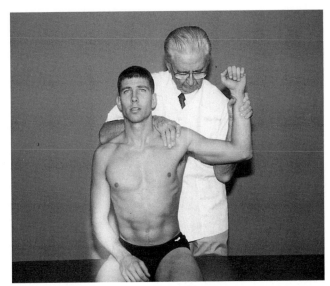

Figure 18.37.

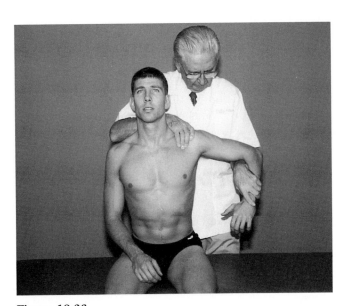

Figure 18.36.

Glenohumeral Joint (Green's) Glenoid Labrum Technique

This technique enhances movement of the humeral head within the glenoid and glenoid labrum.

1. Patient prone with the involved arm off the edge of the table, and operator sits at side facing dysfunctional shoulder (Fig. 18.38).
2. Operator grasps distal humerus in both hands and applies caudad and anterior traction with internal and external rotation two to three times (Fig. 18.39).
3. Operator next grasps patients humeral neck with thumbs on the greater tuberosity, the index and middle fingers on the attachment of the rotator cuff, and the ring and little fingers surrounding the proximal shaft, controlling the humeral shaft against the thenar eminences (Fig. 18.40).
4. Operator applies movement through the humeral head in an anterior-posterior, cephalic-caudad, and medial and lateral traction distraction directions.
5. Operator induces circular and figure of eight motions, enhancing range in all directions.
6. Operator emphasizes increase in caudad translatory movement of the humeral head on the glenoid.
7. Retest.

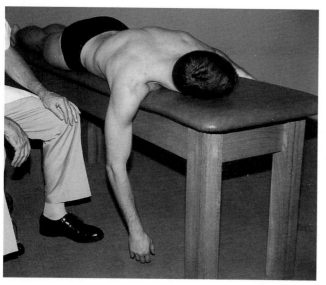

Figure 18.38.

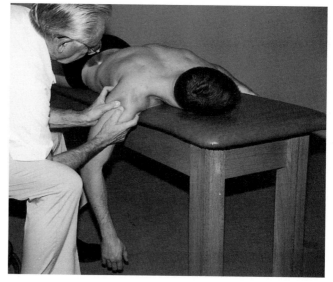

Figure 18.40.

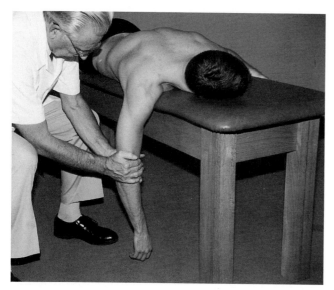

Figure 18.39.

Glenohumeral Seven Step Spencer Technique

The principle is sequential, direct action, mobilization without impulse (articulatory) technique against motion resistance.

1. Patient in lateral recumbent position with affected shoulder uppermost, head supported, knees flexed.

2. Operator stands facing patient.

3. Operator's proximal hand stabilizes the shoulder girdle, including the clavicle and scapula.

4. (Step 1) Operator gently flexes (Fig. 18.41) and extends arm (Fig. 18.42) in the sagittal plane with the elbow flexed. Repetitions are made within limits of pain provocation.

5. (Step 2) Operator flexes patient's arm in the sagittal plane with elbow extended in a rhythmic swinging movement, increasing range so that patient's arm covers the ear (Fig. 18.43).

6. (Step 3) Operator circumducts patient's abducted humerus with the elbow flexed. Clockwise and counterclockwise concentric circles with gradual increase in range are made within limits of pain (Fig. 18.44).

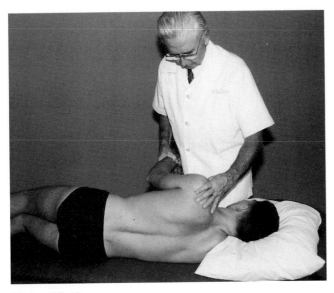

Figure 18.41.

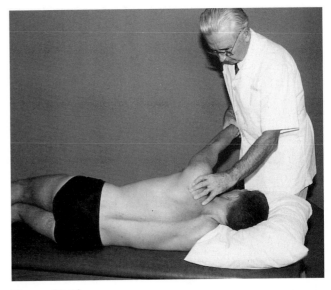

Figure 18.43.

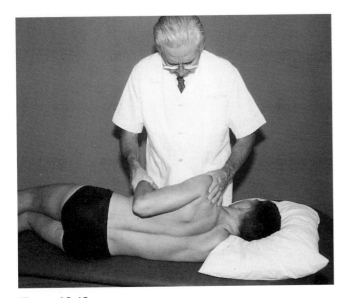

Figure 18.42.

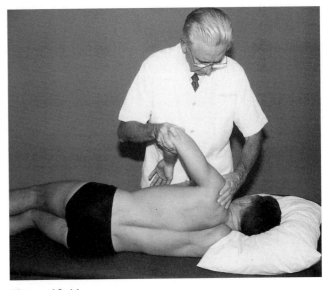

Figure 18.44.

7. (Step 4) Operator circumducts patient's humerus with elbow extended in clockwise and counter-clockwise circles, increasing range permitted by pain (Fig. 18.45).

8. (Step 5) Operator abducts patient's arm with elbow flexed with gradual increases of range of abduction against the stabilized shoulder girdle (Fig. 18.46).

9. (Step 6) Operator places patient's hand behind the rib cage and gently springs elbow forward and inferior, increasing internal rotation of the humerus (Fig. 18.47).

10. (Step 7) Operator grasps patient's proximal humerus with both hands and applies lateral and caudad traction in a pumping fashion (Fig. 18.48).

11. Retest.

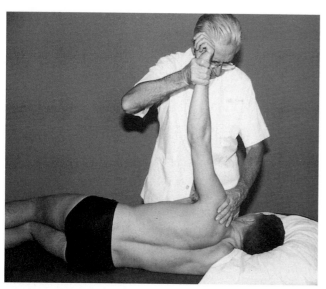

Figure 18.45.

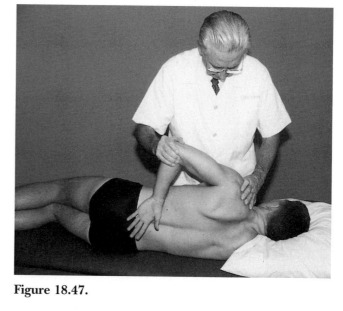

Figure 18.47.

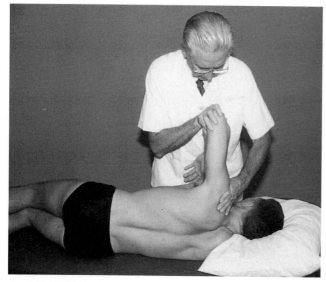

Figure 18.46.

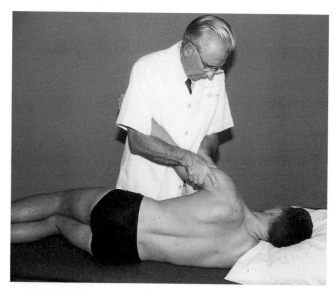

Figure 18.48.

ELBOW REGION

There are three joints at the elbow region: the ulnohumeral joint, the radiohumeral joint, and the proximal radioulnar joint. The primary movements are flexion and extension, pronation and supination, and a small amount of abduction-adduction. All joints participate in elbow function. Flexion-extension is the primary movement at the ulnohumeral joint, and pronation-supination is a combined radiohumeral and proximal radioulnar joint movement. Abduction-adduction movement is primarily a joint play movement at the ulnohumeral joint and, when dysfunctional, reduces the flexion-extension range. The elbow region has a number of related pain syndromes frequently described as "tennis elbow." Many of these patients present with pain on the lateral aspect of the elbow, radiating into the forearm and aggravated by activity. Dysfunction of the radial head, involving the proximal radioulnar and the radiohumeral joint, is a frequent finding. Radial head dysfunction is the most common somatic dysfunction within the elbow region.

Elbow Region

Diagnosis: Restricted Abduction-Adduction (Ulnohumeral joint)

1. Patient sitting on table with operator standing in front.
2. Operator's two hands circumferentially grasp proximal radioulnar region.
3. Operator supports patient's hand and wrist between lateral elbow and trunk.
4. Operator's hands introduce translatory movement medially (Fig. 18.49) and laterally (Fig. 18.50)

through the arc from flexion to extension, testing for resistance.

5. Comparison made with the opposite side.
6. A direct action mobilization without impulse, carried through to mobilization with impulse, has operator engage either the adduction or abduction barrier while extended (Fig. 18.51). Mobilization without impulse repetitions are made against resistant barrier with final mobilization with impulse performed.
7. Retest.

Note: Adduction restriction is more common than abduction.

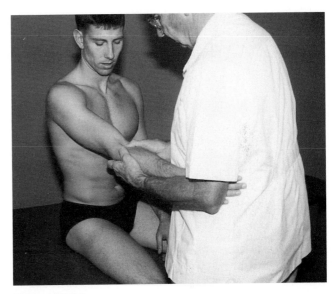

Figure 18.50.

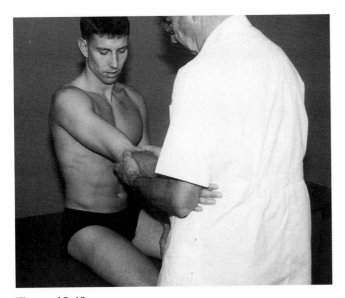

Figure 18.49.

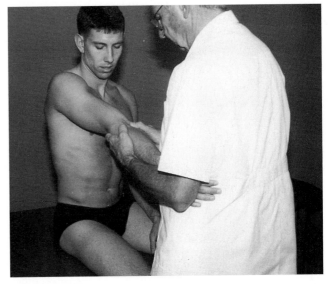

Figure 18.51.

Elbow Region

Muscle Energy Technique
Restricted Elbow Extension

1. Patient sitting on table with operator standing in front.
2. Operator medial hand grasps patient's distal supinated forearm with lateral hand stabilizing the elbow.
3. Elbow extension barrier is engaged (Fig. 18.52).
4. Patient performs a series of three to five muscle contractions for 3–5 seconds against operator's resistance.
5. Operator progressively engages elbow extension barrier after each muscle contraction (Fig. 18.53).

6. Retest.
7. An alternate technique has patient perform three to five series of isotonic contractions of the triceps muscle through full flexion to extension arc.
8. Operator fully flexes elbow, stabilizing elbow with lateral hand and grasping distal forearm to provide resistance to isotonic contraction (Fig. 18.54).
9. Patient performs three to five repetitions with progressive increasing resistance by the operator's medial hand until full elbow extension is achieved (Fig. 18.55).
10. Retest.

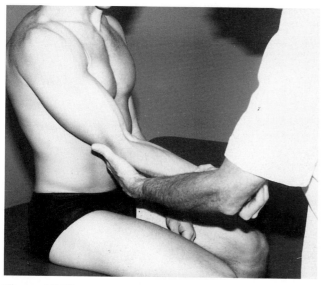

Figure 18.52.

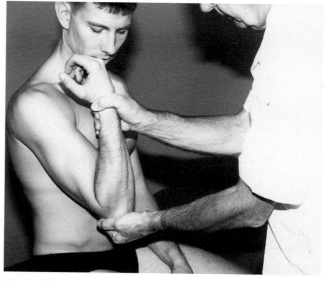

Figure 18.54.

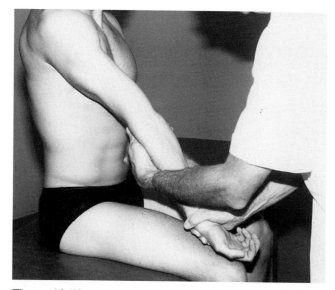

Figure 18.53.

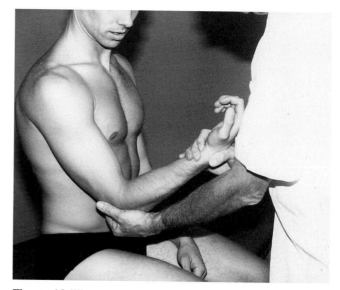

Figure 18.55.

Elbow Region

Muscle Energy Technique
Restricted Pronation and Supination

1. Patient sitting on table with operator standing in front.

2. Operator's medial hand stabilizes patient elbow flexed to 90°. Lateral hand grasps distal forearm, wrist, and hand with patient's thumb pointing vertically (Fig. 18.56).

3. Operator introduces supination (Fig. 18.57) and pronation (Fig. 18.58), testing for restriction.

4. Comparison is made with the opposite side.

5. Treatment of restricted supination has operator's lateral hand stabilizing the flexed elbow and monitoring the radial head while medial hand supinates forearm to resistant barrier (Fig. 18.59).

6. Patient performs three to five muscle contractions for 3–5 seconds against resistance offered by operator's medial hand.

7. Operator engages new supination barrier after each patient effort.

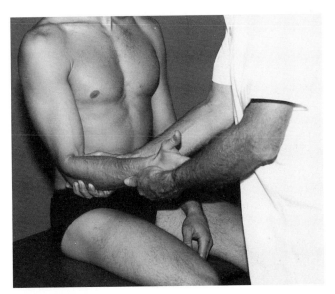

Figure 18.56.

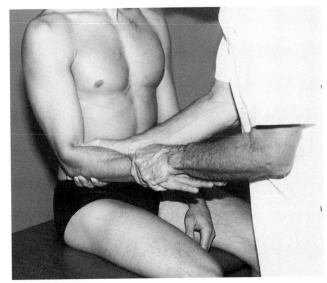

Figure 18.58.

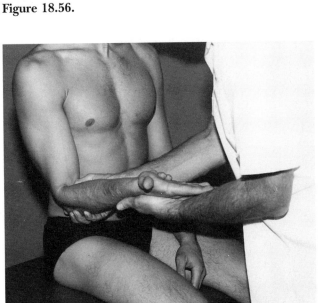

Figure 18.57.

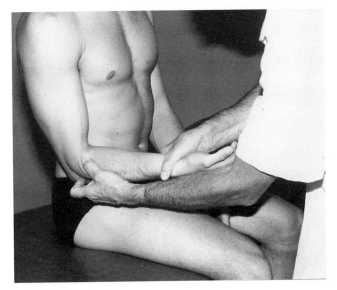

Figure 18.59.

8. Treatment of restricted pronation has operator's two hands in same location but engaging pronation barrier (Fig. 18.60).

9. Patient performs three to five muscle contractions for 3–5 seconds against operator resistance.

10. Operator engages new pronation barrier after each muscle contraction.

11. Retest.

Note: Restricted pronation and supination of the forearm combines motion of the radiohumeral, proximal radioulnar, and distal radioulnar articulations. Supination is the most common restriction.

Elbow Region

Diagnosis of Radial Head Dysfunction
Test 1: Palpation for Asymmetry

1. Patient sitting on table with elbows flexed to 90° and forearms supinated and supported in lap.

2. Operator stands in front and palpates the radial head posteriorly with the index fingers and the soft tissues anteriorly with the thumbs (Fig. 18.61).

3. Operator assesses the symmetrical relation of the radial head to the capitulum of the humerus.

4. In addition to asymmetry, the dysfunctional side is usually tender with tension of the periarticular tissues.

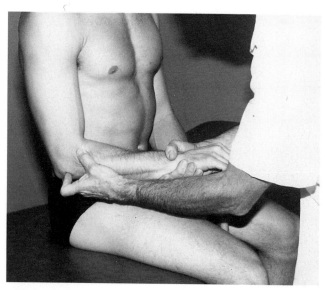

Figure 18.60.

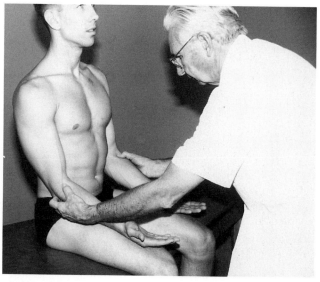

Figure 18.61.

Elbow Region

Diagnosis of Radial Head Dysfunction
Test 2: Motion of the Radial Head

1. Patient sitting on table with elbow flexed to 90°.

2. Operator stands in front with lateral hand palpating the radial head at the radiohumeral articulation with the index finger posteriorly and the thumb anteriorly.

3. Operator's medial hand grasping distal radius and ulna introduces supination (Fig. 18.62) and pronation (Fig. 18.63).

4. Comparison is made with the opposite side. In dysfunction, asymmetry is identified between the radial head and the capitulum.

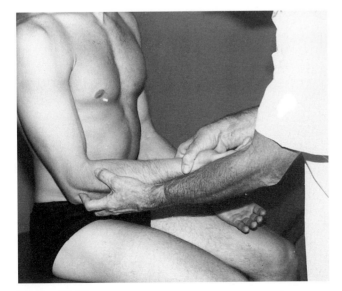

Figure 18.62.

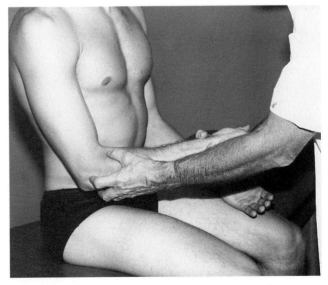

Figure 18.63.

Elbow Region

Diagnosis of Radial Head Dysfunction
Test 3: Motion Test

1. Patient sits on table with forearms supinated.

2. Patient flexes and brings elbows to front of chest with medial margins of forearm and hand approximated (Fig. 18.64).

3. Patient attempts to extend elbows while maintaining forearms together (Fig. 18.65).

4. Dysfunction of the radial head is identified by forearm pronating during elbow extension.

Elbow Region

Muscle Energy Technique
Diagnosis
        Position: Radial head posterior
        Motion restriction: Supination

1. Patient sitting on table with elbow flexed to 90°.

2. Operator stands in front with lateral hand supporting the proximal forearm and index finger over the posterior aspect of the radial head.

3. Operator's medial hand grasps distal forearm and introduces supination to the barrier (Fig. 18.66).

4. Patient pronates the hand against operator resistance for 3–5 seconds and three to five repetitions.

5. Operator engages new supination barrier after each patient effort.

6. With last patient muscle effort, an attempt is made to flex the elbow in addition to pronation.

7. Retest.

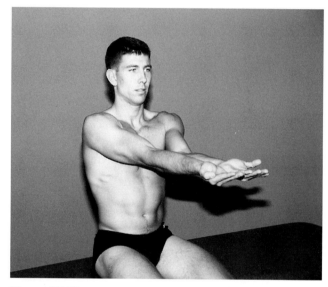

Figure 18.65.

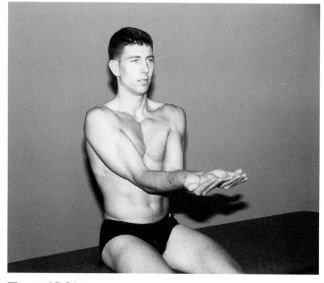

Figure 18.64.

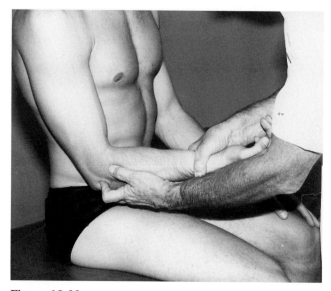

Figure 18.66.

Elbow Region

Mobilization with Impulse Technique
Diagnosis
Position: Radial head posterior
Motion restriction: Supination

1. Patient sitting on the table.

2. Operator stands in front grasping proximal forearm with index finger of lateral hand overlying posterior aspect of radial head (Fig. 18.67).

3. Operator controls patient's distal forearm, hand, and wrist between elbow and chest wall.

4. Operator engages barrier of extension, supination, and slight adduction (Fig. 18.68).

5. Operator performs mobilization with impulse thrust in a lateral and anterior direction.

6. Retest.

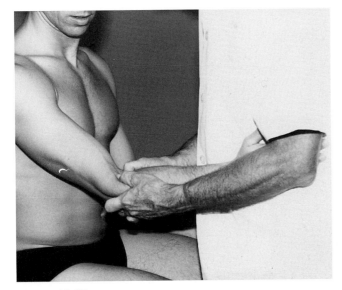

Figure 18.67.

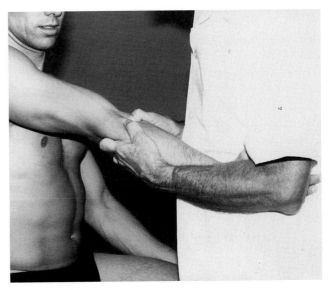

Figure 18.68.

Elbow Region

Mobilization with Impulse Technique
Diagnosis
Position: Radial head anterior
Motion restriction: Pronation

1. Patient standing or sitting on table.

2. Operator stands in front with medial hand grasping proximal forearm and thumb of lateral hand over the anterior aspect of the radial head (Fig. 18.69).

3. Operator pronates and flexes patient's forearm while thumb holds radial head posteriorly (Fig. 18.70).

4. When barrier is engaged, a mobilization with impulse thrust is made by increasing elbow flexion.

5. Retest.

WRIST AND HAND REGION

Like the elbow, the wrist is not a single articulation but a combination of many. They include the radiocarpal joint with the distal radius articulating with the carpal scaphoid and lunate, the distal radioulnar joint, the ulnar-meniscal-triquetral, the intercarpal joint, and the carpometacarpal joints. Movements at the wrist region include dorsiflexion, palmar flexion, adduction (ulnar deviation), abduction (radial deviation), and pronation and supination. Pronation and supination occur primarily at the distal radioulnar joint and are related to similar pronation-supination movement at the elbow region.

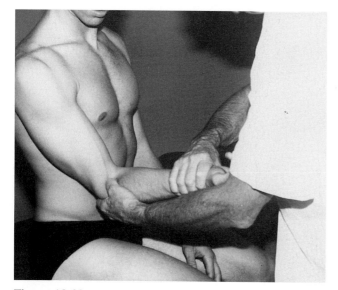

Figure 18.69.

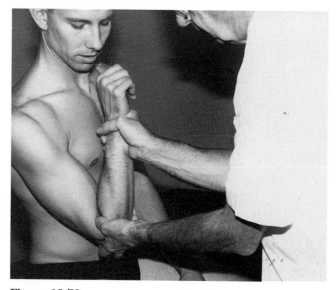

Figure 18.70.

Wrist and Hand Region

Diagnosis

1. Patient sitting on table with operator standing in front.
2. Patient's arms at the side with elbows flexed to 90°.

3. Operator introduces palmar flexion (Fig. 18.71), dorsiflexion (Fig. 18.72), ulnar deviation pronated (Fig. 18.73), radial deviation pronated (Fig. 18.74), radial

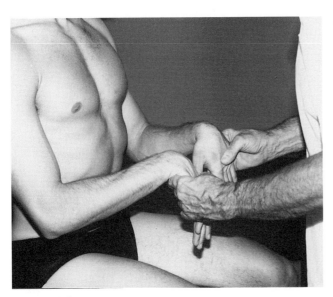

Figure 18.71.

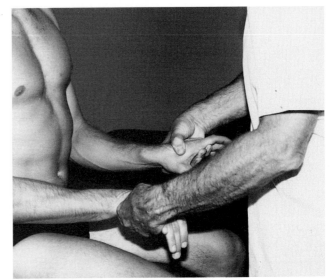

Figure 18.73.

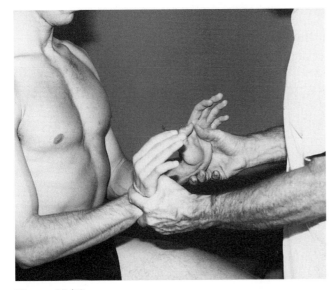

Figure 18.72.

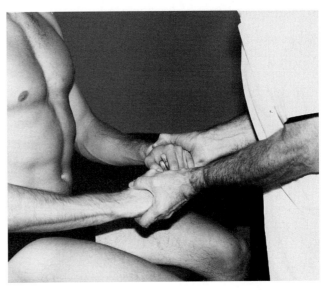

Figure 18.74.

deviation supinated (Fig. 18.75), and ulnar deviation supinated (Fig. 18.76) testing for restricted range of movement.

4. Muscle strength testing can be performed in the same directions.

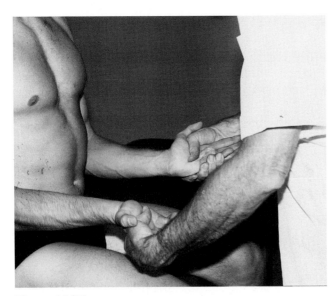

Figure 18.75.

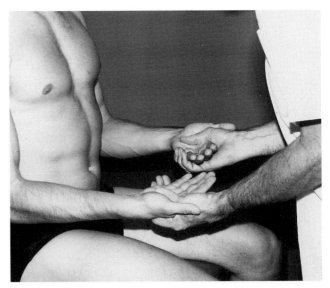

Figure 18.76.

Wrist and Hand Region

Muscle Energy Technique

1. Patient sitting on table with operator standing in front.

2. Operator's proximal hand stabilizes patient's distal forearm while distal hand engages resistant barrier of wrist and hand motion.

3. Operator engages resistant barriers in palmar flexion (Fig. 18.77), dorsiflexion (Fig. 18.78), pronated radial deviation (Fig. 18.79), pronated ulnar deviation (Fig. 18.80),

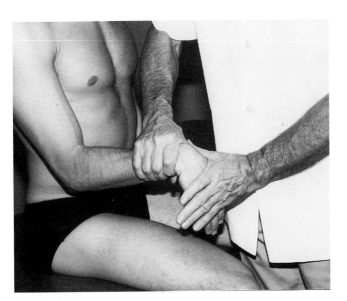

Figure 18.77.

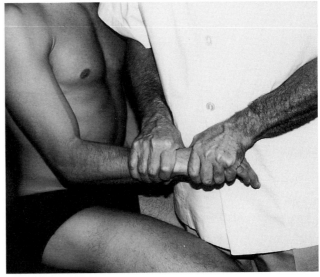

Figure 18.79.

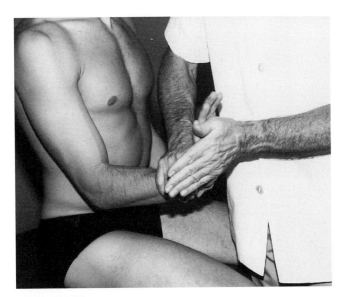

Figure 18.78.

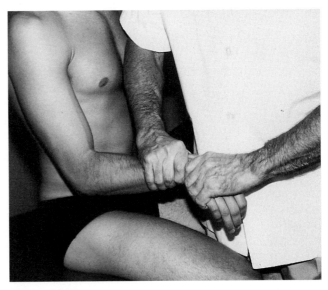

Figure 18.80.

supinated radial deviation (Fig. 18.81), and supinated ulnar deviation (Fig. 18.82).

4. Patient performs 3- to 5-second muscle contraction against operator resistance with three to five repetitions.

5. Operator engages new barrier after each patient effort.

6. Retest.

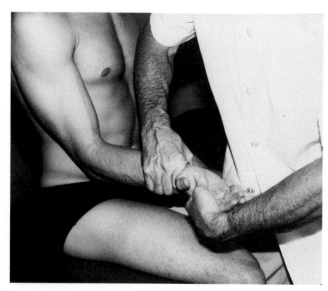

Figure 18.81.

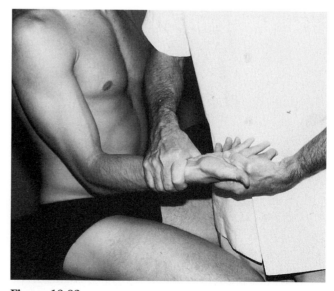

Figure 18.82.

Wrist and Hand Region

  Mobilization with Impulse Technique
1. Patient sitting on table with operator standing in front.
2. Operator's two hands grasp patient's hand and wrist with operator's thumbs contacting dorsal aspect of the scaphoid and lunate (Fig. 18.83) and with index fingers grasping volar aspect of the scaphoid and lunate (Fig. 18.84).
3. Operator engages dorsiflexion barrier and applies mobilization with impulse thrust by taking patient's wrist toward the floor (Fig. 18.85).
4. Operator engages palmar flexion barrier and provides a mobilization with impulse thrust by carrying wrist toward the ceiling (Fig. 18.86).

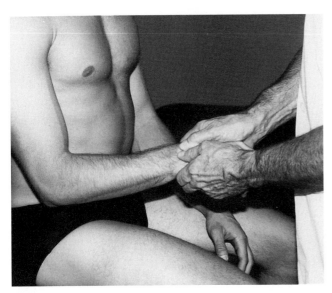

Figure 18.83.

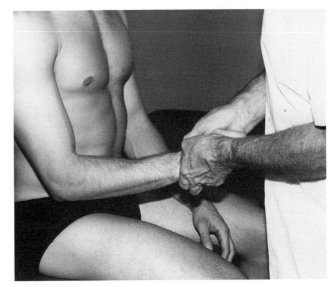

Figure 18.85.

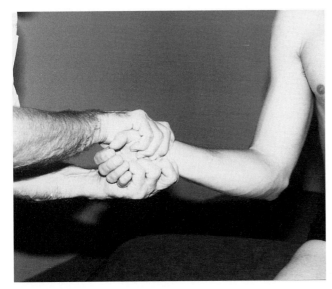

Figure 18.84.

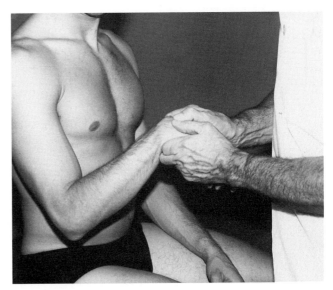

Figure 18.86.

5. Operator engages radial deviation barrier and performs mobilization with impulse thrust while taking the wrist laterally (Fig. 18.87).

6. Operator engages ulnar deviation barrier and provides mobilization with impulse thrust by taking the wrist medially (Fig. 18.88).

7. Retest.

Wrist and Hand Region

   Joint Play
      Radiocarpal Joint

1. Patient sitting or standing on table with operator in front.

2. Operator's proximal hand stabilizes patient's elbow flexed to 90°.

3. Operator's distal hand grasps radiocarpal joint just distal to the radial and ulnar styloid processes (Fig. 18.89).

4. Operator takes up long axis extension to barrier.

5. A long axis extension thrust is performed by the distal hand.

6. Retest.

   Note: This technique also performs joint play movement at the proximal radioulnar and radiohumeral joint.

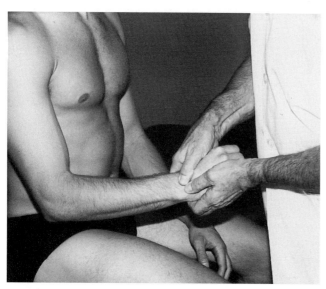

Figure 18.87.

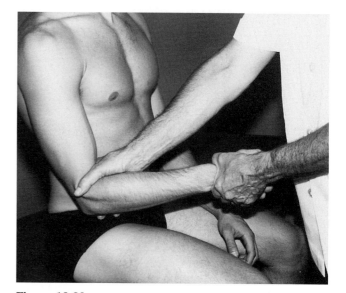

Figure 18.89.

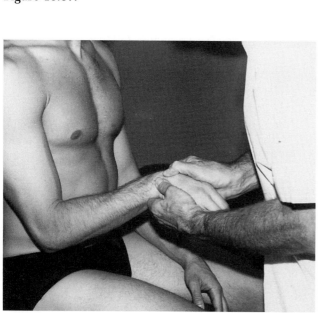

Figure 18.88.

Wrist and Hand Region

Joint Play
Distal Radioulnar and Ulna-Meniscal-Triquetral Articulations

1. Patient standing or sitting on table with operator in front.

2. Operator stabilizes patient's hand and radiocarpal region by placing index finger in the web of the patient's thumb (Fig. 18.90) and with the thenar eminences and middle ring and little fingers grasping the distal radius and proximal carpals (Fig. 18.91).

3. Operator grasps distal ulna between thumb and pads of the fingers (Fig. 18.92).

4. Operator provides anteroposterior glide and medial and lateral rotary joint play movements of the distal ulna (Fig. 18.93).

5. With the same hand hold to stabilize the distal radius and carpals, operator places the right thumb

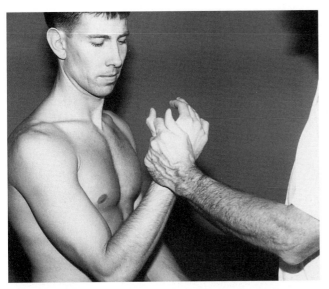

Figure 18.90.

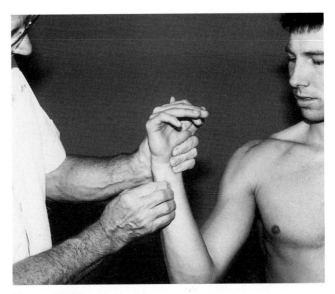

Figure 18.92.

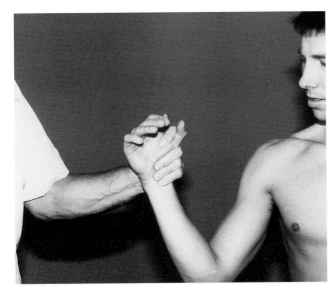

Figure 18.91.

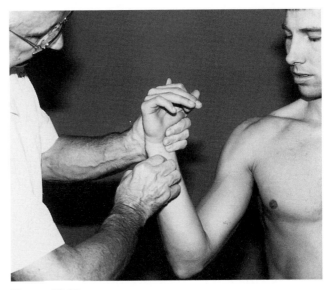

Figure 18.93.

over the dorsal surface of the distal ulna and the proximal interphalangeal joint of the right index finger over the pisiform bone (Fig. 18.94).

6. Operator squeezes thumb and index finger providing an anteroposterior glide joint play movement at the ulnar-meniscal-triquetral joint (Fig. 18.95).

7. The maneuver is a squeeze and release process through operator's right hand.

8. Retest.

Wrist and Hand Region

Joint Play
Midcarpal Joint

1. Patient standing or sitting on table with operator at side.

2. Operator's proximal hand grasps distal radius and ulna, and fingers contact the proximal row of the carpal bones.

3. Operator's distal hand controls patient's hand and distal row of carpal bones.

4. Operator's knuckles of the index fingers and thumbs are together.

5. Operator introduces approximately 15° of palmar flexion to loose pack the midcarpal joint (Fig. 18.96).

6. While maintaining stability with the proximal hand, the distal hand moves toward the ceiling and to the floor, providing an anteroposterior glide of the midcarpal joints.

7. Retest.

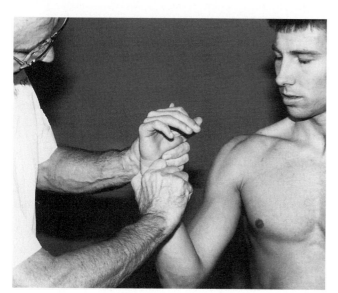

Figure 18.94.

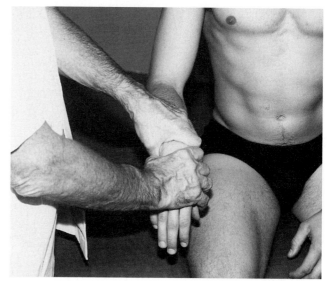

Figure 18.96.

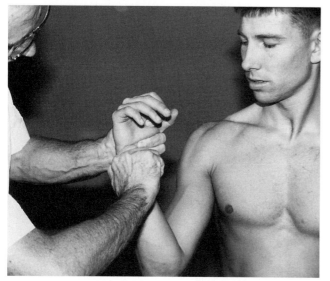

Figure 18.95.

Wrist and Hand Region

Joint Play
Midcarpal Joint Dorsal Tilt

1. Patient standing or sitting on table with operator standing in front.

2. Operator's right thenar eminence is placed transversely across the proximal crease of the patient's wrist, stabilizing the distal radius, ulna, and proximal row of carpals (Fig. 18.97).

3. Operator identifies dorsal aspect of head of capitate by coursing left index finger proximally between the shafts of the patient's second and third metacarpal bones (Fig. 18.98).

4. Operator places left pisiform over head of patient's capitate with the rest of the hand stabilizing patient's hand (Fig. 18.99).

5. Operator's two arms are parallel with each other, and by moving both elbows medially, a joint play dorsal tilt of the head of the capitate is performed.

6. Retest.

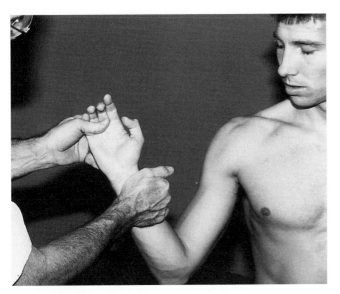

Figure 18.97.

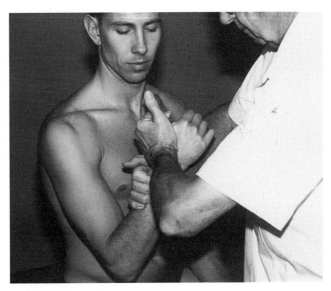

Figure 18.99.

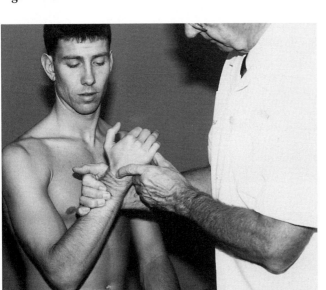

Figure 18.98.

Wrist and Hand Region

Joint Play

First Metacarpal-Carpal Joint

1. Operator's left hand stabilizes patient's wrist and hand (Fig. 18.100).

2. Operator grasps patient's thumb and first metacarpal bone, placing operator's to patient's first metacarpals (Fig. 18.101).

3. Operator performs joint play mobilizing thrust by tilting with the right hand toward the patient, resulting in an anterposterior tilt of the first metacarpal carpal joint.

4. Retest.

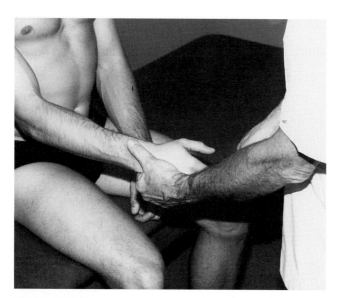

Figure 18.100.

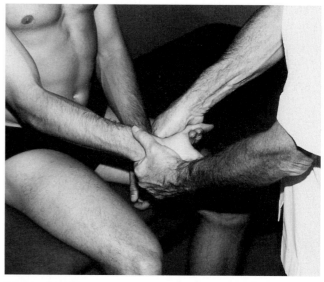

Figure 18.101.

Wrist and Hand Region

Myofascial Release

1. Patient sitting on table with operator standing in front.

2. Operator's two hands grasp patient's hand with one hand holding the thumb (Fig. 18.102) and the other holding the ulnar side of the patient's hand (Fig. 18.103).

3. Operator's hand applied abduction and extension load to the thumb while the other hand introduces radial-ulnar deviation and palmar-dorsi flexion loads in a circular fashion, seeking direct and indirect barriers.

4. Operator localizes to individual carpal bones by contacting dorsal surface with the tip of the thumb and the volar surfaces with the finger pads (Fig. 18.104).

5. Retest.

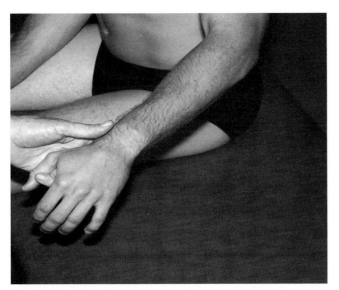

Figure 18.102.

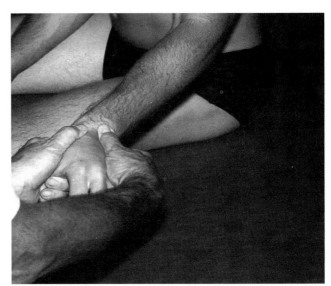

Figure 18.104.

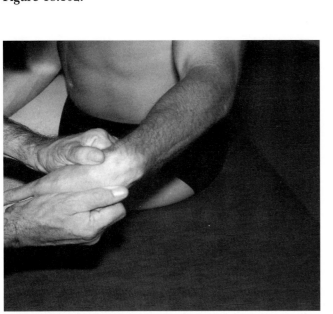

Figure 18.103.

Wrist and Hand Region

Myofascial Release
Wrist Retinaculum

1. Patient sitting on table with operator standing in front.

2. Operator's two hands grasp the patient's hand with the thumbs over the lateral attachments of the wrist retinaculum (Fig. 18.105). Fingers overlie the dorsal aspect of the wrist.

3. Operator's hands introduce dorsiflexion of the patient's wrist (Fig. 18.106).

4. Operator applies lateral distraction load until release is achieved (Fig. 18.107).

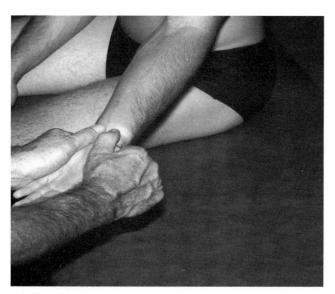

Figure 18.105.

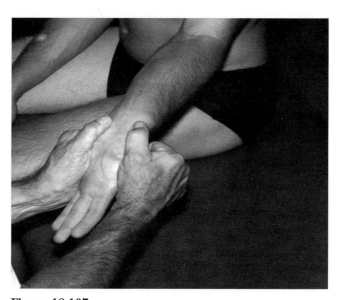

Figure 18.107.

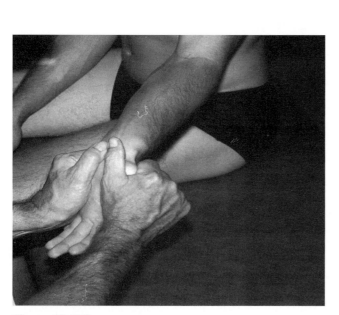

Figure 18.106.

Wrist and Hand Region

Flexor Retinaculum and Flexor Tendons

1. Patient sitting on table with operator standing in front.

2. Operator interlaces the fingers of both hands, applying a thenar eminence contact across distal radius and ulnar on the dorsal side and the wrist retinaculum on the volar side (Fig. 18.108).

3. Operator maintains anteroposterior compression over wrist while patient actively flexes and extends fingers (Fig. 18.109).

4. Patient repeats flexion and extension efforts several times, mobilizing flexor tendons under flexor retinaculum while operator's two hands maintain compression and resulting in distraction.

5. Retest.

SUMMARY

Frequent complaints in the upper extremity include bursitis, tendonitis, epicondylitis, tennis elbow, golfer's elbow, carpal tunnel syndrome, and many others. Dysfunction in the symptomatic joint regions are commonly found, as well as dysfunctions proximal and distal. The identification and appropriate treatment of dysfunctions within the entire upper extremity are helpful in the management of these patients.

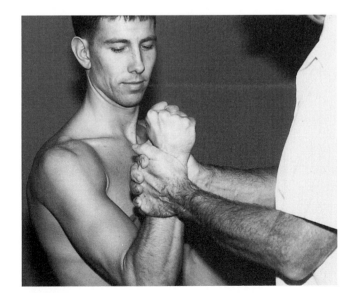

Figure 18.108.

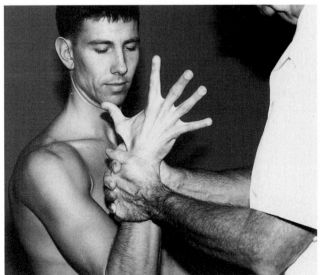

Figure 18.109.

19

The primary function of the lower extremity is ambulation. The complex interactions of the foot, ankle, knee, and hip regions provide a stable base for the trunk in standing and a mobile base for walking and running. Dysfunction in the lower extremities alters the functional capacity of the rest of the body, particularly the pelvic girdle. The screening examination (see Chapter 2) evaluated the lower extremities while standing; during walking; and while performing the squat test, the straight leg raising test (for hamstring length), the standing flexion test, and one-legged stork test. A positive finding of any of these screening tests requires that the examiner further evaluates the hip, knee, foot, and ankle. This chapter deals with the lower extremity from the hip to the distal regions. From the functional perspective, the lower extremity begins at the sacroiliac joint rather than the hip joint. The innominate bone functions as a lower extremity bone during the walking cycle. Assessment of lower extremity function must include the pelvic girdle.

As with the upper extremities, evaluation should proceed from proximal to distal for several reasons. First, when considering the respiratory circulatory model, it is appropriate to proceed from proximal to distal for enhancement of venous and lymphatic return. If edema and inflammation are part of the restrictive process, this sequence assists fluid movement. Second, proceeding from proximal to distal provides the examiner a point of reference for evaluating one bone in relation to another at an articulation. Structural examination of the lower extremities should be combined with standard orthopedic and neurological tests and particularly some of the newer neural and dural tension signs found within the system of mobilization of the nervous system. The ultimate goal of evaluation and treatment of the lower extremities is to return the most symmetrical walking cycle that is possible. Anatomical variation in the bones of the lower extremity can result in the "short leg" and pelvic tilt syndrome that has clinical significance in somatic dysfunction of the vertebral column and pelvic girdle. Alteration in the mechanics of the foot with flattening of the medial, transverse, and lateral arches; of the knee region, including the tibiofemoral and proximal tibiofibular articulation; and the hip may alter function within the vertebral axis and pelvic girdle.

As with the upper extremity, several of Mennell's diagnostic and therapeutic joint play techniques are presented, but a thorough study of that system can be found in the publications by Mennell, including *Joint Pain* and *Foot Pain*.

HIP JOINT

The hip joint is a ball-and-socket articulation that has polyaxial movement. There is a cartilaginous lip surrounding the acetabulum, and the hip capsule is intimately related to the extensive musculature surrounding the hip joint. Hip joint movement includes flexion-extension, abduction-adduction, and internal rotation-external rotation. The musculature surrounding the hip joint can be divided into six groups, each being responsible for one of the movement directions. In addition to dysfunction of muscle, there are joint play dysfunctions and capsular restrictions that need to be assessed and treated to achieve muscle balance surrounding the hip joint.

Hip Joint

Supine

Assessment of Hip Capsular Pattern

1. Patient supine with operator standing at side of table.

2. Operator's distal hand grasps the ankle region while the proximal hand controls the flexed hip and flexed knee.

3. Operator introduces circumduction in a clockwise (Fig. 19.1) and counterclockwise direction (Fig. 19.2).

4. Operator increases the circumduction arc to see whether the capsular pattern is smooth in all directions.

5. A positive finding is to have a hitch or delay in movement during the circumduction arc that frequently is reported by the patient as being pinching and painful.

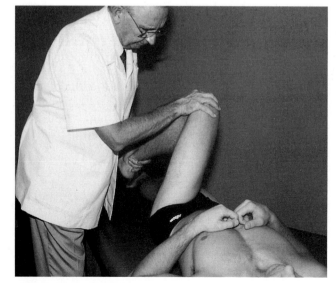

Figure 19.1.

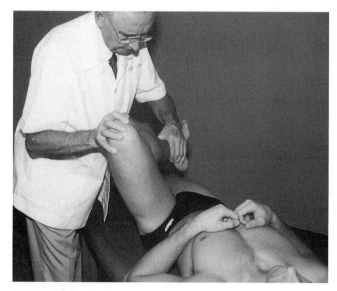

Figure 19.2.

Hip Joint

Supine

Joint Play

1. Patient supine with operator standing at side of table.

2. Operator flexes hip and knee to 90°.

3. Operator drapes flexed knee over shoulder and grasps with interlaced hands the anterior aspect of the proximal femur.

4. When all slack is taken up, a mobilizing joint play distraction thrust is applied in a caudad direction by the two hands (Fig. 19.3).

5. Operator drapes knee over the neck and with interlaced fingers grasps medial side of proximal femur.

6. When slack is taken out in a medial to lateral direction, a joint play thrust is applied in lateral distraction by the two hands (Fig. 19.4).

7. Reassess.

Hip Joint

Supine

Acetabular Labrum and Posterior Capsule Stretch Technique (Example: Left Hip)

1. Patient supine with operator standing at side of table.

2. Operator flexes knee and hip and controls left lower extremity with the left arm, axilla, and trunk.

3. Heel of right hand is placed against the lateral aspect of the left greater trochanter (Fig. 19.5).

4. Operator applies a series of impaction compressive forces through the right arm in the direction of the femoral head and hip joint while alternately providing an anteroposterior compressive force through the left arm contact and with some cephalic to caudad distraction as well.

5. Various degrees of adduction-abduction and internal-external rotation are used to fine-tune against the resistant barrier.

6. Particular attention to the posterior hip capsule occurs with an anterior to posterior compression load through the left arm with the hip in an internally rotated and adducted position.

7. The activating forces are mobilization without impulse.

8. Retest.

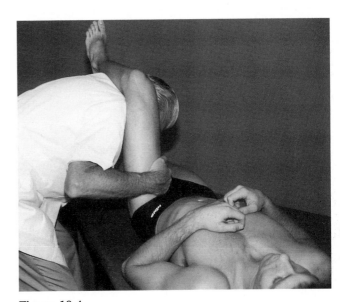

Figure 19.4.

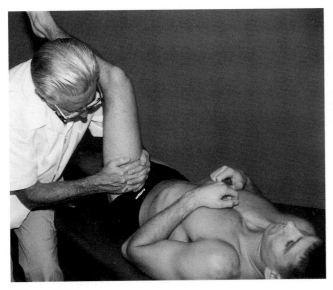

Figure 19.3.

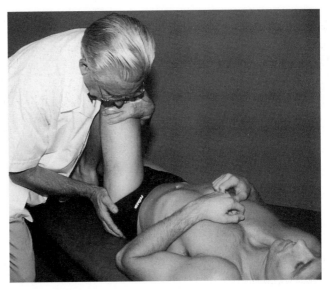

Figure 19.5.

Hip Joint

Prone

Mobilization of Anterior Capsule (Example: Right Hip)

1. Patient prone with operator standing at side of table.

2. Operator flexes right knee and grasps anterior aspect of distal right femur with the right hand and arm.

3. Operator's left hand contacts the posterior aspect of the proximal right femur with the left arm fully extended (Fig. 19.6).

4. Operator gently lifts the right knee off the table and applies a series of mobilizing without impulse forces in an anterior direction against the proximal femur.

5. Operator fine-tunes against resistant barrier by internally and externally rotating the right femur and by applying both medial and lateral directional forces through the left hand.

6. Retest.

The primary dysfunctions of the hip joint are imbalance of length and strength of the six muscle groups. Structural diagnosis and muscle energy technique for these muscle imbalances are as follows:

1. Operator passively takes the hip joint through a range of motion, evaluating quantity of range, quality of movement during the range, and quality of the end feel.

2. Comparison is made on the opposite side.

3. Asymmetry may be due to shortening of the muscle group on the restricted side or weakness of the contralateral muscle group with increased range.

4. Strength testing is performed by asking the patient to maximally contract the muscle against equal and opposite resistance, comparing one side with the other.

5. Treatment of short and tight muscle groups is achieved by a 3- to 5-second isometric contraction against operator's equal and opposite resistance. After each patient effort, the operator engages the next resistant barrier with gradual lengthening of the shortened muscle by the principle of postisometric relaxation.

6. Treatment of functional weakness of a muscle group is accomplished by asking the patient to perform a series of three to five concentric isotonic contractions made through the total range of movement against an operator counterforce that is yielding in nature but with progressive increase in resistance with each effort.

7. Retest for length and strength of comparable muscle groups.

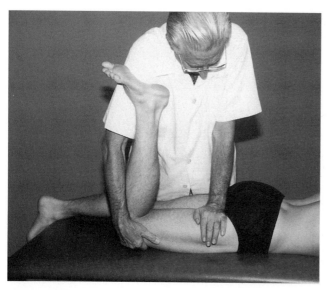

Figure 19.6.

Hip Joint

Muscle Energy Technique

Motion Tested: Abduction
Muscles Tested: Adductors (Adductor Magnus, Adductor Brevis, Adductor Longus)

1. Patient supine on table with operator standing at end grasping lower extremity at the ankle.

2. Operator abducts extended lower extremity to end point, evaluating total range and quality of movement during the range (Fig. 19.7). During motion testing, the operator prevents the extended leg from moving into external rotation.

3. Adductor strength is tested by the operator offering resistance against the patient's extended leg with the knee fully extended. Operator's resistance is above the knee joint to protect the medial collateral ligament (Fig. 19.8).

4. Treat either shortness or weakness as appropriate.

5. Retest.

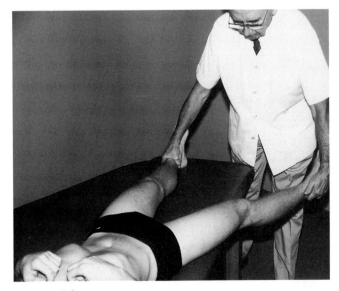

Figure 19.7.

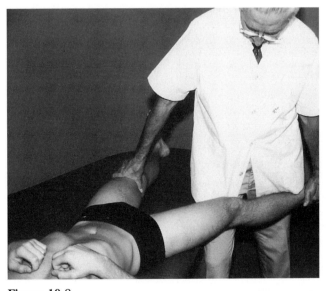

Figure 19.8.

Hip Joint

Muscle Energy Technique

Motion Tested: Adduction

Muscles Tested: Abductors (Gluteus Medius, Gluteus Minimis)

1. Patient supine on table with operator standing at end.

2. Operator adducts the extended leg across the front of the opposite leg, testing for range and quality of movement (Fig. 19.9).

3. Strength testing is performed by asking the patient to maximally abduct the leg against resistance offered by the operator, holding the leg in the adducted position (Fig. 19.10).

4. Comparison is made with the opposite leg.

5. Treatment for shortness or tightness is accomplished as appropriate.

6. Retest.

Note: An alternate method is to lift the leg not being tested and adduct the extended leg being tested beneath it. Testing in this position also evaluates the tensor fascia lata muscle.

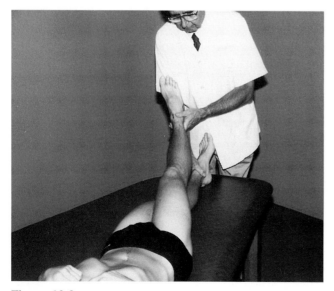

Figure 19.9.

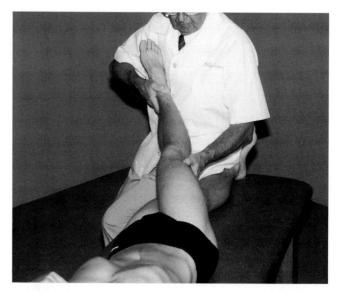

Figure 19.10.

Hip Joint

Muscle Energy Technique

Motion Tested: External Rotation with Hip Flexed to 90°

Muscles Tested: Internal Rotators (Gluteus Medius, Gluteus Maximus)

1. Patient supine on table with operator standing at side next to extremity being tested.

2. Operator holds lower extremity with 90° flexion at both the hip and the knee (Fig. 19.11).

3. Operator externally rotates the femur by carrying the foot and ankle medially, evaluating range and quality of movement (Fig. 19.12).

4. Strength testing is made by patient internally rotating the femur against equal and opposite resistance offered by the operator (Fig. 19.13).

5. Comparison is made with the opposite side.

6. Shortness or weakness are treated as appropriate.

7. Retest.

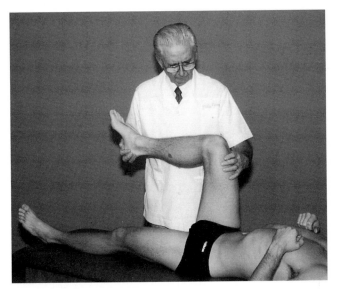

Figure 19.11.

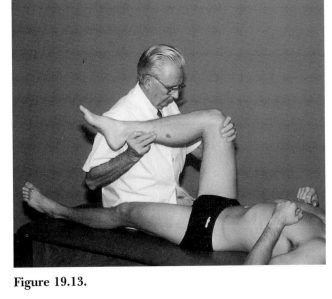

Figure 19.13.

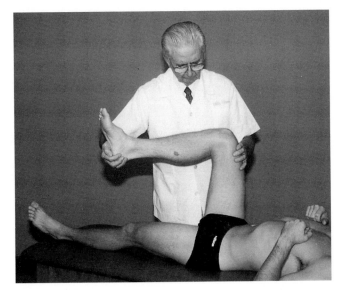

Figure 19.12.

Hip Joint

Muscle Energy Technique

Motion Tested: Internal Rotation with Hip Flexed to 90°

Muscles Tested: External Rotators (Primarily Piriformis)

1. Patient supine on table with operator standing at side next to extremity being tested.
2. Operator holds the lower extremity with 90° flexion at both the hip and knee (see Figure 19.11).

3. Operator introduces internal rotation, testing for range and quality of movement (Fig. 19.14).
4. Strength testing is performed by asking the patient to externally rotate against resistance offered by the operator (Fig. 19.15).
5. Comparison is made with the opposite side.
6. Shortness and tightness are treated as appropriate.
7. Retest.

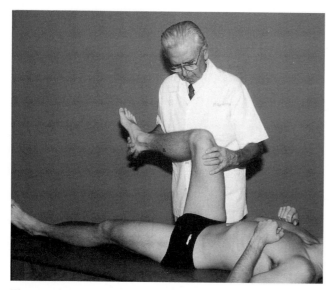

Figure 19.14.

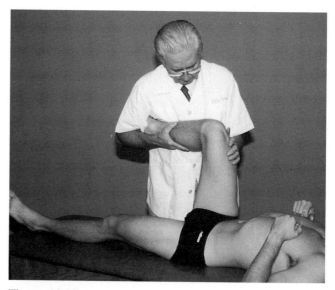

Figure 19.15.

Hip Joint

Muscle Energy Technique

Motion Tested: Partial Hip Flexion (Straight Leg Raising)

Muscles Tested: Hip Extensors, Primarily Hamstring Muscles (Semitendinosus, Semimembranosus, Biceps Femoris)

Note: Gluteus maximus and adductor magnus become hip extensors when thigh is flexed

1. Patient supine on table with operator standing at side of table.

2. Operator monitors anterior superior iliac spine on side opposite leg being tested.

3. Operator lifts extended leg introducing hip flexion, testing for range and quality of movement with the end point being the first movement of the opposite anterior superior iliac spine (Fig. 19.16).

4. Shortness and tightness are treated by a series of isometric contractions against resistance with the patient effort being to pull the heel toward the buttock (Fig. 19.17).

Note: An alternative position has the patient holding the posterior aspect of the distal thigh while the operator extends the knee and resists a knee flexion effort by the patient against the operator's resistance (Fig. 19.18).

5. Strength testing is performed by having the patient prone on the table with the operator resisting patient attempts at knee flexion in a bilateral fashion.

6. Weakness is treated by a series of concentric isotonic contractions through the full range of knee flexion against progressively increasing operator resistance.

7. Retest.

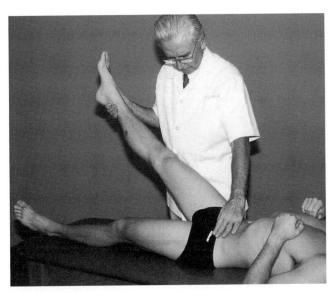

Figure 19.16.

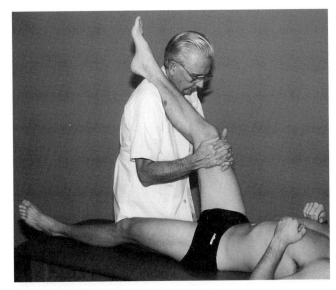

Figure 19.17.

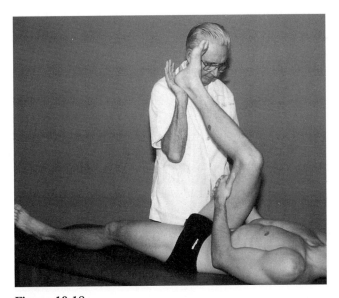

Figure 19.18.

Hip Joint

Muscle Energy Technique

Motion Tested: Hip Extension
Muscle Tested: Iliopsoas

1. Patient supine with pelvis close to the end of the table so that lower extremity below the knee is free of the table.

2. Operator stands at end of table facing patient.

3. Both hips and knees are flexed.

4. Patient holds leg opposite that being tested in a flexed position while operator passively extends the leg being tested (Fig. 19.19).

5. Normal range is for the back of the thigh to strike the table with the knee fully flexed (Fig. 19.20).

6. Strength testing is performed by having the patient attempt to lift the knee to the ceiling against operator resistance.

7. Comparison is made with the opposite side.

8. Shortness is treated by isometric contraction against operator resistance. Patient is instructed to perform hip flexion. Operator also resists attempts at external rotation of the hip by offering a resistance with leg against the medial side of the patient's foot and ankle (Fig. 19.21).

9. Weakness is treated by a series of concentric isotonic contractions of hip flexion and external rotation.

10. Retest.

Note: Before testing for length and strength of the iliopsoas, the lumbar spine should be evaluated and treated appropriately. The iliopsoas test puts stress on the lumbar spine, particularly the lumbosacral junction.

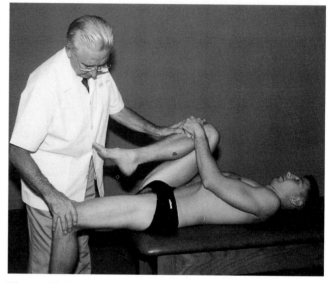

Figure 19.20.

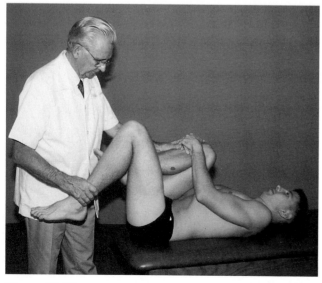

Figure 19.19.

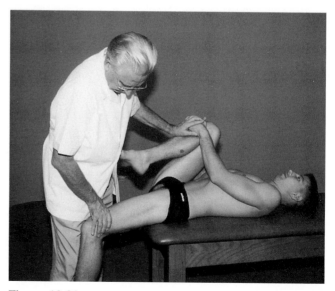

Figure 19.21.

Hip Joint

Muscle Energy Technique

Motion Tested: Knee Flexion
Muscles Tested: Quadriceps Group (Rectus Femoris, Vastus lateralis, Vastus intermedius, Vastus medialis)

1. Patient prone on table with operator standing at foot facing patient.

2. Operator flexes both knees while holding patient's ankles (Fig. 19.22).

3. Test is made for range and quality of movement.

4. Strength testing is performed by asking the patient to extend the knees against resistance with both sides contracting simultaneously.

5. Shortness is treated by a series of isometric contractions against resistance (Fig. 19.23).

6. Weakness is treated by a series of concentric isotonic contraction against progressively increasing operator resistance.

7. Retest.

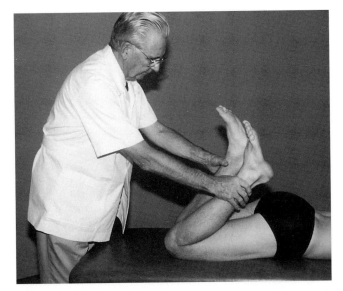

Figure 19.22.

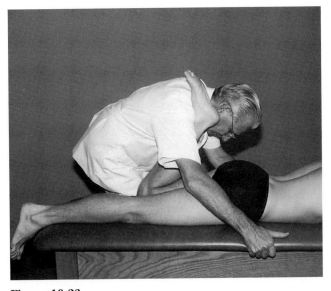

Figure 19.23.

Hip Joint

Muscle Energy Technique

Motion Tested: Internal Rotation with Hips in Neutral

Muscles Tested: External Rotators (Obturator Internus, Obturator Externus, Gemellus Superior, Gemellus Inferior, Quadratus Femoris, and Piriformis)

1. Patient prone on table with operator standing at foot of table facing patient.

2. Operator flexes patient's knees to 90° (Fig. 19.24).

3. Operator tests for range and quality of internal rotation by allowing the feet to drop laterally (Fig. 19.25).

4. Strength testing is performed by asking the patient to bilaterally pull the feet together against resistance.

5. Shortness is treated by operator holding the opposite leg with the knee flexed and hip internally rotated while the patient performs external rotation of the leg in the 90° flexed position against operator resistance (Fig. 19.26).

6. Weakness is treated by a series of concentric isotonic contractions through a range of external rotation with the knee at 90°.

7. Retest.

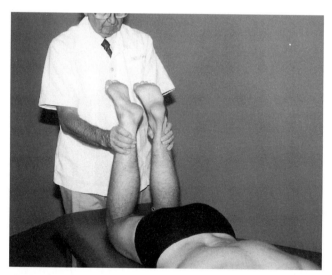

Figure 19.24.

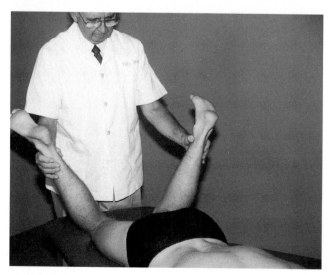

Figure 19.25.

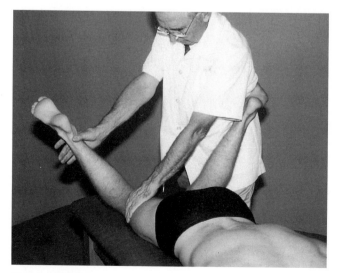

Figure 19.26.

Hip Joint

Muscle Energy Technique

Motion Tested: External Rotation with the Hips at Neutral

Muscles Tested: Internal Rotators (Gluteus Medius, Gluteus Minimis, Tensor Fascia Lata)

1. Patient prone on table with operator standing at foot facing patient.

2. Operator fixes leg opposite one being tested with slight knee flexion and hip external rotation.

3. Leg being tested is flexed to 90° and externally rotated, looking for range and quality of movement (Fig. 19.27).

4. The opposite side is tested in a similar manner (Fig. 19.28).

5. Strength is tested by asking the patient to internally rotate against resistance.

6. Shortness and tightness are treated by a series of isometric contractions of internal rotation against resistance (Fig. 19.29).

7. Weakness is treated by a series of concentric isotonic contractions against increasing operator resistance.

8. Retest.

The balancing of the hip musculature is an important part of the treatment of the patient's musculoskeletal system, particularly those patients with lower back and lower extremity pain syndromes. The exact treatment sequence is debated by many authors, but this author has found it most effective to treat shortness and tightness before treating weakness. Clinical observation finds that the short tight group of muscles reflexively inhibit the antagonist, resulting in apparent weakness of the antagonist muscle. Once the shortness and tightness of the agonist is removed, the apparent weakness of the antagonist is frequently no longer present. If a muscle still appears to be functionally weak after treating the shortness and tightness of its antagonist, then it should be treated for weakness using the techniques described. Muscle imbalance patterns are frequently seen in the six muscle groups. It is common to find the right adductors tight with apparent weakness of the left adductors and weakness of the right abductors. The psoas and rectus femoris muscles are frequently tight and need to be stretched so that appropriate hip extension can occur during the walking cycle. The imbalance of tightness and weakness between agonist and antagonist is consistent with the tight loose concept found when using the myofascial release system of diagnosis and treatment.

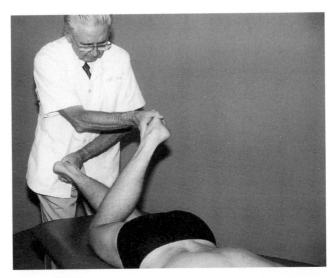

Figure 19.28.

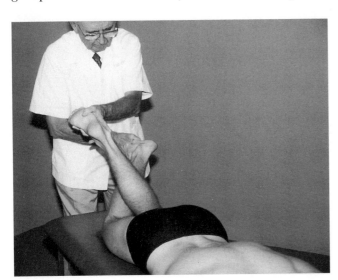

Figure 19.27.

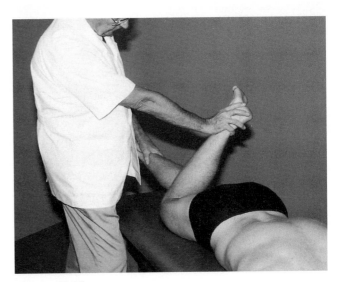

Figure 19.29.

KNEE JOINT

The primary movement at the knee joint is flexion and extension of the tibia under the femur. The length of the medial and lateral femoral condyles is different, resulting in an internal-external rotational component to the flexion-extension arc. During extension, the tibia rotates externally, and during flexion, the tibia rotates internally. Dysfunction of the internal-external rotation interferes with normal flexion-extension. The flexion-extension and the internal-external rotation movements depend on a small anteroposterior glide and medial to lateral gapping of the opposing joint surfaces. These minor joint play movements are present within the constraints of normal ligamentous stability. The movements are increased when there is ligamentous or cartilage damage within the knee. The primary somatic dysfunctions of the knee joint are at the medial meniscus and internal-external rotation of the tibia on the femur.

Knee Joint

Supine

Medial Meniscus Technique
Mobilization Without Impulse

1. Patient supine on table with operator standing at side near dysfunctional knee.

2. Operator holds patient's distal leg between upper arm and chest with both hands surrounding the proximal tibia.

3. Operator's thumbs are placed over the medial joint space with the knee in flexion (Fig. 19.30).

4. Operator's lateral hand exerts a medial compression on the distal femur while operator's thumbs maintain posterolateral compressive force on the medial meniscus and the leg is carried into extension (Fig. 19.31).

5. Several repetitions of this procedure may be necessary to release restriction of the medial meniscus.

6. Retest.

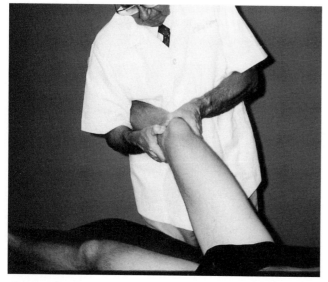

Figure 19.30.

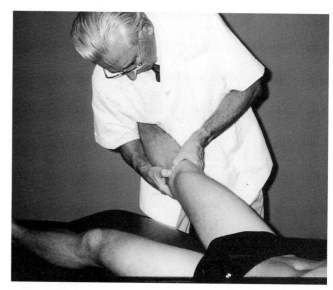

Figure 19.31.

Knee Joint

Supine

Medial and Lateral Meniscus Technique
Mobilization Without Impulse Technique

1. Patient supine on table with operator standing at caudal end facing patient.

2. Operator supports the patient's dysfunctional leg between the thighs over the edge of table.

3. Operator's two hands grasp proximal tibia with the thumbs over the anteromedial or anterolateral joint space, depending on whether the restriction is of the lateral or medial malleolus (Fig. 19.32).

4. For medial meniscus dysfunction, a circumduction movement begins in flexion and includes medial translation with thumb compression over the medial meniscus while carrying the knee into full extension (Fig. 19.33).

5. For restriction of the lateral meniscus, the thumbs overlay the anterolateral aspect of the knee and the circumduction movement begins in flexion and includes lateral translation while carrying the distal leg into extension.

6. Several repetitions may be necessary.

7. Retest.

Note: Restriction of the medial meniscus is much more common than that of the lateral meniscus.

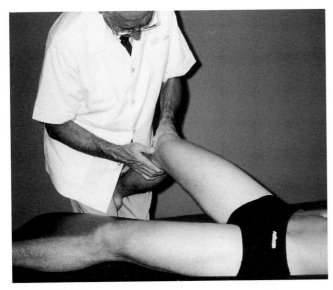

Figure 19.32.

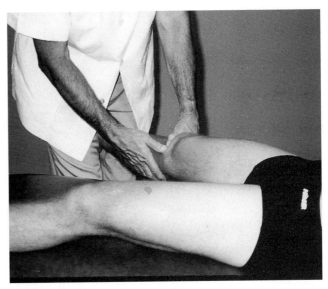

Figure 19.33.

Knee Joint

Supine

Medial and Lateral Meniscal Tracking
Joint Play

1. Patient supine on table with operator standing at side closest to dysfunctional knee.

2. Operator controls dysfunctional leg at a 90° hip and 90° knee flexion position with the distal hand controlling dorsiflexion of the ankle for close packing while the proximal hand controls the distal femur with the thumb over the lateral meniscus and the index and middle fingers over the medial meniscus (Fig. 19.34).

3. Operator medially and laterally rotates the tibia through the close packed ankle joint with progressive extension of the hip and knee (Fig. 19.35).

4. Several repetitions are necessary. The amount of medial and lateral rotation gradually decreases as the knee extends.

5. Retest.

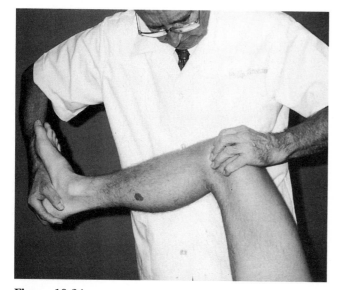

Figure 19.34.

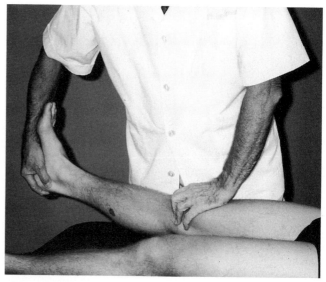

Figure 19.35.

Knee Joint

Supine

Extension Compression Test

1. Patient supine on table with operator standing at side of dysfunctional leg.

2. Operator's proximal hand stabilizes the distal femur.

3. Operator's distal hand grasps patient's heel (Fig. 19.36).

4. Operator carries the distal leg into increased extension at the knee against the stabilizing proximal hand.

5. Comparison is made with the opposite side.

6. Restriction of extension with pain provocation is a positive test and indicates restriction of external rotation and extension of the knee joint or meniscal injury.

Knee Joint

Sitting

Diagnosis: Restriction of Internal-External Rotation

1. Patient sits on edge of table with lower legs dangling with operator sitting in front of patient.

2. Operator grasps feet and dorsiflexes ankles to close pack position.

3. Operator introduces external rotation (Fig. 19.37) and internal rotation (Fig. 19.38), testing for range, quality of range, and end feel.

4. Strength testing is performed by asking the patient to internally and externally rotate tibia against resistance.

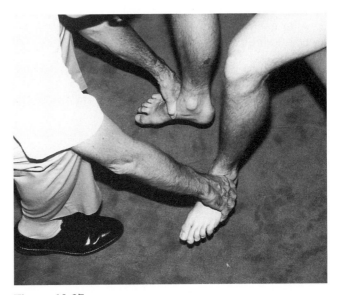

Figure 19.37.

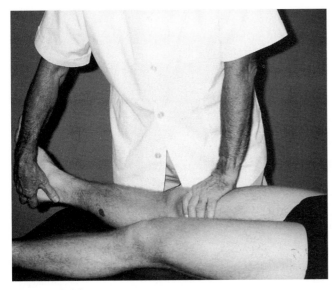

Figure 19.36.

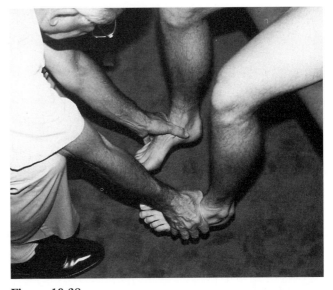

Figure 19.38.

Knee Joint

Sitting

Muscle Energy Technique
Diagnosis
   Position: Tibia internally rotated
   Motion restriction: External rotation of tibia

1. Patient sitting on edge of table with lower legs dangling and operator sitting in front of patient.

2. Operator grasps heel of foot in one hand and forefoot in the other.

3. Operator dorsiflexes foot at ankle and introduces external rotation to barrier (Fig. 19.39).

4. Patient internally rotates forefoot against operator resistance for 3–5 seconds and three to five repetitions.

5. After each patient effort, operator externally rotates tibia to the new barrier.

6. Retest.

Knee Joint

Sitting

Muscle Energy Technique
Diagnosis
   Position: Tibia externally rotated
   Motion restriction: Internal rotation of the tibia

1. Patient sits on edge of table with lower legs dangling with operator sitting in front of patient.

2. Operator grasps heel of foot in one hand and forefoot in the other.

3. Operator dorsiflexes foot at ankle and introduces internal rotation to barrier (Fig. 19.40).

4. Operator externally rotates forefoot against operator resistance for 3–5 seconds and three to five repetitions.

5. After each patient effort, operator internally rotates tibia to the new barrier.

6. Retest.

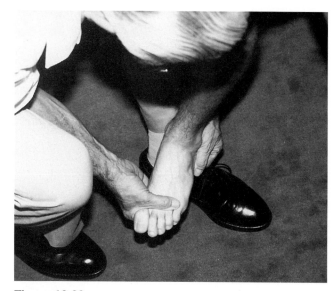

Figure 19.39.

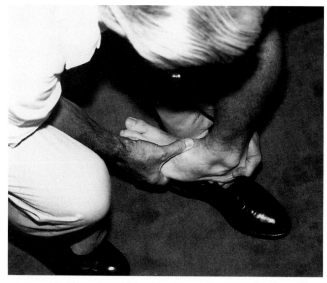

Figure 19.40.

Knee Joint

Prone

Muscle Energy Technique
Diagnosis of Internal-External Rotation

1. Patient prone on table with knees flexed to 90° and operator standing at end of table grasping each foot in each hand.

2. Operator introduces dorsiflexion of the ankle and externally rotates (Fig. 19.41) and internally rotates tibia (Fig. 19.42), testing for range, quality of range, and end feel.

3. Strength testing is performed by asking the patient to internally or externally rotate the foot against resistance offered by the operator.

Knee Joint

Prone

Muscle Energy Technique
Diagnosis: Tibia Internally Rotated
Motion restriction: External rotation of the tibia

1. Patient prone on table with operator standing on side of dysfunctional extremity.

2. Operator flexes knee to 90° and grasps heel and forefoot in each hand.

3. Operator dorsiflexes ankle and externally rotates foot to barrier (Fig. 19.43).

4. Patient internally rotates forefoot against operator resistance for 3–5 seconds and three to five repetitions.

5. After each patient effort, operator externally rotates foot to new barrier.

6. Retest.

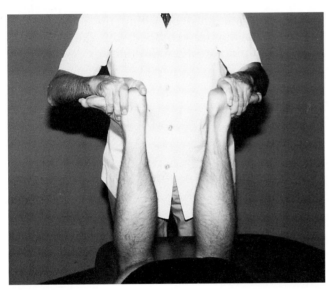

Figure 19.41.

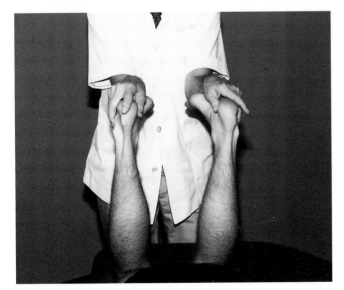

Figure 19.42.

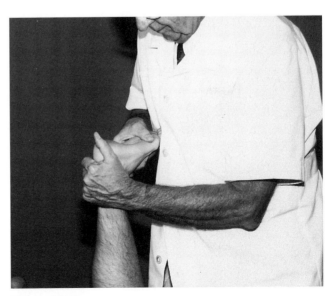

Figure 19.43.

Knee Joint

Prone

Muscle Energy Technique
Diagnosis
Position: Tibia externally rotated
Motion restriction: Internal rotation of tibia

1. Patient prone on table with operator standing at side of dysfunctional extremity.

2. Operator flexes knee to 90° and grasps heel and forefoot of patient.

3. Operator dorsiflexes ankle and internally rotates the tibia to the barrier (Fig. 19.44).

4. Patient externally rotates forefoot against operator resistance for 3–5 seconds and three to five repetitions.

5. After each patient effort, operator internally rotates foot to new barrier.

6. Retest.

PROXIMAL TIBIOFIBULAR JOINT

This articulation is intimately related to the knee joint and is equally important in its relation to the ankle. The proximal tibiofibular joint has an anteroposterior glide and is influenced by the action of the biceps femoris muscle inserting at the fibular head. The proximal tibiofibular joint can be restricted either anteriorly or posteriorly. Restoration of the normal anteroposterior glide and its normal relationship to the tibia are the goals of treatment.

Restoration of normal internal-external rotational movement of the tibia on the femur is accomplished before addressing the proximal tibiofibular joint.

The plane of the joint is approximately 30° from lateral to medial and from before backward. Testing for the anteroposterior movement of the proximal tibiofibular joint must be within the plane of the joint and can be accomplished with the patient in either the supine or sitting positions.

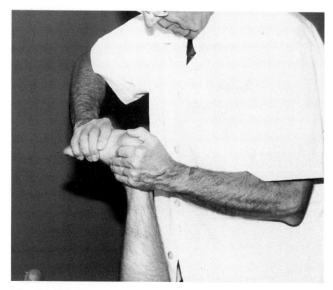

Figure 19.44.

Proximal Tibiofibular Joint

Testing for Anteroposterior Glide

1. Patient sits on table with both feet flat for fixation (Fig. 19.45) or patient sits on edge of table with the operator sitting in front holding the medial sides of both feet together (Fig. 19.46).

2. Operator grasps the proximal fibula between the thumb or thenar eminence and the fingers of each hand being careful not to compress the peroneal nerve against the fibular head.

3. Operator translates the fibular head anteriorly and posteriorly within the plane of the joint, testing for comparable range on each side, the quality of movement, and end feel.

4. A fibular head that resists anterior translatory movement is positionally a posterior fibular head, and a fibular head that resists posterior translatory motion is positionally an anterior fibular head.

Proximal Tibiofibular Joint

Sitting

Muscle Energy Technique
Diagnosis
    Position: Fibular head posterior
    Motion restriction: Anterior glide of the fibular head

1. Patient sits on edge of table with dysfunctional leg dangling and operator sitting in front with the medial hand grasping the patient's forefoot.

2. Operator inverts and internally rotates the patient's foot while the lateral hand exerts an anterolateral force on the posterior aspect of the fibular head (Fig. 19.47).

3. Patient is instructed to evert and dorsiflex the foot against resistance offered by the operator's medial hand for 3–5 seconds and three to five repetitions.

4. Operator engages new barrier after each patient effort.

5. Retest.

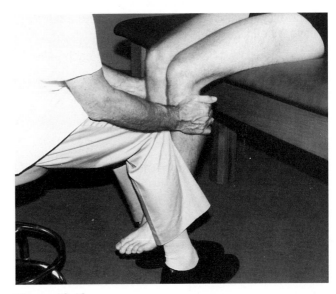

Figure 19.46.

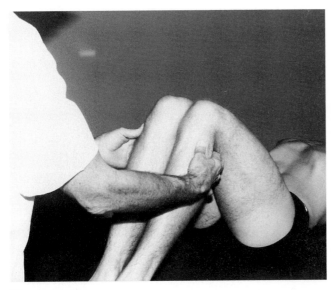

Figure 19.45.

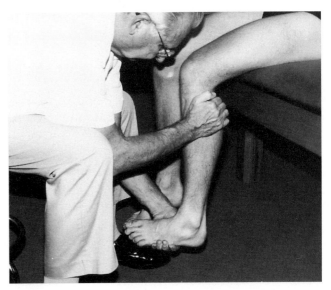

Figure 19.47.

Proximal Tibiofibular Joint

Sitting

Muscle Energy Technique
Diagnosis
    Position: Fibular head anterior
    Motion restriction: Posterior glide of the fibular head

1. Patient sitting on edge of table with dysfunctional leg dangling and operator sitting in front with the medial hand grasping the patient's forefoot.

2. Operator inverts and externally rotates the patient's foot while the lateral thumb exerts a posteromedial force against the anterior aspect of the fibular head (Fig. 19.48).

3. Patient everts and plantar flexes the foot against operator resistance for 3–5 seconds and three to five repetitions.

4. Operator engages a new barrier after each patient effort.

5. Retest.

Proximal Tibiofibular Joint

Supine

Mobilization with Impulse Technique
Diagnosis: Posterior fibular head
    Motion restriction: Anterior glide of fibular head

1. Patient supine on table with operator standing at side of dysfunction with caudal hand controlling patient's foot and ankle.

2. Operator's cephalic hand supports the flexed knee with the metacarpophalangeal joint of the index finger posterior to the fibular head (Fig. 19.49).

3. Operator engages barrier by externally rotating the flexed knee and pinching the metacarpophalangeal joint between the distal femur and the fibular head.

4. A mobilization with impulse thrust is performed by exaggerating the knee flexion, bringing the fibular head anterior (Fig. 19.50).

5. Retest.

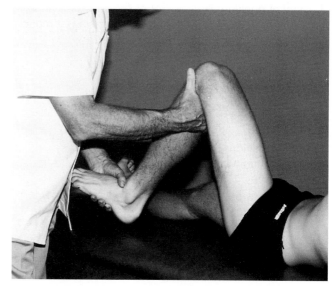

Figure 19.49.

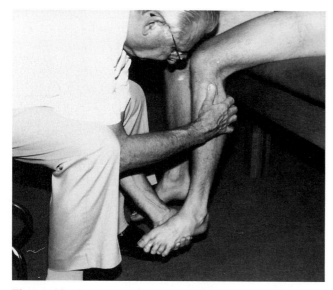

Figure 19.48.

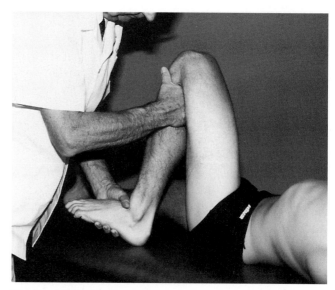

Figure 19.50.

Proximal Tibiofibular Joint

Prone

Mobilization with Impulse Technique
Diagnosis
    Position: Posterior fibular head
    Motion restriction: Anterior glide of the fibular
    head

1. Patient prone on table with operator standing at side of dysfunction with distal hand controlling the foot and ankle.

2. Operator's proximal hand is laid over the popliteal space with the metacarpophalangeal joint of the index finger posterior to the fibular head (Fig. 19.51).

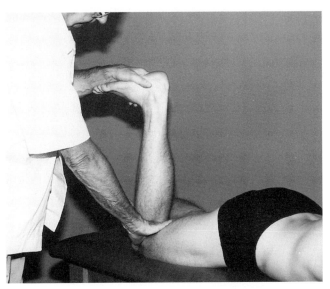

Figure 19.51.

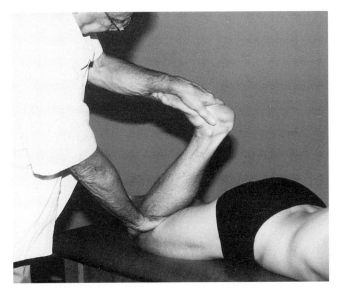

Figure 19.52.

3. Operator's knee is flexed, pinching the metacarpophalangeal joint between the fibular head and the femur.

4. The barrier is engaged by slight external rotation to the leg and flexion of the knee and a mobilization with impulse thrust is performed by exaggerating knee flexion (Fig. 19.52).

5. Retest.

Proximal Tibiofibular Joint

Supine

Mobilization with Impulse Technique
Diagnosis
    Position: Fibular head anterior
    Motion restriction: Posterior glide of the fibular head

1. Patient supine on table with operator standing on side of dysfunction.

2. Operator's distal hand controls the lower leg in knee extension and internally rotates to approximately 30°.

3. The thenar eminence of the operator's proximal hand is placed over the anterior aspect of the proximal fibula (Fig. 19.53).

4. Operator engages barrier of the anteroposterior motion of the fibular head by downward compression through the extended arm.

5. When barrier is engaged, a mobilization with impulse thrust is performed by dropping the body weight of the operator through the extended arm onto the anterior aspect of the fibular head.

6. Retest.

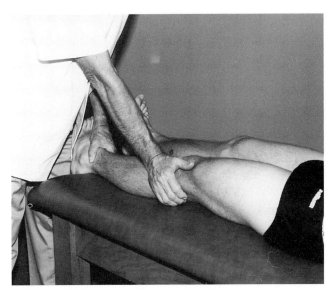

Figure 19.53.

ANKLE REGION

The ankle region consists of the distal tibiofibular articulation, the articulation of the superior aspect of the talus with the tibiofibular joint mortice, and the talocalcaneal (subtalar) articulation. Although the talocalcaneal joint is frequently classified as being in the foot, it is the key to functional movement of the talus. Talar restriction from either above or below significantly restricts ankle motion. The talus is of interest because it has no direct muscular attachments. Its movement is determined by muscle action on bones above and below. Dysfunction of the talus at the tibiofibular joint mortice is one of the more common dysfunctions in the lower extremity. Another important anatomical feature of the talus is that its superior surface is wedge-shaped, with the posterior aspect being narrower than the anterior, as it articulates with the tibiofibular joint mortice. The ankle is more stable when dorsiflexed than plantar flexed. The most common dysfunction at this joint is restricted dorsiflexion.

The distal tibiofibular joint is quite stable and is infrequently dysfunctional. The distal tibiofibular joint is associated with the function of the proximal tibiofibular articulation. Appropriate treatment at the proximal tibiofibular articulation frequently restores function at the distal tibiofibular articulation. Appropriate evaluation and treatment of the proximal and distal tibiofibular articulations should be performed before addressing the talotibiofibular mortice articulation.

Distal Tibiofibular Joint

Supine

Diagnosis
1. Patient supine on table with operator standing at foot with the medial hand grasping the posterior and medial aspects of the patient's ankle and heel.
2. Operator's lateral hand grasps the lateral malleolus between the thumb and index finger (Fig. 19.54).
3. Operator's left hand glides the lateral malleolus anteriorly and posteriorly against the fixed foot and ankle.
4. Restriction of anterior movement is a posterior distal tibiofibular joint, and restriction of posterior movement is an anterior distal tibiofibular joint.
5. Comparison is made with the opposite side.

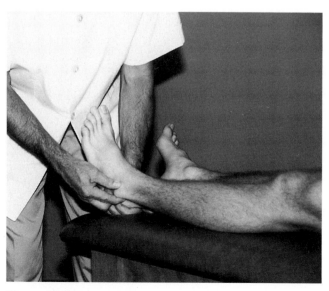

Figure 19.54.

Ankle Region: Distal Tibiofibular Joint

Supine

Mobilization with Impulse Technique
Diagnosis
Position: Anterior distal tibiofibular joint
Motion restriction: Posterior movement of the
lateral malleolus

1. Patient supine on table with operator standing at foot.

2. Operator's medial hand grasps the patient's heel and maintains the ankle at 90° flexion. The thumb is placed over the anterior aspect of the lateral malleolus (Fig. 19.55).

3. The thenar eminence of the operator's lateral hand is superimposed on the thumb with the fingers curled around the posterior aspect of the ankle (Fig. 19.56).

4. When the barrier is engaged, a mobilization with impulse thrust is performed in a posterior direction against the anterior aspect of the lateral malleolus by a combined effort of the thenar eminence of the lateral hand and the thumb of the medial hand.

5. Retest.

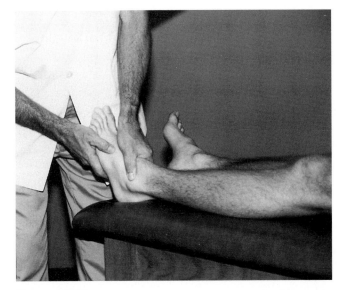

Figure 19.55.

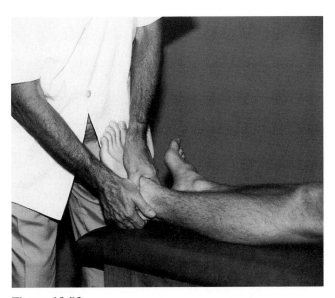

Figure 19.56.

Ankle Region: Distal Tibiofibular Joint

Prone

Mobilization with Impulse Technique
Diagnosis
Position: Posterior distal tibiofibular joint
Motion restriction: Anterior movement of the lateral malleolus

1. Patient prone with feet over edge of table with operator standing at foot facing cephalward.

2. Operator's medial hand grasps the foot and ankle, maintaining dorsiflexion at the ankle. The thumb is placed over the posterior aspect of the lateral malleolus (Fig. 19.57).

3. Operator's lateral hand places the thenar eminence against the opposing thumb (Fig. 19.58).

4. The barrier is engaged in an anterior direction, and a mobilization with impulse thrust is performed by combined activity of the lateral hand thenar eminence and the medial hand thumb carrying the lateral malleolus toward the floor.

5. Retest.

Ankle Region: Talotibial Joint

Diagnosis

1. Patient sitting on table with legs dangling and operator sitting in front of patient.

2. Operator grasps forefoot and plantar flexes to the barrier, evaluating each side for restriction.

3. Each thumb is placed on the anterior aspect of the neck of the talus with the fingers under the forefoot and the operator passively swings the foot toward

the table, resulting in dorsiflexion of the talotibial joint (Fig. 19.59). Restriction of dorsiflexion is compared from side to side. Frequently, the neck of the talus on the dysfunctional side will be tender.

4. A frequent cause of restricted dorsiflexion of the talotibial joint is shortness and tightness of the gastrocnemius-soleus muscles in the calf.

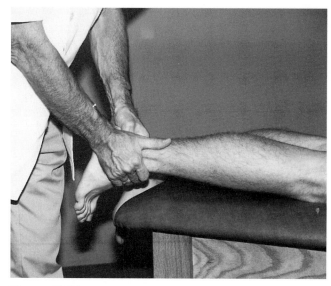

Figure 19.58.

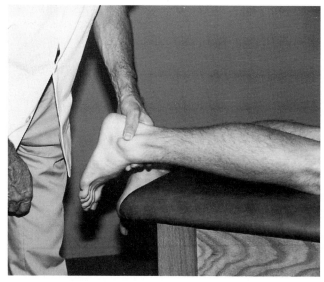

Figure 19.57.

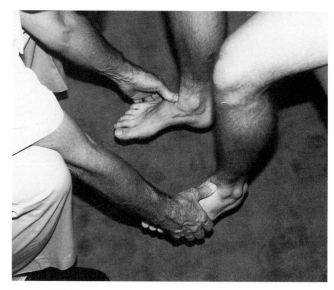

Figure 19.59.

Ankle Region: Talotibial Joint

Sitting

Muscle Energy Technique
Diagnosis
    Position: Talus plantar flexed
    Motion restriction: Dorsiflexion of the talus

1. Patient sitting on edge of table with feet dangling and operator sitting in front of the dysfunctional talus.
2. Operator places medial hand under the plantar surface of the forefoot with the web of the lateral hand overlying the neck of the talus (Fig. 19.60).

3. The dorsiflexion barrier is engaged through a combined dorsiflexion movement of the foot and a posterior force on the talar neck.
4. Patient performs plantar flexion muscle effort against equal and opposite resistance for 3–5 seconds and three to five repetitions (Fig. 19.61).
5. After each patient effort, additional dorsiflexion is introduced against the resistant barrier.
6. Retest.

Note: It is helpful to have the operator cross the lower legs under the patient's forefoot to assist in resistance of plantar flexion.

Ankle Region: Talotibial Joint

Supine

Mobilization with Impulse Technique
Diagnosis
    Position: Talus plantar flexed
    Motion restriction: Dorsiflexion of the talus

1. Patient supine with operator standing at foot of table.
2. Operator's hands encircle patient's foot with middle fingers overlapping the superior aspect of the talar neck and the thumbs on the sole of the foot (Fig. 19.62).
3. Operator engages barrier by dorsiflexing and long axis traction.
4. A mobilization with impulse thrust is made by long axis extension through both hands.
5. Retest.

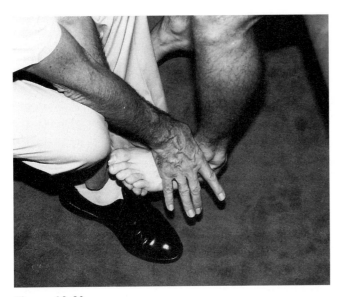

Figure 19.60.

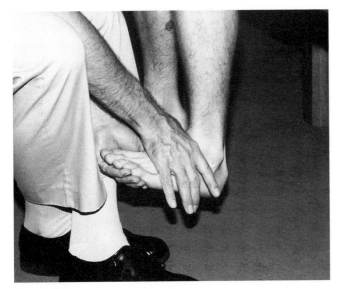

Figure 19.61.

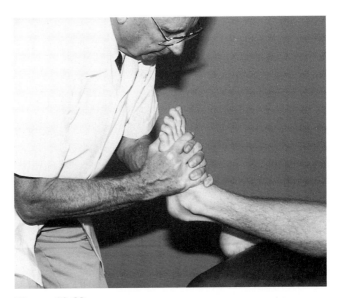

Figure 19.62.

Ankle Region: Talotibial Joint

Mobilization with Impulse Technique
Diagnosis

Position: Dorsiflexed or plantar flexed talus
Motion restriction: Dorsiflexion or plantar flexion of talus

1. Patient supine on table with operator sitting on edge on dysfunctional side facing caudad.

2. Patient's hip is flexed to 90° and externally rotated. The thigh is flexed to 90° with the thigh against the operator's posterior trunk.

3. The webs of operator's thumb and index fingers are placed on the neck of the talus anteriorly and the tubercle of the talus posteriorly through the achilles tendon (Fig. 19.63).

4. The talus is dorsiflexed or plantar flexed against the resistant barrier.

5. When the barrier is engaged, a direct action mobilization with impulse thrust is made in a long axis distraction direction.

6. Retest.

Ankle Region: Talocalcaneal (Subtalar) Joint

Testing for anteromedial to posterolateral glide.

1. Patient supine on table with operator standing at end facing dysfunctional ankle.

2. Operator's proximal hand grasps the ankle region with the web of the thumb and index finger over the neck of the talus, the fingers grasping the medial malleolus and the thumb over the lateral malleolus stabilizing the talus.

3. Operator's distal hand grasps the calcaneus, maintains the foot and ankle at 90°, and translates the calcaneus anteromedially and posterolaterally under the talus, sensing for restricted movement (Fig. 19.64).

4. Comparison is made with the opposite side.

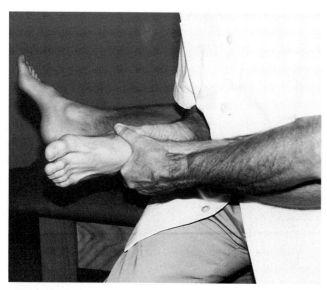

Figure 19.63.

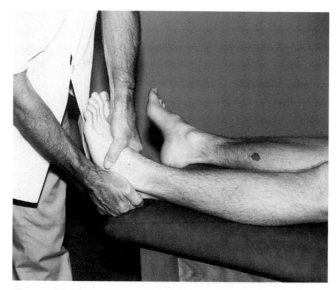

Figure 19.64.

Ankle Region: Talocalcaneal (Subtalar) Joint

Supine

Mobilization with Impulse Technique
Diagnosis
Position: Anteromedial or posterolateral talus
Motion restriction: Posterolateral or anteromedial glide of the talus

1. Patient supine on table with operator sitting on table facing caudally.

2. Patient's hip is flexed to 90° and externally rotated with the knee flexed to 90° and the posterior aspect of the thigh being against the operator's trunk.

3. The web between the thumb and index finger of the operator's medial hand contacts the superior aspect of the calcaneus.

4. The web of the thumb and index finger of the operator's lateral hand grasps the anterior and lateral aspect of the calcaneus and incorporates the cuboid. The thumb is on the tarsal navicular.

5. In the presence of an anteromedial talus (calcaneus posterolateral), the calcaneus is medially rotated (inverted to the barrier) (Fig. 19.65).

6. In the presence of a posterolateral talus (calcaneus anteromedial), the calcaneus is laterally rotated (everted) (Fig. 19.66).

7. When the barrier is engaged, a mobilization with impulse thrust is performed through both hands by a long axis distraction maneuver.

8. Retest.

FOOT

The foot is a complex structure incorporating the tarsals, metatarsals, and the phalanges. There are four arches within the foot. The lateral weight-bearing arch runs from the calcaneus, through the cuboid, to the fourth and fifth metatarsal bones, and to the fourth and fifth toes. The key to the lateral weight-bearing arch is the cuboid, which rotates medially and laterally around the anterior articulation of the calcaneus. The medial spring arch includes the talus, the navicular, the medial cuneiform, the first metatarsal, and the great toe. The medial and lateral rotation of the navicular around the head of the talus determines the function of the medial spring arch. The transverse arch includes the cuboid laterally and the navicula medially and the accompanying cuneiforms.

The major restrictors of the transverse arch are dysfunction of the cuboid laterally and the navicula medially. The most common dysfunction of the transverse arch is the cuboid being rotated internally and pronated.

The metatarsal arch is not a true arch but refers to the relation of the heads of the five metatarsals. Restrictions of the metatarsal heads at the metatarsal arch are usually secondary to dysfunction of the other arches of the foot and are accompanied by restriction of the soft tissues of the foot, primarily the plantar fascia.

Dysfunction at the navicula is either internal or external rotational restriction. Dysfunction usually accompanies that of the cuboid and the most common

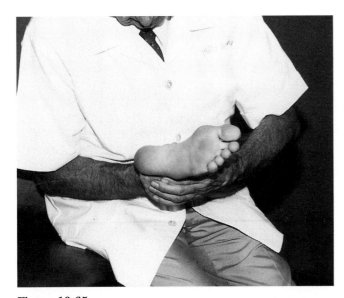

Figure 19.65.

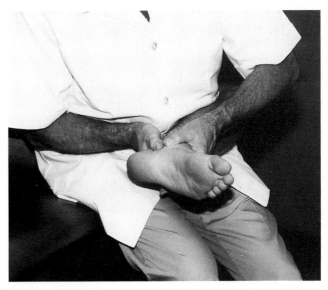

Figure 19.66.

is for the navicula to rotate externally with elevation of its medial tubercle. A less common dysfunction is with the navicula rotating internally with depression of the medial tubercle.

The cuneiforms respond to normal motion or dysfunction of the navicula and the cuboid. The first cuneiform rotates internally and externally on the navicula. The remaining cuneiforms glide upon each other, and when dysfunctional, there is usually depression with flattening of the transverse arch.

The first tarsometatarsal joint has similar movement to the navicula on the talus and the first cuneiform on the navicula. The remaining tarsometatarsal joints have a dorsal to plantar joint play glide motion in response to the transverse tarsal arch. A second joint play movement is medial and lateral rotation.

The metatarsal heads form the pseudometatarsal arch. The second metatarsal appears to be the axis of the forefoot, and the first metatarsal is moved on the second, the third on the second, the fourth on the third, and the fifth on the fourth. The joint play movements present are dorsal and plantar glide as well as rotation. The most common area of restriction is between the second and third metatarsal heads. When the metatarsal heads are restricted, there is frequent tension and tenderness of the interosseous muscles.

The metatarsophalangeal joints and the interphalangeal joints have primary motions of dorsiflexion and plantar flexion. There are also minor play movements of these joints with medial and lateral tilt and rotation. Reestablishment of the joint play movements frequently restores pain free flexion and extension of the metatarsophalangeal and interphalangeal joints.

The primary goals of manual medicine treatment of the foot are to restore functional capacity of the entire mechanism, particularly of the cuboid laterally, the navicula medially, the tarsometatarsal joints, the metatarsal heads, and the joints of the phalanges. Appropriate diagnosis and treatment of dysfunctions of the foot frequently restore pain free movement. Treatment of these dysfunctions strongly influences the remaining lower extremity joints and trunk during the walking cycle.

Calcaneocuboid Joint

Supine

Diagnosis
1. Patient supine on table with operator standing at end.
2. Operator palpates plantar surface of each cuboid looking for prominence of the tuberosity on the dysfunctional side.
3. Operator palpates plantar surface of each cuboid for tenderness and tension.
4. Operator motion tests cuboid on each side by having the medial hand grasp the calcaneus and holding the foot in 90° at the ankle. The lateral hand grasps the lateral side of the forefoot encircling the cuboid. Internal and external rotation of the forefoot is performed while monitoring for movement at the cuboid calcaneal joint (Fig. 19.67).

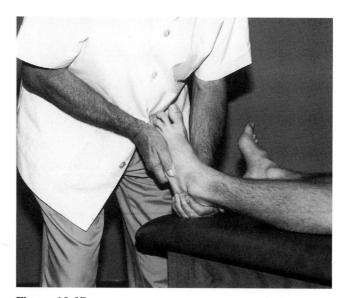

Figure 19.67.

Calcaneocuboid Joint

Prone

Mobilization with Impulse Technique
Diagnosis
  Position: Cuboid pronated (internally rotated)
  Motion restriction: Cuboid supination (external rotation)

1. Patient prone with dysfunctional leg off side of table with operator standing at side on dysfunctional side facing cephalad.
2. Operator's two hands grasp the forefoot.

3. The thumb of the lateral hand is placed over the plantar surface of the cuboid and is reinforced with the thumb of the medial hand (Fig. 19.68).
4. Operator swings the foot in a series of oscillating movements plantar flexing the forefoot.
5. With engagement of the barrier the foot is "thrown" toward the floor with acute plantar flexion of the forefoot and with the reinforced thumbs carrying the cuboid dorsally and into external rotation (Fig. 19.69).
6. Retest.

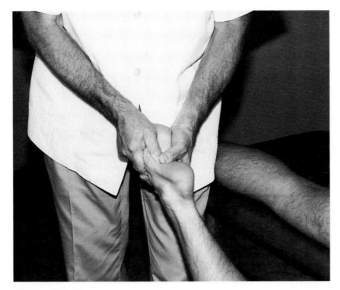

Figure 19.68.

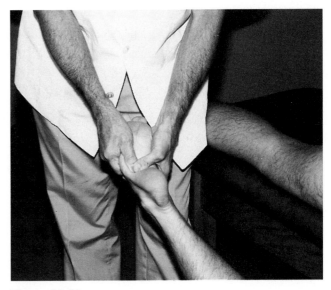

Figure 19.69.

Calcaneocuboid Joint

Supine

Muscle Energy Technique and Mobilization with Impulse Technique

Diagnosis

Position: Cuboid pronated (internally rotated)

Motion restriction: Supination (external rotation) of the cuboid

1. Patient supine on table with operator standing at foot facing dysfunctional foot.

2. Medial hand grasps the calcaneus and maintains the foot in 90° of flexion.

3. Operator's lateral hand grasps the lateral aspect of the foot with the middle and ring fingers overlying the plantar aspect of the cuboid and the hypothe-nar eminence over the dorsal aspect of the fourth and fifth metatarsal shafts (Fig. 19.70).

4. The resistant barrier is engaged by lifting with the middle and ring fingers and depressing the metatarsals with the hypothenar eminence.

5. Patient is instructed to perform dorsiflexion of the little toe against resistance for three to five repetitions of 3–5 seconds.

6. Operator engages a new barrier after each effort.

7. With the same localization, a mobilization with impulse thrust can be performed by an acute lifting maneuver with the reinforced middle and ring fingers and depression of the fourth and fifth metatarsals (Fig. 19.71).

8. Retest.

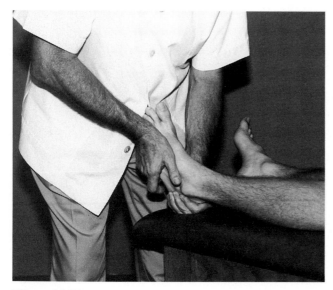

Figure 19.70.

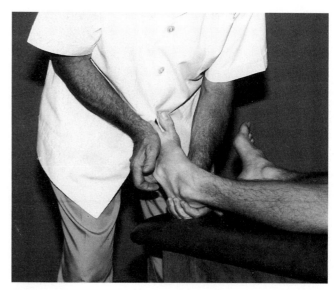

Figure 19.71.

Talonavicular Joint

Diagnosis: Internal or External Rotation of the Navicula

1. Patient supine on table with operator standing at end facing cephalward.

2. Operator palpates the medial tubercle of each navicula for symmetry, tension, and tenderness of the medial and plantar surface.

3. Operator's proximal hand grasps the neck of the talus between the web of the thumb and index finger. The web and index finger of the distal hand surrounds the tarsal navicula. Operator stabilizes the proximal hand and internally and externally rotates with the distal hand in a "wringing" motion, testing for the capacity for internal rotation (Fig. 19.72) and external rotation (Fig. 19.73).

4. Comparison is made with the opposite side.

Talonavicular Joint

Muscle Energy Technique and Mobilization with Impulse Technique

Diagnosis

Position: Navicula internally rotated or externally rotated

Motion restriction: Internal or external rotation of the navicula

1. Patient and operator position the same as for the diagnostic procedure.

2. With the navicula externally rotated, the operator's distal hand internally rotates the navicula against the resistant barrier (Fig. 19.72). Patient is instructed to invert the foot against resistance for 3–5 seconds and repeat three to five times.

3. After each muscle effort, the new barrier is engaged.

4. With the navicula internally rotated, the distal hand externally rotates the navicula to the resistant barrier. The patient is instructed to evert the foot against resistance for 3–5 seconds and three to five repetitions (Fig. 19.73).

5. Operator engages new barrier after each patient effort.

6. A mobilization with impulse thrust activating force can be substituted for the muscle energy activity by mobilizing the distal hand against the proximal.

7. Retest.

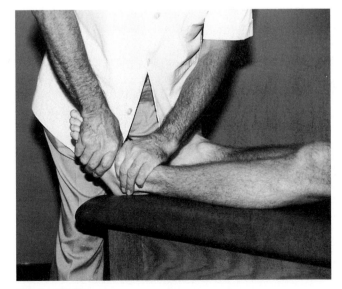

Figure 19.72.

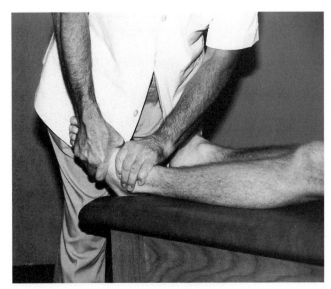

Figure 19.73.

Cuneiform Bones (Intertarsal Joints)

Diagnosis

1. Patient supine on table with operator standing at foot facing cephalward.

2. Each cuneiform is grasped between the thumb and index finger. While stabilizing one cuneiform the other is tested for dorsi to plantar joint play movement (Fig. 19.74).

3. With the thumbs on the dorsum of the cuneiforms and the fingers of both hands on the plantar surface of the foot, a plantar force is exerted through the thumbs, ascertaining the presence or absence of springing movement.

4. Both sides are tested for comparison.

5. A joint play treatment procedure can be performed by grasping cuneiform and moving the adjacent one in a dorsal to plantar joint play direction.

Cuneiform Bones (Intertarsal Joints)

Muscle Energy Technique
Diagnosis
    Position: Depression of cuneiforms
    Motion restriction: Dorsal arching of the cuneiforms

1. Patient supine on table with operator standing at foot facing cephalward.

2. Operator's proximal hand stabilizes the hind foot with the thumb against the plantar surface of the dysfunctional cuneiform exerting a dorsal force.

3. Operator's distal hand stabilizes the forefoot with the hypothenar eminence over the dorsal aspect of the metatarsal shafts.

4. The barrier is engaged by plantar flexing the forefoot (Fig. 19.75).

5. Patient is instructed to perform a muscle effort of lifting the toes cephalward against equal and opposite resistance for 3–5 seconds and three to five repetitions (Fig. 19.76).

6. A new barrier is engaged after each patient effort.

7. Retest.

Note: In the presence of dysfunction of the first cuneiform to the navicula, the muscle energy and mobilization with impulse technique of the navicula on the talus can be modified by the proximal hand grasping the navicula and the distal hand the first cuneiform.

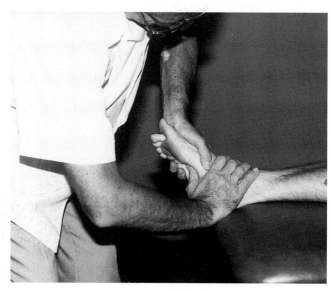

Figure 19.75.

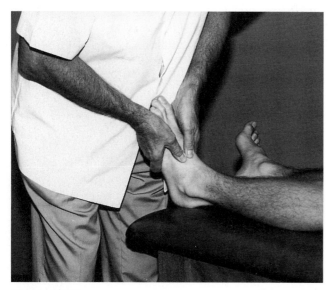

Figure 19.74.

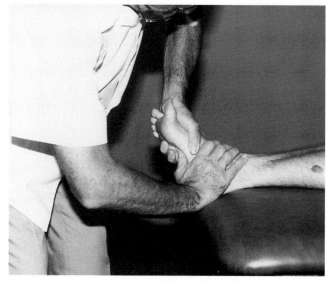

Figure 19.76.

Tarsometatarsal Joints

Joint Play
Diagnosis: Restoration of Dorsal to Plantar Glide

1. Patient supine with operator standing at foot of table.

2. Operator's two thumbs are on the plantar surface of adjacent metatarsal bases with the fingers on the dorsal side of the proximal metatarsal shafts.

3. One metatarsal is held while the other is moved in a dorsal to plantar glide fashion (Fig. 19.77).

4. If restriction is noted, a mobilizing without impulse joint play maneuver is performed, enhancing gliding movement between the bases of the metatarsal bones and the tarsometatarsal articulations.

5. Each metatarsal base and shaft is evaluated and treated sequentially.

6. Comparison is made with the opposite side for symmetry.

Tarsometatarsal Joints

Joint Play
Diagnosis: Evaluation and Restoration of Medial and Lateral Rotation

1. Patient supine with operator standing at foot of table.

2. Operator's proximal hand stabilizes the cuneiform bones through the web of the thumb and index finger.

3. Operator's distal hand dorsiflexes forefoot and introduces eversion of the forefoot (Fig. 19.78) and inversion of the forefoot (Fig. 19.79).

4. Comparison of eversion and inversion of each foot is made.

5. In the presence of restriction in either direction, a mobilizing with impulse joint play maneuver is performed against the resistant barrier.

6. Retest.

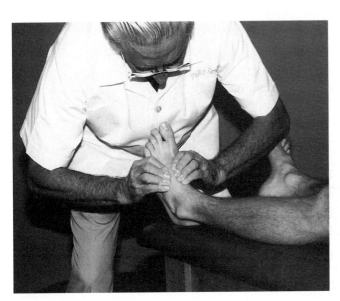

Figure 19.77.

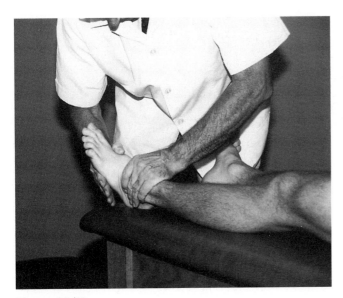

Figure 19.78.

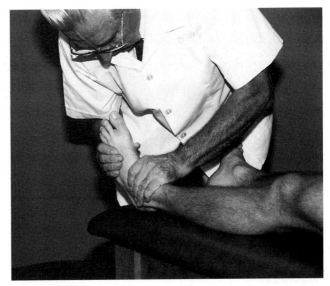

Figure 19.79.

Metatarsal Heads

Joint Play
Diagnosis: Restriction of Joint Play at Metatarsal Heads

1. Patient supine with operator standing at end of table.

2. Operator's medial hand grasps the shaft of the second metatarsal while the lateral hand grasps the shaft of the third metatarsal (Fig. 19.80).

3. While stabilizing the second metatarsal, operator's lateral hand dorsi and plantar moves the metatarsal head, seeking resistance to motion. Comparison is made with the opposite side.

4. Operator's medial hand holds the shaft of the second metatarsal and the lateral hand the shaft of the third metatarsal. The lateral hand is rotated medially and laterally, testing for rotary capacity of the metatarsal heads. Comparison is made with the opposite side.

5. Sequentially, the fourth metatarsal is moved on the third, the fifth metatarsal is moved on the fourth, and the first metatarsal is moved on the second in similar fashion.

Metatarsal-Phalangeal Joints and the Interphalangeal Joints

Motion Testing and Joint Play
Example: First Metatarsal-Phalangeal Joint

1. Patient supine with operator standing at foot of table.

2. Operator stabilizes proximal bone (first metatarsal) with thumb and fingers.

3. Operator grasps distal bone (proximal phalanx of the first toe).

4. Flexion-extension, anterior posterior glide, medial and lateral rotation, and medial and lateral tilt are performed, testing for resistance to movement (Fig. 19.81).

5. Comparison is made with the opposite side.

6. Sequential joint play motions are performed to restore all joint play movements.

7. All other interphalangeal joints can be treated in similar fashion by stabilizing the proximal bone and moving the distal upon it.

CONCLUSION

The foot of the lower extremity is the bottom block of the postural structural model. Intrinsic dysfunction within the foot or secondary to other dysfunctions within the lower extremity can influence the biomechanical function of the total musculoskeletal system. Lower extremity joint function is essential for symmetrical gait. The sole of the foot is a sense organ for sensory motor balance. Evaluation and restoration of function to the foot and lower extremity is an essential component in the management of patients with musculoskeletal problems.

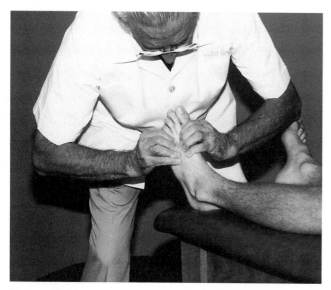

Figure 19.80.

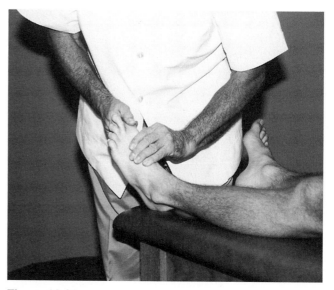

Figure 19.81.

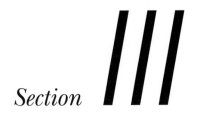

Section **///**

CLINICAL INTEGRATION
AND CORRELATION

20

EXERCISE PRINCIPLES AND PRESCRIPTION

Exercise has a long history in the healing arts and has been used for the maintenance of general health and for the prevention of disease by both Eastern and Western cultures. The ancient Greeks originated the Olympics to honor those with exceptional athletic skills. Modern Olympians continue that tradition, spending enormous time and energy enhancing their level of expertise and maximizing their performance potential.

Today there is an ever-increasing interest in exercise and sporting activities. An increase continues in the numbers of health spas, athletic centers and clubs dedicated to the principle that exercise is a fundamental good that is not only essential for one's health but also an enjoyable leisure pastime.

Exercise is increasingly used by health professionals of many disciplines, particularly physical therapists. In the area of low back pain, William's flexion exercises and Mackenzie's extension program have been widely used. There is more to the William's program than flexion and more to the Mackenzie program than extension, but these systems, and many similar programs, are designed to enhance the strength and flexibility in the patient who suffers from low back pain from a variety of causes.

There are numerous texts on procedures for manual muscle testing, stretching, and strengthening. More recently, video series have been developed both for health professionals and lay persons to assist in the maintenance of health and therapeutic treatment plans.

Numerous diagnostic and therapeutic exercise equipment systems have been developed and are currently on the market. This equipment objectively measures range of motion and strength of muscle in various physical activities. Machines have been developed to exercise various areas of the body and related muscle groups, whereas other equipment has been designed for the maintenance of aerobic capacity and restoration of fitness after bouts of injury or disease.

Despite all of the activities described, it has been this author's observation that many health professionals, in a variety of disciplines, have limited knowledge and understanding of how to prescribe exercises that are appropriate for their patients. Although there are a number of programs that have generic value, each patient is an individual and requires an exercise program specific for their problem. The practitioner needs the skill to identify problems of the patient's neuromusculoskeletal system and prescribe appropriate exercises just as they prescribe appropriate medication, manual medicine, or surgical intervention. The following principles and procedures are those that this author has found effective and are the results of the contributions of numerous authors and colleagues.

PRINCIPLES OF MUSCLE IMBALANCE

As stated in Chapter 1, the goal of manipulation is to restore maximal pain free movement of the musculoskeletal system in postural balance. When the manipulative intervention has achieved maximum mobility, the question remains, how is it maintained? The obvious answer is an appropriate exercise program the patient can perform that maintains the functional capacity of the musculoskeletal system within the constraints of the available anatomy. The manual medicine practitioner is limited by the available anatomy that may be altered by genetic development, single or repetitive trauma, and surgical intervention. Despite the altered anatomy and pathology present, it is most surprising and satisfying to both the practitioner and the patient to see the amount of functional capacity that can be restored and maintained by an appropriate exercise program.

An appropriate exercise prescription provides the patient with the ability and responsibility to maintain a high level of neuromusculoskeletal health. It is important that the patient understand, and commit to perform, the necessary exercise program. While being as comprehensive as necessary, it should be simple and be performed without depending on specialized equipment or facilities. Obviously, if appropriate equipment is available, its use can be most beneficial. Of utmost importance is the patient understanding that after a disabling musculoskeletal condition, it is imperative to continue an active exercise program for the rest of their lives.

PRINCIPLES OF MOTOR CONTROL
Muscle Pathology

Functional pathology of muscle results from perturbation of a highly complex neurological control system. A disturbance of musculoskeletal function initiates a series of events, beginning with stimulation to mechanoreceptors and nociceptors and resulting in afferent neural activity that initiates a variety of reflexes both at the cord, brainstem, and cortical levels. The final common pathway is the α motor neuron, which stimulates muscle fiber to contract, and through the γ system the muscle spindle to adapt, resulting in alteration in muscle tone. Chronic articular or muscle dysfunction feeds the afferent loop with more nociception and abnormal mechanoreceptor information, perpetuating ongoing aberrant muscle tone. The more this vicious cycle can be interrupted and reprogramed, the better is the overall muscle tone and balance maintained.

Morphology

The morphology and functional characteristics of articular receptor systems have been well appreciated since the work of Wyke and his colleagues.

Receptors

There are basically four different types of receptors (Fig. 20.1). These receptors are found in joint capsules, ligaments, and articular fat pads. They have different sizes, shapes, clusters, and different nerve fibers, from small unmyelinated to very small, small, medium, and large myelination. Their different behaviors include response to static and dynamic change, with low or high thresholds, and range from rapidly adapting to slow adapting to nonadapting. In simplistic terms, this system provides to the central nervous system information on the three-dimensional position of joints and the rate of change in relationship. This articular information, combining impulses from muscle spindles and golgi tendon organs reporting on muscle length and tension, is transmitted to the spinal cord for central processing. Afferent fibers from nociceptors and mechanoreceptors enter the dorsal horn where numerous neuronal reflexes are initiated and mediated.

Neurons

There are numerous combinations of neuronal connections acting on the motor neuron of the final common pathway. Divergence describes the process of a single neuron synapsing with several target end organs, either directly or through interneurons. Convergence describes the process where a motor neuron receives and summates inputs from a variety of fibers, including afferents, interneurons, and descending fibers from other spinal and supraspinal regions. Gaiting is the process of altering the output from the motor neuron via inhibitory interneurons or inhibiting neurons from descending control signals. Occasionally, the gait can be initiated by presynaptic inhibition, an example being a descending inhibitory control signal acting on the presynaptic terminals of afferent fibers.

Four Components of Motor System

There are four hierarchically organized components of the motor system. From above downward they include the premotor cortical regions, the motor cortex, the brainstem, and the spinal cord. It is through the spinal cord that many activities of the motor system are initiated and maintained. The cord is programed to respond to both peripheral and central stimulation. The spinal cord has the capacity to learn. Preprogramed normal behavior can be replaced by abnormal response if the cord has repetitive aberrant stimulation. This process can be viewed as both good and bad, because the cord that learns to perpetuate abnormal mechanical behavior through persistence of structural and functional pathology can be reprogramed to more normal activity through appropriate manual medicine and exercise procedures.

All four components of the motor system are functionally interrelated. A stimulus from the periphery initiates afferent input to segmental spinal reflexes and carries information centrally to the brainstem and cortical areas. The cord level information proceeds through spinal pathways to muscle groups, resulting in force generation to displace a load. The responses to this activity return by afferent loops joining with the original afferent stimulation to continue information processing at the cord level. The initial afferent input stimulates cortical and brainstem levels, initiating descending pathways from both the

Shape:	Nerve:	Characteristic:
1. Globular	Small myelinated	Static and dynamic mechanoreceptors
2. Conical	Large myelinated	Dynamic mechanoreceptor
3. Fusiform	Medium myelinated	Mechanoreceptor
4. Plexus	Unmyelinated	Nociceptor

Figure 20.1.
Four types of articular receptors.

brainstem and the motor cortex. These complex descending pathways are modulated through the basal ganglion and cerebellar systems, changing brainstem activity that descends through the cord, modulates cord reflexes, and ultimately influences muscle activity.

Spinal Cord

The spinal cord has intricate neuronal interconnections through long and short propriospinal pathways, influencing motor neuron pools to the muscles of the axial skeleton and the extremities. The neuronal pools for the axial muscles are oriented medially, those for the extremities more laterally, with the proximal limb being central and the distal limb more lateral. These neuronal pathways occur both ipsilaterally and contralaterally and course up and down through several levels of the spinal cord.

Brainstem Pathways

There are two groups of descending brainstem pathways. The first is the ventral medial group, which includes the reticulospinal, the vestibulospinal, and the tectospinal tracts. The dorsolateral pathways are primarily those related to the red nucleus. The rubrospinal tract crosses centrally and descends in the contralateral dorsolateral funiculus of the cord. Much of the central control of cord and spinal column activity results from information in these descending brainstem pathways.

Cortical Pathways

The descending cortical pathways include the crossed and uncrossed systems. The lateral cortical spinal tract crosses in the pyramidal desiccation and terminates in the lateral aspect of the cord. This system has considerable input to the rubrospinal tracts of the brainstem. The ventral cortical spinal tract is uncrossed and terminates more centrally in the ventral portion of the cord. Influence from this tract occurs through the ventral medial brainstem pathways. Most cortical influence on cord activity occurs through the brainstem pathways rather than directly at cord level. The information descending from the cortex and brainstem is designed to initiate muscle action and modulate it based on response. Much of the descending information is inhibitory to the programed cord response so that the resultant action is controlled, smooth, and appropriate for the desired result.

α Motor Neuron

Stimulation to the α motor neuron, the final common pathway, results in muscle activity. The resultant action is reported through a complex feedback system to determine both muscle length and muscle tension. Control of muscle length is primarily determined by the response of the muscle spindle. When the muscle is stretched, increasing discharge from the spindle reports to the cord that the muscle is lengthening. When the muscle contracts with shortening of the extrafusal fibers, there is initially electrical silence from the spindle, followed by rapid stimulation to the spindle to shorten in response to the shortening of the extrafusal fibers. The spindle has both nuclear bag and nuclear chain fibers, each having their own afferent control. The spindle responds to change in static length as well as dynamically in the rate of change in length. Control of muscle tension is primarily mediated through the golgi tendon apparatus. Although the muscle spindles are parallel to the extrafusal fibers, the golgi tendon organs are in series. The golgi tendon organ responds to muscle stretch and contraction. It discharges most actively during muscle contraction and initiates an inhibitory reflex arc, preventing overload of the muscle and the musculotendinous junction.

The α motor neuron is controlled by central demand and through feedback loops. The central control of the γ motor neuron establishes the length of the muscle spindle and sets the anticipated activity of the positive stimulation to the α motor neuron. After the α motor neuron is stimulated, changes in muscle length and tension occur. The response is then compared by the spindle as to the anticipated activity. Feedback loops to the spinal cord modulate the continued central control of the α motor neuron. Differences between anticipated and actual change result in appropriate muscle length and tension through the activity. Feedback loops from the spindle report difference in length, whereas the golgi tendon organ reports difference in force. Feedback loops can be either excitatory or inhibitory to the α motor neuron so that the final action of muscle is appropriate.

Another Reflex Pathway

Another basic reflex pathway governs reciprocal innervation and inhibition. Stimulation to both limb flexor and extensor muscles is called cocontraction and stabilizes a joint and restricts its movement. During joint flexion, the flexor contracts and, by reciprocal inhibition, the extensor muscle group relaxes, allowing for controlled flexion activity. The reverse is true for extension: the extensor contracts and the flexor is inhibited and relaxes. This reciprocal inhibition occurs contralaterally as well as ipsilaterally. When the ipsilateral flexor contracts, there is reflex inhibition of the contralateral flexor. The harder one muscle contracts, the more it inhibits its antagonist. This phenomena occurs both ipsilaterally and contralaterally. Through this reflex pathway, facilitated muscle contracts and is maintained in a shortened position, resulting in inhibition of its antagonist, which becomes weakened.

Muscle Fiber Type

Muscle is characterized by its fiber type, either slow or fast twitch. Slow-twitch muscle uses oxidative metabolism and has a high capillary density, giving it its characteristic red color. The twitch speed is slow, and the function of these muscles is that described as being tonic or postural. Muscles that have high density slow-twitch fibers react to functional disturbance by shortening and tightening. Fast-twitch fibers use a glycolytic metabolic pathway, fatigue rapidly, and have low capillary density that results in a white color. Muscles of this type are described as phasic in function and react to disturbance by weakening.

All muscles have a mixture of slow- and fast-twitch fibers, but some muscles have more slow twitch, whereas others have more of fast twitch. Muscles with primary postural or tonic function in the pelvic and hip regions include the hamstrings, iliopsoas, rectus femoris, tensor fascia lata, thigh adductors, and piriformis. Phasic muscles in the pelvic and hip region include the vastus medialis and lateralis of the anterior thigh and the gluteus medius, maximus, and minimis. In the trunk, the postural tonic muscles are the erector spinae group, primarily in the lumbar and cervical regions, the quadratus lumborum, and the scalenes. The phasic muscles of the trunk are the erector spinae muscles in the midthoracic region. In the lower extremity, the gastrocnemius and soleus muscles are tonic and tibialis anterior and perineal muscles are phasic. In the shoulder girdle, the postural tonic muscles are pectoralis major, levator scapulae, upper trapezius and biceps brachii. The phasic muscles are the rhomboids, lower trapezius, and triceps brachii. An understanding of muscle function, either phasic or tonic, is important for the prescription of an appropriate exercise program.

THEORETICAL CAUSES OF MUSCLE IMBALANCE
Malregulation by the Central Nervous System

Muscle imbalance consists of shortening and tightening of muscle groups (usually the tonic muscles), weakness of certain muscle groups (usually the phasic muscles), and loss of control on integrated muscle function. Alteration in length, strength, and motor control can occur from a variety of causes. Muscle balance is continually adapting the body's posture to gravity. Faulty posture results in alteration of the center of gravity, which initiates mechanical responses requiring muscle adaption. Change in mechanical behavior of a joint causes neuroreflexive alteration in muscle function through aberrant afferent mechanoreceptor stimulation of articular reflexes. Long-term activation of abnormal articular reflexes cause change in cord memory from normal to an abnormal adaptive program, resulting in muscle imbalance. Muscle imbalance results from malregulation by the central nervous system, either at the cord level or higher centers, from altered agonist and antagonist reactions and responses to dysfunction of the limbic system.

Muscle balance is altered in response to noxious stimuli through central mediated pathways and segmental reflexes. Central mediation through the lateral reticular system alters activity of γ motor neurons, resulting in hyperreflexia and altered time activation sequences of muscle action. At a segmental level, nociception facilitates α motor neurons to the flexors in the limbs and to the extensors in the neck and trunk. Muscle balance responds to the physical demand placed on it. Depending on its metabolic pathway, muscle responds to fatigue in different ways. Tonic muscles fatigue more slowly than phasic muscles. In the presence of altered movement patterns through chronic overuse, some muscles will become tight, and abnormal muscle pattern habits result. It is for this reason that motor programing through appropriate exercise is so important. Psychological factors can influence muscle balance and tone. Who is not aware of the tightness and fatigue that result when we are "uptight"? Muscle imbalance is clearly a multifactorial problem and can be highly complex. In simplistic terms, the result of muscle imbalance is that tight muscles become tighter, weak muscles become weaker, and motor control becomes more asymmetric. Each of these factors need to be addressed in an exercise program.

Scientific-Clinical Theory of Janda

Much of the following material is based on the work of Janda, a specialist in rehabilitation medicine at the University of Charles, Prague, Czechoslovakia, who has researched normal and abnormal muscle function at both the basic science and clinical levels. He has determined that muscle dysfunction is not a random occurrence but that muscles respond in characteristic patterns.

Pseudoparesis. Postural-tonic muscles respond to dysfunction by facilitation, hypertonicity, and shortening. Dynamic-phasic muscles respond to dysfunction by inhibition, hypotonicity, and weakness. Janda described this weakness as being pseudoparesis. The weakness of the muscle is due to inhibition rather than being intrinsically weak. There are multiple patterns of muscle response to dysfunction in which certain muscles become inhibited and weak, whereas others become facilitated and tight. In the hip region, the weak muscles are the gluteus medius and maximus, whereas the facilitated tight muscles are the iliopsoas, piriformis, adductors, and tensor fascia lata. In shoulder dysfunction, the weak muscles are the supraspinatus, deltoid, infraspinatus, rhomboids, lower trapezius, and serratus anterior, whereas the facilitated tight muscles are the levator scapula, upper trapezius, and pectorals.

Muscle Firing Patterns. Muscle dysfunction is not only characterized by facilitation and inhibition but also in the manner in which muscles sequentially fire. Altered muscle firing pattern shows delay in activation and in the amplitude of electromyographic activity of the dynamic-phasic muscles. Continued exercise in the presence of abnormal muscle firing sequence perpetuates hypertonicity, tightness, and shortening of the tonic muscles with continued and progressive inhibition of the phasic muscles.

Janda's research work identified the normal and abnormal muscle firing patterns in the movement patterns of hip extension, hip abduction, and shoulder abduction. The normal firing pattern of prone hip extension is hamstrings, gluteus maximus, contralateral lower lumber erector spinae, and ipsilateral lower erector spinae. The most common alteration of this normal pattern is failure of activation and weakness of the gluteus maximus with substitution by the hamstrings and erector spinae musculature, particularly in the upper lumbar and lower thoracic regions (Fig. 20.2, a and b).

The muscle firing sequence for hip abduction in the sidelying posture is gluteus medius, tensor fascia lata, ipsilateral quadratus lumborum, and erector spinae. The most common substitution pattern is for weakness of the gluteus medius with early firing the tensor fascia lata or the quadratus lumborum. Early firing the tensor fascia lata results in internal rotation and flexion of the hip during hip abduction. The worst scenario is that the motion is initiated by the

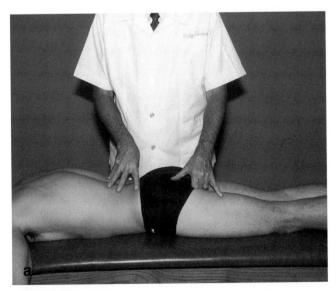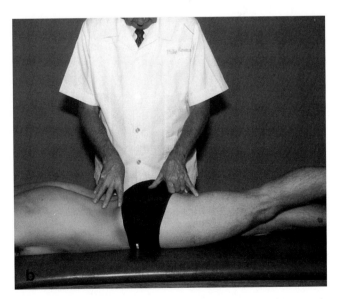

Figure 20.2.
(a) Hip extension firing pattern beginning position. (b) Hip extension firing pattern during patient muscle contraction.

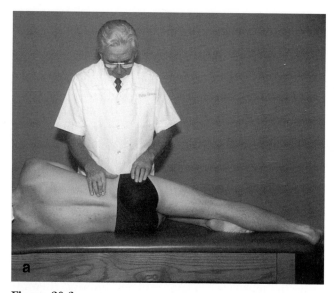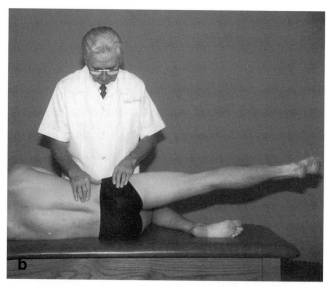

Figure 20.3.

(a) Hip abduction firing pattern beginning position. (b) Hip abduction firing pattern during patient muscle contraction.

firing of the quadratus lumborum (Fig. 20.3, a and b).

The firing sequence for shoulder abduction while seated is supraspinatus, deltoid, infraspinatus, middle and lower trapezius, and contralateral quadratus lumborum. The most common substitution pattern is for shoulder elevation by the levator scapulae and upper trapezius and early firing of the quadratus lumborum, even on the ipsilateral side (Fig. 20.4, a and b).

Muscle Imbalance Syndromes. Janda also de-

scribed three different syndromes resulting from muscle imbalance. They are the lower crossed syndrome in the pelvic girdle, the upper crossed syndrome in the shoulder girdle, and the layer syndrome from caudad to cranial. The upper and lower cross syndromes are described subsequently. The layer syndrome is characterized by alternate bands of muscle tightness and weakness on the dorsal surface of the body beginning from below upward (Fig. 20.5, a–d). It is usually characterized by tightness of the gastrocsoleus muscles, tightness of the hamstrings,

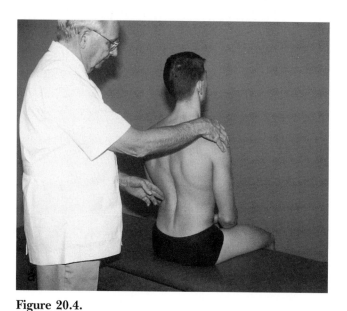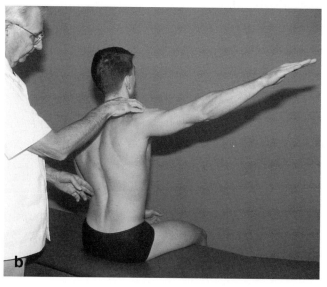

Figure 20.4.

(a) Shoulder abduction firing pattern beginning position. (b) Shoulder abduction firing pattern during patient muscle contraction.

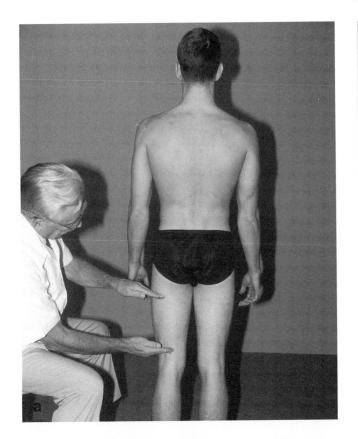
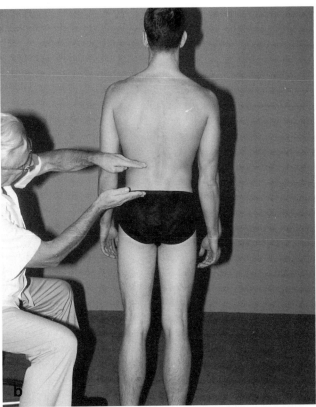
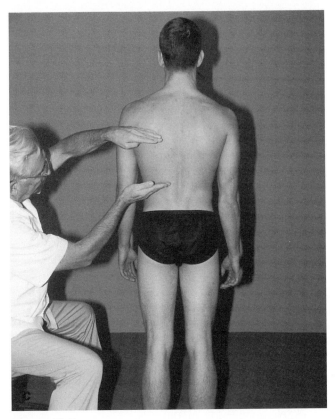
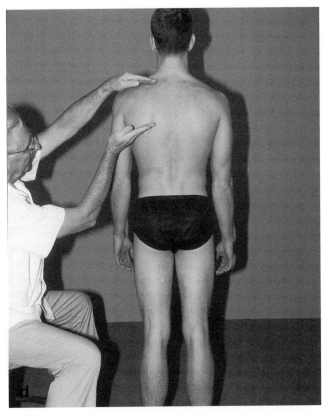

Figure 20.5.
(a) Layer syndrome, hamstrings. (b) Layer syndrome, lumbar spine. (c) Layer syndrome, thoracolumbar spine. (d) Layer syndrome, upper thoracic spine.

weakness of the glutei and the lower erector spinae, tightness of the lower thoracic and upper erector spinae, weakness of the rhomboids and lower trapezii, and tightness of the upper trapezius and levator scapulae. Another feature of the layer syndrome is "banding" in erector spinae musculature. With close observation, the examiner can identify sequential areas of hypertonicity and inhibition in various groups of the erector spinae muscle mass, particularly the longissimus. These reflect themselves as layers of fullness and small divots when observing tangentially along the erector spinae mass (Fig. 20.6).

PRINCIPLES IN TREATMENT OF MUSCLE IMBALANCES

In treating muscle imbalances, the fundamental principles are to restore length, strength, and control of muscle function. Many systems of exercise deal with length and strength, but few deal with the issues of motor control. A successful exercise program restores nervous system control of muscle function as much as possible. Of fundamental concern is the sequence of muscle firing. To achieve this result, the sequence that has been found most useful is as follows:

1. Sensory motor balance training;
2. Stretching of short, tight, hypertonic muscle to symmetry;
3. Strengthening of inhibited weak muscles to balance;
4. Restoration of symmetrical movement patterns; and
5. Aerobic conditioning.

GOALS OF TREATMENT OF MUSCLE IMBALANCES

In manual medicine practice, the goal for an exercise program is to maintain the enhanced functional capacity of the musculoskeletal system that has been achieved by appropriate manual medicine intervention. Appropriate exercise assists the patient in assuming control of their musculoskeletal system and its associated painful conditions. Improved muscle balance helps protect the osteoarticular system and reduce the strain on joints, their capsule, and ligaments. Appropriate muscle balance of agonist and antagonist provides shock absorption and prevents impact loading of joint surfaces. Lewit noted that dysfunction of the musculoskeletal system appeared earlier than degenerative morphological change. It is hypothesized that the establishment and maintenance of length and strength of the hip flexors and extensors might well prevent degenerative hip joint disease.

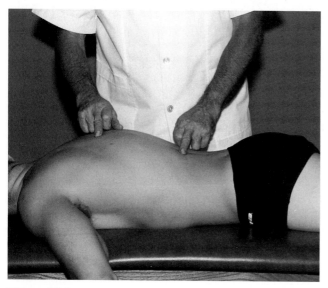

Figure 20.6.
Muscle banding.

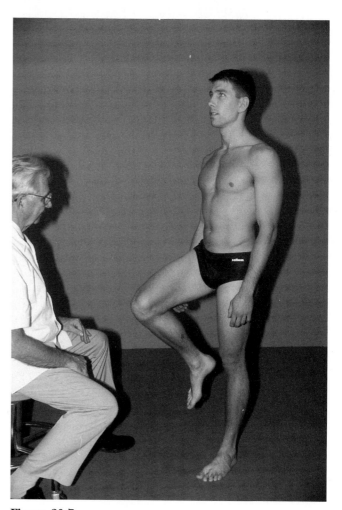

Figure 20.7.
Balance testing, level one.

SENSORY MOTOR BALANCE TRAINING

Sensory motor balance training restores symmetrical muscle firing patterns for control of motor function. Restoration of normal muscle firing sequences provides opportunity to successfully stretch hypertonic shortened muscle and to strengthen inhibited muscle.

Body balance is a complex function and is the result of three primary afferent systems. Our orientation in three-dimensional space results from the visual system, the vestibular system, and the proprioceptive input from the soles of the feet. The body adapts to loss of vision by enhanced proprioception from the extremities and greater dependence on the vestibular mechanism. The visual system compensates for reduced efficiency of proprioceptive input from contact with the ground by the soles of the feet.

Indications for Training

The first indication that a patient may need sensory motor balance training occurs during the screening and scanning examinations, particularly the function of the pelvic girdle. During the one-legged stork test, the patient stands on a single foot. If the patient is so unsteady that it is impossible to perform the test smoothly, an index of suspicion is high that the patient has deficit of proprioceptive sensitivity of the sole of the foot. Initial diagnostic testing includes asking the patient to stand in bare feet, first on one foot and then on the other to see whether there is equal balance right to left (Fig. 20.7). A second level of difficulty of this test is to ask the patient to stand on one leg with arms crossed (Fig. 20.8). This removes the balancing assistance of the upper trunk and extremities. A third level of difficulty is to ask the patient to stand on one leg with arms crossed and then close the eyes (Fig. 20.9). The removal of visual perception greatly increases the difficulty. Ideally, the patient should be able to symmetrically stand on one leg with arms crossed and eyes closed for 30 seconds.

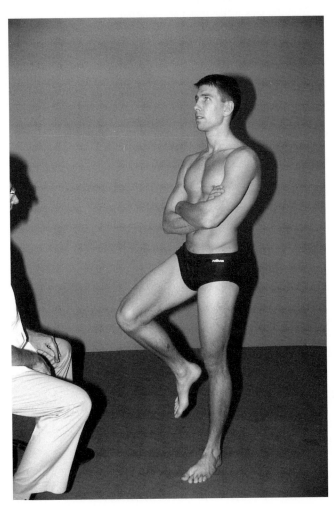

Figure 20.8.
Balance testing, level two.

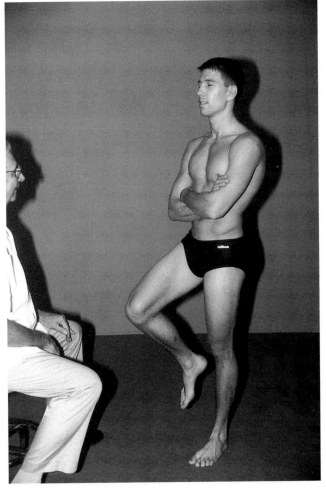

Figure 20.9.
Balance testing, level three.

Retraining

Sensory motor retraining should be done with bare feet on a carpeted surface. One of the primary goals is to stimulate the proprioceptors of the sole of the foot. One begins by practicing to shorten the foot. The "short foot" is obtained by attempting to grasp the floor with the sole of the foot without excessive curling of the toes. The shortened foot elevates the medial longitudinal arch and enhances the sensitivity of the sole of the foot. All exercises should be done with a shortened foot. A simple home program for sensory motor retraining is shown in Figure 20.10.

The goal of sensory motor balance training is the capacity to symmetrically stand on one leg with arms crossed and eyes closed for 30 seconds. The more severe the deficit, the more difficult it will be to achieve the goal. Symmetry right to left is the primary objective, and the highest level of difficulty with arms crossed, eyes closed, and length of time is the ultimate goal. The presence of neurological deficit of a lower extremity, which frequently follows a lumbar radiculopathy, can make this exercise difficult. Even in the presence of neurological deficit, it is advisable to achieve the maximum possible functional capacity to assist in the restoration of more normal muscle firing pattern sequences.

EVALUATION AND TREATMENT OF THE LOWER QUARTER

The muscle imbalances of the lower extremity include facilitation, hypertonicity, and shortening of the iliopsoas, rectus femoris, tensor fascia lata, quadratus lumborum, short thigh adductors, piriformis, hamstrings, and lumbar erector spinae. The dynamic muscles involved with inhibition, hypotonicity, and weakness are the gluteus maximus, medius, and minimis; rectus abdominis; external and internal obliques; peroneals; vastus medialis and lateralis; and tibialis anterior.

Janda's lower crossed syndrome includes weakness of the gluteus maximus and tightness of the hip flexors, weak abdominals, and short erector spinae, weak gluteus medius and minimis with short tensor fascia lata and quadratus lumborum, increased lumbar lordosis and anterior pelvic tilt, with hypermobility of the lower lumbar levels and altered functional activities that include curling up and sitting up from a supine and forward-bent posture.

SIX DIAGNOSTIC TESTS

Diagnosis of muscle imbalance and faulty postural control of the lower quarter uses six tests.

Test 1

The evaluation begins with three-dimensional assessment of pelvic control by the use of a pelvic clock

Figure 20.10.
Sensory motor examination and retraining program.

DO ALL ACTIVITIES WITH BARE FEET

1. Sitting—practice shortening both feet
2. Standing—feet aligned with the hips, neutral pelvis, trunk erect, both knees slightly flexed, practice shortening both feet

DO THE FOLLOWING ACTIVITIES WITH A NEUTRAL PELVIS, ERECT TRUNK, AND SHORTENED FEET

1. Standing on one leg
   A. Eyes open, arms down
   B. Eyes open, arms crossed
   C. Eyes closed, arms down
   D. Eyes closed, arms crossed
2. Standing—feet aligned with the hips, practice slight squatting, keep heels on surface, gradually increase to semi-squat (up to 90°)
3. Standing on one leg—practice squatting
   A. Eyes open, arms down
   B. Eyes open, arms crossed
   C. Eyes closed, arms down
   D. Eyes closed, arms crossed
4. Standing on a rocker board or rebounder
   A. Feet parallel about one foot apart; shift weight from side to side, bringing trunk over each foot
   B. One foot placed a short step in front of the other, shift weight from back to front, alternate feet
   C. Do both with arms crossed
   D. Do both with eyes closed and arms crossed
5. Standing on one foot on a rocker board or rebounder, repeat with arms crossed and then eyes closed
6. Walk on the floor/balance beam—place one foot directly in front of the other (heel to toe), done first with eyes open and then with eyes closed
7. Walk on the floor/balance beam—place one foot directly behind the other (toe to heel), done first with eyes open and then with eyes closed

---

maneuver in the supine position (Fig. 20.11, a–f). The examiner monitors the patient's anterior superior iliac spine with thumb contact while the patient moves the pelvis from 12 o'clock to 6 o'clock through a range of anterior and posterior pelvic tilt. In the presence of good pelvic control, the anterior superior iliac spine stays symmetric from neutral to 12 o'clock and to 6 o'clock. In the presence of poor pelvic control, the anterior superior iliac spine becomes more asymmetric at the 12 o'clock or 6 o'clock position. A dysfunctional pattern is to find

Figure 20.11. (facing page)
(a) Pelvic clock, beginning position. (b) Pelvic clock, posterior tilt to 12 o'clock. (c) Pelvic clock, anterior tilt to 6 o'clock. (d) Pelvic clock, rotation left to 3 o'clock. (e) Pelvic clock, rotation right to 9 o'clock. (f) Pelvic clock, body orientation.

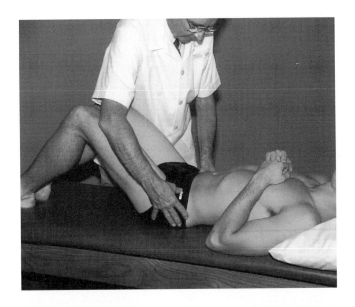

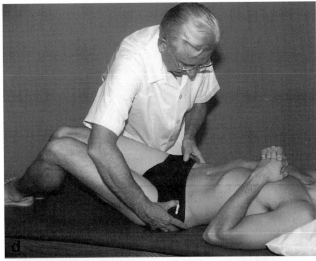

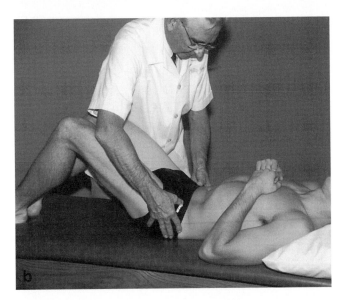

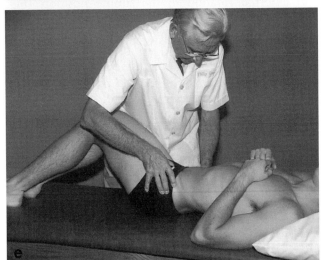

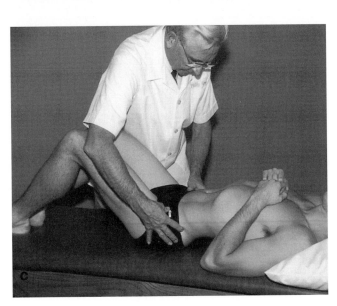

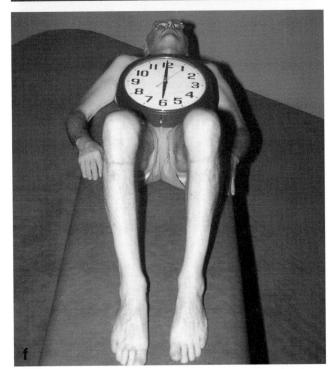

that the right anterior superior iliac spine does not proceed as far cephalically as the left at 12 o'clock and the left anterior superior iliac spine does not travel as far caudally as the right at 6 o'clock. This is followed by assessment of the anterior superior iliac spine as the pelvis is moved from 3 o'clock to 9 o'clock. This maneuver frequently reproduces low back pain. Good pelvic control finds that the pelvis rolls symmetrically across the horizontal plane from 3 o'clock to 9 o'clock and 9 o'clock to 3 o'clock. Poor trunk control is identified when there is elevation of one anterior superior iliac spine by hip hiking and substitution by lumbar spine extension.

Test 2

The second test is to evaluate passive hip abduction and external rotation in the supine position (Fig. 20.12). The examiner places the thumbs under the anterior superior iliac spines and asks the patient to do a posterior pelvic tilt in the 12 o'clock maneuver. While holding the posterior pelvic tilt, the patient is asked to drop the knees apart. Loss of control in maintaining the posterior pelvic tilt is indicative of muscle imbalance, particularly tightness of the short hip abductors. One of the most common patterns is that the right anterior superior iliac spine cannot be maintained in a cephalic direction during hip abduction and external rotation and travels in a caudad direction during the maneuver. This muscle imbalance is commonly seen in pubic dysfunction.

Test 3

The third test is the performance of a pelvic tilt and heel slide in the supine position (Fig. 20.13, a and b). The patient is asked to lie supine with the knees flexed, maintain a posterior pelvic tilt, and slowly extend first one leg and then the other, ascertaining whether it is possible to maintain a posterior pelvic tilt during eccentric lengthening of the iliopsoas. In the presence of a tight iliopsoas muscle, the patient is unable to maintain the lumbar spine flat on the examining table. This test also assesses the strength of the abdominal musculature in a lengthened position.

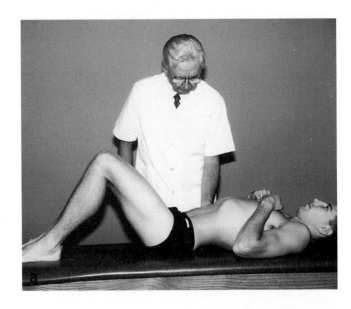

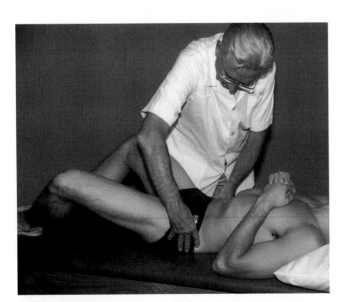

Figure 20.12.
Hip abduction, external rotation holding 12 o'clock position.

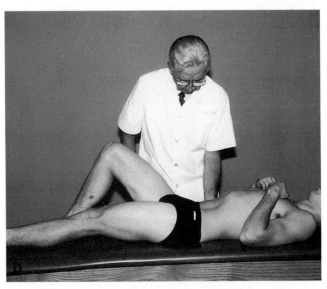

Figure 20.13.
(a) Pelvic tilt and heel slide, beginning position. (b) Patient slides heel while holding 12 o'clock position.

Test 4

The fourth test is active trunk rotation in the supine position (Fig. 20.14, a and b). With the knees and hips flexed, the patient is asked to maintain the knees and feet together and drop the knees first to one side and then to the other. With the trunk fully rotated, the patient is asked to return the knees to the midline by the use of abdominal control and not hip rotation. The patient is asked to bring the back to the table from above downward without any arching of the lower thoracic and lumbar spine. This test assesses the control of the abdominal obliques and short deep lumbar musculature. Loss of this lumbar spine segmental control is frequently associated with nonneutral lumbar spine dysfunctions and may cause exacerbation of lower back pain.

Tests 5 and 6

The fifth and sixth tests are the muscle firing pattern sequence of hip extension and hip abduction previously described.

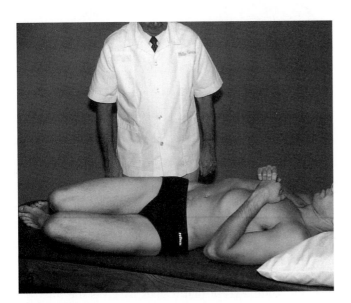
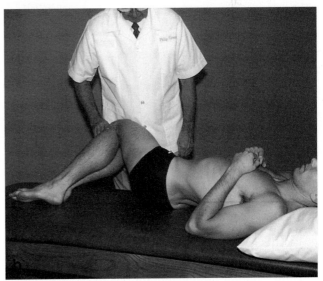

Figure 20.14.
(a) Active trunk rotation right. (b) Active trunk rotation left.

MUSCLE ASSESSMENT

Assessment is made of muscle length, and shortness and tightness are treated by manual stretching followed by self-stretches at home. The commonly tight muscles can be treated by a sustained stretch in the test position for 20–30 seconds with two or three repetitions. A second process can be postisometric relaxation. A 5- to 7-second muscle contraction against resistance is followed by a slow sustained stretch to engage a new motion barrier. Test position and manual stretching are shown in Figures 20.15 through 20.22. Self-stretches with a 20- to 30-second hold with two to three repetitions are in Figures 20.23 through 20.33.

After short and tight muscles are stretched, muscles that are inhibited can undergo retraining. Lower quadrant retraining exercises are found in Figures 20.34 through 20.44. As in all manual medicine procedures, after assessment, stretching, and strengthening, reevaluation of faulty movement patterns of the lower quadrant is done.

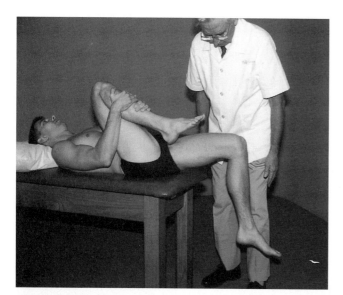

Figure 20.15a.
Psoas muscle.
Length test and manual stretch position supine.
1. Patient supine sitting at end of table with operator standing at end of table.
2. Patient holds leg not being tested in a flexed position.
3. Operator extends leg being tested. The back of the thigh should contact the table. If not, psoas shortness is present.
4. If short and tight, operator resists a 5- to 7-second contraction of hip flexion, for five to seven repetitions, with the operator increasing hip extension after each effort.

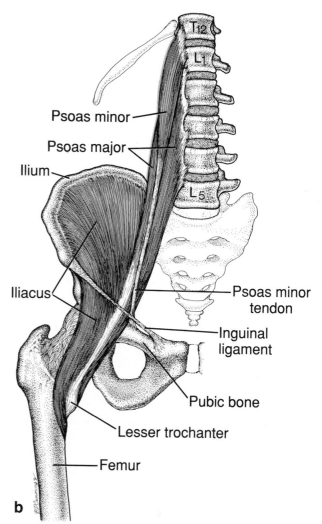

Figure 20.15b.
Attachments of the right psoas major, psoas minor and iliacus muscles. The psoas major crosses many articulations including those of the lumbar spine and the lumbosacral, sacroiliac, and hip joints. The psoas minor does the same, except that it does *not* cross the hip joint. The iliacus, on the other hand, crosses only the hip joint.

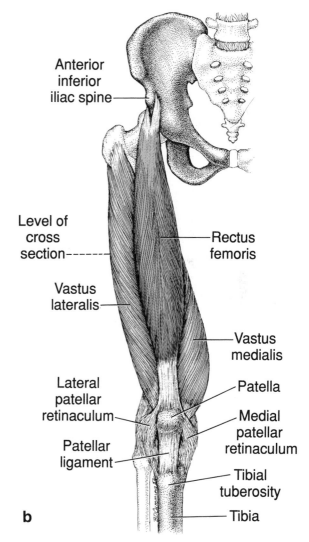

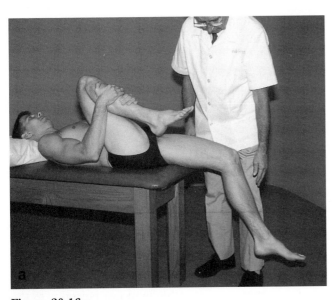

Figure 20.16a.
Rectus femoris muscle.
Length test and manual stretch position supine.
1. Patient supine sitting on end of table with operator standing at end of table.
2. Patient holds leg not being tested in a flexed position with thigh of the tested leg on the table.
3. Operator assesses flexion at the knee. If less than 90°, rectus femoris shortness is present.
4. If short and tight, operator resists a 5- to 7-second contraction of knee extension, for five to seven repetitions, with the operator increasing knee flexion after each patient effort.

Figure 20.16b.
Attachments (front view) of the right rectus femoris muscle in relation to the vastus lateralis and vastus medialis muscles.

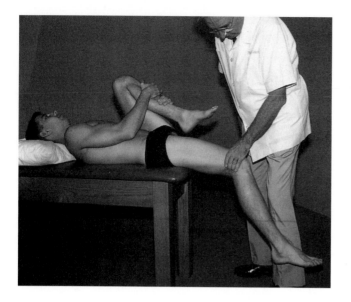

Figure 20.17a.
Tensor fascia lata muscle. Length test and manual stretch position supine.

1. Patient supine on end of table with operator standing at end of table.
2. Patient holds leg not being tested in the flexed position with the thigh of the tested leg on the table.
3. Operator introduces internal rotation of the thigh and external rotation of the tibia sensing for resistance and monitors the contour of the lateral thigh. If resistance is encountered and the lateral thigh shows a groove, tightness of the tensor fascia lata muscle is present.
4. If short and tight, operator maintains internal rotation of the femur, external rotation of the tibia, adduction of the femur, and resists a 5- to 7-second patient effort of hip flexion, for five to seven repetitions. The operator engages a new barrier after each patient effort.

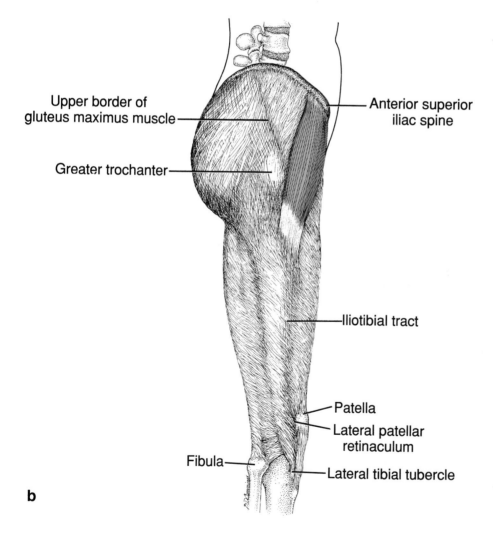

Upper border of gluteus maximus muscle

Greater trochanter

Anterior superior iliac spine

Iliotibial tract

Patella

Lateral patellar retinaculum

Fibula

Lateral tibial tubercle

b

Figure 20.17b.
Side view of attachments of the right tensor fasciae latae muscle. The muscle attaches along and below the crest of the ilium just posterior to the anterior superior iliac spine. The anteromedial tendinous fibers attach to the fascia at the knee, and the posterolateral tendinous fibers anchor to the iliotibial tract, which continues down to the lateral tubercle of the tibia.

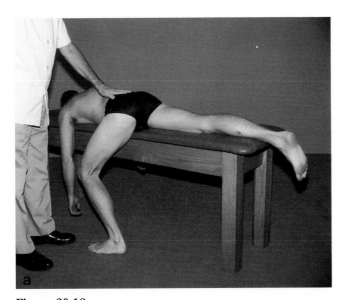
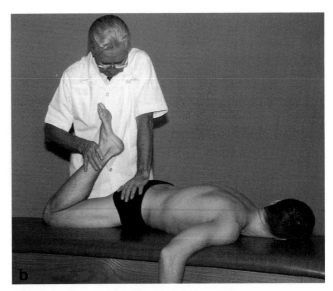

Figure 20.18.
Rectus femoris muscle.
Testing and manual stretch position prone.
1. Patient prone with leg not tested flexed at the hip and the foot on the floor (Fig. 20.18a).
2. Operator stands at side of table and flexes knee until resistance is felt. Normally, the heel of the tested leg touches the buttock. If not, tightness of the rectus femoris muscle is present (Fig. 20.18b).
3. If short and tight, operator maintains leg at the flexion barrier and resists a 5- to 7-second effort of knee extension, with five to seven repetitions. The operator engages a new barrier after each patient effort.
4. An on and off pumping maneuver by the operator can be substituted for the patients contract relax effort.
5. Operator care in knee flexion must be made to avoid abnormal stretch on the femoral nerve. If this causes severe pain to the patient with an empty end feel, be suspicious of a femoral nerve problem and not rectus femoris tightness.

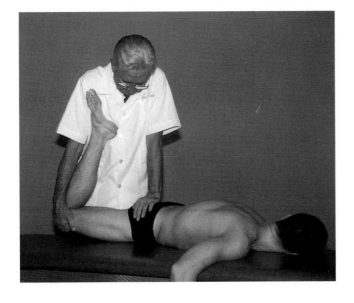

Figure 20.19.
Psoas muscle.
Length test and manual stretch position prone.
1. Patient and operator is same position as for testing rectus femoris muscle.
2. Operator lifts patient leg with knee flexed, while blocking pelvic motion at the ischial tuberosity, until engaging barrier. Normally the knee can be lifted 6 inches off the table. If less, tightness and shortness of the psoas is present.
3. In the presence of shortness and tightness, operator resists a 5- to 7-second patient effort of hip flexion (knee to table) for five to seven repetitions, with re-engagement of the barrier after each effort.

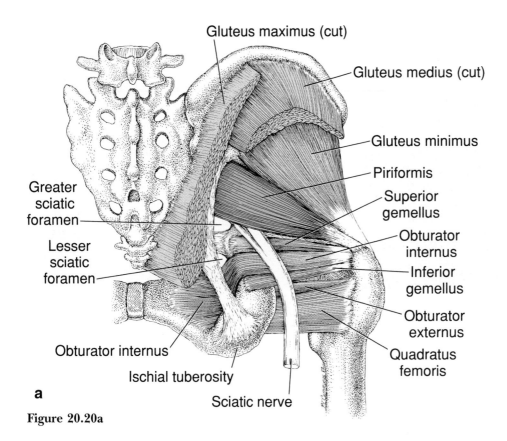

Gluteus maximus (cut)

Gluteus medius (cut)

Gluteus minimus

Piriformis

Superior gemellus

Greater sciatic foramen

Obturator internus

Lesser sciatic foramen

Inferior gemellus

Obturator externus

Obturator internus

Quadratus femoris

Ischial tuberosity

Sciatic nerve

a

Figure 20.20a

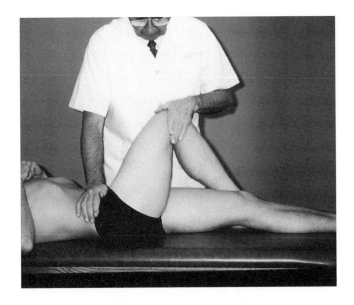

Figure 20.20b.
Piriformis muscle.
Length test and manual stretch position below 90°, supine position.
1. Patient supine on table with operator standing on opposite side of leg being tested.
2. Operator flexes tested leg at the hip and knee and places the foot outside of the opposite knee. Operator stabilizes anterior superior iliac spine on side being tested.
3. Operator introduces internal rotation and adduction of the tested leg to the barrier and compares with the opposite side. Reduced range and a tight end feel indicate shortness and tightness of the piriformis muscle being tested.
4. If short and tight, operator resists a 5- to 7-second patient effort of knee abduction and external rotation for five to seven efforts with the operator engaging a new barrier after each effort.
5. Operator maintains a compressive force toward the hip joint while stabilizing the anterior superior iliac spine.
6. This technique is also of value in stretching the posterior hip capsule.

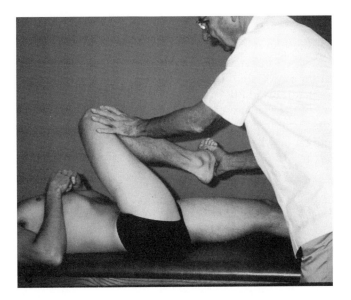

Figure 20.20c.
Psoas muscle.
Length test and manual muscle stretch above 90° supine.
1. Patient supine with operator standing on same side as leg being tested.
2. Operator grasps patients knee and ankle of leg being tested and introduces hip flexion and external rotation.
3. Resistance to further hip flexion and external rotation, compared with the opposite side, indicates shortness and tightness of the piriformis muscle. Normally the knee should touch the chest.
4. In the presence of shortness and tightness, operator resists a 5- to 7-second patient effort of extending the leg against operators two hands for five to seven repetitions. Operator engages a new barrier after each effort.

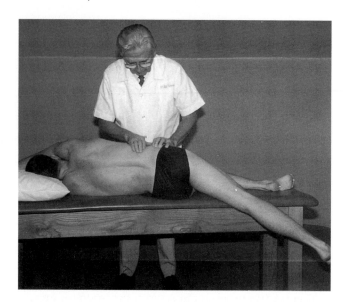

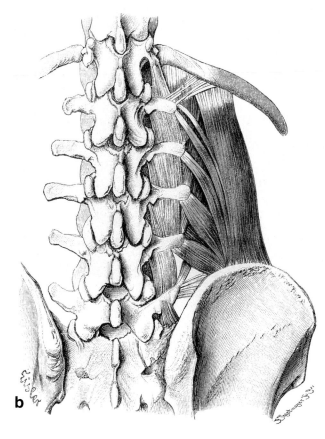

Figure 20.21 a and b.
Quadratus lumborum muscle.
Length test and manual stretch position lateral recumbent.

1. Patient in the lateral recumbent position with the leg not being tested in the flexed position and the leg being tested straight and slightly behind the trunk.
2. Operator stands in front monitoring the quadratus lumborum muscle and the iliac crest. If hip adduction is less on one side compared with the other, tightness of the quadratus lumborum is present. The operator also palpates tension in the muscle and reduced caudad motion of the iliac crest.
3. If shortness and tightness are present, operator resists at the distal femur a 5- to 7-second patient hip abduction effort for five to seven repetitions with the operator engaging a new barrier after each effort.

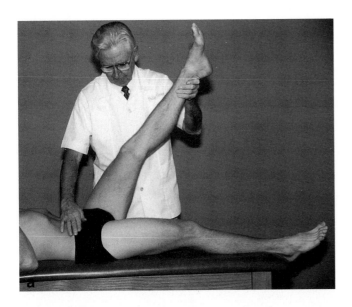

Figure 20.22 a and b.
Hamstring muscles.
Length test and manual stretch position supine.
1. Patient supine on table with operator standing on same side as leg being tested.
2. Operator monitors the opposite anterior superior iliac spine while lifting the tested leg to the barrier of hip flexion. Comparison is made with the opposite side. If asymmetric, shortness and tightness is present in the involved hamstring muscles.
3. Operator performs the test with the leg adducted and abducted to test the difference in tightness of the medial and lateral hamstrings.
4. If short and tight, operator resists a 5- to 7-second patient effort of hip extension for five to seven repetitions with the operator engaging a new barrier after each effort.

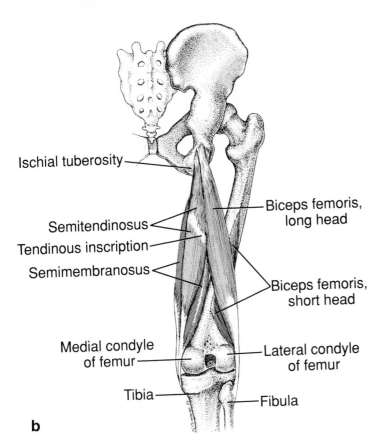

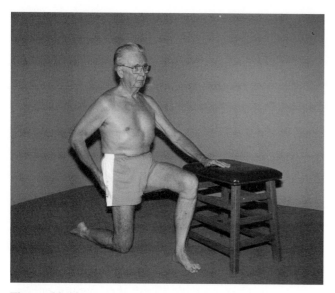

Figure 20.23.
Psoas muscle.
Self-stretch position kneeling.
1. Patient kneels and internally rotates femur on side to be stretched with the opposite hip and knee flexed to 90°.
2. Patient places hand on buttock, flattens stomach, and maintains a 12 o'clock posterior pelvic tilt.
3. Patient maintains trunk in an upright position, uses the opposite leg to pull the body forward, leading with the involved hip, and maintaining contraction of the glutei muscles throughout the stretch which is felt in the front of the hip and thigh.
4. A series of contract relax stretches for 1–2 minutes or a sustained 30-second stretch repeated two to three times is performed. The opposite side should be stretched in the same manner to achieve balance.
5. This position can be modified to stretch the tensor fascia lata by externally rotating the femur and side-bending the trunk away from the side being stretched before leading forward with the hip.

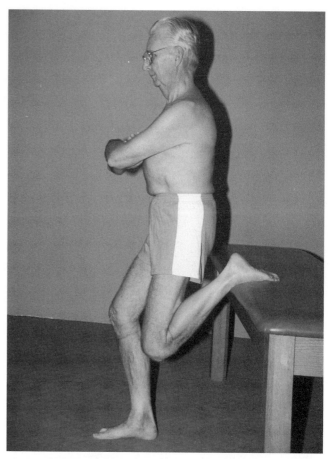

Figure 20.24.
Rectus femoris muscle.
Self-stretch standing.
1. Patient stands with foot of leg to be stretched on a table or chair with the knee flexed.
2. Patient contracts abdominal and gluteal muscles in the 12 o'clock position. If stretch is felt in the anterior thigh, it is maintained for 10–15 seconds and repeated three times.
3. As length increases, additional stretch is obtained by flexing the opposite knee and is felt in the anterior thigh.
4. This is repeated on the opposite for muscle balance.
5. A dual outcome results with stretching of one side, while strengthening on the side of active knee flexion.

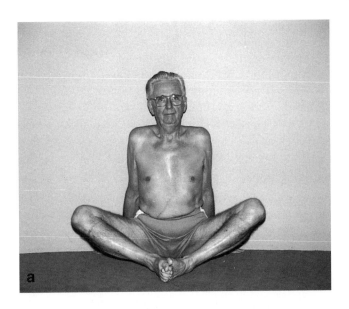

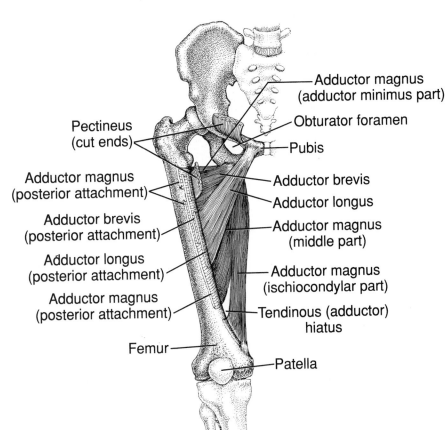

Figure 20.25 a and b.
Hip Adductor muscles.
Self-stretch sitting.

1. Patient sits with the buttocks as close to the wall as possible with the lumbar spine in neutral. A pillow or towel may be placed beneath the ischial tuberosities to provide an anterior pelvis tilt. The patient may begin by sitting on a low step.
2. Patient places soles of feet together, pulls the feet toward body, and actively externally rotates and abducts both legs.
3. Patient places both hands behind hips to assist in lifting and anteriorly rotating the pelvis.
4. Stretch is held for 10–15 seconds and repeated three to four times with increasing external rotation and abduction with each effort.

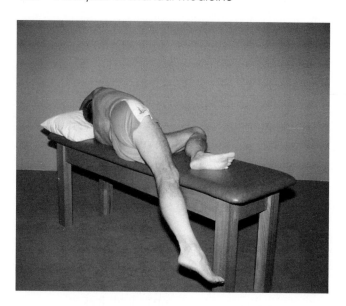

Figure 20.26

Quadratus lumborum muscle.

Self-stretch position lateral recumbent.

1. Patient lies in the lateral recumbent position with the involved side uppermost.
2. The bottom leg is flexed to 90°, with the involved leg extended and adducted off the side of the table or bed.
3. Patients arm on involved side reaches overhead, adding to the stretch by the weight of the leg.
4. Stretch is held for 10–15 seconds repeated three times or a sustained 30-second stretch.
5. The opposite side is stretched to balance.

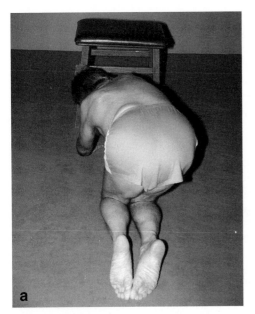

Figure 20.27 a and b.
Quadratus lumborum and Latissimus dorsi muscles.
Self-stretch position kneeling.
1. Patient on hands and knees reaches forward with the hand on the side to be stretched and grasps a chair or stool.
2. Patient shifts pelvis laterally and then sits back, elongating the involved side with each repetition and increasing the diagonal drop of the pelvis.
3. Externally rotating the hand adds an increase in the stretch of the latissimus dorsi.
4. Stretch is held for 10–15 seconds and repeated three to four times.
5. The opposite side is stretched to balance.

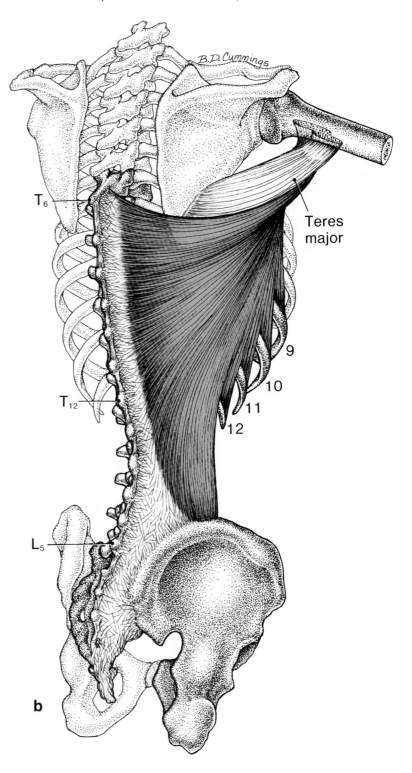

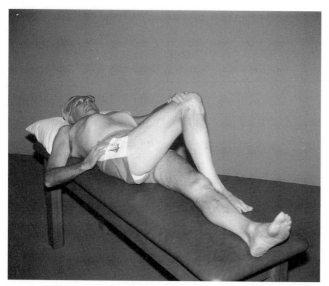

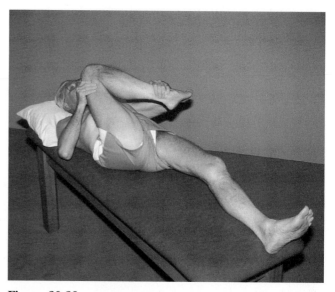

Figure 20.28

Psoas muscle below 90°.

Self-stretch position supine.

1. Patient supine with leg on involved side flexed at the hip and knee and with the foot lateral to the opposite knee.
2. Patient grasps distal thigh and maintains adduction and internal rotation of the leg, while stabilizing the pelvis with the other hand on the anterior superior iliac spine. If the arm is too short, a belt or towel can be placed around the distal thigh to offer resistance.
3. Patient pushes knee laterally against resistance and without rotating pelvis.
4. A series of contract relax muscle efforts of 5–7 seconds with five to seven repetitions is performed.
5. This also stretches the posterior hip capsule. Compression through the femur during the stretch assists in stretching the hip capsule.

Figure 20.29.

Piriformis muscle above 90°.

Self-stretch position supine.

1. Patient lies on back and grasps with both hands the ankle and knee of involved side.
2. The knee is pulled toward the opposite shoulder until a stretch is felt in the buttock.
3. A sustained 30-second stretch repeated twice or a series of 5- to 7-second contract relax muscle efforts repeated five to seven times are performed.
4. The opposite side is stretched to balance.

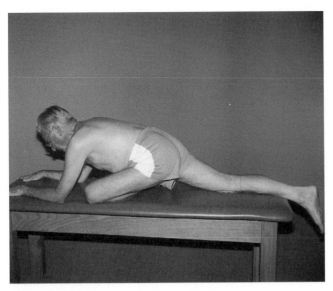

Figure 20.30.
Piriformis muscle.
Self-stretch position prone.
1. Patient begins on hands and knees and places foot of involved side in front of the opposite knee, with the foot pointing toward the ceiling and the knee lateral to the trunk. The involved leg is flexed, externally rotated, and abducted.
2. The opposite leg is stretched distally while keeping the pelvis level until stretch is felt in the buttock.
3. A sustained 30-second stretch is repeated twice.
4. The position is reversed to stretch the opposite side to balance.

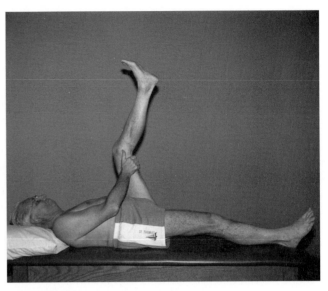

Figure 20.31.
Hamstring muscles.
Self-stretch position supine.
1. Patient lies on back with lumbar spine in neutral. A towel or small pillow may be necessary.
2. Patient grasps the back of the thigh with both hands with the hip at 90°.
3. Patient actively extends the knee, reaching with the foot to the ceiling.
4. Dorsiflexion of the ankle increases the stretch.
5. A series of contract relax muscle efforts for 5–7 seconds repeated five to seven times is performed.
6. This procedure can also be used to mobilize the sciatic nerve complex.

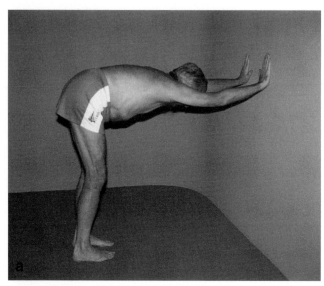 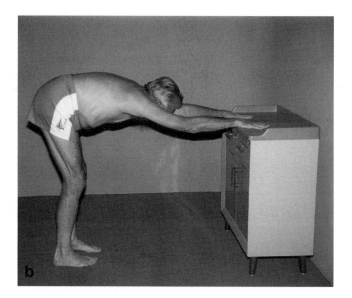

Figure 20.32.
Hamstring muscles.
Self-stretch position standing.
1. Patient stands with the feet 6 inches apart with the hands on the wall (Fig. 20.32a) or on a table or stand (Fig.20.32b).
2. Patient bends hips to 90° and flexes knees so that trunk can become straight and arms fully extended.
3. Patient extends knees in an attempt to lift the buttock toward the ceiling and elongate the spine.
4. A series of contract relax knee extension muscle efforts for 5–7 seconds repeated five to seven times is performed.
5. Patient pushes against the wall or the table during knee extension efforts, keeping the spine in neutral mechanics and without dropping the head.
6. The patient may have to begin with the hands farther up the wall to maintain neutral spine mechanics. As progress is made, the hands are lowered on the wall until trunk is horizontal to the floor.

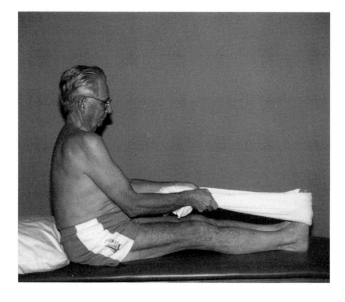

Figure 20.33.
Hamstring muscles.
Self-stretch position sitting.
1. Patient sits with the buttock on a pillow or rolled towel to assist in maintaining pelvis in anteriorly rotated (6 o'clock) position.
2. A belt or towel is placed on the forefoot.
3. Beginning with the knees flexed, patient actively extends knees, feeling stretch in the posterior leg. It is important to maintain neutral lumbar mechanics during the stretch.
4. A series of contract relax knee extension muscle efforts of 5–7 seconds repeated five to seven times is performed.
5. The patient may need to begin by sitting on a step to maintain neutral spinal mechanics.

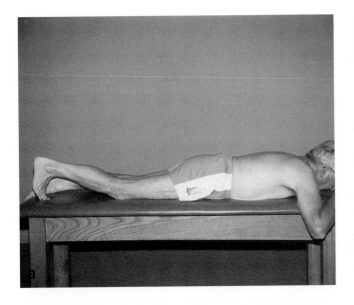

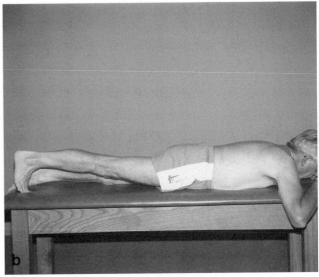

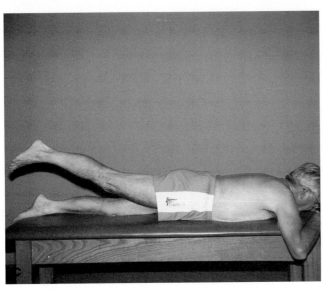

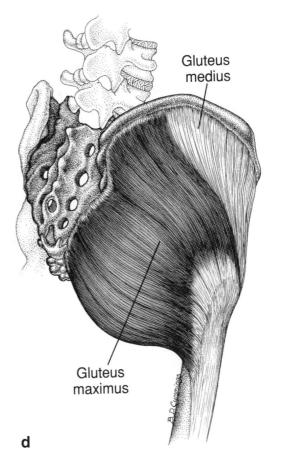

Figure 20.34

Gluteus maximus muscle.

Retraining.

1. Patient prone and places toe on table (Fig. 20.34a).
2. Patient actively contracts the buttock to straighten the knee (Fig. 20.34b).
3. Patient lifts knee from table, extends foot, and slowly returns the leg to the table (Fig. 20.34c).
4. Patient holds lifted leg for 5–7 seconds and repeats five to seven times.
5. Patient cannot proceed to step 3 until able to sustain a voluntary contraction of the gluteus maximus muscle (Fig. 20.34d). There should be no rotation of the trunk or pelvis by substitution of other muscle effort.

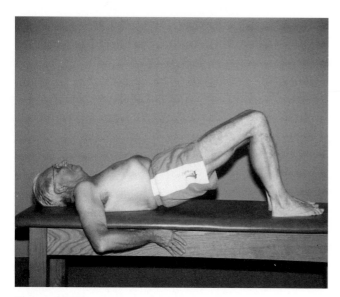 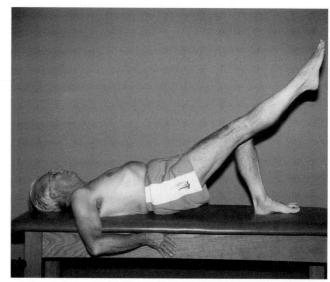

Figure 20.35
Gluteus maximus muscle.
Retraining.
1. Patient lies on back with knees flexed and feet flat.
2. Patient assumes posterior pelvic tilt to 12 o'clock and then lifts buttocks from the table while squeezing the bottom (Fig. 20.35a). The pelvis should remain level and there should be no lumbar extension.
3. Patient holds position for 5–7 seconds, slowly returns to the table, and repeats five to seven times.
4. When able to perform easily, patient progresses to straighten one leg while in the bridged position (Fig. 20.35b) and repeats the 5- to 7-second hold for five to seven repetitions on each side.

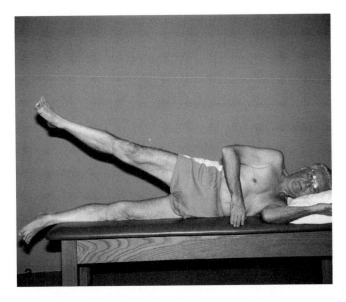

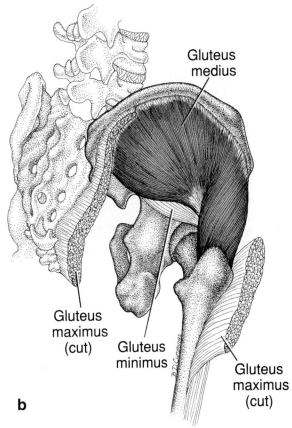

Gluteus
medius

Gluteus
maximus
(cut)

Gluteus
minimus

Gluteus
maximus
(cut)

b

Figure 20.36 a and b.
Gluteus medius muscle.
Retraining.
1. Patient in lateral recumbent position with the shoulders and pelvis perpendicular to the table and knees extended.
2. Patients upper arm is placed on and pushes into the table while dorsiflexing the upper foot.
3. Patient slowly raises upper leg to hip level, holds for 5–7 seconds, and lowers leg slowly. This is repeated five to seven times.
4. Externally rotating the leg reduces the influence of the tensor fascia lata muscle and isolates action more to the gluteus medius.
5. Repeat on opposite side for balance.
6. As patient progresses, exercise may be done with knees at 90°. Added difficulty is to raise both legs to the ceiling.

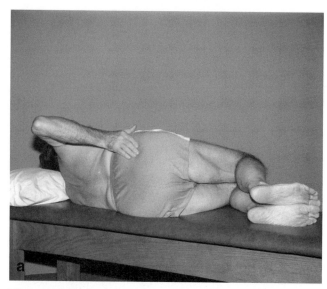 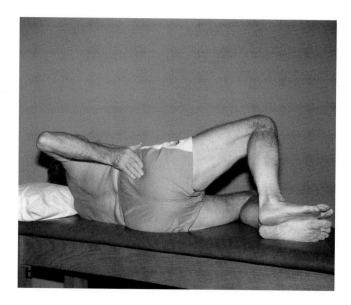

Figure 20.37

Gluteus medius muscle.

Retraining.

1. Patient lies in the lateral recumbent position with the knees flexed to 45–60° and upper hand overlying the gluteus medius muscle (Fig. 20.37a).
2. Maintaining the feet together, patient lifts top knee toward the ceiling, holds for 5–7 seconds, slowly lowers leg, and repeats five to seven times (Fig. 20.37b).
3. This muscle may fatigue rapidly with this exercise, and the patient must be cautious about the number of repetitions.
4. Repeat on the opposite side for balance.

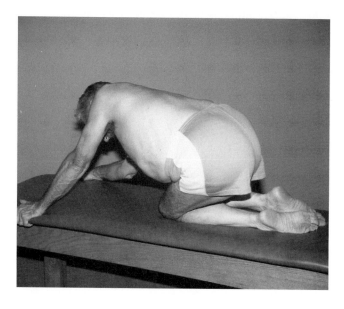

Figure 20.38

Gluteus medius muscle.

Retraining.

1. Patient begins in the hands and knees position and diagonally sits back. The pelvis should translate laterally and the spine of the side being stretched should elongate.
2. Patient holds position for 5–7 seconds, returns to the starting position, and repeats on the opposite side. This is repeated five to seven times.
3. As strength returns, patient can sink further back. The direction and distance should be symmetrical on each side.
4. The arms should be passive and the control should come from the buttocks.

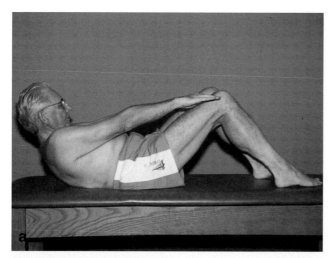

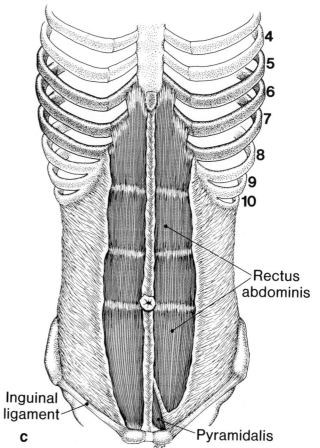

Figure 20.39 a, b, and c.
Abdominal muscles.
Retraining with curl-up.

1. Patient lies supine with hips and knees flexed.
2. Patient extends arms in front and slowly curls up beginning in the cervical spine and to the upper back while reaching toward the knees. Position is held for 5–7 seconds and then spine is slowly lowered segmentally to the start position. Repeat five to seven times.
3. To increase the difficulty, the hands may be placed behind the neck.

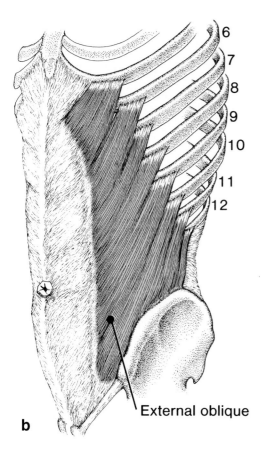

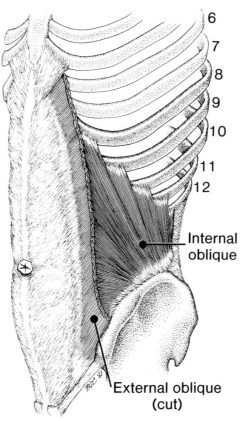

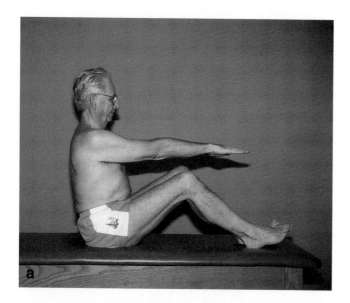

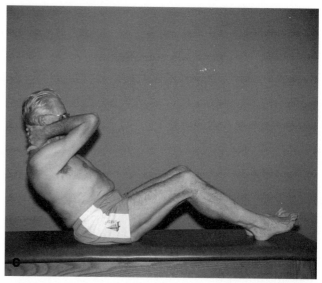

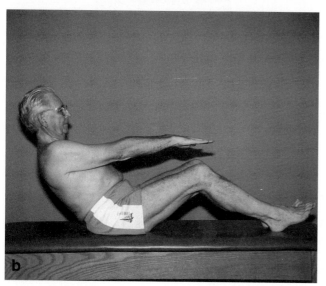

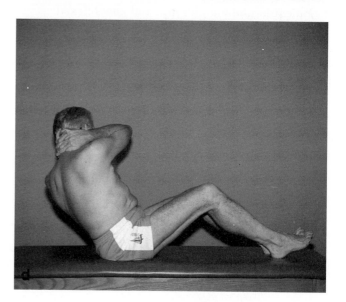

Figure 20.40

Abdominal muscles.

Retraining with sit backs.

1. Patient sits with heels digging in and toes flexed.
2. With knees flexed and spine in neutral mechanics, arms are extended over the knees (Fig. 20.40a).
3. From this position, patient sits back as far as possible without lifting feet and while maintaining a neutral spine (Fig. 20.40b). This is held for 5–7 seconds and then returned to starting position. This is repeated five to seven times (Step 1).
4. Increased difficulty has the hands behind the neck (Fig. 20.40c) and performing the sit back for five to seven repetitions of a 5- to 7-second hold (Step 2).
5. When proficient at step 2, patient now performs a sit back with the beginning position of the right elbow over the left knee (Fig. 20.40d) and reversing with the left elbow over the right knee. The spine must be in neutral. Again, five to seven repetitions of a 5- to 7-second hold are made on each side (Step 3).
6. This exercise works the abdominals, including the obliques, in a lengthened position and with a neutral spine.

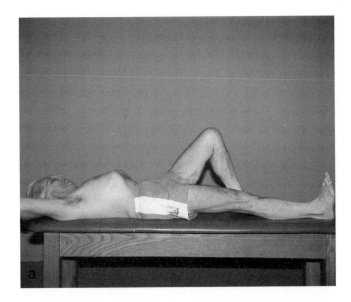

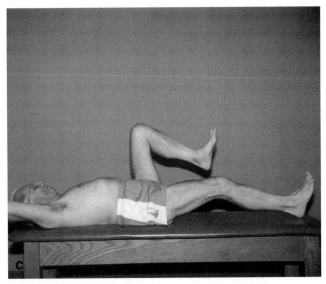

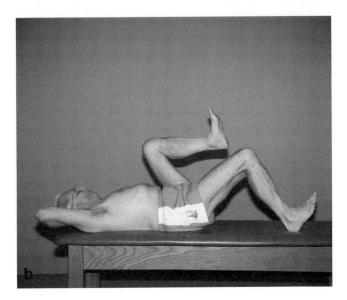

Figure 20.41
Abdominal muscles.
Retraining. Heel slides and Norwegian.
1. Patient lying with knees and hips bent and feet on table or floor.
2. Patient flattens back by abdominal contraction and assumes the 12 o'clock pelvic position.
3. Patient slowly slides one heel down the table or floor without allowing lumbar spine to flex. Each leg is alternately extended with 6–10 repetitions (Fig. 20.41a).
4. Beginning in the same starting position, both hips and knees are flexed and one leg at a time alternately touches the table or floor (Fig. 20.41b).
5. An advanced level has the patient touch the heel with more extension of the hips and knees (Fig. 20.41c).
6. The back must be kept flat throughout the exercise. It is frequently useful to place a hand under the lumbar area and maintain pressure on the hand.
7. The goal is to perform the Norwegian leg extensions for two minutes while counting aloud to prevent holding the breath.

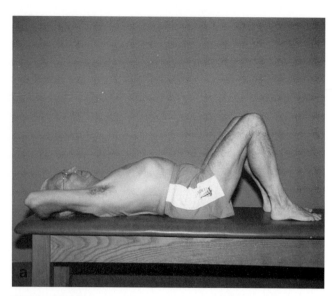 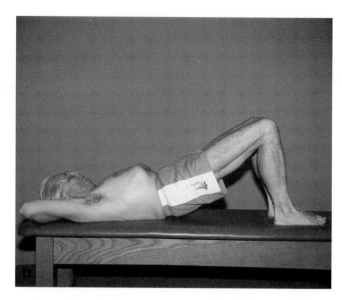

Figure 20.42

Pelvic see-saw (Lewit).

Trunk control exercise.

1. Patient lies supine with knees bent and feet flat on the table or floor.
2. Patient contracts erector spinae muscles introducing a lumbar lordosis (Fig. 20.42a).
3. Patient contracts abdominals and gluteal muscles, flattening the lumbar lordosis one segment at a time from caudal to proximal until pelvis is lifted from the table (Fig. 20.42b).
4. After a 5- to 7-second hold, the process is reversed by dropping each vertebral segment to the table one by one from above downward, again introducing a lumbar lordosis by contraction of the erector spinae muscles.
5. The process is repeated five to seven times to increase flexion-extension control of the trunk.

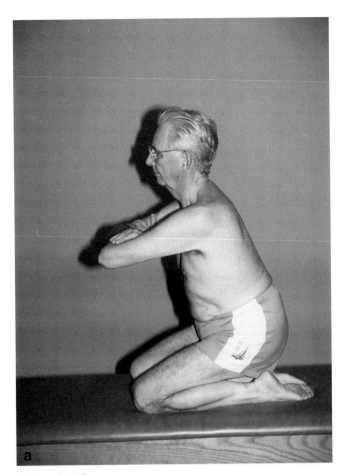 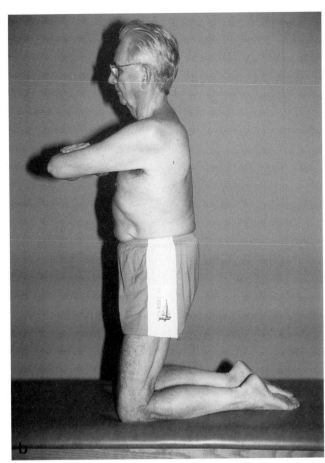

Figure 20.43
Sitting to kneeling (Lewit).
Trunk control exercise.
1. Patient sits on heels with erect trunk and flexes and extends until a neutral spine is identified (Fig. 20.43a).
2. While maintaining a neutral spine, patient lifts body to an erect kneeling position using the gluteal and thigh muscles (Fig. 20.43b).
3. Patient returns to beginning position slowly and repeats five to seven times.
4. This exercise strengthens abdominals, gluteals, and provides trunk stability and trunk motor control.

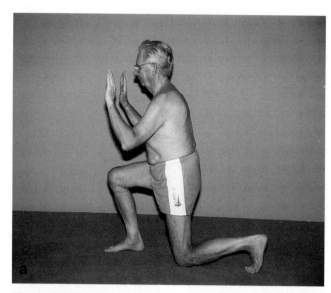 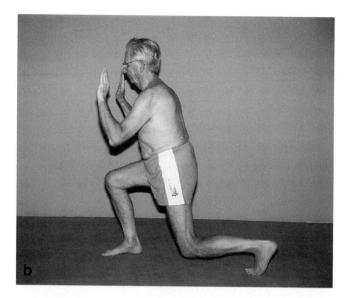

Figure 20.44

Trunk lift exercise.

1. To maintain good body posture and trunk control for a lifting effort, the patient begins the exercise by kneeling on one knee with the other leg flexed at the hip and knee to 90°. The spine is held in neutral mechanics with the arms in front (Fig. 20.44a).

2. The toe of the leg in the kneeling position is placed on the floor.

3. Patient lifts the body so that the knee is off the floor while maintaining upper body posture in neutral position and holds for 5–7 seconds (Fig. 20.44b).

4. Five to seven repetitions are performed when patient is capable.

5. Patients ability to do this exercise is of value in restoration of lifting capacity without adverse effect on the back.

EVALUATION AND TREATMENT OF THE UPPER QUARTER

In the upper quarter, the postural muscles that are facilitated, hypertonic, and short include the levator scapulae, upper trapezius, sternocleidomastoid, scalenes, pectorals, and flexors of the upper extremity. The dynamic muscles that are inhibited, hypotonic, and weak include the middle and lower trapezius, serratus anterior, rhomboids, supraspinatus and infraspinatus, deltoid, deep neck flexors, and extensors of the upper extremity.

Janda's upper crossed syndrome finds the upper trapezius, levator scapulae, and the scalenes shortened and hypertonic with weakness and inhibition of the lower trapezius and serratus anterior. The pectorals are short and tight and the interscapular muscles, the serratus anterior and rhomboids, are weak and inhibited. The sternocleidomastoid and suboccipital muscles functioning as neck extensors are short, whereas the deep neck flexors are weak and inhibited. The upper crossed syndrome pattern affects the functional capacity of the cervical spine and the upper extremities and results in a forward head posture, straightening of the cervical lordosis, extension of the upper cervical spine, increased kyphosis of the cervical thoracic junction, and internal rotation of the shoulder girdles. Resultant alteration in shoulder mechanics can contribute to strain of the shoulder joints.

IDENTIFICATION OF UPPER QUADRANT FAULTY MOVEMENT PATTERNS

Four tests are used to identify faulty movement patterns of the upper quarter.

Test 1

The first is the supine cervical flexion test (Fig. 20.45, a–c). The patient lies supine and is asked to look down to the feet. In the presence of strong deep neck flexors, the chin tucks down and rolls forward, whereas in weakness of the deep neck flexors, the sternocleidomastoid and scalene muscles substitute and the head is carried forward before looking downward.

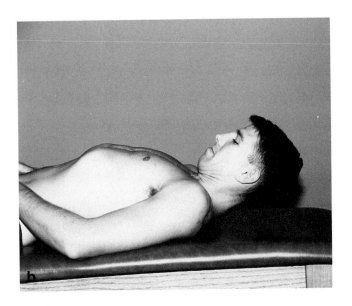

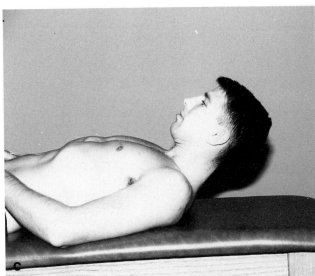

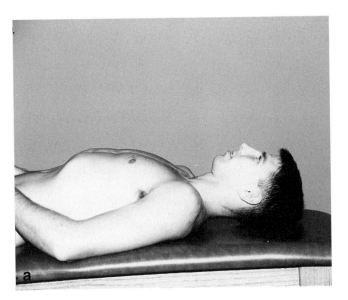

Figure 20.45.
(a) Cervical flexion test supine starting position. (b) Cervical flexion test normal with neck flexion curl. (c) Cervical flexion test showing weak neck flexors with forward head posture.

Test 2

The second test is the bilateral shoulder abduction maneuver (Fig. 20.46). The firing pattern of the upper extremity is evaluated (Fig. 20.4). Weakness of the supraspinatus and deltoid result in substitution by levator scapulae and upper trapezius muscles, which excessively elevate the shoulder and is associated with loss of scapular stabilization by the lower trapezius and serratus anterior. This condition may well result in impingement syndrome of the shoulder and further strain on the cervical spine.

Test 3

The third test is for scapular stabilization on the hands and knees. Excessive winging of the medial border of the scapula occurs because of weakness and lack of stabilization by the lower trapezius, serratus anterior, and rhomboid muscles (Fig. 20.47).

Test 4

The fourth test is for scapular depression (Fig. 20.48). In the prone position the patient is asked to push the inferior angle of the scapula in a medial and caudal direction against operator resistance.

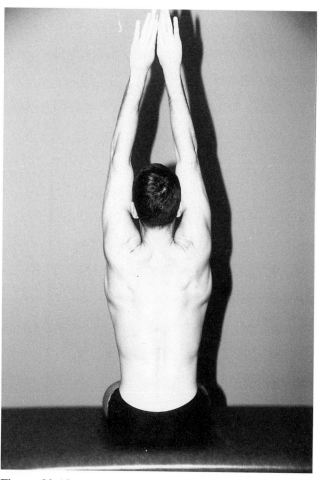

Figure 20.46
Shoulder abduction test.

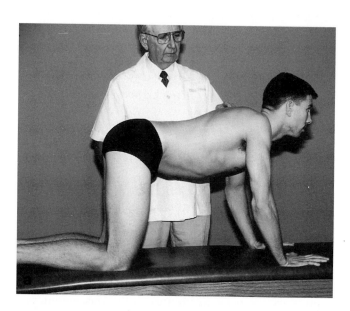

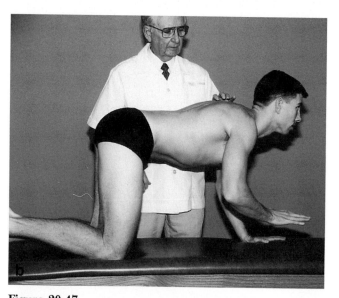

Figure 20.47
(a) Scapular stabilization test hands and knees position. (b) Scapular stabilization test lifting one hand.

ASSESSMENT OF MUSCLE LENGTH AND TREATMENT BY MANUAL STRETCHING

The tight muscle groups of the upper quadrant can be treated in a similar fashion to those in the lower quarter and include static stretches of 20–30 seconds with two to three repetitions or postisometric relaxation after a 5-second contraction. Muscles to be assessed include the levator scapulae and splenius capitis, upper trapezius and sternocleidomastoid, scalenes, pectoralis major and minor, and latissimus dorsi (Figs. 20.49 through 20.55).

Self-stretching exercises for the same group of muscles are found in Figures 20.56 through 20.60.

Upper quarter retraining is similar to that described for the lower quarter and includes modification of the testing procedures and repetitive action of the inhibited muscle group. These procedures are shown in Figure 20.61 through 20.69.

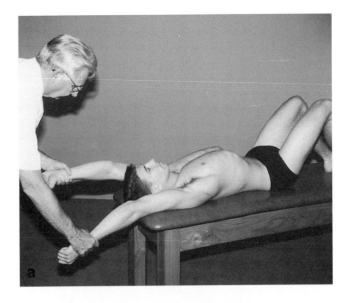

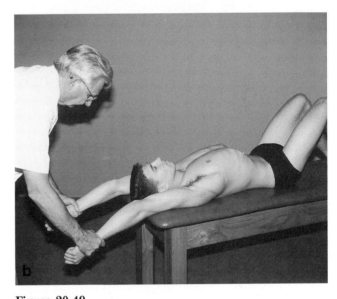

Figure 20.49
Latissimus dorsi muscle.
Length test and manual stretch position.
1. Patient supine with operator at the head of the table.
2. Patient's knees are flexed and operator grasps both wrists and introduces upper extremity flexion (Fig. 20.49a).
3. Asymmetric arms elevation indicated tight latissimus dorsi muscle.
4. Operators resists patient effort of arms extension for 5–7 seconds and with five to seven repetitions until arm flexion is symmetric (Fig. 20.49b).
5. If another operator is available, a pumping on and off maneuver of hip and pelvic flexion, while traction is held on both arms, enhances the latissimus stretch.

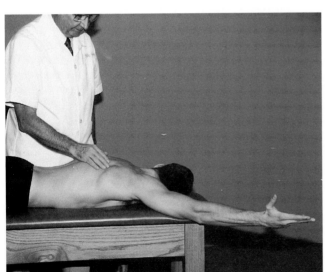

Figure 20.48
Scapular depression test.

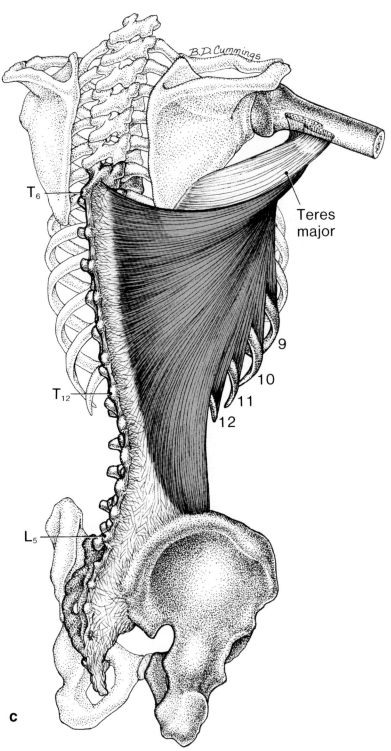

Figure 20.49c.
Latissimus dorsi muscle.

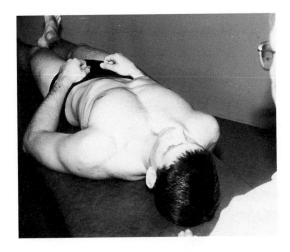

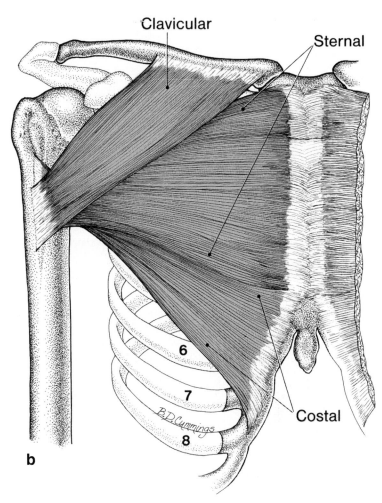

Figure 20.50 a and b.
Pectoral muscles.
Test position supine.
1. Patient supine with operator sitting at head of table.
2. Operator assesses whether both shoulder girdles are symmetric.
3. If one shoulder is held in an anterior position in relation to the thoracic cage, shortness and tightness of the pectoral muscles is present.

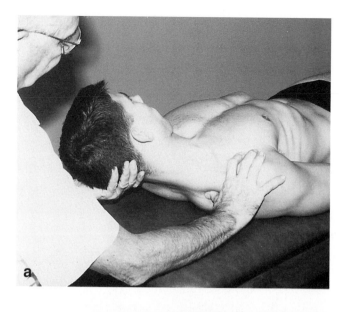

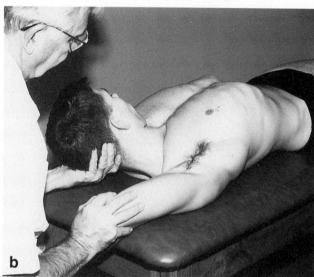

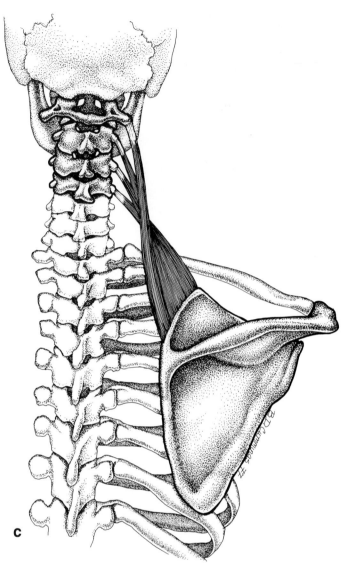

Figure 20.51

Levator scapulae muscle.

Test and manual stretch position.

1. Patient supine with operator sitting at head of table.
2. Operator's lateral hand stabilizes shoulder girdle with the thumb on the superior medial angle of the scapula.
3. Operator's medial hand supports the occiput and introduces flexion, sidebending, and rotation away to the barrier (Fig. 20.51a).
4. An alternate position is to elevate the patient's arm above the head and place caudad compression on the elbow while flexing, sidebending, and rotating the head away (Fig. 20.51b).
5. Shortness and tightness is present if the range of motion is asymmetric.
6. Shortness and tightness is treated by a series of 5- to 7-second contract relax muscle efforts of shoulder elevation by the patient against operator resistance at the barrier repeated five to seven times.
7. The opposite side is stretched to balance.

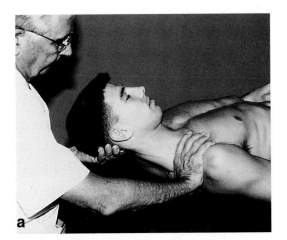

Figure 20.52 a and b.
Upper trapezius muscle.
Testing and manual stretch position.

1. Patient supine with operator sitting at head of table.
2. Operator's lateral hand stabilized patient's scapula and clavicle on the side being tested.
3. Operator's medial hand controls the occiput of the skull and introduces flexion, sidebending away, and rotation toward the side being tested.
4. If range is asymmetric, shortness and tightness is present.
5. To stretch tightness and shortness, patient attempts to elevate the shoulder toward the ear against operator resistance for 5–7 seconds with five to seven repetitions, with the operator increasing the flexion and sidebending after each effort.

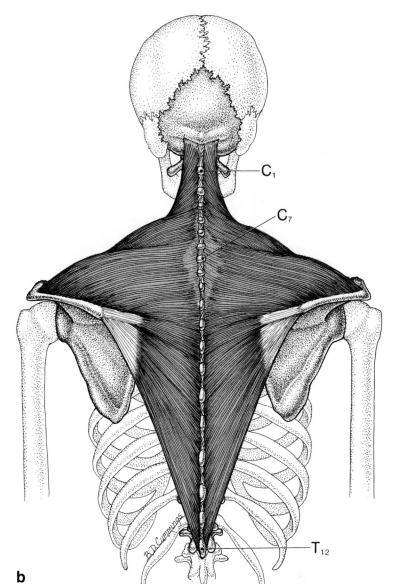

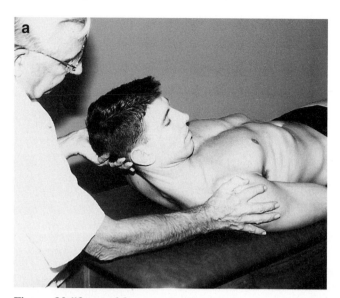

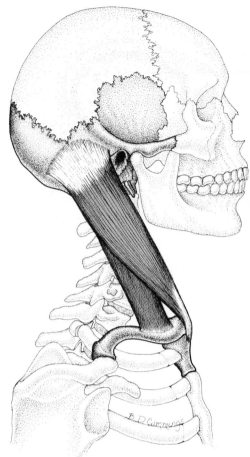

Figure 20.53 a and b.
Sternocleidomastoid muscle.
Test and manual stretch position.

1. The sternocleidomastoid and upper trapezius muscles are synergistic and can be tested and treated together.
2. Patient supine and operator sitting at head of table.
3. Operator's lateral hand stabilizes the scapula and clavicle.
4. Operator's medial hand controls the occiput of the skull and introduces flexion, sidebending away, and rotation to the side being tested.
5. Comparison is made with the opposite side. If asymmetric, shortness and tightness are present.
6. Stretching of shortness and tightness is performed by asking the patient to chin tuck and elevate the shoulder girdle against operator resistance for 5–7 seconds and five to seven repetitions.

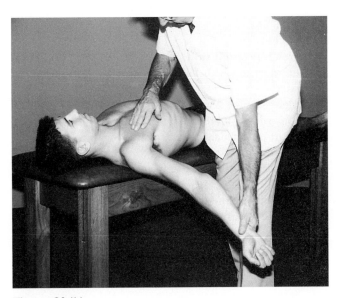

Figure 20.54

Pectoral muscles.

Length test and manual stretch position supine.

1. Patient supine with operator standing at side.
2. Operator controls patient upper arm at the wrist and extends the elbow.
3. Operator monitors tightness in the pectoral region as the upper extremity is abducted and horizontally extended until barrier is reached.
4. Comparison is made with the opposite side.
5. Stretching for shortness and tightness has patient perform a series of five to seven contract relax efforts for 5–7 seconds with the operator engaging new barrier after each effort.

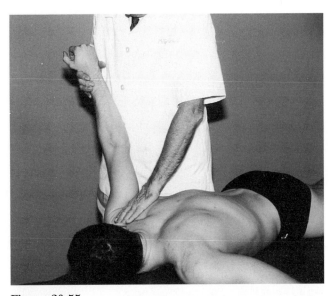

Figure 20.55

Pectoral muscles.

Length test and manual stretch position prone.

1. Patient prone with operator standing at the side of the table.
2. Operator grasps wrist, extends elbow, and horizontally extends arm while stabilizing the scapula with the other hand.
3. Comparison is made with the other side. The normal range is 90° of horizontal extension.
4. Stretching of shortness and tightness can be obtained by a sustained operator stretch supplemented by 5- to 7-second contract relax patient efforts.
5. This stretch also stretches the anterior shoulder capsule and can be used for that purpose. Caution must be used with a history of anterior dislocation.

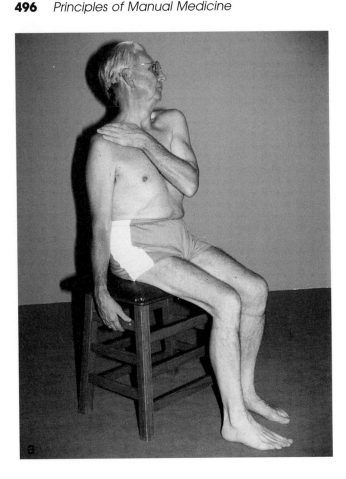

Figure 20.56a
Scalene muscles.
Self-stretch position sitting.
1. Patient sitting with hand on treated side holding chair.
2. Patient's other hand is placed over the clavicle and upper rib to stabilize the first and second ribs.
3. Patient posteriorly translates head with a chin tuck, sidebends the head and neck away, and rotates toward and away until tightness is felt.
4. A sustained 10- to 15-second hold is repeated three to five times, fine-tuning the rotation with added sidebending after each stretch.

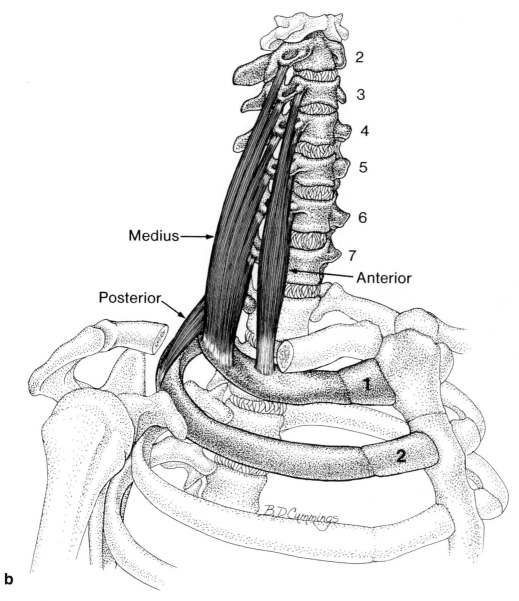

Figure 20.56b.
Scalene muscles.

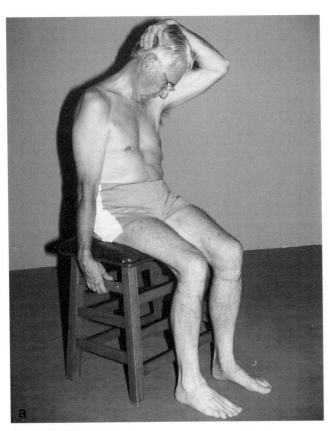

Figure 20.57a
Levator scapulae muscle.
Self-stretch position sitting.
1. Patient sitting with hand on treated side holding chair.
2. Patient flexes, sidebends, and rotates the head away and supports that position with the other hand.
3. Patient leans trunk away for stretch. The head and neck are not pulled by the contact hand.
4. The stretch can be enhanced by a contraction of the lower trapezius muscle on the same side.
5. The stretch is held for 10–15 seconds and repeated three to five times with increased sidebending away each time.

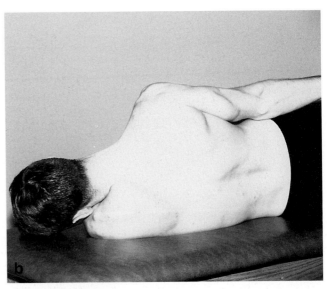

Figure 20.57b
Levator scapulae muscle.
Self-stretch position lateral recumbent.
1. Patient in lateral recumbent position without a pillow.
2. Patient flexes and rotates the head away with the sidebending introduced by body position.
3. Stretch position is held for 30 seconds and repeated twice.
4. Stretch can be enhanced by active contraction of the lower trapezius on the same side.
Note: In the same patient position, the operator can perform a manual stretch, stabilizing the head and neck with one hand and resisting with the other at the medial angle of the scapula as the patient attempts to elevate the scapula. A series of contract relax efforts can be performed by the patient.

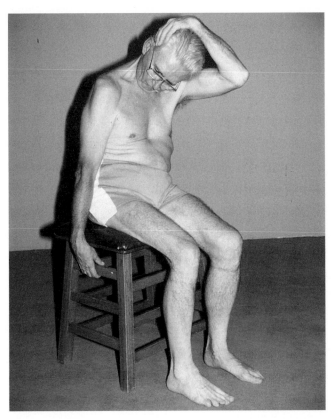

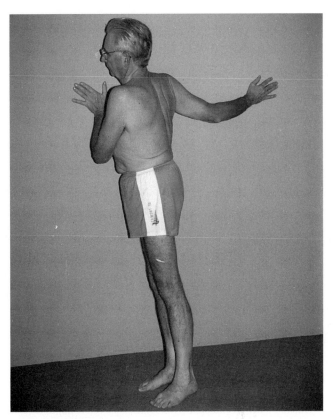

Figure 20.58
Upper trapezius and Sternocleidomastoid muscles.
Self-stretch position.
1. Patient sitting with one hand grasping chair.
2. Patient flexes, sidebends away, and rotates toward the head and neck. The other hand holds the head in this position but does not pull.
3. Patient leans body away until a stretch is felt. A chin tuck increases the stretch on the sternocleidomastoid.
4. Stretch is held for 10–15 seconds and is repeated three to five times.
5. The opposite side should be stretched to balance.

Figure 20.59
Pectoral muscles.
Self-stretch position.
1. Patient stands facing wall and places both hands on wall at shoulder height.
2. Patient turns body away from the involved side, keeping the shoulder from elevating until a stretch is felt in the pectoral area.
3. By using the other hand, patient leans the body toward the wall, increasing the pectoral stretch.
4. Patient maintains a neutral spine throughout the stretch.
5. Stretch is held for 10–15 seconds and is repeated three to five times. The shoulders should be able to be perpendicular to the wall.
6. The opposite side should be stretched to balance.

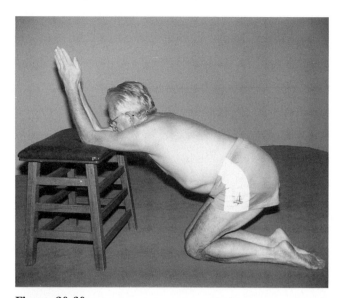

Figure 20.60
Latissimus dorsi muscle.
Self-stretch thoracic spine elongation position.
1. Patient kneels with elbows together and placed on a stool or chair.
2. Patient separates the scapulae by externally rotating the arms and maintaining the elbows together.
3. Patient drops chest to floor and sits back toward heels.
4. When stretch is felt, an increase in lumbar lordosis adds to the stretch.
5. Stretch is held for 30 seconds and repeated twice.
6. It is advisable to perform this exercise after any trunk rotational exercise to restore trunk elongation.

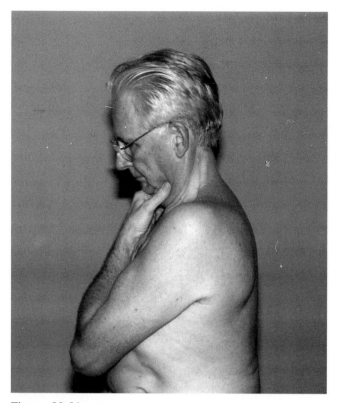

Figure 20.61
Cervical flexor muscles.
Retraining in sitting position.
1. Patient sits and palpates superficial anterior cervical muscles.
2. Patient nods head forward, using deep neck flexors by a chin tuck and without contracting superficial muscles.
3. Hold for 5–7 seconds with five to seven repetitions.
4. Patient should be capable of performing this exercise before proceeding to the supine position.

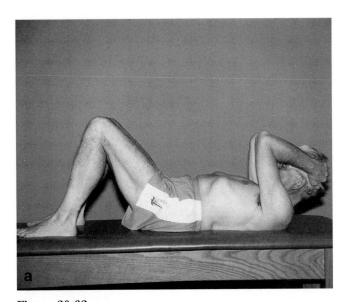 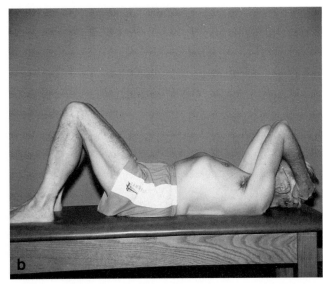

Figure 20.62

Cervical flexor muscles.

Assisted eccentric strengthening supine.

1. Patient supine with hands behind the head passively flexes head and tucks the chin to the chest, stretching the posterior cervical muscles (Fig. 20.62a).
2. After holding for 10 seconds, the head is slowly lowered, keeping the chin tucked, until head returns to the table (Fig. 20.62b).
3. As neck flexors become stronger, less assistance is provided by the hands on the head.
4. Repeat five to seven times.
5. Patient should be capable of performing this exercise before proceeding to unassisted strengthening.

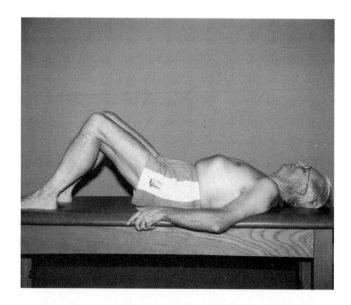

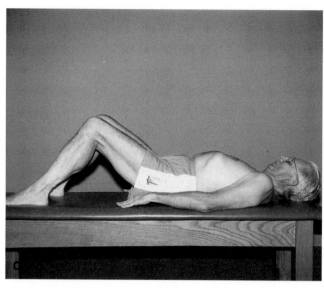

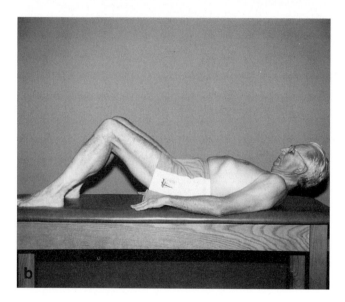

Figure 20.63
Cervical flexor muscles.
Unassisted eccentric strengthening supine.
1. Patient is supine (Fig. 20.63a) and rolls head forward by a chin tuck, lifting the head from the table to look down at the feet (Fig. 20.63b).
2. Position is held for 5–7 seconds and the head is slowly returned to the table, attempting to touch one vertebra at a time (Fig. 20.63c).
3. Repeat five to seven times.

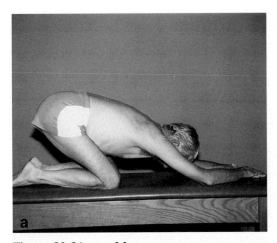

Figure 20.64 a and b.
Lower trapezius muscle.
Retraining position hands and knees.
1. Patient on hands and knees, resting head on table, sits back on heels.
2. Patient pulls scapulae in a medial and caudad direction without pulling the shoulder blades together.
3. Position is held for 5–7 seconds with five to seven repetitions.
4. Patient should be capable of performing this exercise before proceeding to the prone position.

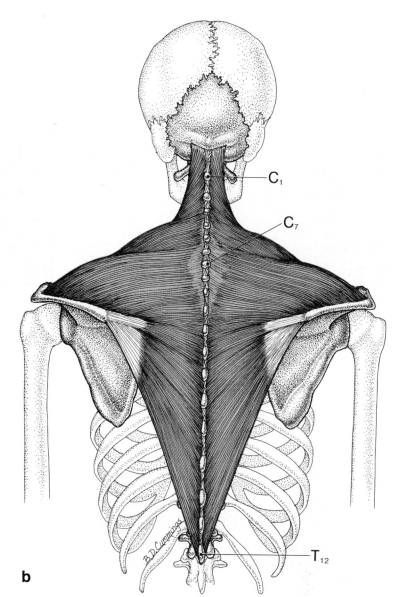

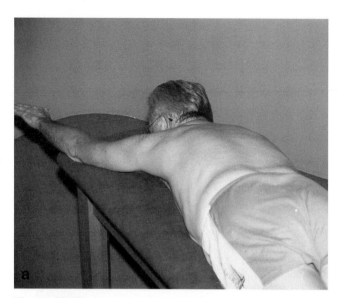
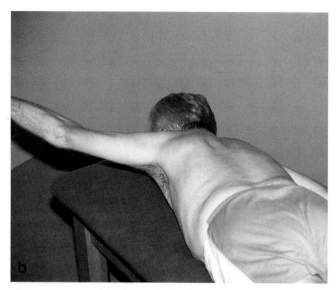

Figure 20.65
Lower trapezius muscle.
Retraining position prone.
1. Patient prone with arm extended above head (Fig. 20.65a).
2. Patient lifts arm from table and pulls the medial border of the scapula caudally and holds for 5–7 seconds (Fig. 20.65b).
3. Repeat five to seven times.

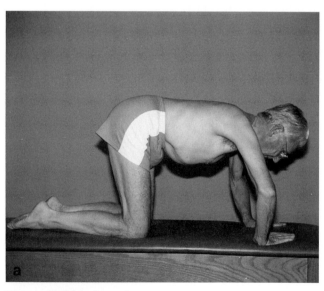
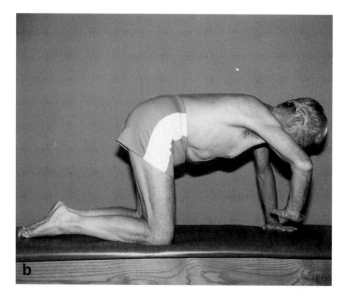

Figure 20.66 a, b, and c.
Serratus anterior muscle.
Retraining position hands and knees.
1. Patient on hands and knees with elbows flexed so that spine is parallel to the table and in neutral position (Fig. 20.66a).
2. Patient raises one hand 1–2 inches off the table while maintaining trunk position (Fig. 20.66b).
3. Position is held for 5–7 seconds with five to seven repetitions.
4. Both sides are strengthened to balance.
Note: If excessive winging of the scapula occurs, this exercise may be too strenuous and should be preceded by the standing and facing wall position.

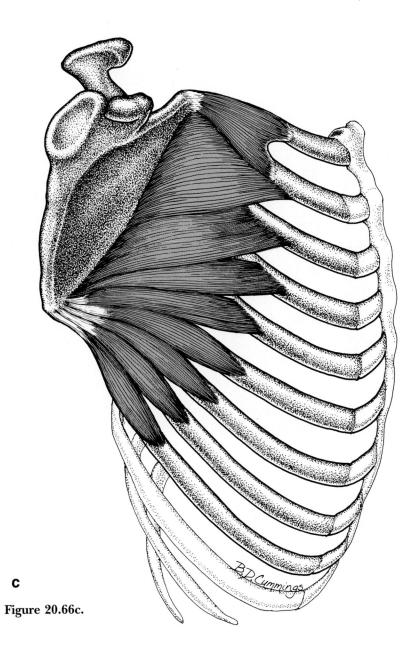

c

Figure 20.66c.

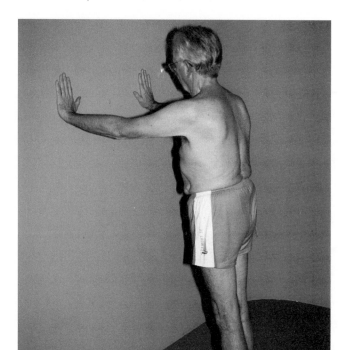

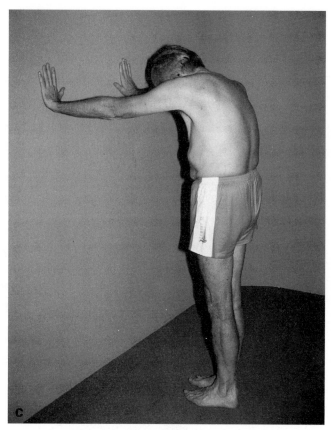

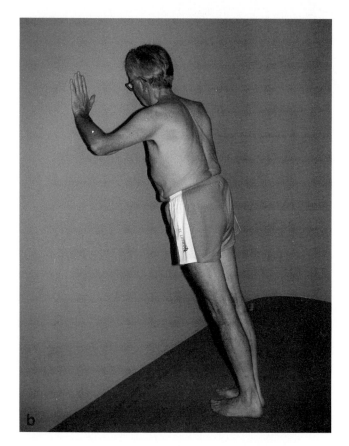

Figure 20.67
Serratus anterior muscle.
Retraining position standing.
1. Patient stands with hands on the wall at shoulder height, arms extended, and with spine in neutral (Fig. 20.67a).
2. Patient touches the nose to the wall while keeping the scapulae depressed (Fig. 20.67b) and holds for 5–7 seconds.
3. Patient performs a standing push-up while dropping the head to the floor with cervical flexion and pushing the upper thoracic spine posteriorly and superiorly (Fig. 20.67c) and holds for 5–7 seconds.
4. Exercise is repeated five to seven times.
Note: When proficient when standing, serratus anterior strengthening can be performed in the prone position in a similar manner.

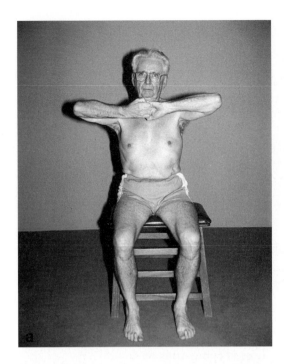

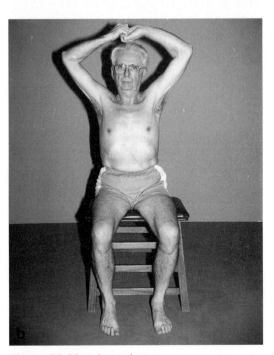

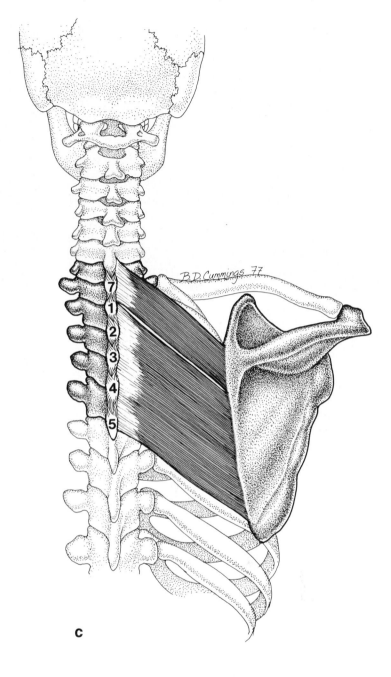

Figure 20.68 a, b, and c.
Rhomboid and Lower trapezius muscles.
Isometric strengthening position sitting.
1. Patient sitting with feet on floor.
2. Patient grasps fingers together with hands in front of upper sternum and arms parallel to the floor (Fig. 20.68a).
3. Patient attempts to pull elbows backward to the wall for a 5- to 7-second isometric contraction and repeats five to seven times to strengthen rhomboids.
4. Patient grasps fingers together with hands over top but not in contact with the head (Fig. 20.68b).
5. Patient attempts to pull elbows down to the floor for a 5- to 7-second isometric contraction and repeats five to seven times to strengthen lower trapezius.

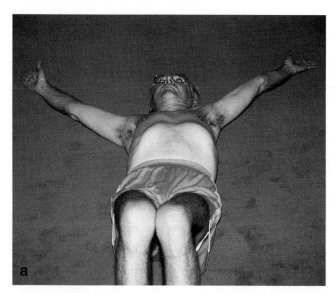 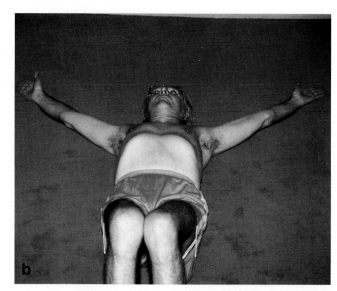

Figure 20.69
Shoulder abduction.
Retraining position supine.
1. Patient lies supine with hands at side, palms up, and slowly abducts arms keeping arms on floor.
2. If one shoulder elevates higher than the other (Fig. 20.69a), patient has gone too far and arms are brought back down to the side.
3. Exercise is repeated only as far as both arms can be abducted without elevating the shoulders (Fig. 20.69b).
4. Repeat five to seven times, being careful that increasing abduction is symmetrical on both sides.

SELF-MOBILIZING EXERCISES FOR SPECIFIC JOINT DYSFUNCTION

Exercise can be used by the patient to maintain correction of joint dysfunction or to self-treat in the presence of recurrence. It assists the patient in taking control of their musculoskeletal system. In the pelvis, the symphysis pubis can be self-mobilized with isometric activation of the hip adductor musculature (Fig. 20.70). Appropriate balancing of the abdominal musculature above and the hip adductor musculature below the symphysis pubis should follow (Figs. 20.25 and 20.39).

Sacroiliac dysfunctions are frequently associated with asymmetric tone of the piriformis muscles. Self-correction for a forward sacral torsion is the same exercise as stretching a tight piriformis (Fig. 20.29). In the presence of a posterior sacral torsion or unilateral posteriorly nutated sacrum (extended), a unilateral prone press-up is used. Frequently, it is necessary to have mobilized this dysfunction adequately before the patient is able to perform this exercise (Fig. 20.71). Because trunk backward-bending in the presence of a posterior nutated sacral base and flexed, rotated, and sidebent (FRS) dysfunction of the lumbar spine are frequently painful, this procedure must be done cautiously and under strict supervision.

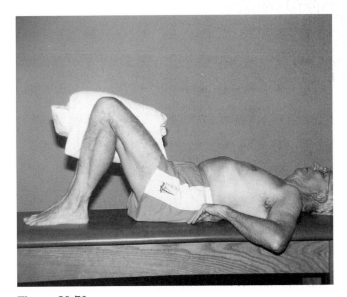

Figure 20.70
Symphysis Pubis.
Self-correction position supine.
1. Patient supine with feet together.
2. Patient abducts knees and places a noncompressible object between them.
3. Patient performs a symmetrical 5- to 7-second isometric activity of both legs trying to bring the knees together.
4. Repeat five to seven times.

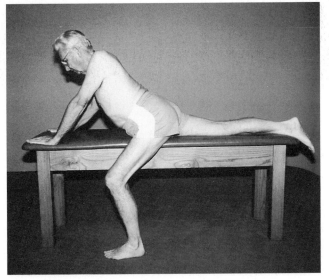

Figure 20.71.
Posterior nutated (extended) sacrum.
Self-correction position prone.
1. Patient prone with involved leg slightly abducted and externally rotated on the table and opposite foot placed on the floor.
2. Patient performs a push-up and maintains a sagging abdomen while forcefully exhaling.
3. Five to seven respiratory cycles are made with an attempt to increase the push-up with each effort.

For the correction of iliosacral rotational dysfunctions, the self-correction procedures are as follows. In the presence of an anterior innominate dysfunction, the patient lies supine and posteriorly rotates the right innominate (Fig. 20.72). For a posterior innominate, the supine patient drops the dysfunctional leg over the edge of the table and uses muscle contraction to extend the hip on the side of the dysfunction (Fig. 20.73).

Self-correction procedures for lumbar spine dysfunctions of the FRS type are modifications of Mackenzie's procedure to reduce the lateral shift and then incorporate extension. Procedures found useful include standing and side gliding into the wall (Fig. 20.74) and while facing the wall (Fig. 20.75, a and b). This procedure allows for fine-tuning the amount of lateral shift and extension. These procedures can be followed by prone press-ups (Fig. 20.76) and backward-bending while standing (Fig. 20.77). Lumbar spine rotational strengthening and control can be performed with trunk rotational reeducation (Fig. 20.78, a and b).

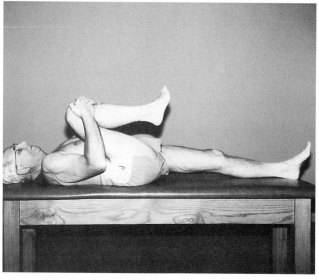

Figure 20.72
Anteriorly rotated innominate.
Self-correction position supine.
1. Patient supine on table with involved hip and knee flexed.
2. Keeping the opposite leg straight, patient grasps with both hands below the knee and attempts hip extension by a 5- to 7-second muscle contraction.
3. After each relaxation, patient increases hip flexion and repeats five to seven times.

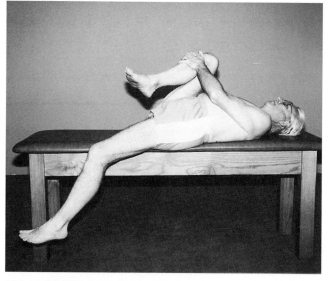

Figure 20.73
Posteriorly rotated innominate.
Self-correction position supine.
1. Patient supine with the involved leg off the edge of the table or bed.
2. Patient flexes the opposite hip and knee bringing the leg to the chest.
3. At full exhalation, patient contracts the gluteal muscles to further extend the leg and holds for 5–7 seconds.
4. Five to seven repetitions are made with increasing amounts of hip extension.

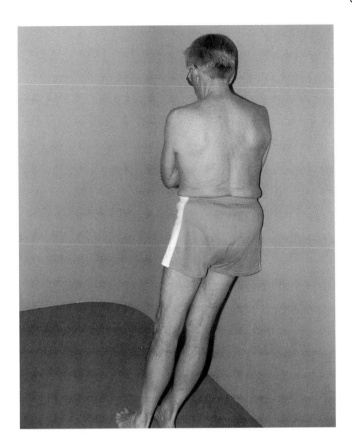

Figure 20.74
Hip shift.
Self-correction position standing.
1. Patient stands about 2 feet away from the wall with one shoulder, upper arm, and elbow against the wall.
2. Patient translates the pelvis toward the wall but avoids side bending of the spine.
3. Patient's other hand can assist by pushing the pelvis to the wall.
4. Position is held for 5–7 seconds and repeated five to seven times.
5. This exercise deals with the sidebending component of an FRS lumbar dysfunction.

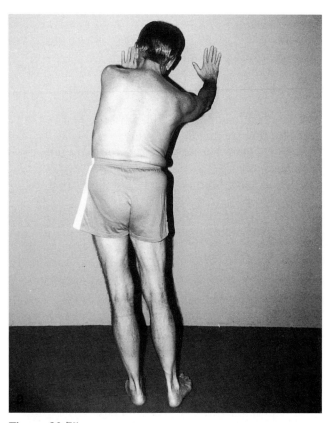 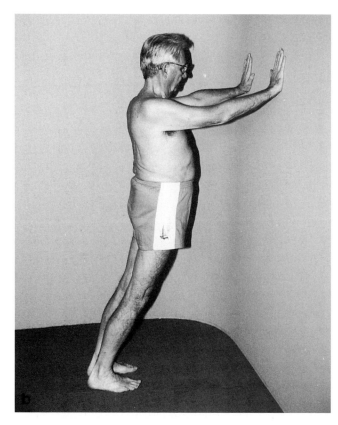

Figure 20.75

Lumbar Spine FRS dysfunction.

Self-correction position standing.

1. Patient stands facing wall with feet acetabular distance apart and hand on wall at shoulder height.
2. Patient shifts hips laterally from side to side toward restriction four to five times with increasing movement into the restrictive barrier (Fig. 20.75a).
3. Patient then introduces extension by sagging the trunk forward while maintaining the arms straight (Fig. 20.75b).
4. The side shifting and extension components are gradually increased with five to seven repetitions.

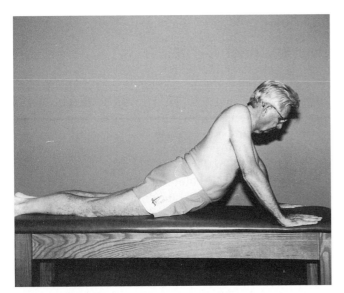

Figure 20.76
Lumbar Spine extension restriction.
Self-correction position prone.
1. Patient prone with hands on table or floor.
2. Patient straightens elbows and extends trunk from above downward.
3. Spinal muscles are relaxed, and the stretch should be felt in the front of the chest and abdomen.
4. Position is held for 3–5 seconds and is repeated five to seven times.

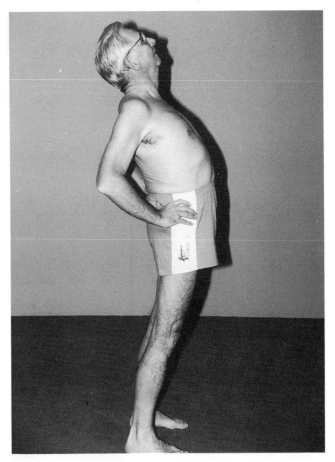

Figure 20.77
Lumbar Spine extension restriction.
Self-correction position standing.
1. Patient standing with hands on posterolateral buttock, feet acetabular distance apart and slightly externally rotated.
2. Patient extends trunk from the head and neck downward and the hips shift anteriorly.
3. Repeat five to seven times with increase in trunk extension each time.
4. This exercise can be added to the hip shift (Fig. 20.74) to correct the extension component of an FRS lumbar dysfunction.

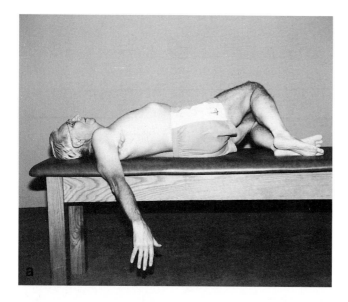

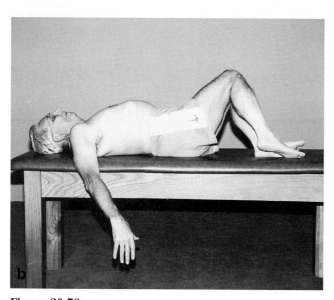

Figure 20.78

Trunk rotation

Reeducation position supine.

1. Patient lies with knees and hips flexed, with feet together and flat on table or floor. Arms are extended laterally with palms up.
2. Patient's knees are slowly dropped to one side and held for a 5- to 7-second stretch (Fig. 20.78a).
3. Knees are slowly brought back to neutral by touching each segment from above downward to the table or floor. Hip and thigh muscles are passive; the motion comes from the trunk muscles (Fig. 20.78b).
4. The other side is exercised in a like manner. Repeat five to seven times.
5. This exercise is good for the rotational component of lumbar nonneutral dysfunctions.

Self-correction for extended, rotated, sidebent (ERS) dysfunctions first needs to restore flexion. This can be performed by single and double bilateral knees to chest in the supine position. Another very effective exercise is a prayer stretch in the hands and knees position (Fig. 20.79). To restore flexion, rotation and sidebending together, the diagonal hip sink in the hands and knees position has been found effective (Fig. 20.80). This exercise is also useful for stretching of the quadratus lumborum and strengthening of the gluteus medius and minimis muscles. Forward-bending in step standing (Fig. 20.81) is also effective in self-correcting ERS lumbar dysfunctions.

The pelvic clock (Fig. 20.11) can be used as a self-correction procedure for both ERS and FRS dysfunctions. The patient performs a clockwise and counterclockwise exercise, touching one number of the clock at a time and graduates to full circle rotation both clockwise and counterclockwise.

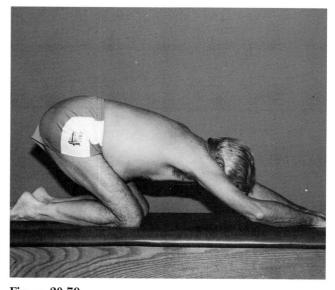

Figure 20.79

Lumbar Spine "Prayer Stretch."

Self-correction position prone.

1. Patient begins in hands and knees position with feet and knees hip width apart.
2. Patient sinks back, attempting to touch buttocks to heels.
3. Patient's head and neck are dropped into flexion, allowing the spine to flex and the chest to drop to the floor.
4. The hands remain in contact with the floor.
5. Stretch is held for 10–15 seconds and is repeated three to four times.
6. This stretch deals with the flexion component of lumbar nonneutral dysfunctions.

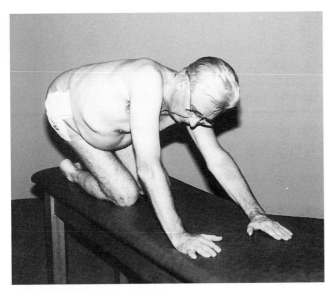

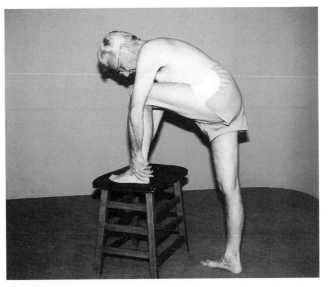

Figure 20.80
Lumbar Spine ERS dysfunctions.
Self-correction position "Diagonal Hip Sink"
1. Patient begins in hands and knees position.
2. Patient sits back diagonally, introducing flexion, sidebending, and rotation toward the dysfunctional facet.
3. Position is held for 5–7 seconds and repeated five to seven times.
4. With each repetition, an increased amount of " hip sink" is done, increasing the mobility in the dysfunctional facet.
5. This exercise also strengthens the gluteal muscles. The operator may offer resistance alternately to the buttocks and the opposite shoulder as the gluteal muscles are asked to work eccentrically and concentrically.
6. This exercise is useful for self-correction of the anteriorly nutated sacrum, which is frequently combined with an ERS dysfunction at L5. Deep inhalation respiratory activating force is combined with the stretch position.

Figure 20.81
Lumbar Spine ERS dysfunction.
Self-correction position standing.
1. Patient stands and places one foot on a chair or stool with the other leg straight.
2. Patient places both hands on the sides of the knee and bends forward, drawing chest toward the knee as the hands slide down the leg to the ankle.
3. Position is held for 5–7 seconds and repeated five to seven times with increased trunk flexion with each effort.

In the thoracic spine, stacked ERS and FRS dysfunctions are not uncommon. These should be successfully treated so that the patient can maintain correction at home. In the thoracic region, exercises to elongate the spine are always helpful. One exercise that is most useful is the wall stretch (Fig. 20.32). Another helpful elongation exercise is the kneeling prayer latissimus dorsi stretch (Fig. 20.82). For correction of restrictions of extension, a hands and knees rocking procedure (Fig. 20.83, a and b) and a supported extension during kneel stand (Fig. 20.84) are effective. For correction of restrictions of flexion, a variant to the classic cat back exercise is used (Fig. 20.85). Specific location of flexion need can be isolated and flexion motion enhanced. A wall press-up exercise promotes flexion in the upper thoracic spine as well as neuromuscular reeducation of scapular control, particularly weakness of the serratus anterior and lower trapezius (Fig. 20.86, a–c). To restore rotation, the procedure identified for the lumbar spine (Fig. 20.75) is useful, particularly in the lower thoracic region. A seated trunk rotation exercise uses respiratory assist as part of the rotary maneuver, beginning from above downward or from below upward, to isolate the region most in need of rotary enhancement (Fig. 20.87). In the cervical spine, the FRS and ERS dysfunctions that are found in the typical cervical segments can be treated as individual segments. Exercises for FRS dysfunctions (Fig. 20.88) and ERS dysfunctions (Fig. 20.89) are useful. The long restrictors of the cervical spine should be stretched before attempts at self-mobilization. In the C1-2 area, the primary motion to be restored is rotation. This is accomplished in the seated position with neck in full flexion and rotated to the restricted side (Fig. 20.90). At the occipitoatlantal junction, the primary motion of flexion-extension is specificity enhanced to one occipitoatlantal joint by rotating 30° and introducing flexion and extension to the side to be mobilized (Fig. 20.91, a and b).

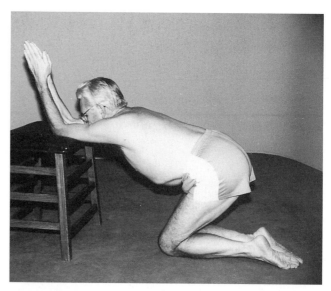

Figure 20.82
Thoracolumbar and Lumbar Spine.
Self-correction position kneeling.
1. Patient kneels with elbows together on a stool or chair.
2. With the lumbar spine in neutral, patient sits back with the buttocks toward the heels.
3. Position is held for 30 seconds and repeated twice.
4. Patient performs a series of deep inhalation/exhalation efforts to mobilize vertebral segments while in an elongated position.
5. This is the same as the latissimus dorsi stretch (Fig. 20.60) but is included here as a self-correction stretch to be used after any self-correction procedures for FRS or ERS lumbar dysfunctions.

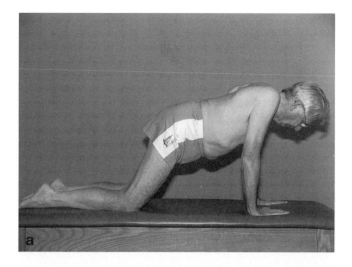

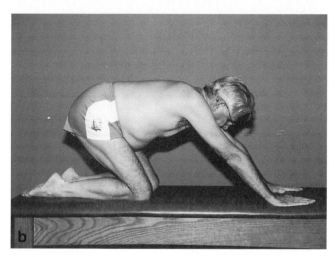

Figure 20.83

Thoracolumbar and Lumbar Spine.

Self-correction position for extension restriction.

1. Patient on hands and knees shifts weight over the hands while sagging the abdomen to extend into the lumbar spine (Fig. 20.83a).
2. While maintaining extension, the weight is transferred over the hips, increasing extension into the thoracic spine.
3. Each extreme of the position is held for 5–7 seconds and repeated five to seven times.
4. This "hands and knees rocking" procedure is used after treatment of FRS dysfunctions to enhance extension movement.

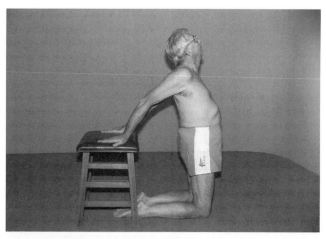

Figure 20.84

Thoracolumbar and Lumbar Spine.

Self-correction position for extension restriction.

1. Patient kneels with back to stool or chair and places hands on stool.
2. Patient extends hips with a strong gluteal contraction.
3. Patient pushes down on the hands and lifts the sternum by bringing scapulae down and back. (Hands may point forward or backward.)
4. Spinal extension is enhanced by anterior translation and lifting of the trunk.
5. Position is held for 5–7 seconds and repeated five to seven times.

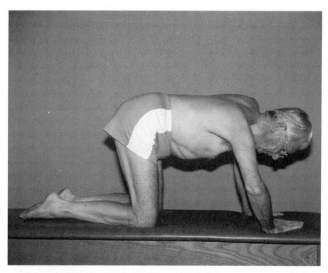

Figure 20.85

Thoracolumbar Spine.

Self-correction position (cat back).

1. Patient on hands and knees.
2. Patient arches back at location of segmental restriction and rocks forward and backward, enhancing flexion movement.
3. Patient lifts segment to the ceiling and holds for 5–7 seconds and repeats five to seven times.

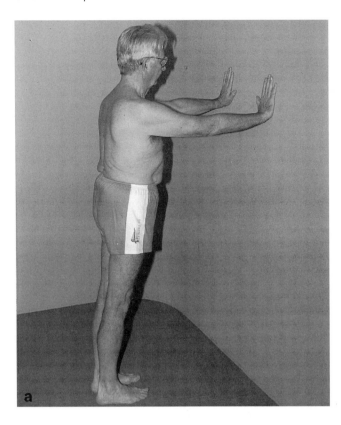

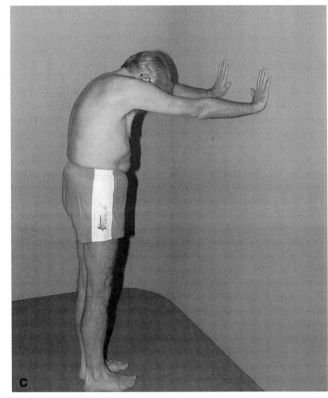

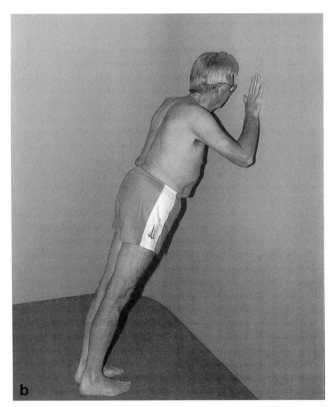

Figure 20.86
Upper Thoracic Spine.
Self-correction position (wall press).
1. Patient stands facing the wall with hands at shoulder height and maintains a neutral lumbar lordosis (Fig. 20.86a).
2. Patient retracts and depresses scapulae and touches the nose to the wall (Fig. 20.86b).
3. Patient holds position for 5–10 seconds and then slowly pushes back from the wall, dropping the head and neck into flexion, protracting the shoulders, and lifting the upper thoracic spine toward the ceiling (Fig. 20.86c).
4. Patient holds position for 5–10 seconds and repeats the procedure five to seven times.

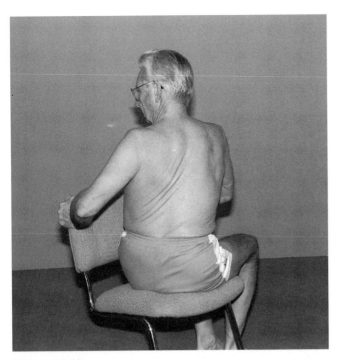

Figure 20.87
Thoracic Spine.
Self-correction position for rotation restriction.
1. Patient sits sideways in a chair holding the back with both hands.
2. Patient inhales deeply, straightening the spine, and during deep exhalation introduces rotation from above downward for three to four segments. Position is held for 5–7 seconds and repeated with increased rotation each time.
3. The arms may assist in the rotational effort.
4. As the rotation gets lower in the thoracic spine, the weight is shifted to the buttock opposite to the rotation.
5. Repeat three to five times on each side for symmetrical balance.

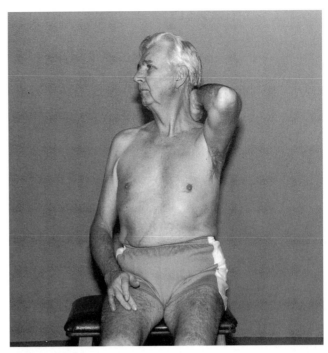

Figure 20.88
Cervical Spine FRS dysfunction.
Self-correction position sitting.
(Example: FRS Left)
1. Patient sits and grasps the articular pillar of the lower vertebra of the dysfunctional segment.
2. While stabilizing lower pillar, patient extends, side-bends, and rotates the cervical spine to the right and looks up with the eyes.
3. Position is held for 5–7 seconds and repeated five to seven times.

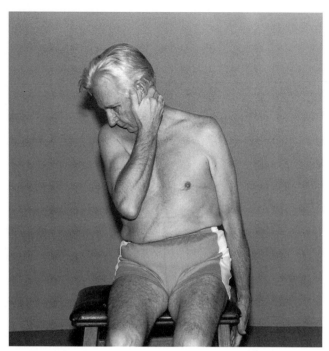

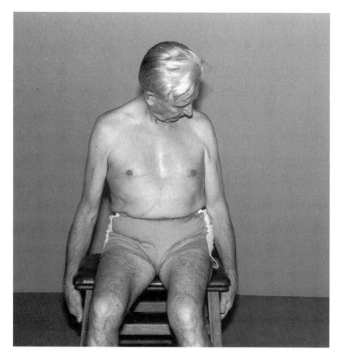

Figure 20.89
Cervical Spine ERS dysfunction.
Self-correction position sitting.
(Example: ERS Left)
1. Patient sits and grasps the articular pillar of the superior vertebra of the dysfunctional segment.
2. Patient flexes, sidebends, and rotates the cervical spine to the right and looks down with the eyes.
3. Position is held for 5–7 seconds and repeated five to seven times.

Figure 20.90
Cervical Spine (atlantoaxial).
Self-correction position sitting.
1. Patient sits and grasps stool or chair with both hands.
2. Patient flexes neck to 45° and introduces rotation in the direction of motion loss.
3. Position is held for 5–7 seconds and repeats five to seven times with increased rotation after each effort.
4. Inhalation/exhalation effort at the barrier assists in the correction.

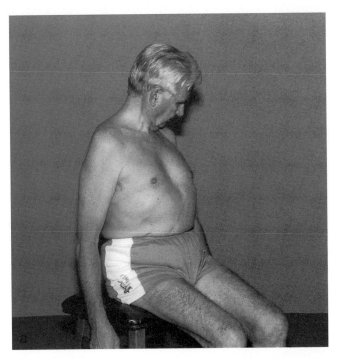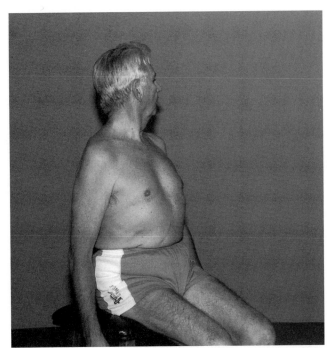

Figure 20.91

Cervical Spine (occipitoatlantal).

Self-correction position sitting.

1. Patient sitting with both hands grasping chair or stool.
2. Patient turns head 30°.
3. Patient nods head while translating backward, introducing flexion movement to the condyle (Fig. 20.91a).
4. Patient translates head forward, leading with the chin, introducing extension movement to the condyle (Fig. 20.91b).
5. The position engaging the restriction is held for 5–7 seconds and repeated five to seven times.

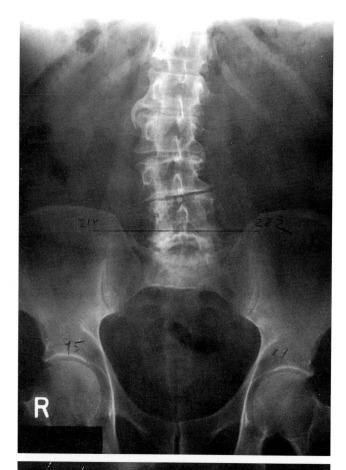

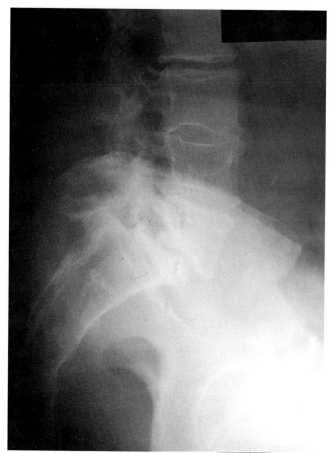

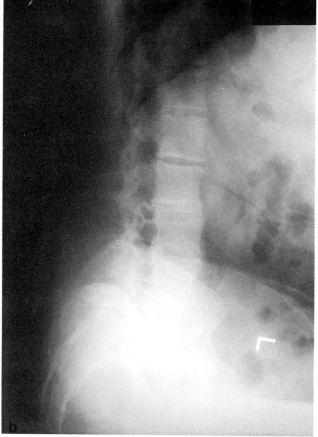

This author's enthusiasm for exercise results from personal experience. With over a 40-year history of recurrent back and right lower extremity pain and with significant pathology identified on x-rays, the best control of these symptoms occurred after the exercise principles identified in this chapter. Figure 20.92 shows plane films that demonstrate significant spondylosis, degenerative disc disease, lateral recess stenosis, and second-degree spondylolisthesis with ischemic defect bilaterally at L5. Despite this osseous pathology, the author demonstrated many of the exercises advocated in this chapter, highlighting the functional capacity of significant osseous pathology in the lumbar spine. In the clinic, the author challenges patients to perform exercises as demonstrated. It is a powerful motivational tool.

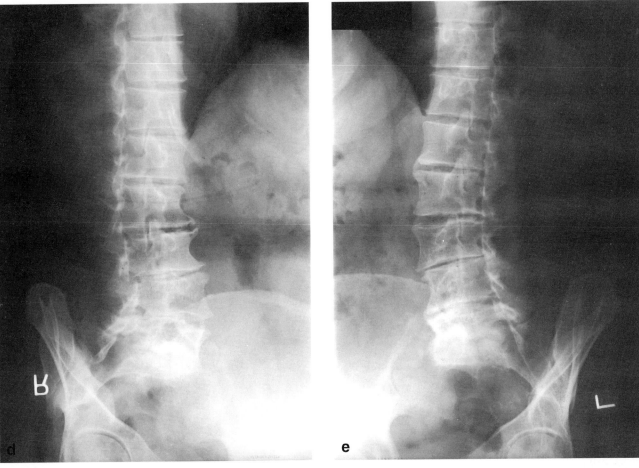

Figure 20.92.
(a) AP erect lumbar spine. (b) Lateral lumbar spine. (c) Lateral spot film lumbosacral junction. (d) Left oblique lumbar spine. (e) Right oblique lumbar spine.

SUMMARY

Exercise is a powerful tool in the management of patients with chronic musculoskeletal disorders and enhances the effectiveness of manual medicine interventions. The principles enumerated here, focusing on centrally mediated and controlled motor balance, followed by stretching, and subsequently with strengthening, have been found to be most effective. Each exercise program must be individualized for the patient, and patient compliance is of utmost importance if the exercise is to be effective. A properly designed and executed exercise program gives the patients control of their level of musculoskeletal health and is very cost effective.

21

ADJUNCTIVE DIAGNOSTIC PROCEDURES

The manual medicine practitioner primarily uses the structural diagnostic process to determine the presence or absence of somatic dysfunction, and its clinical significance, before instituting a manual medicine treatment. Adjunctive diagnostic procedures are frequently of assistance in determining the presence or absence of organic pathology of the musculoskeletal system in addition to the dysfunction. It is helpful to know whether the symptom presentation is due to organic pathology, dysfunction, or a combination of both. In most instances, it is a combination of both, and the practitioner needs to deal with all components of the patient's presentation. Manual medicine must be practiced within the context of total patient care.

IMAGING PROCEDURES

The appropriate use, and inappropriate abuse, of imaging procedures remains controversial within the health care system. Imaging procedures can be expensive, carry some risk, demonstrate both false-positive and false-negative results, and provide information that may be of little assistance in patient management. An admonition for all musculoskeletal medicine practitioners is to treat patients and not images. The following sections are not designed to be comprehensive but to share with the reader the opinions of this author on the assistance imaging procedures can have in manual medicine practice.

Plain Films

Plain films of the lumbar spine and pelvis are not necessary before performing a manual medicine intervention. If the history and physical examination leads the practitioner to a high index of suspicion of organic bone or joint disease, plain films are indicated because they are relatively inexpensive, demonstrate osseous and joint anatomy, and can be of assistance in ruling out major traumatic, neoplastic, and inflammatory disease. Plain films should include as a minimum an anteroposterior (AP) (Fig. 21.1) and lateral projection (Fig. 21.2). Right oblique (Fig.

21.3) and left oblique (Fig. 21.4) studies, although not routinely performed, provide good visualization of the zygapophysial joints and of the pars interarticularis. These views visualize the "Scottie dog" appearance of the posterior elements of the lumbar spine. Scottie dog's eye is the pedicle, the associated transverse process is the nose, the superior facet joint is the ear, the inferior facet joint is the front leg, and the neck is the pars interarticularis. Defect through the pars interarticularis is identified as spondylolysis, and separation of the defect is termed spondylolisthesis. Another commonly used view is a spot lateral

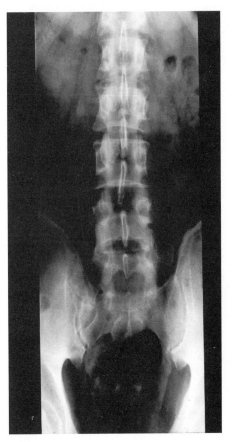

Figure 21.1.
AP lumbar spine (supine).

projection of the lumbar sacral junction, particularly to look at the L5–S1 disc space. Preference is given to a 30° cephalic angled study (sunshine view) (Fig. 21.5) because it provides excellent visualization of the lumbosacral disc space, both sacroiliac joints, and is of great assistance in the detailed assessment of transitional lumbosacral vertebra. Note the bat-wing transverse process with a pseudoarthrosis to the sacrum and to the ilium in Figure 21.5. This structural variation is one of the few predictors of future pathology and disability within the lumbar spine. The disc above the transitional vertebra is statistically at risk for herniation and the development of discogenic radiculopathy.

Plain Film Postural Study. If the practitioner has suspicion of a short leg pelvic tilt syndrome based on the clinical finding of unleveling of the iliac crest and greater trochanter in the standing position, plain film postural study is useful in confirming the diagnosis and determining the exact amount of the leg inequality and the unleveling of the sacral base. The postural study includes an AP projection of the lumbar spine and pelvis with the patient standing (Fig. 21.6) and in the lateral projection (Fig. 21.2). Great

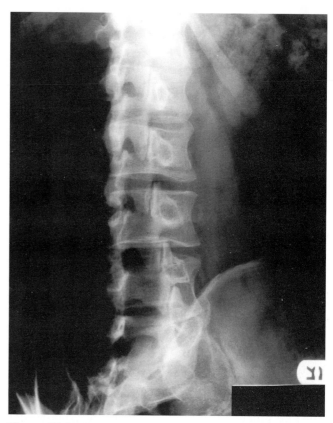

Figure 21.3.
Right oblique lumbar spine.

care by the technician is necessary to obtain quality images for postural analysis. The important technical factors are as follows:

1. An upright bucky level with floor or foot rest of the table;
2. 14 × 17 film loaded level in the cassette;
3. Cassette loaded level in bucky;
4. Patient standing erect with equal weight distribution on feet 15 cm (6 inches) apart at the medial malleolus;
5. One meter (40 inches) target to film distance; and
6. Vertical film centered at iliac crest;
7. Central ray projected at center of film.

The AP and erect films are measured in the following fashion:

1. AP Projection
   a. A horizontal line is drawn across the top of each femoral head.
   b. A horizontal line is drawn across the sacral base. Three variations are provided in the order of their reliability:

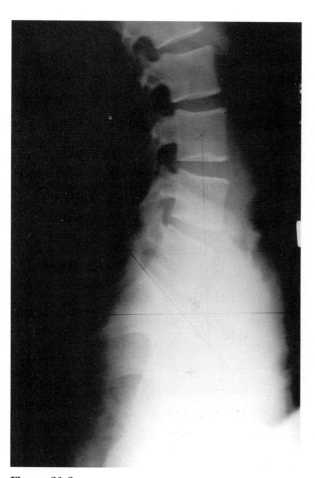

Figure 21.2.
Lateral lumbar spine (erect).

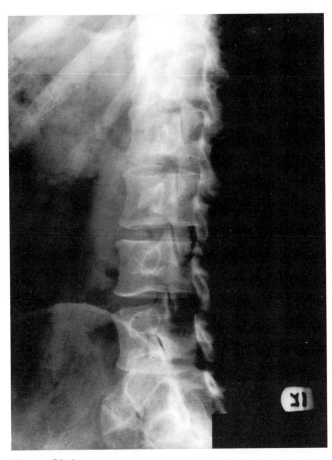

Figure 21.4.
Left oblique lumbar spine.

1. Across the most posterior aspect of the posterior margin of S1 body;
2. Inferior aspect of sacral notch (transverse process S1);
3. Medial corner of S1 facet at junction with sacral body.

   c. Two vertical lines are drawn from the bottom of the film through the highest point of the femoral head to the line drawn across the sacral base.

   d. The difference in the distance from the femoral head to the bottom of the film is the leg length deficit.

   e. The difference in distance from the sacral base line and the bottom of the film on each side is the amount of sacral base unleveling.

2. Lateral Projection

   a. A line is drawn across the superior aspect of the body of S1 to meet a horizontal line drawn parallel to the bottom of the film at the level of the anterior aspect of S1. The resultant acute angle is called the

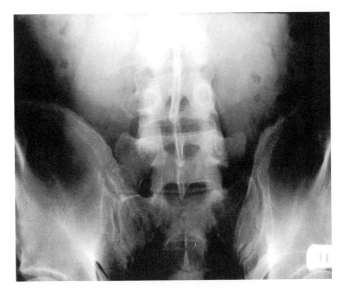

Figure 21.5.
Sunshine view of the sacroiliac and lumbosacral joints.

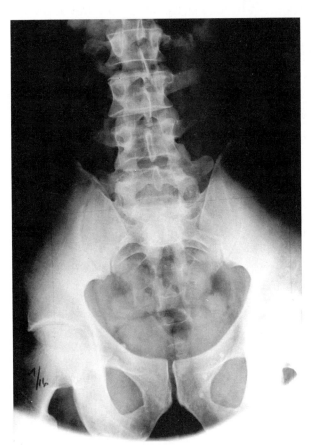

Figure 21.6.
AP lumbar spine erect for postural analysis.

"sacral base angle." In the erect position, the normal sacral base angle is 40 ± 2°.

    b. The midportion of the third lumbar body is identified and a vertical line dropped from the midthird lumbar body. Normally, this line should strike upon the superior aspect of S1.

3. Lumbar Scoliosis

    a. Assessment is made of the lumbar scoliosis in the AP projection. The normal adaptive process should show a lumbar convexity toward the side of sacral base unleveling.

Experience has shown that interrater and intrarater reliability using this methodology is 1 mm of difference. Unless the history and physical examination requires plain film study before the initiation of treatment, it is advisable to treat the lumbar spine and pelvis to maximum biomechanical balance before performing a postural radiographic study. Occasionally, dysfunction of the lumbar spine and pelvis, particularly associated with major muscle imbalance, makes the study technically difficult and the measurements less than reliable. The study is best performed with the patient at maximum biomechanical function of the lumbar spine, pelvis, and lower extremities.

Dynamic Studies

Plain films are frequently supplemented by dynamic studies in the erect position performing AP right sidebending (Fig. 21.7), left sidebending (Fig. 21.8), backward-bending (Fig. 21.9), and forward-bending lateral projection (Fig. 21.10). Assessment is made of the dynamic changes in both the AP and lateral projections and compared with the neutral AP and lateral views. In the sidebending dynamic films, assessment is made of the presence or absence of neutral or nonneutral lumbar vertebral coupling. Figure 21.7 demonstrates sidebending to the right with rotation of the vertebra into the concavity consistent with nonneutral vertebral mechanics in the lumbar spine. Figure 21.8 shows sidebending to the left with rotation of lumbar vertebra to the right consistent with neutral vertebral motion in the lumbar spine. By overlying one film on another, it is frequently possible to identify which segment within the lumbar spine resists sidebending to the right or to the left. In the forward-bending and backward-bending, lateral projections analysis is made of intersegmental mobility. Again, by overlaying one film on the other, in reference to the neutral lateral projection, identification can be made of the vertebral segment that resists forward-bending or backward-bending. Coupling the neutral or nonneutral behavior of the lumbar spine in sidebending, with intersegmental

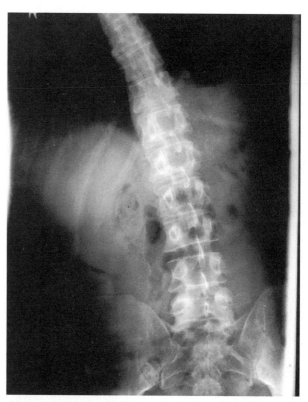

Figure 21.7.
AP erect, right sidebending dynamic film.

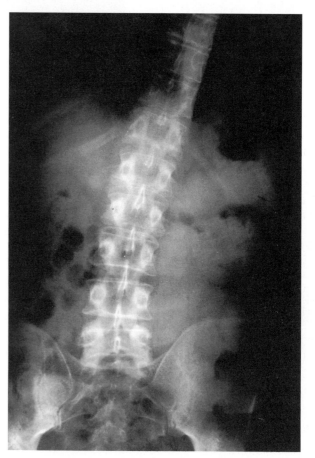

Figure 21.8.
AP erect, left sidebending dynamic film.

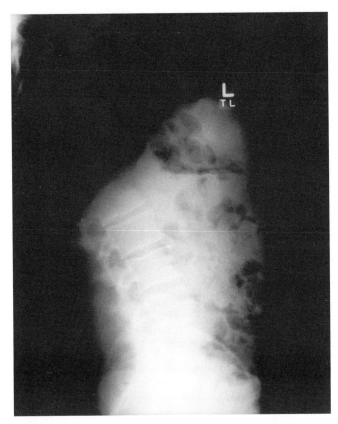

Figure 21.9.
Lateral backward-bending dynamic film.

restriction of flexion or extension, can assist in the evaluation of nonneutral vertebral dysfunction within the lumbar spine. The role of dynamic studies remains controversial because of difficulty in the biomechanical research of the methodology. Despite this concern, clinical experience has shown them to be of assistance in cases and in the collaboration of the structural diagnostic finding.

Special Imaging Studies

There are a number of special imaging studies that have use in musculoskeletal problems, particularly in lower back and lower extremity pain syndromes. Before ordering a special imaging study, the practitioner should show care in selecting a procedure that will provide the information desired. Different imaging studies provide different information. Special imaging studies should be done to confirm impressions gained from the clinical examination. Special images such as magnetic resonance imaging (MRI) should not be used as a screening tool to look for pathology in a patient presenting with back pain. MRI has many advantages in the diagnostic process and provides the best information about the soft tissues of the musculoskeletal system. It has become the image of choice for diagnosis of disc herniation, cord lesions, brain lesions, and many of the less common development variants like syringomyelia and tethered cord (Fig. 21.11). MRI can provide images that demonstrate the nucleus of the disc similar to a discogram and outline the spinal canal and its contents

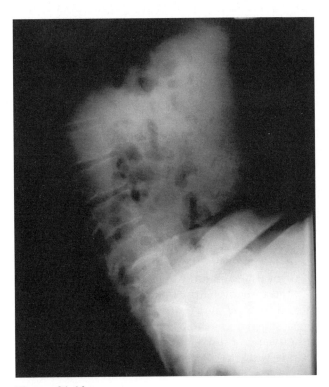

Figure 21.10.
Forward-bending, lateral, dynamic film.

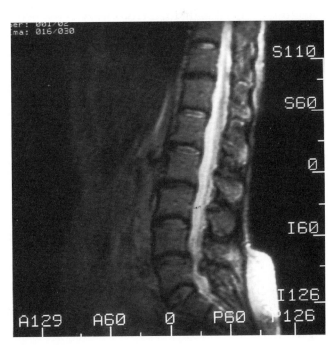

Figure 21.11.
MRI, lumbar spine, sagittal view.

similar to myelogram. The procedure involves no ionizing radiation, is noninvasive, and has few contraindications, namely metal implants and pacemakers. MRI gantries are becoming larger so that the patient is less likely to become claustrophobic in the machine. One drawback to MRI studies is the difficulty in obtaining dynamic studies because of the dimension of the gantry and the fact that the patient is in an unloaded position. With special technical effort, it is possible to obtain some dynamic flexion and extension studies of the cervical spine. Dynamic studies of the lumbar spine are much more difficult.

Computed Tomography

Computed tomography (CT) studies have a longer history than MRI. CT is the image of choice when looking for morphology of the osseous system. It is also useful in identifying disc disease, including herniation with extrusion of nuclear material into the central and lateral vertebral canals as well as lateral and interior herniation (Fig. 21.12). This technology is particularly useful in the assessment of central and lateral recess stenosis, as seen in Figure 21.12. CT can be combined with discography and myelography to provide additional diagnostic information (Fig. 21.13). Plain CT is noninvasive but does require the patient to be exposed to ionizing radiation. Metallic implants are not a contraindication, but the images are frequently distorted by artifact. A discography CT and myelography CT require an accompanying invasive procedure.

Myelography

Myelography is one of the older special images in the diagnosis of spinal pathology. Historically, it has been

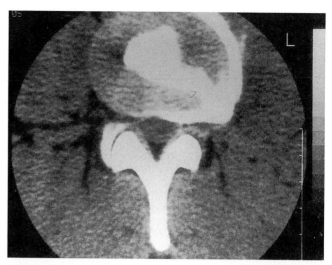

Figure 21.13.
Lumbar spine, discogram CT.

used for localization of disc pathology, neurocompression, blockage of cerebral spinal fluid, and intraspinal pathology such as cord tumor. It is an invasive procedure, and some of the older dye material was toxic and lead to complications. There is a statistically significant increase in arachnoiditis with pantopaque myelography. Currently, water soluble contrast materials are much less toxic, but in a few individuals who are iodine sensitive they are contraindicated. False negatives in myelography are common for disc disease at the L5–S1 level. Myelography occasionally becomes a procedure of choice, particularly in association with CT imaging in certain diagnostic challenges.

Discography

Discography continues to have its advocates and detractors. It is an invasive procedure with considerable technical difficulty. Radiopaque material is injected into the nucleus of the disc and images are made for interdiscal pathology (Fig. 21.14). Discography also provides the opportunity to assess whether a disc is a pain generator. Injections into a normal disc are usually nonpainful. Injections of a diseased disc are frequently painful and, if it replicates the patient's pain complaint, gives some corroboration of the disc as the site of pain generation. Commonly in the presence of disc herniation, there is exacerbation of the associated radiculopathy. Like myelography, the procedure is invasive and requires the introduction of a foreign substance, which carries some allergic risk. Another value of discography is the ability to perform the study with the patient loaded and unloaded. In the erect loaded position, flexion and extension can be performed to further assist in the diagnostic pro-

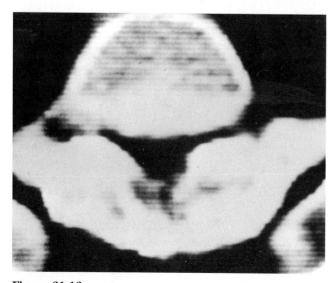

Figure 21.12.
CT scan, lumbar spine, bone window.

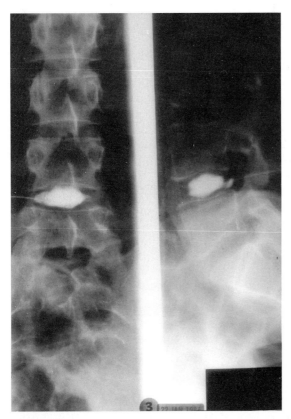

Figure 21.14.
Discogram AP and lateral projections.

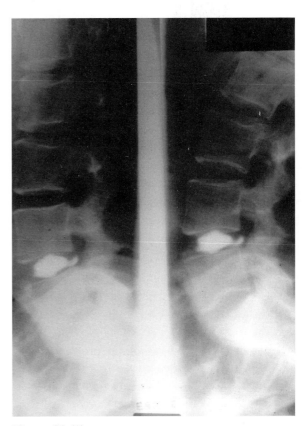

Figure 21.15.
L4–5 lumbar discogram, erect, forward-bending and backward-bending.

cess (Fig. 21.15). Note in Figure 21.15 that there was additional extrusion of the opaque nuclear material in a posterior direction during trunk backward-bending. Like discography, myelography can be performed in the standing loaded position and can be subjected to dynamic stress of forward-bending, backward-bending, and right to left sidebending.

Diagnostic Blocks and Injections

On occasion, additional special studies can be of assistance in determining the location of the pain generator and the significance of altered anatomy. These procedures include zygapophysial and sacroiliac joint injections, selected nerve blocks, and the previously discussed discography. These procedures require fluoroscopic control, the use of contrast material, and the installation of anesthetic agents to see whether the structure is painful and responds to a local block (Figs. 21.16 and 21.17). Figures 21.16 and 21.17 demonstrate the role of a zygapophysial injection to determine whether the spondylolisthesis at this level was symptomatic. Note the needle is placed in the L4–5 joint, but with installation of contrast material there its delineation of the pars defect and the zygapophysial at L5–S1. The procedure was totally pain free for the patient, and the conclusion was that this defect was not pain producing. The sacroiliac

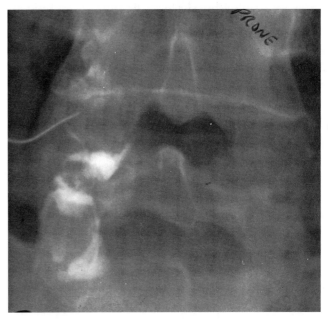

Figure 21.16.
L4–5 joint block, AP projection.

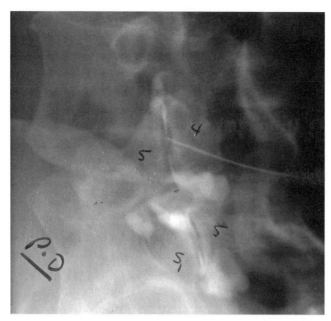

Figure 21.17.
L4–5 zygapophysial joint block, oblique projection.

joint can be challenged and visualized by arthrography (Figs. 21.18–21.20). Under fluoroscopic control, the inferior margin of the synovial portion of the sacroiliac joint can be entered and contrast material injected. Like zygapophysial joint injection, if the joint is contributing to pain generation, the injection is painful to the patient. Installation of local anesthetic with relief of concordant pain identifies this structure as a pain generator. Figures 21.18–21.20 show an example of anterior capsular diverticuli in the presence of a joint that was positive to the challenge of injection and resulted in complete removal of concordant pain after installation of local anesthetic. This confirmed the left sacroiliac joint as a pain generator contributing to the patient's presentation. Figure 21.21 is a special CT view of the sacroiliac joints in the case represented in Figures 21.18–21.20. Note the asymmetric relationship of the anterior aspects of the sacrum to the posterior aspects of the ilium as shown by the horizontal lines. This finding was imaging confirmation of the palpatory assessment of sacral torsion in this patient. Occasionally, information can be obtained about the functional capacity of the anatomy so well displayed by such imaging techniques. Selective nerve blocks require fluoroscopic guidance and again seek to identify whether a specific nerve root and its sheath are contributing to pain generation. This technology has greater value in the diagnosis of acute discogenic radiculopathy than it does in the dysfunctional pathology dealt with by manual medicine.

Special MRI Studies

MRI is an excellent technology to distinguish difference in soft tissues. For the past 2 years, a special protocol for MRI of the upper cervical spine has identified selective fatty replacement of rectus capitis posterior minor and rectus capitis posterior major muscles. This fatty replacement is seen in 87% of patients presenting with posttraumatic cervical cranial pain syndromes and is not found in 100% of a normative population (Figs. 21.22 and 21.23). Figure 21.22 shows good definition of both the rectus capitis posterior major and minor with muscle density at arrows in a patient with no history of trauma and asymptomatic. Figure 21.23 shows fatty replacement of rectus capitis posterior major and minor muscles

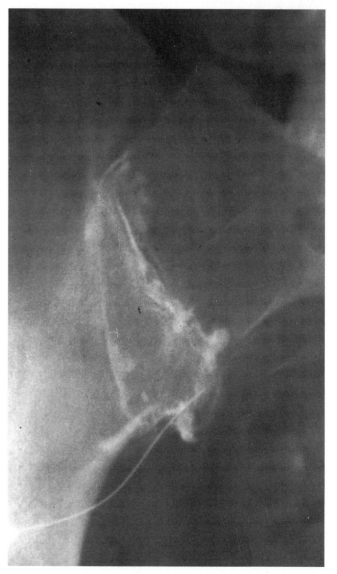

Figure 21.18.
Left sacroiliac arthrogram, AP view.

at the arrows in a patient who was 2 years post-motor vehicle injury with flexion extension of the cervical spine and resultant pain in the upper cervical region with radiation of headache anteriorly from the cranial base. The exact cause of the fatty replacement continues under study, and the overall significance is yet to be determined. Intuitively, one would assume that if muscle has been replaced by fat and has lost its contractile properties, this may contribute to persistent symptoms and the lack of response to manual medicine using muscle energy activating force.

Electrodiagnostic Studies

The use of electromyography and nerve conduction studies can be of assistance in the differential diagnosis of cervicobrachial and lower extremity pain syn-

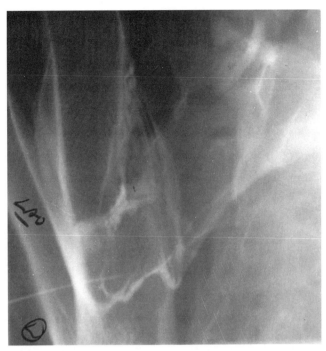

Figure 21.20.
Left sacroiliac arthrogram, left anterior oblique.

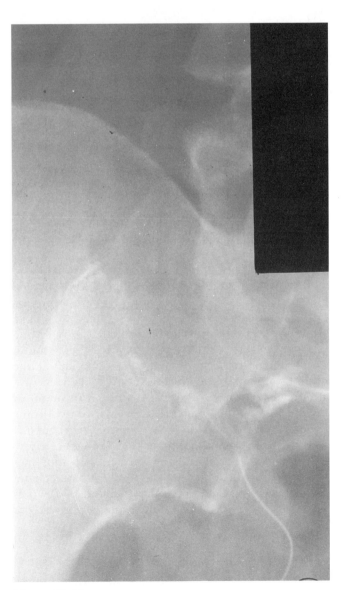

Figure 21.19.
Left sacroiliac arthrogram, right anterior oblique.

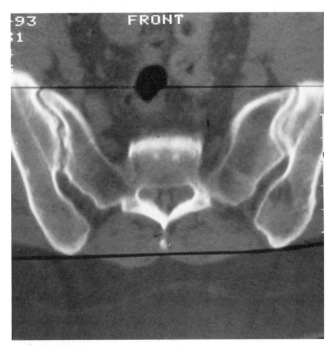

Figure 21.21.
CT of sacroiliac joints.

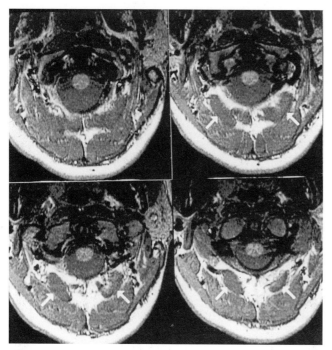

Figure 21.22.
Cervical spine MRI in nontraumatic nonsymptomatic patient.

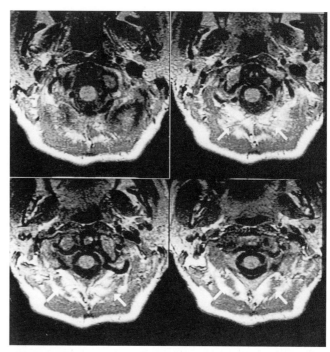

Figure 21.23.
Cervical spine MRI in posttraumatic symptomatic patient.

dromes to rule in or rule out the presence of significant radiculopathy from discogenic disease or from other causes. Nerve conduction studies are particularly of value in documenting the presence of the carpal tunnel or tarsal tunnel syndromes. There are many sophisticated neurophysiological tests available, but seldom are they needed in the practice of manual medicine. Electromyogram (EMG) study in the presence of acute radiculopathy is not diagnostic for the initial 3–week period. A negative study in an early presentation does not rule out the presence of radiculopathy. A positive EMG with acute changes can help confirm the diagnosis of discogenic radiculopathy in a patient who presents with classical clinical findings and has an associated positive image that is consistent. This author uses confirmatory EMG studies before subjecting patients to surgical intervention for disc disease.

Surface EMG is of diagnostic assistance in the determination of normal or abnormal muscle firing pattern sequences. Janda has described normal muscle firing sequences for hip extension, hip abduction, and shoulder abduction (see Chapter 20). These aberrations can be documented by surface EMG study, and the technology can be of assistance in documenting the response to treatment interventions.

LABORATORY TESTING

The practitioner has a vast array of laboratory diagnostic tests available. In musculoskeletal medicine, there are a few that can be of assistance, particularly in ruling out rheumatological conditions in addition to identifying general systemic illness. It has been said that the sedimentation rate takes the temperature of the musculoskeletal system. It is a valuable screening test requiring additional laboratory testing if positive. Basic rheumatological tests are found within the arthritic profile and, depending on the findings, directs the clinician toward more extensive antinuclear antibody and DNA study. Assessment of thyroid function is frequently of assistance in chronic patients. Borderline hypothyroidism is frequently seen in patients with primary and secondary fibromyalgia. Not all patients who present with musculoskeletal pain syndromes are the result of biomechanical dysfunction. The alert practitioner uses all tools available, including laboratory testing, to assess the total patient.

PSYCHOLOGICAL EVALUATION

Psychological assessment of patients with musculoskeletal pain syndromes, particularly of the chronic nature, is frequently of assistance in patient management. Psychosocial factors play a large role in back pain disability. A number of standardized tests, such as the Minnesota Multiphasic Personality Inventory, have had extensive use in assessing the psychological and psychiatric status of a patient. A one-on-one psychological evaluation by a trained clinical psychologist conversant with musculoskeletal pain syndromes can be of great assistance. Psychological evaluation, particularly the neuropsychological examination, is of considerable value in identifying the presence and severity of traumatic brain injury. Traumatic brain injury is frequently seen in patients with chronic pain syndromes and is probably underdiagnosed. A probing history will frequently identify trauma resulting in transient unconsciousness and disorientation.

OCCUPATIONAL THERAPY ASSESSMENT

A cognitive perceptual motor evaluation by a skilled occupational therapist is another test useful in the diagnosis of traumatic brain injury. Assessment of the work site, particularly in those patients presenting with repetitive strain injuries, can be most useful in total patient management. Work site modification is of frequent assistance in the rehabilitation of disabled patients as well as in the prevention of injuries in the future.

NUTRITIONAL EVALUATION

The services of a skilled nutritionist can be of assistance in the rehabilitation process. Many patients with musculoskeletal pain syndromes have poor nutrition with heavy use of caffeine, alcohol, and fast foods. A poor diet contributes to an unhealthy musculoskeletal system and interferes with normal neurological control of motor system function. Obesity continues to be a societal problem, particularly in those patients with chronic musculoskeletal problems that reduce the patient's activity level. Smoking contributes to poor response to both nonoperative and operative care of spinal problems. Reduction in smoking, alcohol, and drugs, plus a well-balanced diet resulting in appropriate weight, can be of major significance in the recovery of patients with musculoskeletal problems.

CONCLUSION

The manual medicine practitioner should be aware of the role of adjunctive diagnostic procedures in patient assessment. Knowledge of the attributes, as well as the shortcomings of many of the aforementioned diagnostic procedures, is necessary for their appropriate use. The practitioner should become acquainted with the expertise of other disciplines that can be included in the patient management process. Such knowledge will lead to the appropriate use and not the inappropriate abuse of medical technology.

22

ADJUNCTIVE THERAPEUTIC PROCEDURES

Manual medicine is a powerful tool in the management of many health problems, particularly those involving the musculoskeletal system. Manual medicine might well be the primary therapeutic intervention used. Other therapies may be used in conjunction with manual medicine. When using manual medicine techniques, it is essential that it be done within the context of total patient care, and the practitioner must see that the manual medicine interventions are appropriate for the patient's physical condition.

Comments follow on a variety of other therapeutic interventions that this author has found to be most useful.

MEDICATION

In using an oral or injectable medication, the practitioner should be knowledgeable about the actions, reactions, and iatrogenic effects of any substance used. The more simple the medication protocol, the better. A general observation is that the more potent the medication is for its effectiveness, the more common are its side effects and reactions.

Medication for pain control is of great importance in the management of musculoskeletal conditions. The longer the nociceptive process is ongoing, the more likely there is for sensitization of pain pathways and deprograming of motor control. The management of pain associated with acute tissue injury is quite different from the management of pain that has been present for months to years. Acute pain is characterized by its specific localization, lancinating quality, and associated tissue damage in a specific structure of the musculoskeletal system. Chronic musculoskeletal pain is quite different. It is characterized by being less well localized, more diffuse in nature, and frequently has a burning quality.

Analgesics and Narcotics

Analgesics and narcotics are most useful for the acute painful condition. In acute pain, it is advisable to determine that the dose is adequate in strength and availability to truly control the painful perception. The persistence of nociceptive pathway stimulation is negative for the patient's nervous system and can lead to chronicity. The dosage should be adjusted to avoid peaks and valleys of pain relief and increased pain perception.

It is currently unknown when acute pain changes to chronic pain. Some view chronicity as being related to time, with the changeover from 3 to 6 months. Some believe that pain pathway stimulation for 30 days is sufficient to change central pain processing pathways. In chronic pain, the patient continues to perceive pain despite the lack of ongoing tissue damage. This is commonly frustrating for both the attending physician and the patient because of the absence of an identifiable cause of persistent pain. However, to the patient, the pain is reality and needs appropriate attention just as the more commonly recognized acute pain associated with acute tissue damage. Chronic pain in the absence of identifiable tissue damage is managed quite differently from patients with chronic pain associated with diseases such as malignancy, inflammatory joint disease, and associated rheumatological conditions. In these conditions, appropriate mix of medications to assist the patient in the control of pain is clearly indicated. In the chronic pain patient without ongoing tissue damage or disease process, medications are mainly contraindicated. Analgesics and narcotics seems to contribute to, rather than ameleriorate, the chronic pain system. These patients need to be weaned off potent medications as rapidly as possible. During their rehabilitative process, particularly with increasing activity during an exercise program, there may be exacerbation of tissue reaction, resulting in short bursts of acute pain. Appropriate acute pain medication at this time is clearly beneficial but needs to be discontinued as rapidly as possible. Acetaminophen in adequate doses seems to work well in these instances. The management of the chronic pain syndrome patient requires an integrated team approach with only one physician responsible for the medication prescriptions.

Antiinflammatory Agents

Another group of medications of great adjunctive use in the management of musculoskeletal conditions is antiinflammatory agents. The nonsteroidal antiinflammatory drugs are quite popular and available over the counter. The several classes of nonsteroidal antiinflammatory drugs differ primarily in the balance of analgesic and antiinflammatory effect and in the length of action. Almost all are irritating to the gastrointestinal tract, and caution must be used in prescribing these agents with peptic ulcer disease, gastritis, and irritable bowel syndromes. Aspirin is the oldest and cheapest of this group. If tolerated by the patient, it is as good as any. In general, it is most effective to use short-acting nonsteroidal antiinflammatory drugs (NSAIDs) in adequate antiinflammatory doses and then wean the patient off of the medication as rapidly as possible. This author has found that 2400–3200 mg of ibuprofen in divided doses for 7–10 days is very useful in dealing with the acute patient, as well as the acute exacerbation in the chronic patient undergoing active manual medicine intervention and early exercise programing. Caution should be used for the longer acting NSAIDs because patients metabolize these drugs differently, and toxic levels can be achieved with little warning. Injectable ketorolac tromethamine (Toradal) is frequently of value in achieving control of acute pain, particularly that associated with acute tissue injury and the acute flare after an active manual medicine intervention. In the long-term management of patients by NSAIDs, careful monitoring of gastrointestinal, hepatic, renal, and hematological function is prudent.

Corticosteroids

Corticosteroids have a place in the management of musculoskeletal conditions, particularly during the acute phase. They can be used both orally and injectably and have particular value in the management of acute radiculopathy. Spinal and caudal epidural steroids have long been used in the management of acute radiculopathies, and both have their advocates and critics. The problem with caudal installation is the difficulty in achieving high enough levels to deal with radiculopathies above S1. Spinal epidurals can be more precise in localization of steroid effect. Both of these invasive procedures should be done under fluoroscopic control to ensure the needle placement and the appropriate installation of therapeutic material.

Oral Steroids

Oral steroid use in the presence of radiculopathy has been effective for many years. A regimen beginning with 60–80 mg of prednisone in divided doses, decreasing daily by 10-mg increments, has been found to be quite effective and inexpensive. Again, caution must be expressed about the patient's tolerance to steroids, particularly from the perspective of the gastrointestinal tract. Cardiovascular and psychic alterations from long-term steroid use are always a cau-

tion, as is the danger of aseptic necrosis in both the shoulder and hip joints. A guiding principle can be that steroids are useful in short-term application for acute conditions. They are much less useful in chronic conditions. Those patients requiring long-term steroid use for the management of systemic disease should be monitored closely for deleterious side effects.

Antidepressants

Another class of drugs found useful in musculoskeletal conditions are those that deal with depression associated with chronic pain and in the restoration of the sleep cycle. The tricyclics benefit these patients. There are a number of tricyclic antidepressants, but this author has found amitriptyline (Elavil) to be useful if the patient can tolerate the drug. Doses from 10 to 150 mg may be necessary to restore a normal sleep cycle. There is some evidence that tricyclics have a positive effect on chronic pain pathways.

Muscle Relaxants

Muscle relaxants are very popular in the treatment of both acute and chronic musculoskeletal conditions. This author has found their use to be quite disappointing. Many of them are central-acting depressants rather than local muscle relaxants. Oral and injectable diazepam (Valium) is somewhat useful in dealing with acute muscle spasm, and if a muscle relaxant is deemed necessary, it is probably the drug of choice.

Medication use requires that the patient understand the drugs prescribed beneficial effects, side effects, length of action, and allergy potential. The more simple a medication program, the better. The prescribing physician must know what over-the-counter medications the patient is taking, as well as drugs prescribed by other physicians for other health problems. Iatrogenic drug interactions contribute greatly to health care cost and should always be on the physician's mind when picking up a pen and prescription pad.

INJECTIONS

Different injection techniques have been found useful in musculoskeletal conditions. They have their indications, as well as their contraindications, and require that the practitioner be skilled in their use. Various injection techniques have both diagnostic and therapeutic indications. The use of epidural steroids in radiculopathy has been referred to above. Concurrent selective nerve blocks are of assistance in identifying the nerve root involved as part of pain generation. These procedures require adequate training and sufficient volume to maintain the skill for the procedure. They all require fluoroscopic control.

Acupuncture

One of the oldest injection procedures is classic acupuncture. There are a number of different schools of acupuncture that can all be classified as peripheral stimulating treatment. In selected cases, acupuncture has been found to be very useful in assisting in pain control. Not all patients are responders to acupuncture. Selection of the patient, as well as the practitioner, is essential for success.

Triggerpoints

Treatment of primary and secondary triggerpoints has long been advocated by Simon and Travell. Spray and stretch techniques have been found useful by some practitioners. This author has found the injection technique of classic Travell triggers more effective than spray and stretch. A clear relationship between the presence of somatic dysfunction and myofascial triggerpoints has been observed. Adequate treatment of the somatic dysfunction frequently relieves the triggerpoints. In other instances, the triggerpoints persist despite adequate treatment of the somatic dysfunction. Appropriate treatment of the triggerpoint would then seem indicated. The reverse is also true. Primary treatment of triggerpoints has reduced observable somatic dysfunction in related parts of the musculoskeletal system, but that is not a 100% rule. This author prefers to treat them in an integrated fashion and will use dry needling or xylocaine injection to triggerpoints if they are present after adequate treatment of somatic dysfunction or if they are viewed as being a primary contributor to the patient's presentation. Follow-up treatment of triggerpoint therapy requires adequate and appropriate exercise whether spray and stretch or injection technique is used.

Sacroiliac Injections

The use of injections in the sacroiliac syndrome is useful from the diagnostic and therapeutic perspective. Injection into the capsular portion of the joint requires fluoroscopic guidance and is best done from the inferior aspect of the joint. Both pain generation and arthrographic appearance can be used in diagnosing the painful sacroiliac joint. Occasionally, injection of the capsular portion of the joint demonstrates extravasation of contrast material in an anterior direction, outlining the L5 and S1 nerve roots. This mechanism may account for the lower extremity pain seen in the sacroiliac syndrome. From a therapeutic perspective, injection into the posterior ligamentous portion of the sacroiliac joint can be useful. If local analgesic infiltration of the posterior sacroiliac joint results in reduction or relief of the patient's pain, the sacroiliac joint is likely the pain generator. Steroid injection into the posterior sacroiliac ligaments for the antiinflammatory effect has been found useful in the management of the sacroiliac syndrome, coupled with appropriate manual medicine and exercise programs. Infiltration of the posterior sacroiliac ligamentous structures can be done without fluoroscopic control if one is familiar with the anatomy and skilled in the procedure. Installation of steroids into the posterior sacroiliac ligaments is usually done no more than twice.

A similar, but less commonly used, procedure is the infiltration of local anesthetic and steroid into the posterior aspect of the zygapophysial joint in the lower lumbar spine. This is not a classic facet injection that requires fluoroscopic control to ensure that you are in the posterior facet. Without fluoroscopy, it is possible to walk a spinal needle along bone to the base of the transverse process, and by moving slightly above and below, one can instill local anesthetic and steroid into the posterior aspect of the capsule of the joint. This can be useful in short-term management of an acute zygapophysial joint pain syndrome. Again, adequate training and practice is essential to perform this procedure. Complications are exceedingly rare but must always be considered.

Prolotherapy

A number of musculoskeletal medicine practitioners advocate the injection of proliferant solutions into ligaments. This procedure was popularized by Gedney in the osteopathic profession and Hackett in the medical profession. The principle concept is to inject material that stimulates proliferation of collagen in ligament to strengthen the ligament and to reduce ligamentous related pain. Historically, a number of solutions have been advocated. The most popular current solution is that advocated by Ongley and consists of hypertonic glucose, glycerine, phenol, diluted with water and then combined with zylocaine for injection. The reader is referred to the text *Diagnosis and Injection Techniques in Orthopaedic Medicine* by Dorman and Ravin for definitive information on this system. Prolotherapy, as it is currently called, has undergone basic and clinical research study. The methodology appears to have value in selected cases. As with all injection techniques, there is a learning curve, and adequate instruction and practice is essential. This author has found prolotherapy to be of use in selected patients with recurrent sacroiliac syndrome, particularly those with hypermobility associated with innominate shear dysfunction and chronic recurrent anteriorly nutated sacroiliac dysfunction with a significant inferior translatory component. Fluoroscopic control is not necessary but is advisable if available. Recently, some researchers have injected proliferant material into the intervertebral disc for the treatment of annular tear. This requires high level skill and fluoroscopic control. Prolotherapy is quite uncomfortable to the patient, and preinjection medication is frequently useful. Like many technologies, prolotherapy can be overused in the hands of an enthusiastic practitioner. For the right patient with the right diagnostic criteria, it is clearly a technology that can be useful.

ORTHOTIC DEVICES

There are numerous orthopedic devices available to the manual medicine practitioner. Those that have been found most useful by this author follow.

Lumbar Corsets

There are numerous lumbar corsets and supporting belts. A contoured belt individualized to the patient by heating of the material can be useful in acute conditions. It stabilizes the patient's trunk during the acute phase but should be replaced as rapidly as possible by an exercise program of trunk stabilization and control. Dependency on supporting corsets can easily occur. The patient should be cautioned that they are for temporary use only and appropriate exercise is the long-term goal of the treatment plan.

Sacroiliac Cinch Belt

The orthotic device found most useful is the Hackett sacroiliac cinch belt manufactured by Brooks Company (Marshall, MI). These varying sized belts without padding over the sacrum provide dynamic tension around the pelvis and assist in stability during the rehabilitative process (Fig. 22.1). All patients with innominate shear dysfunction use them while weight bearing for a minimum of 6 weeks. If the innominate shear does not recur within a 6-week period, the belt is discontinued except during strenuous exercise and long motor vehicle trips. Occasionally, the same device is used for the chronic recurrent low back pain syndrome associated with an anteriorly nutated sacrum, a posteriorly rotated innominate, and a superiorly displaced pube. This device allows for free mobility of the pelvis during the walking cycle. Other devices that restrict the sacrum by a compressive pad have limited value in this author's experience.

Heel Lift

The most commonly used orthotic device is a heel lift for the long-term management of the short leg/pelvic tilt syndrome. The amount of shortness of a lower extremity and the amount of pelvic tilt that is clinically significant differ greatly from author to author. This author has found that sacral base unlevel-

ing of 6 mm or more is clinically significant in patients with lower back and lower extremity pain syndromes, particularly those recurrent in nature. The methodology for the diagnosis of the short leg and pelvic tilt syndrome has been described in Chapter 21. There are times when one does not wish to expose the patient to additional x-ray procedures. Clinical assessment of short leg and pelvic tilt can be quite accurate if plane films are available showing the shape and symmetry of the two innominate bones and the sacrum. The practitioner can use a series of shims placed under the supposed short lower extremity to restore functional balance to the pelvis and lumbar spine. One-eighth-, 1/4-, 3/8-, and 1/2-inch shims can be easily obtained from a lumbar dealer. When the adequate manual medicine intervention has restored mobility to the lumbar spine and pelvis, the patient is evaluated in the erect position sequen-

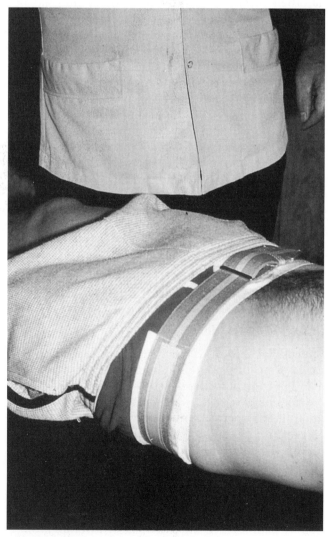

Figure 22.1.
Sacroiliac cinch belt.

tially using shims to achieve a level of greater trochanter height, level iliac crest, and symmetrical trunk sidebending behavior of the lumbar spine (Fig. 22.2, a–c). When the amount of lift needed has been identified, either by radiographic study or by clinical assessment as described above, temporary lifts can be placed inside the heel of the shoe to be followed by permanent additions to the heel and sole to balance lumbopelvic mechanics. In most cases, any shoemaker can add the appropriate amount of lift to the heel and sole. In some instances, a specialized prescription to an orthotist or pedorthist is necessary. Both heel and sole lift should ideally be used so that the device does not alter foot and ankle mechanics. It has been found empirically that most people can tolerate a 3/8-inch heel lift without additional sole

lifting, but this must be individualized for each patient.

The following is a suggested prescription sequence for the use of lift therapy. If the ultimate goal is 3/8 inch or less, a single addition of a heel lift to the short leg/pelvic tilt side is sufficient. Despite past recommendations that lifts be increased in 1/8-inch increments, most patients tolerate 3/8 inch in a single application. If the sacral base angle is greater than 42° or clinical assessment shows an increased lower lumbar lordosis, it is advisable that the heel on the long leg be reduced by the appropriate amount rather than adding to the short leg. One does not want to increase the anterior tilt of the pelvis more than necessary. If the lift needed is greater than 3/8 inch but less than 3/4 inch, it should be applied in

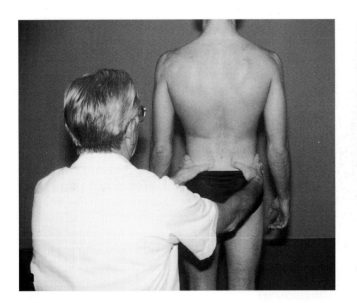

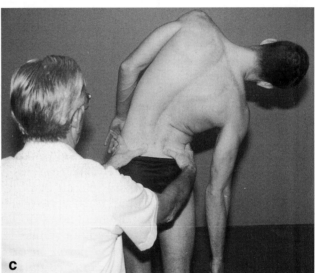

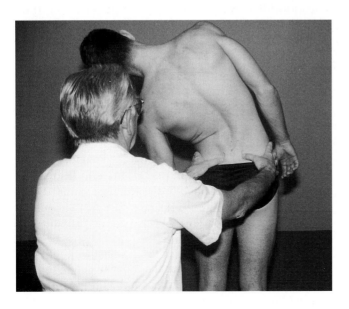

Figure 22.2.
(a) Iliac crest height. (b) Trunk sidebending left.
(c) Trunk sidebending right.

two stages. First, add half the amount needed to the heel of the short leg, followed in 3–6 weeks by reducing the other half from the heel of the long leg. If the amount of lift needed is greater than 3/4 inch, it should be staged in a maximum of 3/8-inch increments, ultimately resulting in heel and sole lift of the required amount. It is rare that a patient cannot tolerate lift therapy if the condition is appropriately diagnosed and treated. Caution must be used in the presence of significant degenerative joint disease, particularly of the hip. Caution must also be used in the presence of pelvic girdle osseous asymmetry when using a lift to the long leg to level the sacral base declination. This places additional stress on the hip joint and the lateral stabilizers of the hip, particularly the gluteus medius and minimis. The lumbar spine usually adapts to the short leg/pelvic tilt syndrome by scoliosis convex to the side of sacral base declination and short lower extremity. Appropriate lift therapy reduces the severity of the adaptive scoliosis and assists in restoring more normal neutral lumbar mechanics. Complications of lift therapy are rare by occasionally occur. These are usually related to the foot and ankle. Lifting a heel changes talotibial mechanics and potentially increases instability of the joint. This can be prevented by appropriate sole lifting in addition to the heel. The second complication involves the plantar fascia, resulting in heel pain due to stress on the plantar side of the calcaneus. This is alleviated by appropriate heel and sole lift or by using the lift in conjunction with an orthotic device. It usually takes 6–8 weeks for a patient to adjust to lift therapy. Appropriate stretching exercises should be prescribed to assist the patient in achieving myofascial balance. The patient must be cautioned that lift therapy use is continuous and must be incorporated in all footwear. The amount of lift does not change unless there is subsequent fracture or rapidly progressive degenerative joint disease in a lower extremity.

Foot Orthotics

Foot orthotic devices can be used to assist the patient in restoring musculoskeletal balance. A podiatrist can individually customize appropriate orthotic devices for foot mechanics. Orthotic devices should never be prescribed until the joints and fascia of the foot and ankle have been treated maximally by appropriate manual medicine. Great care must be exercised when using lift therapy in conjunction with an orthotic device. Incorporation of the appropriate amount of lift to the orthotic device is frequently sufficient. Occasionally, it is necessary to change the shoe to correct the short leg/pelvic tilt requirement and use appropriate orthotic correction inside of the shoe for foot mechanics.

MODALITIES

Modalities are extensively used in the health care delivery system despite the paucity of research evidence for effectiveness. The opinions expressed here are based on clinical experience of the author.

Ice

Ice packs are frequently used in acute soft tissue injuries. The classic athletic medicine principle of RICE—rest, ice, compression, and elevation—are appropriate for many conditions. Ice packs are used posttreatment to reduce the inflammatory response after stimulating chronic dysfunctional musculoskeletal tissues. Frequent short-term applications are most effective. Caution must be used to not chill the skin.

Heat

External heat has wide acceptance by most patients and, although comforting, is frequently abused. Frequent history for a patient with an acute lower back injury is to continuously apply a heating pad overnight while asleep and find it impossible to get out of bed the next day. Short-term applications of heat does enhance circulation to the body part and can be effective in mobilizing the inflammatory process. However, too much heat, applied for too long a period of time, can overly congest a part and contribute to the inflammatory process. Hot packs, particularly moist heat, is very useful before extensive manual stretching. For home use, the patient is advised to apply heat, either moist or dry, for no longer than 15 minutes and no more frequently than every 2 hours, with a maximum of six applications per day.

Ultrasound

Ultrasound is used for deeper heat penetration to tissue. It is used is mainly in the shoulder region in preparation for more extensive stretching and rehabilitation exercises.

Traction

The application of external traction, either by static devices or machines, has extensive use in musculoskeletal medicine. Research evidence of the effectiveness of traction in the literature is sparse, but the empirical use of traction in certain conditions has been deemed valuable. Pelvic traction of 90–90 in acute lumbar discogenic disease can be helpful. In this instance, the patient's body weight provides the appropriate amount of traction, and distraction, of the lower lumbar spine in a flexed position.

The Natchez Mobil-Trac system is a mechanical table allowing the patient to self-position and apply muscle contraction to provide distraction and mobilization of the spine in the presence of discogenic disease. If this equipment is available, with expertise in its use, it is certainly worth a short-term trial. Traction is more frequently used in the cervical spine, particularly in home programs.

Head halter cervical traction is an effective adjunctive intervention. The patient needs adequate instruction in positioning the head halter to avoid compression on the jaw and irritation to the temporomandibular joint. Five to 8 pounds is the weight recommended and should be maintained up to 20 minutes twice daily. Small increments of flexion-extension and rotation right-left exercises while unloaded seem to assist in the management of both acute and chronic conditions of the cervical spine. More extensive use of traction can be by way of the Gravity Lumbar Traction system for both hospital and home use. A body jacket is applied, and the patient's body weight is the activating force at various levels of inclination from horizontal to semivertical. A variation on this theme is to use the same body jacket to unload some of the patient's weight and then perform exercises, particularly walking on a treadmill. This system has been found useful in the management of acute lumbar discogenic radiculopathy.

TENS

Transcutaneous electrical nerve stimulation (TENS) units are quite popular both with health professionals and the laity. This author has been personally disappointed in their effectiveness. Electrical stimulation therapy has also been helpful to some practitioners. Like the TENS unit, the results have been disappointing.

SURGERY

Spinal surgery has two major objectives. The first is decompressing neural structures compromised by trauma or degenerative disease. The second is to stabilize hypermobile and unstable vertebral segments. There are a vast array of options available for both decompression and stabilization. A successful surgical outcome depends on identifying the right procedure for the right patient at the right level at the right time performed by the right surgeon. The goal of any surgical intervention is to assist in the restoration of maximal functional capacity of the musculoskeletal system in postural balance. Before any surgical intervention is performed, the patient should have adequate and appropriate diagnostic studies and nonoperative care. The diagnostic studies should demonstrate a surgical pathology that contributes to, or causes, the patient's pain complaint. Appropriate nonoperative care should be aggressive and comprehensive and not consist of bed rest, modalities, and analgesics.

Most discogenic radiculopathies will respond to aggressive nonoperative care, including appropriate manual medicine, antiinflammatory agents, analgesics, short-term rest, and exercise. Should the patient not respond to nonoperative care and show evidence of progressive neurological deficit, surgical consultation and intervention should be obtained as soon as possible. The neurological deficits of most concern are the cauda equina syndrome and progressive muscle weakness or increasing dural tension signs despite appropriate nonoperative care. The diagnostic workup should identify a surgical pathology consistent with the patient's presentation and should be confirmed by electrodiagnostic studies.

For successful surgical outcome, the patient should receive both prehabilitation and rehabilitation. Adequate nonoperative care before surgery should prepare the patient's musculoskeletal system for the surgical intervention. Postsurgical rehabilitation occurs as soon as possible. Even in the presence of a stabilization procedure, early isometric stabilization exercise can be done before ambulation. Restoration of mobility, muscle control, and balance are the goals of postoperative rehabilitation. A successful surgical outcome is based on the preparation of the patient for the anticipated outcome. Many patients expect total pain relief and restoration of a normal back after a surgical intervention. They should be cautioned that is not the case. The pathology for which the surgery is performed, coupled with the surgical procedure itself, results in alteration of the anatomy that can never be restored to "normal." Unwarranted patient expectations should be avoided.

The surgical intervention should be the least invasive possible. Every attempt should be made to maintain the integrity of the anatomy. Postsurgical magnetic resonance imaging studies show fatty replacement infiltration of the deep fourth-layer muscles of the spinal complex. After fatty replacement, muscles no longer provide the proprioceptive information essential for muscle control and a good functional outcome. This is the reason an intensive exercise program should be performed by the postoperative patient.

EXERCISE

Of all of the adjunctive therapeutic procedures, the one of most value to this author has been exercise. Exercise is fundamental to maintain the therapeutic effectiveness of manual medicine intervention. The principles identified in Chapter 20 are applicable to all patients and are worth the effort of the practitioner to master.

SUMMARY

Manual medicine practitioners should avail themselves of any adjunctive therapeutic procedure that assists in patient management. The broader the physicians armamentarium, the more likely is success. Each patient must be individually evaluated, and the devised treatment plan should be unique to that individual. Adjunctive therapeutic procedures, like manual medicine, should not be prescribed in a cookbook fashion.

23

COMMON CLINICAL SYNDROMES

Practitioners of musculoskeletal medicine experience patients with similar clinical presentations. Those who use the structural diagnosis and manipulative treatment aspects of manual medicine will notice that many of these patients present with similar structural diagnostic findings. Appropriate treatment of the areas of somatic dysfunction in some instances results in total symptom resolution, whereas another patient's recurrence and persistence occurs. Included here are some of the common presentations seen in manual medicine practice.

COMMON COMPENSATORY (UNIVERSAL) PATTERN

Numerous authors refer to a common "universal" pattern. It is commonly noted that patients are notoriously asymmetric in the functional behavior of their musculoskeletal systems. Symmetrical function is the ideal but is seldom identified. The universal pattern consists of a cluster of findings, including a pronated right foot, an anteriorly rotated right innominate, a posteriorly rotated left innominate, a right inferior pube, a left superior pube, a left on left forward sacral torsion, a lower thoracic scoliosis convex to the right and a left lumbar scoliosis, an anterior and inferior right shoulder girdle, and a left cervical scoliosis. A number of theories have been postulated to account for this pattern, including the coreolis force of gravity. It was originally postulated that this pattern was common in the northern hemisphere and that the reverse would be identified in the lower hemisphere, similar to the differences noted in the way that water runs down a drain. This author has been privileged to assess patients in the lower hemisphere in New Zealand and Australia and finds the same universal pattern found in the northern hemisphere. Obviously, the coreolis effect is not the cause. Another theory is that it results from right handedness. Because right-handed people are a high percentage of the population, this may have some credibility. Our society is dominated by tools and equipment that are made for a right-handed and not a left-handed person, so that even left-handed individuals must live in a right-handed world. Perhaps repetitive

movement in this right-handed environment contributes to this universal pattern. This author has often wondered if the fact that most children are delivered in a vertex presentation with the left occiput anterior might be a factor in the development of the functional asymmetry of the musculoskeletal system. The dilemma remains a subject for future research. It is true that this pattern is frequently seen in patients who are both symptomatic and asymptomatic. The question is of what clinical significance is this common pattern. Observation shows that if the patient's dysfunctions are out of this pattern, they are more clinically significant. A structural diagnostic finding that does not fit the pattern should alert the diagnostician that the presentation is unusual.

In addition to the articular restrictions noted in the universal pattern, there are consistent patterns of asymmetric muscle function with some muscles becoming more tight and others becoming inhibited and weak. These patterns have been described in Chapter 20 and warrant study. It is amazing how the muscle pattern fits the articular dysfunction as well, causing the ever present question of which came first and which contributes to the persistence of the other. Is it joint or muscle? In all probability, it is a combination of both.

The presence of the common universal pattern can result in practitioners treating patients in a cookbook fashion to restore motion to the segments in this universal pattern. That is poor practice. Each patient should be viewed from their individual pattern and how it deviates from that which is more common. Again, dysfunctions out of pattern have been found to be more clinically significant.

FAILED LOWER BACK SYNDROME

Disability from lower back pain continues to be a major societal problem. The cost of care to the industrial back pain patient continues to escalate and frustrates the health care delivery system, the insurance industry (both public and private), and employers. For the patient, it can be catastrophic with loss of income, reduced activities of daily living, loss of self esteem, and dependency. The prevention of the failed lower back syndrome, and the rehabilitation of its sufferers, is indeed a challenge.

Structural diagnostic and manual medicine practice has demonstrated a cluster of findings in patients presenting with the failed lower back pain syndrome. This cluster has been designated the "dirty half dozen." The dirty half dozen consists of dysfunction within the lumbar spine, pelvis, and lower extremities. They are

1. Nonneutral dysfunction within the lumbar spine, primarily flexed, rotated, and sidebent (FRS) dysfunctions in the segments of the lower lumbar and thoracolumbar spine;
2. Dysfunction at the symphysis pubis;
3. Restriction of anterior nutational movement of the sacral base, either a posterior (backward) torsion or a posteriorly nutated (extended) sacrum;
4. Innominate shear dysfunction;
5. Short leg/pelvic tilt syndrome; and
6. Muscle imbalance of the trunk and lower extremities.

This author studied 183 patients with an average age of 40.8 years disabled for an average of 30.7 months and consisting of 79 males and 104 females. All patients had disability, with 53% working less than full-time and disabled for some activities of daily living, 42% were not working and had disability of most of the activities of daily living, and 5% were totally disabled and needed assistance for activities of daily living. Eighteen percent had previous surgical treatment, suggesting that most of the failed lower back syndrome is a failure of previous nonoperative care. The 18% surgical failure rate is close to the national average of 15% failed surgical patients. The primary presentation was of back pain with some radiation to the buttock and thigh and in 38% some radiation below the knee. None of the patients presented with leg pain alone. The primary presentation was back, buttock, and thigh pain. The yield from standard neurological and orthopedic testing was low. Ten percent had some reflex change at the patellar or achilles levels. Less than 5% showed evidence of significant muscle weakness. Seven percent showed some sensory loss. The classic straight leg raising with positive dural response was only identified in 2%. None had the classic crossed straight leg raising sign pathognomonic of discogenic radiculopathy. Assessment of the dirty half dozen found 84% to have FRS dysfunctions in the lumbar spine clustered at the L4 and L5 level. Seventy-five percent had unleveling of the symphysis pubis. A total of 48.6% had restriction of anterior nutation of the posterior sacral base. Twenty-four percent showed the presence of innomi-

nate shear with a 2:1 ratio of females to males. The short leg/pelvic tilt syndrome was found in 63%. This is quite consistent with a number of previous studies showing 2 of 3 people with back and lower extremity disability having inequality of leg length as compared with 8–20% of the asymptomatic population. Muscle imbalance was found in almost all of the patients.

Only five patients (3.7%) failed to demonstrate any of the dirty half dozen. Fifty-five percent of the population showed three or more of the dirty half dozen. Despite an average of 2.5 years of disability, 75% of this population returned to full employment and active activities of daily living after a treatment plan directed toward the findings.

CHRONICALLY RECURRENT LOW BACK PAIN SYNDROME (COCKTAIL SYNDROME)

Victims of this problem present with chronic recurrent disabling back pain with minimal radiation to the lower extremity below the buttock. They find it difficult to stand for any period of time as the back pain progressively increases while standing without being mobile. Hence, the term cocktail party syndrome. It is of major significance in patients who must stand in a confined area for long periods of time such as workers on assembly lines or cashiers at checkout counters. The pain is lessened by walking activities or by sitting. Victims of this problem are frequently one-legged standers who do not bear weight symmetrically on their lower extremities, resulting in chronic postural imbalance.

The structural diagnostic findings in this population usually consist of the problem on the left side with the left pube being superior, the left sacrum being anteriorly nutated (flexed), the left innominate posterior, an L5 with extended, rotated, and sidebent (ERS) dysfunction to the left with tight erector spinae muscles and weak abdominals. Treatment of these patients is difficult and frequently frustrating. Recurrent exacerbations are common. They require appropriate manual medicine treatment for the dysfunctions described and a lifelong exercise program to maintain trunk and abdominal muscle control. The patient must learn to maintain balanced standing posture. Modifications of the work activity may be necessary to provide the patient with the opportunity to move on a frequent basis and not restricted for too long a period of time in the standing nonmobile posture.

SPINAL STENOSIS

Spinal stenosis is becoming an increasing problem as our society ages. Central canal and lateral recess stenosis resulting from spinal spondylosis and spondylarthrosis can be seen at all vertebral levels but particularly in the lumbar spine. The classic presentation is a patient who is in a flexed position with difficulty in spinal extension and who finds it difficult to walk in the upright position for any period of time or distance. Frequently, the patient will relate that they are more comfortable walking behind a shopping cart. Persistent forward-bent posture for comfort leads to many secondary dysfunctions and muscle imbalances. The neurogenic claudication experienced by these patients may well be due to perineural and endoneural passive congestion rather than to compression. A manual medicine treatment plan that maximizes the lumbopelvic mechanics, particularly intersegmental motion, may reduce the inflammatory reaction to the passive congestion and give the patient some relief. Manual medicine will not change the osseous pathology of spinal stenosis.

CASE HISTORY

A 64-year-old female presented in October 1988 with disabling lumbar and bilateral leg pain worse on walking and relieved by sitting. She could not walk from her house to the one next door without disabling lower extremity pain. Physical examination failed to determine any vascular deficits of the lower extremities. The greater trochanters were level, but the left iliac crest was low and there was a long c-curve with convexity to the left in the thoracic and lumbar spine. Global trunk extension restriction was present. A neurological examination was within normal limits (Fig. 23.1–23.6). Plain film radiography of the lumbar spine, including erect films for postural study and flexion-extension dynamic studies, revealed unleveling of the sacral base plane with it being inferior on the left side by 1.9 cm. Oblique studies (Figs. 23.2 and 23.3) demonstrated significant degenerative disease of the zygapophysial joints at L4-5. Lateral view in the erect position revealed a sacral base angle of 36°, a slightly anterior midthird lumbar perpendicular, and a first-degree degenerative spondylolisthesis at L4 on L5 (see Figure 23.4). The dynamic studies (Figs. 23.5 and 23.6) showed some increase in the translatory component of L3 on L4 during the flexion-extension process.

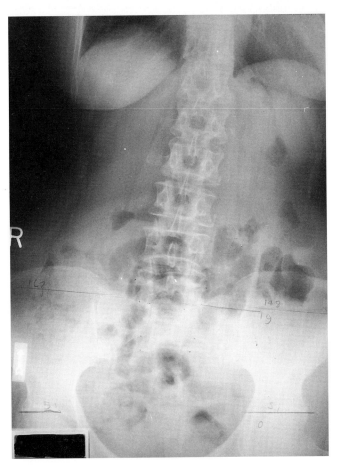

Figure 23.1.
Lumbar spine erect AP projection.

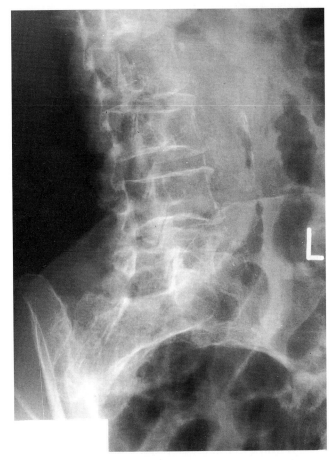

Figure 23.2.
Lumbar spine left oblique projection.

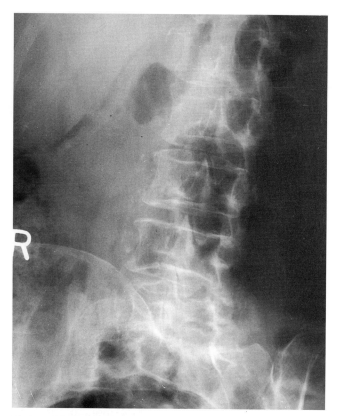

Figure 23.3.
Lumbar spine right oblique projection.

Magnetic resonance imaging (MRI) (Figs. 23.7 and 23.8) showed significant stenosis of the spinal canal at the L4-5 level with other changes consistent with degenerative disc disease.

The patient was placed on a treatment plan consisting of muscle energy and mobilization without impulse directed toward maximizing intersegmental mobility to all elements of the lumbar spine in neutral mechanics. Progressive lift therapy was started in the left shoe, beginning with 6 mm (1/4 inch) with the ultimate goal of 12 mm (1/2 inch), which was accomplished without difficulty. An intensive exercise program, including sensory motor balance training and stretching to symmetry, was used, culminating in a home exercise program the patient performed daily. The acute treatment plan was completed in 3 months. At the end of that time, the patient was able to walk erect for 1 mile in 20 minutes. As she gradually gained functional capacity, she was able to walk 2 miles in 40 minutes without symptoms. She was followed semiannually for the next 3 years and annually since. She is now over 6 years postacute treatment and is asymptomatic but continues to use lift therapy and perform her exercise program.

This patient is an example of the ability to increase functional capacity despite osseous pathology present. The goal of manual medicine to provide maximum pain free movement in postural balance was attempted and achieved in this patient, as well as in many others with similar presentations. The inclusion of mobilization without impulse to the lumbar segments to restore symmetrical zygapophysial joint motion in neutral mechanics is believed to enhance the decongestive process in the lateral spinal canal, reducing the neurogenic claudication. Whether this is the mechanism or not, this treatment plan has been successful in many patients with spinal stenosis. This approach should be aggressively used in patients before being subjected to decompressive surgical procedures that may result in spinal instability.

INTERCOSTAL NEURALGIAS

Pain in the chest wall aggravated by respiration is not an uncommon patient presentation. These patients are given a diagnosis of "intercostal neuralgia" or "pleurisy." The chest wall complaint may be primary or associated with other complaints within the musculoskeletal system.

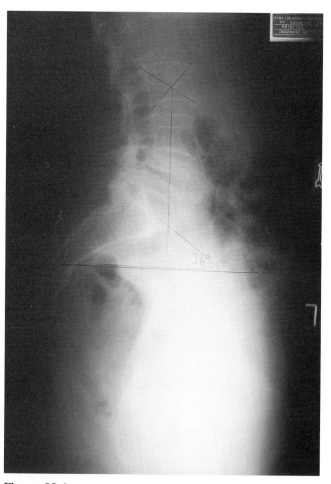

Figure 23.4.
Lumbar spine erect lateral projection.

The common structural diagnostic finding in these patients is a structural rib dysfunction frequently associated with a nonneutral dysfunction of the ERS type in the thoracic spine. External rib torsional dysfunction with an associated ERS dysfunction of the thoracic spine is the most common finding and is associated with exhalation restriction of the ribs superior to the torsional dysfunction. The anterior and posterior subluxations and anteroposterior or lateral compressions can likewise lead to symptoms simulating intercostal neuralgia. These structural rib dysfunctions are also characterized by exquisite tenderness and tissue reactivity at the costochondral junction, the so-called Tzietze's syndrome. If the practitioner does not identify a structural rib pathology in a patient with this presentation, the index of suspicion for organic neurological disease should be high. Tumors of the thoracic cord, herpes zoster infection, and diabetic neuropathy are but a few of those entities in a differential diagnosis. Most "intercostal neuralgias" result from structural rib dysfunctions. If one is not found, a neurologist should be consulted.

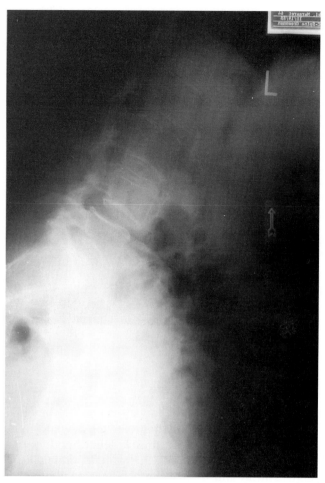

Figure 23.6.
Lumbar spine erect lateral forward-bending projection.

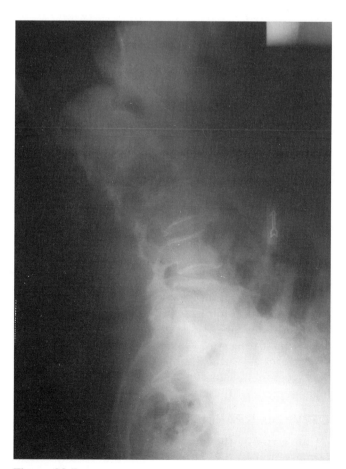

Figure 23.5.
Lumbar spine erect lateral backward-bending projection.

CERVICAL BRACHIALGIAS

Painful stiffness of the cervical spine and associated pain, numbness, and tingling in the upper extremity is a common patient presentation. There are a number of structures that can be involved with structural pathology, dysfunctional pathology, or a combination of both that need to be assessed. From the structural diagnostic process, the following assessment sequence should be performed to identify those dysfunctions amenable to manual medicine intervention that could cause the symptom complex. Obviously, standard neurological and orthopedic testing should also be performed.

The process begins in the cervical spine to assess the mobility characteristics of the zygapophysial joints for their potential involvement in compressive or inflammatory entrapment of a cervical nerve root. Zygapophysial dysfunction of the cervical spine always involves the intertransversarii muscles through which the nerve root passes as it exits the lateral ver-

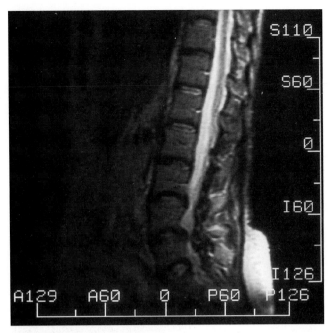

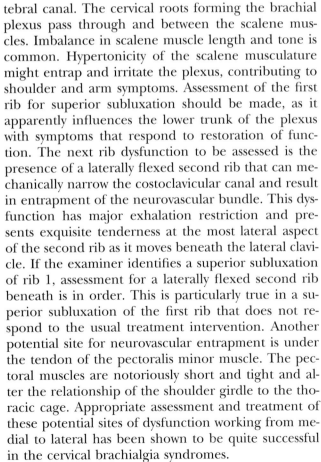

Figure 23.7.
MRI lumbar spine saggital view.

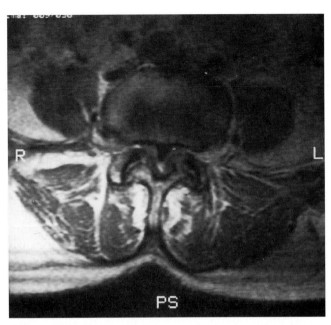

Figure 23.8.
MRI lumbar spine axial view at L4-5.

tebral canal. The cervical roots forming the brachial plexus pass through and between the scalene muscles. Imbalance in scalene muscle length and tone is common. Hypertonicity of the scalene musculature might entrap and irritate the plexus, contributing to shoulder and arm symptoms. Assessment of the first rib for superior subluxation should be made, as it apparently influences the lower trunk of the plexus with symptoms that respond to restoration of function. The next rib dysfunction to be assessed is the presence of a laterally flexed second rib that can mechanically narrow the costoclavicular canal and result in entrapment of the neurovascular bundle. This dysfunction has major exhalation restriction and presents exquisite tenderness at the most lateral aspect of the second rib as it moves beneath the lateral clavicle. If the examiner identifies a superior subluxation of rib 1, assessment for a laterally flexed second rib beneath is in order. This is particularly true in a superior subluxation of the first rib that does not respond to the usual treatment intervention. Another potential site for neurovascular entrapment is under the tendon of the pectoralis minor muscle. The pectoral muscles are notoriously short and tight and alter the relationship of the shoulder girdle to the thoracic cage. Appropriate assessment and treatment of these potential sites of dysfunction working from medial to lateral has been shown to be quite successful in the cervical brachialgia syndromes.

A similar approach of working from central to distal is also of value in patients with symptoms around the elbow and at the wrist. The classic presentation of medial or lateral epicondylitis will most frequently be associated to restriction of pronation and supination of the radial head at the radiohumeral and proximal radioulnar joint. Restoration of function of the radial head is frequently sufficient to treat the "tennis elbow."

Symptoms related to the carpal tunnel have escalated in recent years and appear to be related to repetitive strain injury, particularly associated with hand action at a computer terminal. Any repetitive motion of the hands and wrists can lead to complaints of wrist pain and associated numbness and tingling in the fingers. Although many of these patients will show borderline delay in median nerve conduction, few demonstrate denervation potentials in the hand muscles, particularly the thenar eminence. Structural diagnosis and manual medicine treatment to the joints at the wrist should follow the previously described assessment and treatment process from the cervical spine distally. The joint play procedures and others addressing dysfunction at the wrist region in Chapter 18 can be of assistance in management of these patients.

CERVICAL CRANIAL SYNDROME

Of all areas in the musculoskeletal system and the spinal column, this author finds the craniocervical junction as the most difficult to adequately assess and successfully manage. Patients presenting with pain in the cervical spine with stiffness and an associated headache, usually hemicephalgic and running from the occiput to the retroorbital area, are all too common in clinical practice. Trauma is a frequent initiator of the symptom complex, but it can occur without a single trauma, such as a motor vehicle accident, by chronic postural imbalance affecting the upper cervical musculature. Structural diagnosis of the upper cervical complex is difficult because of the unique anatomy in the region (see Chapter 13). Diagnosis of restricted mobility in the upper cervical complex is more easily accomplished than the assessment of hypermobility. Relative hypermobility on the opposite side of restricted motion is quite common and confusing to the examiner. If there is high suspicion and physical findings consistent with hypermobility, special imaging studies are in order. They should include plain film flexion and extension studies in the lateral projection and rotary stress films with axial views of the cervicocranial and upper cervical regions by either computed tomography or MRI.

The common structural diagnostic findings in these patients is an ERS left dysfunction at C2-3, the atlas rotated to the right, and the occiput flexed sidebent right and rotated left. There is frequently an associated dysfunction of the left occipitomastoid suture (Figs. 23.9 and 23.10).

Figures 23.9 and 23.10 demonstrate the MRI findings in a patient presenting with a 6-year history of cervical cranial pain syndrome after a major motor vehicle accident. Her injuries included fractures of the pelvis and a traumatic brain injury. She had been

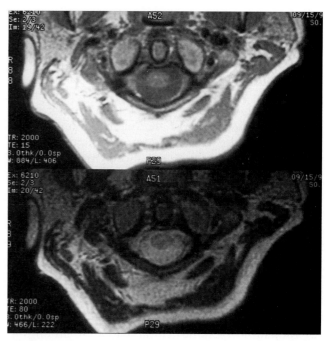

Figure 23.10.
MRI cervical spine axial cuts.

successfully treated and rehabilitated and had returned to full-time work but persisted with recurring upper cervical painful stiffness and an associated hemicephalgia. Her structural diagnostic findings were as described above but were very difficult to manage and sustain in a maximal functional capacity. The sagittal views of the cervical cord and cervical spine (Fig. 23.9) are essentially within normal limits. The axial MRI views (Fig. 23.10) show major loss of muscle density in the region of the rectus capitis posterior minor and major muscles. This finding may account for the difficulty in responding to manual medicine procedures of all types.

CEPHALGIA ASSOCIATED WITH TRAUMATIC BRAIN INJURY

Many patients who have sustained a closed head injury resulting in minimal to mild to moderate brain dysfunction have an associated headache complaint that is very resistant to treatment. Major structural diagnostic findings of the craniosacral mechanism are found in such patients in addition to dysfunctions elsewhere in the system. The craniosacral findings have been remarkably consistent in this population. They all appear to have reduction in the rate and amplitude of the cranial rhythmic impulse with an average in the 6–7 range. They all appear to have some level of sphenobasilar compression, particularly of the anteroposterior type. The sphenobasilar strain patterns most consistently found are the presence of

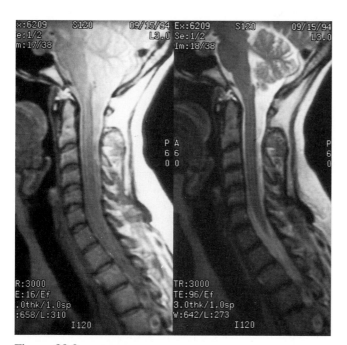

Figure 23.9.
MRI cervical spine sagittal cuts.

a lateral and torsional strain restriction to the same side. Appropriate craniosacral manipulation can be useful in the rehabilitation of these patients. If the craniosacral system responds to treatment by an increase in the rate and amplitude of the cranial rhythmic impulse and with balanced and enhanced mobility of the sphenobasilar junction, then this correlates well with the outcome of the rehabilitation process. Conversely, if the patient does not respond to craniosacral manipulation by an enhanced cranial rhythmic impulse rate and amplitude, the outcome of the rehabilitative process is less satisfactory. Caution is advised in the use of craniosacral manipulation in this population because it does carry an approximate 5% iatrogenic complication rate.

RECURRENT ANKLE SPRAINS

Recurrent ankle sprain is as common with the weekend warrior as with the high level athlete. They do not provide a difficult diagnostic challenge but they are difficult to treat. Structural diagnostic findings in this population consistently show dysfunction at the proximal tibiofibular joint and dorsiflexion restriction of the talus at the talotibial articulation. Altered subtalar gliding movement is common in these patients along with pronation of the cuboid on the same side. Muscle assessment frequently reveals weakness of the tibialis anterior and the peroneal muscles. Adequate treatment for this dysfunctional pattern frequently prevents recurrence of ankle sprain. Another very troublesome outcome of ankle sprains is difficulty with proprioceptive balance, particularly when standing on one leg. This appears to result in altered muscle firing pattern sequence and to contribute to muscle imbalance throughout the total musculoskeletal system.

CONCLUSION

Many of the common clinical syndrome findings from the structural diagnostic and manual medicine perspective are reviewed. Although these are frequently seen, the practitioner is urged to assess each patient on an individual basis in a very comprehensive fashion to determine the exact dysfunctional pattern present and to develop an appropriate treatment plan. The higher the level of structural diagnostic skill and the greater the competence in multiple manual medicine interventions the practitioner has, the better will be the outcome. The manual medicine armamentarium is quite broad, and the practitioner should be familiar with as many as possible. Remember the admonition that if you only have a hammer in your toolbox, most everything begins to look like a nail.

Alderink GJ: The Sacroiliac Joint: Review of Anatomy, Mechanics, and Function. J Orthop Sports Phys Ther. 13:71–84, 1991.

Beal MC: Motion sense. Osteopath Assoc. 53:151–153, 1953.

Beal MC: Spinal Motion. Yearbook of the Academy of Applied Osteopathy Carmel, CA, 1970, pp 11–16.

Beal MC: The Sacroiliac Problem: Review of Anatomy, Mechanics, and Diagnosis. J Am Osteopath Assoc. 81:667–679, 1982.

Bourdillon JF, Day EA, Bookhout MR: Spinal Manipulation, ed 5. Oxford, Butterworth-Heinemann Ltd., 1992.

Bowles CH: Functional Technique: A Modern Perspective. J Am Osteopath Assoc. 80:326–331, 1981.

Buerger AA, Greenman PE (eds): Empirical Approaches to the Validation of Spinal Manipulation. Springfield, IL, Charles C Thomas, 1985.

Buerger AA, Tobis JS: Approaches to the Validation of Manipulation Therapy. Springfield, IL, Charles C Thomas, 1977.

Burton CV: The Sister Kenny Institute, Gravity Lumbar Reduction Therapy Program. Chapter 8 In Finneson B: Low Back Pain. Philadelphia, JB Lippincott Co., 1980.

Butler DS: Mobilization of the Nervous System. Melbourne, Churchill Livingstone, 1991.

Buzzell KA: The Cost of Human Posture and Locomotion. Chapter 4 In: The Physiological Basis of Osteopathic Medicine. New York, The Post Graduate Institute of Osteopathic Medicine and Surgery, 1970.

Cyriax J: Textbook of Orthopedic Medicine, ed 7. East Sussex, England, Bailliere-Tindall. Vol. I, 1978.

DiGiovanna EL, Schiowitz S: An Osteopathic Approach to Diagnosis and Treatment. Philadelphia, JB Lippincott Co., 1991.

DonTigney RL: Function and Pathomechanics of the Sacroiliac Joint. J Am Phys Ther Assoc. 65:35–44, 1985.

Dorman TA, Ravin TH: Diagnosis and Injection Techniques in Orthopaedic Medicine, Baltimore, Williams & Wilkins, 1991.

Dvorak J, Dvorak V: Manual Medicine, Diagnostics. New York, Thieme-Stratton Inc, 1983.

Dvorak J, Dvorak V, Schneider W (eds): Manual Medicine 1984. Heidelberg, Springer-Verlag, 1985.

Dvorak J, Froehlich D, Penning L, Baumgartner H, Panjabi MM: Functional Radiographic Diagnosis of the Cervical Spine: Flexion/Extension. Spine. 13:748–755, 1988.

Dvorak J, Hayek J, Zehnder R: C-T Functional Diagnostics of the Rotary Instability of Upper Cervical Spine. Part 2. An Evaluation on Healthy Adults and Patients with Suspected Instability. Spine. 12:726–731, 1987.

Dvorak J, Orelli F: How Dangerous is Manipulation to the Cervical Spine? Manual Medicine. 2:1–4, 1985.

Dvorak J, Panjabi MM, Gerber M, Wichmann W: C-T Functional Diagnostics of the Rotary Instability of Upper Cervical Spine. Part 1. An Experimental Study on Cadavers. Spine. 12:197–205, 1987.

Evjenth O, Hamberg J: Muscle Stretching in Manual Therapy. A Clinical Manual. Alfta, Sweden. Alfta Rehab Forlag. Vols. 1 & 2, 1984.

Farfan HF: The Scientific Basis of Manipulative Procedures. Clin Rheum Dis. 6(1):159, 1980.

Fisk JW: The Painful Neck and Back. Springfield, IL, Charles C Thomas, 1977.

Friberg O: Clinical Symptoms and Biomechanics of Lumbar Spine and Hip Joint in Leg Length Inequality. Spine. 8:643–651, 1983.

Fryette HH: Principles of Osteopathic Technic. Carmel, CA, American Academy of Osteopathy, 1954.

Gevitz N: The D.O.'s-Osteopathic Medicine in America. Baltimore, Johns Hopkins University Press, 1982.

Good AB: Spinal Joint Blocking. J Manipulative Physio Therapy. 8(1):1–8, 1985.

Greenman PE: Manipulation with the Patient Under Anesthesia. J Am Osteopath Assoc. 92:1159–1170, 1992.

Greenman PE: Clinical Aspects of Sacroiliac Function in Walking. J Manual Medicine. 5:125–130, 1990.

Greenman PE: Lift Therapy: Use and Abuse. J Am Osteopath Assoc. 79:238–250, 1979.

Greenman PE: The Osteopathic Concept in the Second Century: Is it Still Germane to Specialty Practice? J Am Osteopath Assoc. 75:589–595, 1976.

Greenman PE: Layer Palpation. Mich Osteopath J. 47(9):936–937, 1982.

Greenman PE (ed): Concepts and Mechanisms of Neuromuscular Functions. Berlin, Springer-Verlag, 1984.

Greenman PE: Models and Mechanisms of Osteopathic Manipulative Medicine. Osteopathic Medical News. 4(5):1–20, 1987.

Greenman PE, Tait B: Structural Diagnosis in Chronic Low Back Pain. Manual Medicine. 3:114–117, 1988.

Grieve GP: Common Vertebral Joint Problems. Edinburgh, Churchill Livingstone, 1981.

Haldeman S: Modern Developments in the Principles and Practice of Chiropractic. East Norwalk, CT, Appleton-Century-Crofts, 1980.

Hoag JM, Cole WV, Bradford SG: Osteopathic Medicine. New York, McGraw-Hill, 1969.

Hoffman KS, Hoffman LL: Effects of Adding Sacral Base Leveling to Osteopathic Manipulative Treatment of Back Pain: A Pilot Study. J Am Osteopath Assoc. 94:217–226, 1994.

Hoover HW: Functional Technique. Yearbook of the Academy of Applied Osteopathy, Carmel, CA 1958, pp 47–51.

Irwin RE: Reduction of Lumbar Scoliosis by Use of a Heel Lift to Level the Sacral Base. J Am Osteopath Assoc. 91:34–44, 1991.

Janda V: Muscle Function Testing. London, Butterworths, 1983.

Johnston WL, Friedman HD: Functional Methods. Indianapolis, American Academy of Osteopathy, 1994.

Johnston WL, Robertson JA, Stiles EG: Finding a Common Denominator for the Variety of Manipulative Techniques. Yearbook of the Academy of Applied Osteopathy, Carmel, CA, 1969, pp 5–15.

Jones LH: Strain and Counterstrain. American Academy of Osteopathy. Colorado Springs, CO, 1981.

Jull G, Bogduk N, Marsland A: The Accuracy of Manual Diagnosis for Cervical Zygapophyseal Joint Syndromes. Med J Australia. 148:233–236, 1988.

Kendall FP, McCreary EK, Provance PG: Muscles: Testing and Function, ed 4. Baltimore, Williams & Wilkins, 1993.

Kimberly PE: Formulating a Prescription for Osteopathic Manipulative Treatment. J Am Osteopath Assoc. 75:486–499, 1976.

Kirkaldy-Willis WH, Burton, CV: Managing Low Back Pain, ed 3. Edinburgh, Churchill Livingstone, 1992.

Kleynhans AM: Complications of and Contraindications to Spinal Manipulative Therapy. Chapter 16 In Haldeman S (ed): Modern Developments in the Principles and Practice of Chiropractic. New York, Appleton-Century-Crofts, 1980.

Korr IM (ed): The Neurologic Mechanisms in Manipulative Therapy. New York, Plenum, 1978.

Lamax E: Manipulative Therapy: A Historical Perspective from Ancient Times to the Modern Era. In Goldstein M (ed): The Research Status of Spinal Manipulative Therapy. National Institute of Neurological and Communicative Disorders and Stroke Monograph No. 15, pp 11–17, 1975.

Lee D: The Pelvic Girdle. Edinburgh, Churchill Livingstone, 1989.

Lewit K: Manipulative Therapy in Rehabilitation of the Motor System, ed 2. Oxford, Heinemann Ltd, 1991.

Magoun HI: Osteopathy in the Cranial Field, ed 2. Kirksville, MO, Journal Printing Co, 1966.

Maigne R: Orthopedic Medicine. Springfield, IL, Charles C Thomas, 1972.

Maitland GD: Vertebral Manipulation, ed 4. Stoneham, MA, Butterworths, 1980.

Mennell J McM: Back Pain. Boston, Little, Brown & Co, 1960.

Mennell J McM: Joint Pain. Boston, Little, Brown & Co, 1964.

Mitchell FL Sr: Motion Discordance. Yearbook of the Academy of Applied Osteopathy, Carmel, CA, 1967, pp 1–5.

Mitchell FL Jr, Moran PS, Pruzzo NA: An Evaluation and Treatment Manual of Osteopathic Muscle Energy Procedures. Valley Park, MO, Mitchell, Moran, and Pruzzo Associates, 1979.

Mitchell FL: Structural Pelvic Function. Yearbook of the American Academy of Osteopathy, Carmel, CA, 1958, pp 71–90.

Morey LW Jr: Osteopathic Manipulation Under General Anesthesia. J Am Osteopath Assoc. 73:84–95, 1973.

Morey LW Jr: Manipulation Under General Anesthesia. Osteopath Annals. 4:127–135, 1976.

Natchev E: Pain Treatment and Auto-Traction for Back Problems. Stockholm, AB Spiraltryck, 1982.

Nicholas NS: Atlas of Osteopathic Techniques. Philadelphia, Philadelphia College of Osteopathic Medicine, 1974.

Northup G: Osteopathic Medicine. An American Reformation, ed 2. Chicago, American Osteopathic Association, 1979.

Northup GW, Korr IM, Buzzell KA, Hix EL: The Physiological Basis of Osteopathic Medicine. New York, Postgraduate Institute of Osteopathic Medicine and Surgery, 1970.

Northup GW (ed): Osteopathic Research: Growth and Development. Chicago, American Osteopathic Association, 1987.

Page LE: The Principles of Osteopathy. Kansas City, MO, American Academy of Osteopathy, 1952.

Patijn J: Complications in Manual Medicine: A Review of the Literature. Manual Medicine. 6:89–92, 1991.

Retzlaff EW, Mitchell FL Jr: The Cranium and its Sutures. Berlin, Springer-Verlag, 1987.

Romney IC: Manipulation of the Spine and Appendages Under Anesthesia: An Evaluation. J Amer Osteo Assoc. 68:235–245, 1968.

Rush WA, Steiner HA: A Study of Lower Extremity Length Inequality. Am J Roentgenology, Radium Therapy and Nuclear Medicine. 56:616–623, 1946.

Sandoz R: Some Physical Mechanisms and Effects of Spinal Adjustments. Ann Swiss Chiro Assoc. 6:91–141, 1976.

Schiotz EH: Manipulation Treatment of the Spinal Column from the Medical-Historical Viewpoint. Tidsskr Nor Laegeforn 78:359–372, 429–438, 946–950, 1003, 1958. (NIH Library Translation NIH-75–22C, 23C, 24C, 25C).

Schiotz EH, Cyriax J: Manipulation Past and Present. London, William Heinemann Medical Books, 1975.

Schneider W, Dvorak J, Dvorak V, Tritschler T: Manual Medicine, Therapy. New York, Thieme Medical Publishers Inc, 1988.

Stiles EG: Manipulative Techniques: Four Approaches. Osteopath Med. 1(6):27–30, 1976.

Stiles EG, Shaw HH: Functional Techniques Based Upon the Approach of George Andrew Laughin DO. Course Syllabus. Michigan State University College of Osteopathic Medicine, Continuing Education, 1991.

Stoddard A: Manual of Osteopathic Technique. London, Hutchinson Medical Publications, 1959.

Stoddard A: Manual of Osteopathic Practice. New York, Harper & Row, 1969.

Travell JG, Simons DG: Myofascial Pain and Dysfunction: The Trigger Point Manual. The Upper Extremities. Baltimore, Williams & Wilkins. Vol. 1, 1983.

Travell JG, Simons DG: Myofascial Pain and Dysfunction: The Trigger Point Manual. The Lower Extremities. Baltimore, Williams & Wilkins. Vol. 2, 1992.

Tucker C, Deoora T: Fundamental Osteopathic Techniques. Melbourne, Research Publications Pty Ltd, 1995.

Upledger JE, Vredevoogd JD: Craniosacral Therapy. Chicago, Eastland Press, 1983.

Walton WJ: Osteopathic Diagnosis and Technique Procedures, ed 2. Colorado Springs, CO, American Academy of Osteopathy, 1970.

Ward RC: Tutorial on Level I Myofascial Release Technique. Course Syllabus. Michigan State University College of Osteopathic Medicine, 1986.

Ward RC, Sprafka, S: Glossary of Osteopathic Terminology. J Am Osteopath Assoc. 80:552–567, 1981.

Zink JG: Respiratory and Circulatory Care: The Conceptual Model. Osteopath Annals. 5:108–124, 1977.

FIGURE CREDITS

Art has been reproduced with permission from the copyright owners as follows:

Becker RF, Wilson JW, Gehweiler JA: The Anatomical Basis of Medical Practice. Baltimore, Williams & Wilkins, 1971.

Figures 1.1 through 1.6 and 15.1 through 15.5.

Agur AMR, Lee MJ: Grant's Atlas of Anatomy, ed 9. Baltimore, Williams & Wilkins, 1991.

Figures 12.1, 12.2, 12.4, and 12.6.

Anderson JE: Grant's Atlas of Anatomy, ed 8. Baltimore, Williams & Wilkins, 1983

Figure 12.3.

Clemente CD: Anatomy: A Regional Atlas of the Human Body, ed 3. Baltimore, Urban & Schwarzenberg, 1987.

Figures 17.1 and 17.2.

Travell JG, Simons DG: Myofascial Pain and Dysfunction: The Trigger Point Manual. The Upper Extremities. Baltimore, Williams & Wilkins. Vol. 1, 1983.

Figures 20.27B, 20.39B, 20.49C, 20.50B, 20.51C, 20.52B, 20.53, 20.56B, 20.64B, 20.66C, and 20.68C.

Travell JG, Simons DG: Myofascial Pain and Dysfunction: The Trigger Point Manual. The Lower Extremities. Baltimore, Williams & Wilkins. Vol. 2, 1992.

Figures 20.15B, 20.16B, 20.17B, 20.20B, 20.21A-C, 20.22B, 20.25B, 20.34D, and 20.36B.

Aprill C: New Orleans, Louisiana.

Figures 21.16 through 21.21.

INDEX

Page numbers in *italics* indicate figures; those followed by "t" indicate tables.